Hypofractionated and Stereotactic Radiation Therapy

Orit Kaidar-Person • Ronald Chen
Editors

Hypofractionated and Stereotactic Radiation Therapy

A Practical Guide

Second Edition

Springer

Editors
Orit Kaidar-Person
Breast Cancer Radiation Unit
Radiation Department
Sheba Tel Hashomer
Ramat Gan, Israel

Ronald Chen
University of Kansas Cancer Center
Kansas City, KS, USA

ISBN 978-3-031-47700-3 ISBN 978-3-031-47701-0 (eBook)
https://doi.org/10.1007/978-3-031-47701-0

This Springer imprint is published by the registered company Springer Nature Switzerland AG
The registered company address is: Gewerbestrasse 11, 6330 Cham, Switzerland

Prof. Kaidar-Person would like to dedicate this book in memory of her mentor, Prof. Abraham Kuten, who was a compassionate doctor, mentor, researcher, and family man. A national and international leader in oncology. He will be thoroughly missed.

Prof. Chen would like to dedicate this book to his wife Petronella Muresan, an incredible mother and outstanding statistician; and to their children, Luke Chen and Matthew Chen.

Preface

Radiation therapy (RT) continues to evolve rapidly as a result of improvements in imaging, advances in patient immobilization and treatment delivery technologies, and our understanding of radiobiology. There are currently two major trends in RT, shortening treatment (hypofractionation) and use of stereotactic radiosurgery and stereotactic body radiotherapy technologies. As published data continue to rapidly accumulate, these treatments are no longer exclusive to specialized centers. Shortening treatment is also appealing to patients because of increased convenience, less interference with planned systemic therapy, and is often less costly than conventionally fractionated (longer) RT courses. Radiation therapy continues to be, and is increasingly so, an effective and cost-effective cancer treatment that reduces cancer-specific mortality (CSM) and overall mortality for many cancers.

This handbook was developed to summarize the data and techniques for hypofractionation and stereotactic radiation in a clinically accessible way, providing concise information ranging from commonly used dose-fractionation schemes to simulation and treatment specifications to published safety and efficacy data. While hypofractionation and stereotactic radiation are used in almost all cancer sites, we note where there are strong supportive data including randomized trials, and other areas where relatively little data are available to guide treatments. Further, we want to highlight that the development of a stereotactic radiotherapy program requires specialized expertise and quality assurance procedures, which are described in Chap. 3.

We hope that you will enjoy the book as much as we enjoyed the process of developing it. This handbook was written to be practical, with usable information relevant for the clinician. We want to thank all the contributors of this book for their hard work and expertise.

Ramat Gan, Israel — Orit Kaidar-Person
Kansas City, KS, USA — Ronald Chen

Contents

Contributors

Katelyn M. Atkins, MD, PhD Department of Radiation Oncology, Cedars-Sinai Medical Center, Los Angeles, CA, USA

Maoz Ben Ayun, PhD Department of Radiation Oncology, Sheba Medical Center, Ramat Gan, Israel

Marc Bussière, MSc Department of Radiation Oncology, Massachusetts General Hospital, Francis H. Burr Proton Therapy Center, Boston, MA, USA

Ronald C. Chen, MD, MPH Department of Radiation Oncology, KU Medical Center, The University of Kansas, Kansas City, USA

Bhishamjit S. Chera, MD Department of Radiation Oncology, MUSC, Medical University of South Carolina, Charleston, USA

Felix Ehret, MD Department of Radiation Oncology, Charité - Universitätsmedizin Berlin, Berlin, Germany

Achilles J. Fakiris, MD Department of Radiation Oncology, Rex Hospital, University of North Carolina Affiliate Hospital, Raleigh, NC, USA

Brittaney-Belle E. Gordon, BA University of Pittsburgh Medical Center, Pittsburgh, PA, USA

Hillman Comprehensive Cancer Center, Pittsburgh, NC, USA

Kenny Guida, DMP Department of Radiation Oncology, University of Kansas Medical Center, Kansas City, KS, USA

Lia M. Halasz, MD Department of Radiation Oncology, University of Washington School of Medicine, Seattle, WA, USA

Jacob M. Hall Department of Radiation Oncology, University of North Carolina School of Medicine, Chapel Hill, NC, USA

Jordan A. Holmes, MD, MPH Department of Radiation Oncology, Indiana University, Indianapolis, PA, USA

Indiana University Simon Cancer Center, Indianapolis, IN, USA

Ellen Jones, MD, PhD Department of Radiation Oncology, University of North Carolina at Chapel Hill, Chapel Hill, NC, USA

Gregory D. Judy, MD, MS Department of Radiation Oncology, University of North Carolina School of Medicine, Chapel Hill, NC, USA

Lineberger Comprehensive Cancer Center, University of North Carolina School of Medicine, Chapel Hill, NC, USA

Orit Kaidar-Person, MD Breast Cancer Radiation Unit, Radiation Department, Sheba Tel Hashomer, Ramat Gan, Israel

School of Medicine, Tel-Aviv University (TAU), Tel Aviv, Israel

Edward Y. Kim, MD Department of Radiation Oncology, University of Washington School of Medicine, Seattle, WA, USA

Bruce F. Kimler Department of Radiation Oncology, University of Kansas Medical Center, Kansas City, Kansas, USA

Yaccov R. Lawrence Radiation Department, Sheba Tel Hashomer, Ramat Gan, Israel

School of Medicine, Tel-Aviv University (TAU), Tel Aviv, Israel

Harold Li Department of Radiation Oncology, University of Kansas Medical Center, Kansas City, KS, USA

Simon S. Lo, MD, FACR, FASTRO Department of Radiation Oncology, University of Washington School of Medicine, Seattle, WA, USA

Jason Matney, PhD Department of Radiation Oncology, University of California at Davis Cancer Center, Sacramento, CA, USA

Dominic H. Moon, MD Department of Radiation Oncology, UT Southwestern Medical Center, Dallas, TX, USA

Kevin Pearlstein, MD Department of Radiation Oncology, University of North Carolina at Chapel Hill, Chapel Hill, NC, USA

Alex Price, MS Department of Radiation Oncology, University of North Carolina School of Medicine, Chapel Hill, NC, USA

Leith Rankine, MS Department of Radiation Oncology, University of North Carolina School of Medicine, Chapel Hill, NC, USA

Subhrajit Saha, M. Tech., Ph.D. Department of Radiation Oncology, University of Kansas Medical Center, Kansas City, Kansas, USA

Helen A. Shih, MD, MS, MPH Department of Radiation Oncology, Massachusetts General Hospital, Francis H. Burr Proton Therapy Center, Boston, MA, USA

Dima Soultan Department of Radiation Oncology, University of Kansas Medical Center, Kansas City, KS, USA

Joel E. Tepper, MD Department of Radiation Oncology, University of North Carolina Hospitals, Chapel Hill, NC, USA

Yolanda Tseng, MD Department of Radiation Oncology, University of Washington School of Medicine, Seattle, WA, USA

Mahesh Varia, MB, ChB, FACR Department of Radiation Oncology, University of North Carolina School of Medicine, Chapel Hill, NC, USA

Andrew Z. Wang, MD UT Southwestern Medical Center, Dallas, TX, USA

Kyle Wang, MD Cincinnati, OH, USA

Ashley A. Weiner, MD, PhD Department of Radiation Oncology, University of North Carolina School of Medicine, Chapel Hill, NC, USA

Timothy M. Zagar, MD Northeastern Radiation Oncology, PLLC, Saratoga Springs, NY, USA

Elaine M. Zeman, PhD Department of Radiation Oncology, UNC School of Medicine, Chapel Hill, NC, USA

Abbreviations

3D	3-Dimensional
3DCRT	3-Dimensional conformal radiotherapy
4D	4-Dimensional
4DCRT	4-Dimensional conformal radiotherapy
5-FU	5-Fluorouracil
AA	Anaplastic astrocytoma
AAPM	American Association of Physicists in Medicine
Ab	Antibody
ABMT	Autologous bone marrow transplant
ABS	American Brachytherapy Society
abstr.	Abstract
ACOSOG	American College of Surgeon Oncology Group
ACS	American Cancer Society
ACTH	Adrenocorticotropic hormone
ADL	Activity of daily living
ADR	Adverse drug reaction
ADT	Androgen deprivation treatment
AE	Adverse event
AFP	Alpha fetoprotein
AIDS	Acquired immune deficiency syndrome
AJCC	American Joint Committee on Cancer
ALL	Acute lymphocytic leukemia
ALND	Axillary lymph node dissection
ALP	Alkaline phosphatase
ALT	Alanine aminotransferase
AMD	Dactinomycin
AML	Acute myeloid leukemia
AP	Anterior-posterior
APBI	Accelerated partial breast irradiation
APR	Abdominoperineal resection
ARC	Arc therapy

ASCO	American Society of Clinical Oncology
ASTRO	American Society for Radiation Oncology
AUC	Area under the curve
AVM	Arteriovenous malformations
b.i.d	Twice a day (bis in die)
Bcc	Basal cell carcinoma
BCG	Bacillus Calmette-Guerin
BCS	Breast-conserving surgery
BCT	Breast-conserving treatment (lumpectomy and radiotherapy)
BED	Biological effective dose
BEV	Beam's eye view
BMJ	*British Medical Journal*
bPFS	Biochemical progression-free survival
BRCP	Borderline resectable pancreatic cancer
BUN	Blood urea nitrogen
Bx	Biopsy
c	Cycles (e.g., for two cycles)
ca	Cancer
CALGB	Cancer and Leukemia Group B
CaSS	Cancer-specific survival
CBC	Complete blood count
CBCT	Cone beam CT
cc	Cubic centimeter
cCR	Clinical complete response
CEA	Carcinoembryonic antigen
CESS	German Cooperative Ewing's Sarcoma Study
cGy	CentiGray
Chemo	Chemotherapy
CHOP	Cyclophosphamide, doxorubicin, vincristine, and prednisone
CI	Conformity index
CIS	Carcinoma in situ
cm	Centimeter
CN	Cranial nerve (e.g., CN X)
COG	Children's Oncology Group
CR	Complete response
Cr	Creatinine
CRC	Colorectal carcinoma
CRM	Circumferential resection margin
CRT	Chemo-radiotherapy
CSF	Cerebrospinal fluid
CSI	Craniospinal irradiation
CSS	Cause-specific survival
CT	Computed tomography
CTCAE	Common Toxicity Criteria for Adverse Events
CT-SIM	CT simulation

CTV_x	Clinical target volume x = 1, 2, 3,…
Cu	Copper
CXR	Chest X-ray
CY	Cyclophosphamide
CyK	CyberKnife
D&C	Dilation and curettage
DCIS	Ductal carcinoma in situ
DES	Diethylstilbestrol
DFS	Disease-free survival
DIBH	Deep inspiration breath hold
dL	Deciliter
DLBCL	Diffuse large B cell lymphoma
DLCO	Diffusing capacity
DM	Distant metastases
Dmax	Maximum dose
DRE	Digital rectal exam
DRR	Digitally reconstructed radiograph
DSS	Disease-specific survival
DVH	Dose-volume histogram
EBCTCG	Early Breast Cancer Trialists' Collaborative Group
EBRT	External beam radiation therapy
EBUS	Endobronchial ultrasound
EBV	Epstein–Barr virus
ECE	Extracapsular extension
ECOG	Eastern Cooperative Oncology Group
ED	Erectile dysfunction
EDTA	Ethylendiaminetetraacetic acid
EFRT	Extended field radiotherapy
EFS	Event-free survival
EGD	Esophagogastroduodenoscopy
EGJ	Esophagogastric junction
EIC	Extensive intraductal component
ENT	Ear nose throat
EORTC	European Organisation for Research and Treatment of Cancer
EPID	Electronic portal imaging device
ER	Estrogen receptor
ERBB	Epidermal growth factor
ERCP	Endoscopic retrograde cholangiopancreatography
ESR	Erythrocyte sedimentation rate
ESTRO	European Society for Radiotherapy and Oncology
ESRTO ACROP	ESTRO and the Advisory Committee in Radiation Oncology Practice
ETE	Extra-thyroid extension
EtOH	Alcohol
EUA	Exam under anesthesia

EUS	Endoscopic ultrasound
FDA	Food and Drug Administration
FDG	Fludeoxyglucose
FEV_1	Forced expiratory volume in 1 second
FFF	Freedom from failure
FFP	Freedom from progression
FFS	Failure-free survival
FH	Family history
FIGO	International Federation of Gynecology and Obstetrics staging system
FISH	Fluorescence in situ hybridization
FNA	Fine needle aspiration
FOBT	Fecal occult blood test
FSH	Follicle-stimulating hormone
FSRT	Fractionated stereotactic radiotherapy
FSU	Functional subunit
FWHM	Full width half maximum
fx	Fraction(s)
GaK	GammaKnife
GBM	Glioblastoma multiforme
GEC-ESTRO	Groupe Européen de Curiethérapie-European Society for Radiotherapy and Oncology
GERD	Gastroesophageal reflux disease
GH	Growth hormone
GHSG	German Hodgkin's Study Group
GIST	Gastrointestinal stromal tumors
GITSG	Gastrointestinal Tumors Study Group
GOG	Gynecologic Oncology Group
GS	Gleason score
GTR	Gross total resection
GTV	Gross tumor volume
GU	Genitourinary
Gy	Gray
H&E	Hematoxylin and eosin
H&N	Head and neck
H&P	History and physical exam
HAART	Highly active retroviral therapy
Hb	Hemoglobin
Hcc	Hepatocellular carcinoma
hCG	Human chorionic gonadotropin
HCV	Hepatitis C virus
HDR	High dose rate
HER2	Human epidermal growth factor receptor 2
HIV	Human immunodeficiency virus
HNPCC	Hereditary nonpolyposis colon cancer

HNSqCC	Head and neck squamous cell carcinoma
HPV	Human papilloma virus
HRT	Hormone replacement therapy
HSRT	Hypofractionated stereotactic radiotherapy
HT	Helical tomotherapy
HTN	Hypertension
HVL	Half-value layer
Hx	History
IC	Intracavitary
ICRU	International Commission of Radiation Units and Measurements
ICU	Intensive care unit
IDC	Invasive ductal carcinoma
IDL	Isodose line
IE	Ifosfamide and etoposide (VP-16)
IESS	Intergroup Ewing's Sarcoma Study
IFN	Interferon
IFRT I	Involved-field radiotherapy
IGRT	Image-guided radiotherapy
IJROBP	International Journal of Radiation Oncology Biology Physics
ILC	Invasive lobular carcinoma
IM	Internal margin
im	Intramuscular
IMN	Internal mammary nodes
IMRT	Intensity-modulated radiotherapy
INSS	International Neuroblastoma Staging System
Int	Intergroup
IORT	Intraoperative radiation therapy
IS	Interstitial
is	in situ
ISRT	Involved site radiotherapy
ITV	Internal target volume [ITV = CTV + IM]
iv	Intravenous
IVC	Inferior vena cava
IVP	Intravenous pyelogram
JCO	*Journal of Clinical Oncology*
JPA	Juvenile pilocytic astrocytoma
KPS	Karnofsky Performance Status
LAPC	Locally advanced pancreatic cancer
LAR	Low anterior resection
LC	Local control
LCIS	Lobular carcinoma in situ
LCSG	Lung Cancer Study Group
LDH	Lactate dehydrogenase
LDR	Low dose rate
LET	Linear energy transfer

LF	Local failure
LFFS	Local failure-free survival
LFTs	Liver function tests
LH	Luteinizing hormone
LINAC	Linear accelerator
LN	Lymph node(s)
LND	Lymph node dissection
LR	Local recurrence/relapse
LRC	Local-regional control
LRF	Local-regional failure
LRRFR	Locoregional recurrence-free rate
LVEF	Left ventricular ejection fraction
LVSI/LVI	Lymphovascular space invasion
m	Meter
MALT	Mucosa-associated lymphoid tissue
MESCC	Metastatic epidural spinal cord compression
MFH	Malignant fibrous histiosarcoma
mg	Milligram
MHD	Mean heart dose
MLC	Multileaf collimator
MLD	Mean lung dose
mm	millimeter
mOS	Median overall survival
MRA	Magnetic resonance angiography
MRC	Medical Research Council
MRCP	Magnetic resonance cholangiopancreatography
MRI	Magnetic resonance imaging
MRSI	Magnetic resonance spectroscopy imaging
MSKCC	Memorial Sloan Kettering Cancer Center
MTD	Maximal tolerated dose
MU	Monitor unit
MUGA	Multiple gated acquisition scan
N+	Node positive
N0	Node negative
NCCN	National Comprehensive Cancer Network
NCI	National Cancer Institute
NCIC	National Cancer Institute of Canada
NED	No evidence of disease
NEJM	*New England Journal of Medicine*
NHL	Non-Hodgkin's lymphoma
NPV	Negative predictive value
NPX	Nasopharynx
NSABP	National Surgical Adjuvant Breast and Bowel Project
NSCLC	Non-small cell lung cancer
NSGCT	Nonseminomatous germ cell tumor

NTCP	Normal tissue complication probability
NWTS	National Wilms' Tumor Study
OAR	Organ at risk
OD	Oligodendroglioma
OPX	Oropharynx
ORN	Osteoradionecrosis
OS	Overall survival
PA	Posterior-anterior
PALN	Para-aortic lymph node
Pb	Lead
pCR	Pathologic complete response
PDR	Pulsed dose rate
PET	Positron emission tomography
PLAP	Placental alkaline phosphatase
PNET	Primitive neuroectodermal tumor
PNI	Perineural invasion
PORT	Postoperative radiotherapy
Post-op	Postoperative
PPV	Positive predictive value
pR	Partial response
PR	Progesterone receptor
Pre-op	Preoperative
PRL	Prolactin
prn	as required
PRV	Planning organ at risk volume [PRV = OAR + IM + SM]
PS	Performance status
PSA	Prostate-specific antigen
PTV_x	Planning target volume $x = 1,2\ldots$
PUVA	Psoralen and ultraviolet light A
q.d	Once daily
q.i.d	Four times a day (quater in die)
q.o.d	Every other day
QA	Quality assurance
QALY	Quality-adjusted life year
QC	Quality control
QOL	Quality of life
RAI	Radioactive iodine
RBE	Relative biological effectiveness
RCC	Renal cell carcinoma
Rct	Randomized controlled trial
RFA	Radiofrequency ablation
RFS	Relapse-free survival
RILD	Radiation-induced liver disease
RP	Radical prostatectomy
RT	Radiotherapy

RTOG	Radiation Therapy Oncology Group
s/p	Status post
SBRT	Stereotactic body radiotherapy
SCID	Severe combined immunodeficiency
SCLC	Small cell lung cancer
SCV	Supraclavicular
SEER	Surveillance, Epidemiology, and End Results
SGOT	Serum glutamic oxaloacetic transaminase
SGPT	Serum glutamic pyruvic transaminase
SI	Sacroiliac
SIADH	Syndrome of inappropriate antidiuretic hormone
SINS	Spinal Instability Neoplastic Score
SLNB	Sentinel lymph node biopsy
SM	Set up margin
SMA	Superior mesenteric artery
SMV	Superior mesenteric vein
SNUC	Sinonasal undifferentiated carcinoma
SOB	Shortness of breath
SPECT	Single-photon emission computed tomography
SPEP	Serum protein electrophoreses
SqCC	Squamous cell carcinoma
SRS	Stereotactic radiosurgery
STAPLE	Simultaneous Truth and Performance Level Estimation
STD	Sexually transmitted disease
STIR	Short Tau Inversion Recover (MRI)
STLI	Subtotal lymphoid irradiation
STR	Subtotal resection
SWOG	Southwest Oncology Group
T&O	Tandem and ovoid
t.i.d	Three times a day (ter in die)
TACE	Transarterial chemoembolization
TAH/BSO	Total abdominal hysterectomy/bilateral salpingo-oophorectomy
TBI	Total body irradiation
TBNA	Transbronchial needle aspiration
TCC	Transitional cell carcinoma
TCP	Tumor control probability
TG101	AAPM Task Force Group 101
TME	Total mesorectal excision
TMP/SMX	Trimethoprim/sulfamethoxazole
TMZ	Temozolomide
TNM	Tumor node metastasis
TPS	Treatment planning system
TRUS	Transrectal ultrasound
TSH	Thyroid-stimulating hormone
TTP	Time to tumor progression

TURBT	Transurethral resection of bladder tumor
UA	Urinalysis
UCSF	University of California, San Francisco
UKCCCR	United Kingdom Coordinating Committee on Cancer Research
UNC	University of North Carolina
UNC-CH	University of North Carolina Chapel Hill
UPEP	Urine protein electrophoreses
US	Ultrasound
USA	United States of America
USO	Unilateral salpingo-oophorectomy
UVB	Ultraviolet light B
VAC	Vincristine, actinomycin-D, and cyclophosphamide
VAIN	Vaginal intra-epithelial neoplasia
VCR	Vincristine
VDC	Vincristine, doxorubicin, cyclophosphamide
VDCA	Vincristine, doxorubicin, cyclophosphamide, and actinomycin-D
VEGF	Vascular endothelial growth factor
VM	Vincristine and melphalan
VMAT	Volumetric arc radiotherapy
VP-16	Etoposide
WART	Whole abdominal radiotherapy
Wbc	White blood cell count
WBI	Whole breast irradiation
WBRT	Whole brain radiotherapy
WHO	World Health Organization
WLE	Wide local excision

Chapter 1
The History and Radiobiology of Hypofractionation

Elaine M. Zeman

1.1 Introduction

The use of hypofractionation in radiation therapy is not a new concept. In fact, it is a very old one, dating back to the first third of the twentieth century, the earliest days of the field that would evolve into today's specialty of radiation oncology. Since its earliest incarnation, however, hypofractionation has been "repurposed" for today's use, thanks to more than a century of advances in physics and imaging that now allow most normal tissue to be excluded from the radiation field, something arguably inconceivable in 1900.

To better understand why hypofractionation was largely abandoned by the late 1920s, only to re-emerge at the beginning of the twenty-first century, an overview of the histories of both radiation therapy and radiation biology is in order. In many ways, these two disciplines evolved in parallel. With a few notable exceptions, for nearly 60 years advances in radiation therapy were empirically based, and advances in radiobiology were seldom of clinical utility. This began to change during the 1950s.

E. M. Zeman (✉)
Department of Radiation Oncology, UNC School of Medicine, Chapel Hill, NC, USA
e-mail: elaine_zeman@med.unc.edu

O. Kaidar-Person, R. Chen (eds.), *Hypofractionated and Stereotactic Radiation Therapy*, https://doi.org/10.1007/978-3-031-47701-0_1

1.2 Historical Context

1.2.1 The Early History of Fractionation in Radiotherapy

At the turn of the twentieth century, X-rays were discovered by German physicist Wilhelm Röntgen, who described them as invisible, "mysterious" emissions from energized vacuum tubes that were capable of producing fluorescence in platinocyanide salts [1]. The following year, French physicist Henri Becquerel identified similar emanations from natural substances—compounds of the element uranium—that didn't require an external energy source, yet like visible light, could expose photographic film [2]. Another year later, Pierre and Marie Curie identified and isolated some of the elements responsible for this "radioactivity" phenomenon, including radium, thorium, and polonium [3]. That X-rays and radioactive sources (emitting γ-rays) had potential medical applications for both imaging and cancer treatment was immediately obvious, and between 1896 and 1900, the nascent field of radiation therapy, as practiced by dermatologists and surgeons of the day, had already claimed cures of both benign and malignant skin conditions [4–6].

In the earliest days of radiotherapy, both X-ray machines and radium applicators were used for cancer treatment, although the greater availability, convenience, and portability of X-ray tubes afforded them a distinct advantage. Add to this the fact that X-ray machines offered, as the technology improved, much higher intensities of radiation output than low-activity radium sources, radiotherapy using X-rays (termed teletherapy) quickly became the international standard. Nevertheless, the use of radioactive sources continued to be developed and refined by the French, a practice that evolved into modern day brachytherapy.

Lacking an understanding at the time of the physical nature of ionizing radiation and how to quantify radiation dose, let alone an understanding of its biological effects, various "philosophies" developed as how best to treat patients. One fundamental radiotherapy principle was recognized early on: the concept of the therapeutic ratio, a risk-versus-benefit approach applied to treatment planning (Fig. 1.1).

In theory, any malignancy could be eradicated simply by delivering a sufficiently high radiation dose. However, in practice, injury to normal tissues that were necessarily irradiated along with the tumor limited the total dose that could be administered safely. Therefore, a balance had to be struck between what was considered an acceptable probability of radiation-induced damage to normal tissue, and the probability of tumor destruction.

Because surgeons were among the early practitioners of radiation therapy, from about 1900 into the 1920s, a prevailing strategy was to view radiotherapy as akin to surgery; that is, to attempt to eradicate the tumor in a single procedure using a large, "tumoricidal" dose. This massive dose technique [7, 8] became a common way of administering radiation therapy, and a (somewhat arbitrary) biological interpretation was also provided: tumors would become increasingly resistant to radiotherapy if too many doses were given, and normal tissues would be preferentially damaged due to "cumulative injury," so it would be preferable to deliver the radiation therapy

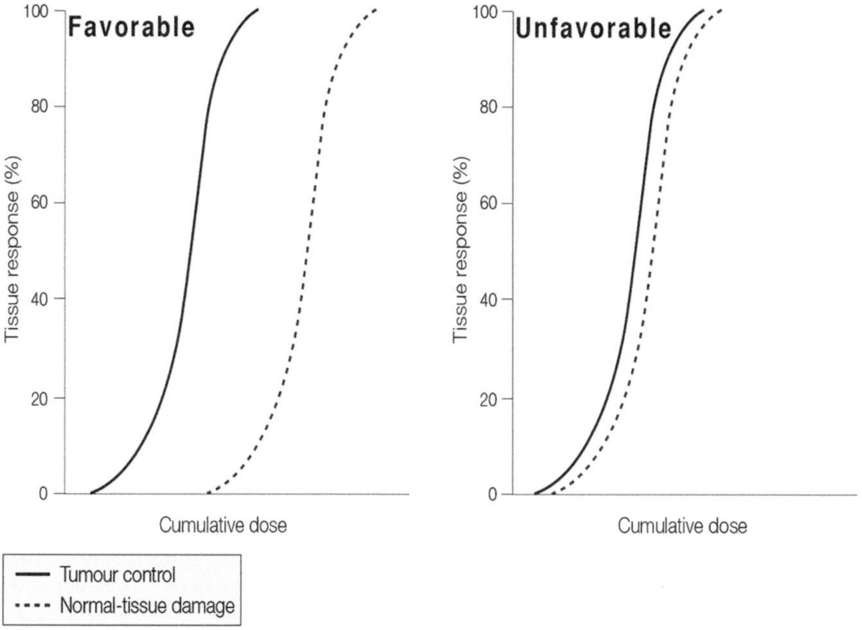

Fig. 1.1 The therapeutic ratio concept, depicted graphically. A favorable therapeutic ratio implies that the radiation response of the tumor is greater than that of the surrounding normal tissue (left panel). In the case of an unfavorable therapeutic ratio (right panel), there is no possibility of obtaining good tumor control without significantly damaging the normal tissue(s) at risk. (Adapted from Bernier et al. [7])

as one or a few large doses over no more than a few days [9]. However, it soon became obvious that this approach did not optimize the therapeutic ratio and that the biological rationale was incorrect; normal tissue complications were typically quite severe, and to make matters worse, the rate of local tumor recurrence was unacceptably high. An early example, in this case involving treatment of a benign hairy nevus, is shown in Fig. 1.2.

As mentioned previously, radium therapy was used more extensively in France. Radium applications involved longer overall treatment times in order to reach total doses comparable to those achieved with X-rays because of the low activity sources. Although multi-day treatments were less convenient in terms of patient throughput, clinical outcomes were often superior for skin and cervix cancers than for X-ray therapy. Brachytherapy proponents also offered a biological rationale, one that was better based on laboratory research than on theory or conjecture. As early as 1906, two French radiation biologists, Bergonié and Tribondeau, observed histologically that undifferentiated, rapidly dividing spermatogonia of the rat testis showed evidence of damage at lower radiation doses than well-differentiated, non-dividing cells of the testicular stroma. Based on these observations, they put forth some basic "laws" stating that radiotherapy was selective for cells that were (1) actively dividing; (2) capable of dividing for extended periods; and (3) poorly or undifferentiated

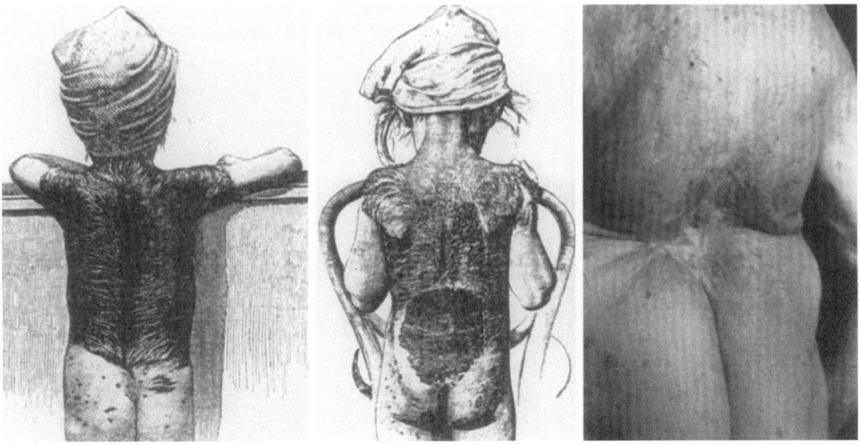

Fig. 1.2 Time course for radiation effects in the skin of a child treated during the "massive dose" era for an extensive hairy nevus before treatment (left), a week after the end of treatment (middle) and 75 years later (right). Acutely, the skin injury consisted of a large area of confluent moist desquamation, but over time, fibrosis, necrosis, and poor wound healing was observed and persisted over the patient's lifetime. Few patients were cured using this large dose, large volume technique, and typically died long before normal tissue damage became manifest. In this particular case, however, the (benign) hairy nevus was eradicated. (Adapted from Kogelnik [5])

[10]. Some tumors were already known at that time to contain cells that were less differentiated and more proliferative than most normal tissues. Accordingly, Bergonié and Tribondeau reasoned that multiple radiation exposures would preferentially kill these tumor cells, while preserving their slowly proliferating, differentiated counterparts in the normal tissues included in the radiation field.

During the 1920s, the massive dose technique began to fall out of favor, particularly in light of the pioneering experiments of Claude Regaud and colleagues, who built on Bergonié and Tribondeau's earlier work [11]. Regaud cleverly used the testes of the rabbit as a model system, reasoning that the process of sperm production (i.e., relatively undifferentiated cells proliferating rapidly and indefinitely) mimicked to a first approximation the behavior of tumors, and that the scrotum could be used as a representative dose-limiting normal tissue. Regaud showed that only through the use of multiple, smaller radiation doses could animals be completely sterilized without producing severe injury to the scrotum [12].

These principles were soon tested in the clinic by French physician Henri Coutard, who used multiple small x-ray doses delivered over extended periods in human patients [13]. Clinical outcomes for patients with head and neck cancer were improved to such an extent that fractionated radiation therapy using many small dose increments spread over several weeks' time soon became the standard of care [13, 14], and has largely remained so to the present day.

Summary: relevance to today's use of hypofractionation

- During the early days of radiotherapy—the first 30 years of the twentieth century—extreme hypofractionation using one or a few very large doses was a treatment standard.
- It was subsequently abandoned when it became clear that tumor control was poor and normal tissue complications severe.
- Early research in radiation biology determined that the best way to optimize the therapeutic ratio was to deliver many small dose fractions over a period of weeks.
- Translating this information into the clinic, fractionated radiotherapy using small doses delivered over several weeks provided much improved outcomes, and became the new standard of care.

1.2.2 Isoeffect Relationships

Once fractionated radiotherapy became the new standard of care a different problem emerged, namely how different practitioners with somewhat different approaches to fractionation, e.g., how many fractions delivered, time between fractions, total dose, overall treatment time, etc., could be inter-compared in terms of tumor control and normal tissue complication probabilities. One approach was to determine "equivalents," that is, treatment combinations that yielded similar outcomes. Time-dose equivalents for skin erythema were published by several investigators [15–18] and these formed the basis for the calculation of equivalents for other normal tissue and tumor responses. By plotting the total dose required for a particular equivalent in a particular tissue, as a function of one of the variable treatment parameters (overall treatment time, number of fractions or dose per fraction), a so-called isoeffect curve could be derived. All time and dose combinations that comprised an isoeffect curve for a certain endpoint would, theoretically, produce tissue or tumor responses of equal magnitude.

Also better appreciated during the 1930s was how and when normal tissue complications occurred after treatment, and their severity as a function of total dose. Presumably, these complications were the result (directly or indirectly) of the killing of critical cells within the tissue, so the higher the radiation dose, the more cells were killed and the more severe the complication. It was also clear that skin, the dose-limiting normal tissue in most cases, could manifest more than one complication and that each seemed to have its own threshold or tolerance dose before the complication occurred, a reflection of the tissue's radiosensitivity. However, the "earliness" or "lateness" of the clinical manifestation of that injury was a separate phenomenon more related to the cellular renewal pattern of the tissue.

The first published isoeffect curves were produced by Strandqvist in 1944 [19], and shown in Fig. 1.3. When plotted on a log–log scale of total dose versus overall treatment time, isoeffect curves for a variety of skin reactions, and the cure of skin cancer, were drawn as parallel lines.

As drawn, Stranqvist's isoeffect curves suggested that there would be *no* therapeutic advantage to using prolonged treatment times and multiple small dose

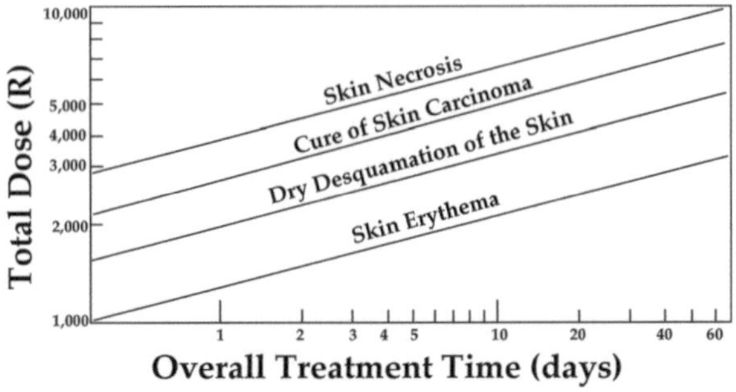

Fig. 1.3 Strandqvist's isoeffect curves, first published in 1944, plotted the log of the total dose to achieve the measured isoeffect as a function of the overall treatment time. The shorter the overall treatment time, the more hypofractionated the schedule, and the lower the dose required to produce the isoeffect. (Modified from Strandqvist [19])

fractions for the preferential eradication of tumors while staying within the tolerance of the normal tissue [20]. Ironically however, it was already known that the therapeutic ratio *did* increase with prolonged, as opposed to very short, overall treatment times. Nevertheless, the reliability of these curves at predicting skin reactions, which were the dose limiting at the time, made them quite popular.

Nearly 25 years after Strandqvist, Ellis [21, 22] revisited his popular isoeffect curves, and armed with new knowledge about the radiobiology underlying fractionation effects in pig skin [23, 24], formulated the NSD concept in 1969. The NSD equation,

$$\boldsymbol{D} = (\mathbf{NSD})\, \boldsymbol{N}^{0.24} \boldsymbol{T}^{0.11},$$

where D is the total dose delivered, N the number of fractions used, T the overall treatment time, and NSD the nominal standard dose (a proportionality constant related to the tissue's tolerance), became widely used, particularly once mathematically simplified derivatives, such as the TDF equation [25] became available. The major innovation of the NSD model was that the influence of the fraction number had been separated from the influence of the overall treatment time, and in fact, the fraction number (and therefore, size) was the more important of the two.

The introduction of the NSD equation allowed radiotherapy treatment practices world-wide to be compared with respect to putative "biological equivalence," provided it was not used for treatments involving extremes of fraction number or overall time outside the range of the data upon which the model was based (i.e., Strandqvist's curves). It also provided a means of revising treatment prescriptions in the event of unforeseen treatment interruptions. However, the NSD formula was ill-equipped to deal with some clinical issues, in particular the prediction of late effects in normal tissues, which, with the advent of megavoltage linear accelerators capable of treating deep-seated tumors, replaced skin as being dose-limiting [26]. In light of the emerging limitations of the NSD model, there was a need for new, radiobiologically based approaches to isoeffect modeling.

Summary: relevance to today's use of hypofractionation

- Isoeffect curves plot the total dose required for a particular tumor or normal tissue endpoint as a function of one of the variable treatment parameters, such as overall treatment time or number of fractions. All time-dose combinations that fell on a particular isoeffect curve were considered biologically equivalent.
- Isoeffects of interest included tumor control and various normal tissue complications, typically in skin, such as desquamation, necrosis, or fibrosis.
- Some complications occurred during or soon after the completion of radiotherapy, "early effects," and others took months or years to manifest, "late effects."
- The total dose required to cause a particular complication was a reflection of the tissue's radiosensitivity, but the time it took for the complication to appear was related to the tissue's natural cell renewal process.
- A mathematical model derived from isoeffect curves, the NSD equation, allowed the calculation of biological equivalents for different treatment schedules. Yet because the model was based on early skin reactions, it was poorly equipped to model late complications in normal tissues. With the advent of megavoltage radiotherapy equipment that allowed treatment of deep-seated tumors, damage to internal organs rather than skin became dose-limiting, and many of these expressed their injuries as late effects.

1.2.3 Tumor Hypoxia

As early as 1909, it was recognized that decreasing blood flow during radiotherapy leads to a reduction in the prevalence or severity of radiation-induced skin reactions [7, 8], although at the time, the mechanism for this effect was unclear. Decades later, chemists and biologists determined that the presence or absence of oxygen was the key, and that the mechanism of oxygen's action was to interact with free radicals produced during irradiation, thereby enhancing the damage to cellular macromolecules. In other words, oxygen acted as a radiation sensitizer. Thus, the relative *absence* of oxygen in an irradiated system meant less molecular damage, and therefore, greater radioresistance.

In 1955, however, Thomlinson and Gray [27] brought this idea to the forefront of radiation biology and radiation therapy by proposing that tumors contained a fraction of oxygen-starved yet still reproductively viable (i.e., "clonogenic") hypoxic cells and that if these persisted throughout the course of fractionated radiotherapy, they would adversely affect the therapeutic ratio. The oxygen enhancement ratio (OER) is a metric developed to quantify how much more radioresistant hypoxic cells were than well-aerated ones. For large, single radiation doses, OER values of 2.5–3.0 were typical, but for conventional radiotherapy using repeated, small dose fractions delivered over several weeks, the OER was lower, typically in the range of 1.5–2.0 [28].

Accordingly, if human tumors contained even a tiny fraction of clonogenic hypoxic cells, simple calculations suggested that tumor control would be nearly impossible [29], even for high doses. The total dose needed to control such tumors would become prohibitive because normal tissues are not hypoxic and therefore would experience higher complication rates if the total dose were increased. In fact, the only way that hypoxic tumor cells would *not* constitute a treatment impediment was if extended periods of hypoxia eventually led to their deaths, that these cells "reoxygenated" during the course of treatment and/or that they were not clonogenic to begin with.

Hypoxia is a consequence of the abnormal vasculature characteristic of tumors. Such blood vessels are the product of abnormal angiogenesis and often are structurally, functionally, physiologically, and/or spatially aberrant which, when combined with the tumor's high oxygen demand and tendency to outgrow its own blood supply, leads to both micro- and macro-regions of hypoxia.

Summary: relevance to today's use of hypofractionation

- Molecular oxygen interacts with free radicals produced during irradiation, enhancing cellular damage. Hypoxic cells that are low in oxygen, but not so low as to result in lethality, can be up to three times more radioresistant than well-aerated ones.
- Vascular abnormalities characteristic of tumors lead to both micro- and macro-regions of hypoxia. Hypoxia is largely absent in normal tissues.
- Simple calculations suggest that tumor control would be impossible—even for the high doses used today in extreme hypofractionation—if human tumors contained even a tiny fraction of clonogenic hypoxic cells, provided they persisted throughout the course of radiotherapy.

1.2.4 The Four R's of Radiotherapy

What was largely lacking during radiotherapy's first half-century was a biological basis for why dose fractionation spared normal tissue complications, and without this information, it was very difficult to determine which biological characteristics of normal or tumor tissues might be exploited to improve the therapeutic ratio. This began to change with the publication in 1975 of a seminal paper entitled "*The Four R's of Radiotherapy*" [30]. The paper was an attempt to explain the biological basis of fractionation by describing in simple terms key radiobiological phenomena thought to affect radiotherapy outcome: *R*epair, *R*epopulation, *R*eoxygenation, and *R*edistribution. In the ensuing years, a fifth "R" was added, *R*adiosensitivity [31], although in some respects, it is inextricably linked to repair. (Redistribution is difficult to measure, yet is assumed to occur in vivo during conventional fractionation. However, it is thought to play only a minor role in treatment outcome and likely has even less of a role for hypofractionation, so will not be discussed further.)

1.2.4.1 Repair and Radiosensitivity

The surviving fraction of cells following a moderate-to-high radiation dose is higher if that dose is split into two increments separated by a time interval than delivered as a single dose, suggesting that cells surviving the initial dose had repaired some of the damage during the radiation-free interval [32]. As such, this damage was no longer available to interact with the damage inflicted by the second dose, so a higher cell surviving fraction resulted. This phenomenon is termed sublethal damage recovery (SLDR). These "split-dose" experiments turned out to be crucial to the understanding of why and how fractionated radiation therapy works, that is, that SLDR was responsible for the greater radiation tolerance of tissues when a large total dose was divided into small dose fractions and protracted over time.

However, this sparing effect of dose fractionation does not continue indefinitely as smaller and smaller (and more numerous) doses are delivered. Instead, a limit is reached where further lowering of the dose per fraction does not produce a further decrease in toxicity. This finding is consistent with the idea that survival and dose response curves have negative initial slopes [33, 34], and that after many, sufficiently small dose fractions are delivered, a "trace" of this initial slope would be obtained.

One important clinical implication of repair and radiosensitivity phenomena is that small differences in shoulder regions of dose response curves for different dose-limiting normal tissues and tumors could be magnified into large differences when many small dose fractions are used compared to a single or a few large fractions. A tissue's radiosensitivity and repair capacity are critically important to the selection of the total dose, dose per fraction and interfraction interval used for radiation therapy, as they govern both the tumor control and normal tissue complication probabilities.

1.2.4.2 Repopulation

Repopulation is defined as an increase in cell proliferation in tissues in response to an injury that produces cell killing. Normal tissues and tumors containing stem or stem-like cells can begin to proliferate during and after a course of radiation therapy, with the timing of this response a function of the proliferation kinetics of the tissue [35, 36], typically during or within 3 months of treatment for "early-responding" normal tissues and most tumors, and more than 6–9 months (if at all) for "late-responding" tissues.

Repopulation is desirable in normal tissues because it facilitates the healing of common radiotherapy complications that develop during or soon after treatment, such as oral mucositis, for example. On the other hand, repopulation of tumor cells is undesirable because it would have the net effect of counteracting ongoing radiation therapy, which in turn would lead to the appearance of tumor "radioresistance" and accordingly, the attendant risk of recurrence. For tumors capable of rapid repopulation that begins during conventional radiotherapy, estimates are that as much as a third (and sometimes more) of the daily dose fraction is wasted simply trying to counteract the production new cells.

Although the killing of cells by ionizing radiation can stimulate repopulation, another radiation effect has the potential to slow or stop it, and that is that radiation exposure introduces blocks and delays in cell cycle transit, which, while transient for lower doses, could become permanent for higher ones. The principal causes of this are dose-dependent blocks in the G_2-to-M phase transition and in the G_1-to-S phase transition, the latter typically more prominent in normal cells than malignant ones.

The critical clinical parameter that determines the influence of repopulation on treatment outcome is the overall treatment time. Shorter overall times—like those used for hypofractionation—would limit the potential for repopulation to negatively affect tumor control, albeit at the risk of exacerbating effects in early-responding normal tissues that depend on repopulation for healing.

1.2.4.3 Reoxygenation in Tumors

The identification of clonogenic, radioresistant hypoxic cells in rodent and human tumors suggests that tumor control with radiotherapy could be compromised, and yet obviously, many therapeutic successes do occur. This suggests that some form of reoxygenation must take place during the course of fractionated radiotherapy.

Are there different types of tumor hypoxia, and by extension, are there also different types of and time scales for reoxygenation? The type of hypoxia initially described by Thomlinson and Gray [27] is termed chronic or diffusion-limited hypoxia, resulting from the tendency of tumors to have high oxygen consumption rates and to outgrow their own blood supply. Cells situated well beyond the diffusion distance of oxygen likely would be dead or dying (of nutrient deprivation and anoxia), yet in regions of chronically low oxygen—on the order of 0.5% oxygen tension, corresponding to about 10 ppm O_2 or less [37]—clonogenic and radioresistant hypoxic cells could persist. Should the tumor shrink as a result of radiation therapy, or, if the cells killed by radiation cause a decreased demand for oxygen, it is likely that this would allow some of the chronically hypoxic cells to reoxygenate. However, such a reoxygenation process would be slow—typically on the order of days or weeks—depending on the regression rates of tumors during treatment. Reoxygenation in some rodent tumors does occur over such time scales, but for others, reoxygenation is considerably faster, on a time scale of minutes to hours [38], and in the absence of either reduced oxygen utilization by tumor cells or tumor shrinkage.

During the late 1970s, Brown and colleagues [39] proposed that a second type of hypoxia must exist in tumors, an acute, intermittent type that occurred secondary to abnormal vascular physiology. Intermittent hypoxia has since been demonstrated unambiguously in rodent tumors [40], and, using hypoxia markers detected noninvasively using PET scanning, in human cancer patients [41]. There are multiple mechanisms to account for intermittent hypoxia including, but not limited to, temporary vessel blockage, vascular shunting, and vessel compression due to high interstitial fluid pressure in the tumor microenvironment [41]. Most of these would cause transient hypoxia of minutes to hours in duration.

Regardless of type or mechanism, the clinical implication of reoxygenation of hypoxic tumor cells is that it would increase the therapeutic ratio, assuming that normal tissues remained well-oxygenated. The overall treatment time would seem critical, with overall times of several weeks in theory allowing "full" reoxygenation to occur and short overall treatment times running the risk of incomplete reoxygenation. Because of this, reoxygenation is thought to be a major factor in the radiosensitization of tumors during conventionally fractionated radiation therapy. Unfortunately, this might not be the case for shorter, hypofractionated schedules.

Summary: relevance to today's use of hypofractionation

- The five R's of radiotherapy are radiosensitivity, repair, repopulation, reoxygenation, and redistribution. These fundamental radiobiological phenomena provide a basis for how best to maximize tumor cell kill and avoid normal tissue toxicity during conventional radiotherapy.
- Radiosensitivity and repair are linked, and to best spare normal tissues, repair must be maximized.
- Accelerated repopulation in response to radiation injury is desirable for early-responding normal tissues, as it facilitates healing. In general, late-responding normal tissues cannot accelerate their proliferation in response to injury, and even among those that can, it would take months to occur, long after the completion of radiotherapy.
- Repopulation in tumors is undesirable, as it counteracts the toxicity of the radiotherapy, possibly culminating in treatment failure. Shorter overall treatment times, like those used for hypofractionation, would provide less time for tumor repopulation.
- Of the five R's, the only one unique to tumors is reoxygenation. In the absence of reoxygenation, tumors containing even a small fraction of clonogenic hypoxic cells would become nearly impossible to cure with radiotherapy. Depending on the type(s) of hypoxia present in tumors, reoxygenation can occur over timescales of minutes, hours, or days.
- The shorter overall treatment times characteristic of hypofractionation may not allow sufficient time for tumor reoxygenation to occur, leading to treatment resistance.

1.2.5 The Linear-Quadratic Isoeffect Model

1.2.5.1 α/β Ratios

The beginnings of the linear-quadratic (LQ) isoeffect model can be traced to the ambitious multifractionation experiments in mice by Douglas and Fowler [42], where a broad range of fraction sizes, numbers, and inter-fraction intervals was used and acute skin reactions in the mouse foot evaluated. They developed a novel method of interpreting their data by creating a new type of isoeffect curve, termed a "reciprocal dose plot," where the reciprocal of the total dose delivered was plotted as a function of the dose per fraction. From such a plot, a fractionation sensitivity metric could be derived for mouse skin which, borrowing the framework of the LQ survival curve expression, was termed the skin's "α/β ratio." Fractionation data that adhered to the LQ formalism would produce a straight line on such a plot. The α/β ratio in turn was used to generate a pseudo dose response curve, the shape of which provided clues as to the tissue's overall radiosensitivity and repair competency. A representative reciprocal dose isoeffect curve is shown in Fig. 1.4.

More widespread use of this technique over time showed that in most cases, there was a systematic difference between early- and late-responding normal tissues in terms of their α/β ratios and significantly, that the majority of tumors behaved like early-responding tissues. The α/β ratios were typically low for late-responding tissues (about 1–6 Gy, with an average of about 3 Gy), and high for early-responding tissues and tumors (about 7–20 Gy, with an average of about 10 Gy). Select α/β ratios for human normal tissues are shown in Table 1.1. It is worth noting that there are exceptions to these general trends, in particular that prostate cancer, and to a lesser extent breast cancer, have low rather than high α/β ratios, meaning that their fractionation sensitivities are more like those of late-responding normal tissues. This finding was a major impetus in the return of hypofractionation.

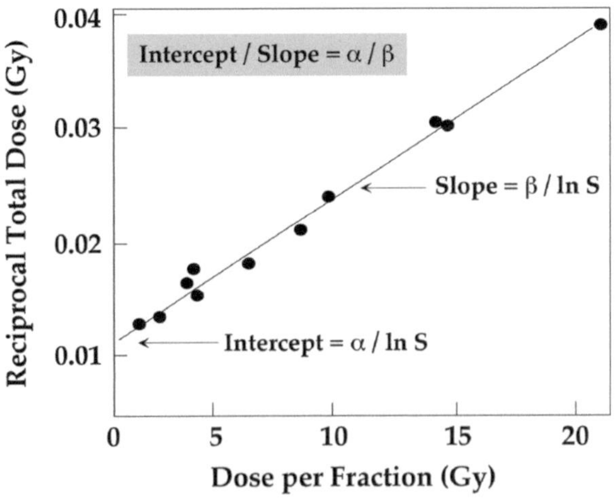

Fig. 1.4 The reciprocal dose plot technique of Douglas and Fowler [42], used to determine a normal tissue's or tumor's α/β ratio. Using this method, the reciprocal of the total dose necessary to reach a given isoeffect is plotted as a function of the dose per fraction. Assuming that the tissue's fractionation response can be modeled using the linear-quadratic expression, $S = e - (\alpha D + \beta D2)$, the α/β ratio can be obtained from the ratio of the isoeffect curve's intercept to its slope. (Modified from Douglas and Fowler [42])

Table 1.1 α/β Ratios for select human normal tissues and tumors

Tissue type (and endpoint)	α/β Ratio (± 95% confidence interval)
Early-responding normal tissues	
Skin	
Erythema Desquamation	10.6 (1.8; 22.8) Gy 11.2 (8.5; 17.6) Gy
Lung: pneumonitis ≤90 days after radiotherapy	>8.8 Gy
Oral mucosa: mucositis	8–15 Gy
Late-responding normal tissues	
Skin	
Telangiectasia Fibrosis	~ 2.7 (−0.1; 8.1) Gy 1.7 (0.6; 3.0) Gy
Breast	
Cosmesis Fibrosis	3.4 (2.3; 4.5) Gy 3.1 (1.8; 4.4) Gy
Lung	
Pneumonitis >90 days after radiotherapy Fibrosis	4.0 (2.2; 5.8) Gy 3.1 (−0.2; 8.5) Gy
Bowel	
Perforation/stricture Various other	3.9 (2.5; 5.3) Gy 4.3 (2.2; 9.6) Gy
Spinal cord: myelopathy	<3.3 Gy
Tumors	
Head and neck	
Vocal cord Tonsil Larynx	~13 Gy 7.2 (3.6; ∞) Gy 14.5 (4.9; 24) Gy
Lung: squamous cell carcinoma	~50–90 Gy
Cervix: squamous cell carcinoma	>13.9 Gy
Skin: squamous cell carcinoma	8.5 (4.5; 11.3) Gy
Prostate	1.8 (−3.3; 5.6) Gy
Breast	4.6 (1.1; 8.1) Gy

Data from Joiner and van der Kogel [43]

1.2.5.2 Steep vs. Shallow Isoeffect Curves

However, many found the use of reciprocal doses confusing and unwieldy, preferring more traditional isoeffect curves like those of Strandqvist. Accordingly, Thames, Withers, Peters, and colleagues [44–46] replotted data obtained from fractionation experiments in rodents as the log of the total dose on the *y*-axis and the log of dose per fraction on the *x*-axis, with this axes reversed to better align with Stranqvist's original curves (where overall time rather than dose per fraction was used). When plotted in this manner, isoeffect curves for late-responding normal tissues were steeper than those for early-responding normal tissues and most tumors. A steep isoeffect curve implied a greater sensitivity to changes in dose per fraction, experiencing greater sparing with decreasing fraction size (i.e., a higher tolerance

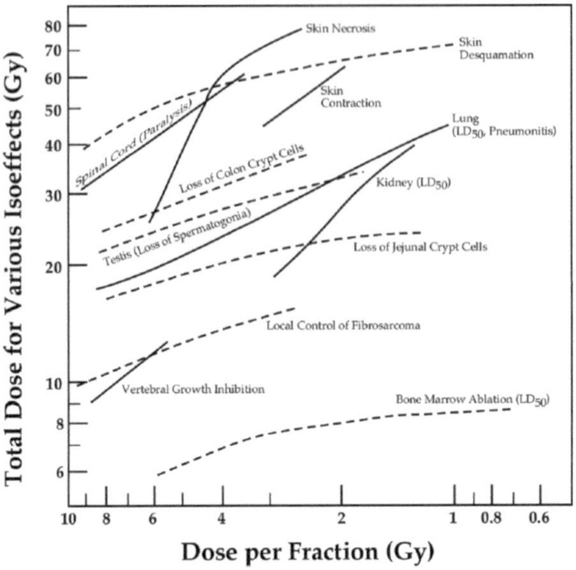

Fig. 1.5 Isoeffect curves in which the total dose to produce a certain normal tissue or tumor endpoint (as indicated on graph) is plotted as a function of the dose per fraction, under conditions where cell proliferation is negligible. Isoeffect curves for late responding normal tissues (solid lines) tend to be steeper than those for early responding normal tissues and most tumors (dashed lines). This suggests that, for the same total dose, late reactions may be spared by decreasing the size of the dose per fraction used (hyperfractionation). However, in the case of a tumor with a steep isoeffect curve, it would be preferentially damaged by using higher doses per fraction (hypofractionation). (Modified from Withers et al. [45])

dose for the isoeffect) and greater damage with increasing fraction size (i.e., a lower tolerance dose for the isoeffect). On the other hand, a shallow isoeffect curve suggested less sensitivity to changes in dose per fraction, that is, less "swing" in tolerance doses when the fraction size was changed. Isoeffect curves plotted in this manner for several normal tissue complications, along with a few corresponding to tumor control doses, are shown in Fig. 1.5.

These authors also discussed in detail the various assumptions implicit in the repurposing of the LQ model for clinical use as a measure of fractionation sensitivity. Perhaps the most egregious of the assumptions was that an isoeffect in a tissue represented an isosurvival of the cells whose deaths precipitated the effect [44, 45]. This is clearly a gross oversimplification of what is now known (and was strongly suspected even then) about the etiology of normal tissue complications, late effects in particular. They develop over extended periods of time as a result of highly complex and dynamic molecular processes involving multiple, interacting cell types rather than a single putative "target cell." Nevertheless, this assumption was necessary in that normal tissue complications were *initiated* by the killing of cells with unique radiosensitivities, in order to justify using a cell survival curve expression to model fractionation effects in vivo.

This assumption is also the probable source of a common misconception about the *LQ isoeffect model*, namely that the α/β ratios quoted for tumors and normal tissues are derived from cell survival curves fitted to the *LQ survival curve model*. This is not and never has been the case; α/β ratios used clinically are derived from multifraction experiments in vivo, and are a reflection of, at best, a composite dose response curve that likely has been further modified by the influence of the five R's. One important corollary is that these dose response curves are *not* quantitative in the same sense cell survival curves are, and treating them as such is, arguably, inappropriate.

Tissue dose response curve shapes consistent with the calculated α/β ratios and steep-vs.-shallow isoeffect curves are shown in Fig. 1.6.

The steeper initial slope in the low dose region for tissues with high α/β ratios (early-responding normal tissues and most tumors) accounts for their reduced sensitivity to changes in dose per fraction. Conversely, the shallower initial slope for late-responding normal tissues and the few tumors with low α/β ratios accounts for their high sensitivity to changes in dose per fraction. The use of low doses per fraction would preferentially spare these tissues, whereas high doses per fraction would be preferentially damaging.

1.2.6 Hyper- vs. Hypofractionation

It was immediately evident that the differences in fractionation response between tumors and normal tissues could be exploited for clinical benefit. For example, it might be possible to increase the therapeutic ratio by sparing late normal tissue complications through the use of larger numbers of smaller fractions to a somewhat

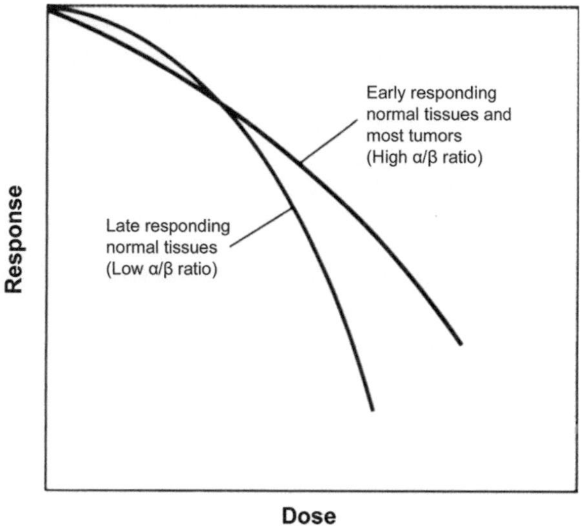

Fig. 1.6 Putative dose response curves for normal tissues and tumors generated from α/β ratios determined in fractionation experiments in vivo. Note that the shapes of these curves, particularly in the low dose region (governed mostly by the α-component), are assumed to account for the differences in fractionation sensitivity of the different tissues. (Modified from Zeman et al. [47])

higher total dose than traditionally used [46, 48, 49], in the hopes that the higher total dose would be sufficient to control a tumor that is relatively insensitive to the change in the dose per fraction. This is termed hyperfractionation. The opposite strategy is also possible, namely, to use fewer, larger dose fractions (typically to a lower total dose compared to conventional treatment) in order to preferentially damage those few tumors with low α/β ratios and steep isoeffect curves. This is called hypofractionation. At the time the LQ isoeffect model was first developed, however, hypofractionation was strongly discouraged because it would likewise exacerbate late effects in incidentally irradiated normal tissues, as had been amply demonstrated during the early days of radiotherapy.

1.2.7 Biologically Effective Doses (BEDs)

The shapes of tissue and tumor isoeffect curves and their associated α/β ratios have a number of clinical applications. For example, α/β ratios can be used to equate treatment schedules employing different-sized doses per fraction in order to match the probability of causing a particular complication [50, 51]. The equation,

$$\boldsymbol{D_2 / D_1 = \left(\alpha / \beta + d_1\right) / \left(\alpha / \beta + d_2\right)},$$

can be used for this purpose, where D_1 and d_1 are, respectively, the total dose and dose per fraction of one treatment prescription, and D_2 and d_2 are the total dose and dose per fraction for an alternate treatment plan designed to be biologically equivalent.

However, it is not sufficient to plan for biological equivalence based on a single normal tissue at risk with its α/β ratio, but rather, in keeping with the concept of therapeutic ratio, it should also be assessed for the tumor with its, presumably different, α/β ratio. In this way, the change in normal tissue tolerance dose *and* tumor control dose can be assessed simultaneously when considering a change in fractionation pattern.

The "biologically effective dose" or BED method [50, 52], another derivative of the LQ model, attempts to address this. Because tissue dose response curves have negative initial slopes, the question may be asked, *"In the limit, for an infinite number of infinitely small dose fractions, what total dose would correspond to normal tissue tolerance or tumor control?"* Clearly, this theoretical dose would be quite large for a tissue characterized by a dose response curve with a shallow initial slope and low α/β ratio, and appreciably smaller for a tissue characterized by a dose response curve with a steep initial slope and high α/β ratio.

The equation,

$$\mathbf{BED} = \boldsymbol{nd\left(1 + d / \alpha / \beta\right)},$$

is used to calculate the BED for tissues with different α/β ratios. In this equation, n is the number of fractions, d is the dose per fraction, and the α/β ratio is specific for the tissue at risk.

In using BEDs to compare likely outcomes for two different fractionation schedules, two important points need to be borne in mind. The first is to understand that BEDs are not real doses, but rather extrapolates based on the α-components of the dose response curves for the tissues at risk. For this reason, the units used to describe these extrapolated doses are, for example, "Gy_3's" and "Gy_{10}'s," rather than "Gy's," where the subscripts 3 and 10 refer to the α/β ratio (in Gy) of the tissue. $Gy_{3's}$ can be compared qualitatively with Gy_3's for different fractionation schedules, and Gy_{10}'s with Gy_{10}'s; however, Gy_3's and Gy_{10}'s cannot be inter-compared.

Representative BED values for conventional, hyperfractionated, and hypofractionated radiotherapy treatments are shown in Table 1.2.

The second important point is that BEDs are somewhat qualitative. By way of example from Table 1.2, a comparison of conventional fractionation (e.g., 30 fractions of 2 Gy) with a hypofractionated regimen (e.g., 3 fractions of 15 Gy), the BEDs for both early (Gy_{10}) and late (Gy_3) endpoints increase, suggesting that the hypofractionated schedule would be "hotter" in terms of complication likelihood, approximately 1.5 times hotter in the case of early effects (and tumor control, in most cases) and almost 3 times hotter for late effects (and a few tumors). However, this does not mean that the normal tissue complication or tumor control frequencies in this example would likewise increase exactly 1.5 or threefold, only that the

Table 1.2 Illustrating the use of BEDs to compare and contrast conventional, hyperfractionated, and hypofractionated treatment schedules for tissues with α/β ratios of 10 Gy versus 3 Gy

30 x 2 Gy = 60 Gy:	BED of 72 Gy_{10} and 100 Gy_3	Conventional
35 x 1.8 Gy = 63 Gy:	BED of 74.3 Gy_{10} and 100.8 Gy_3	
68 x 1.2 Gy = 81.6 Gy:	BED of 91.4 Gy_{10} and 114 Gy_3	Hyperfractionated
70 x 1.15 Gy = 80.5 Gy:	BED of 89.8 Gy_{10} and 111.4 Gy_3	
20 x 2.8 Gy = 56 Gy:	BED of 71.7 Gy_{10} and 108 Gy_3	Hypofractionated
16 x 3.4 Gy = 54.4 Gy:	BED of 73 Gy_{10} and 116.1 Gy_3	
3 x 15 Gy = 45 Gy:	BED of 112.5 Gy_{10} and 270 Gy_3	

probabilities of such complications might be expected to increase by using hypofractionation compared to standard fractionation. In fact, using head and neck cancer as an example, Fowler and colleagues [53, 54] suggested that only increases in BED of more than about 15–20% would yield clinically detectable changes in complication or tumor control frequency.

Summary: relevance to today's use of hypofractionation

- The sensitivity of normal tissues and tumors to changes in dose per fraction can be expressed qualitatively either in terms of an α/β ratio (low for late-responding tissues and high for early responding ones) or isoeffect curve slopes (steep for late-responding tissues and shallow for early responding ones).
- Both metrics use the LQ survival curve model as a conceptual framework, but otherwise are derived solely from multifraction experiments conducted in vivo, not from cells irradiated in vitro.
- A third metric of interest is the biologically effective dose or BED, a theoretical, extrapolated total dose to achieve a particular isoeffect, pegged to a tissue's α/β ratio. BEDs are used to compare and contrast different radiotherapy treatment prescriptions with respect to how both normal tissue tolerance and tumor control change.
- Because BEDs are theoretical and not actual doses, they are expressed in a different dose unit, for example, Gy_3's or Gy_{10}'s, with the subscript identifying which α/β ratio was used to derive it. Gy_3's can be compared qualitatively with Gy_3's, and Gy_{10}'s with Gy_{10}'s, but not with each other.

1.2.8 Hypofractionation Today

The stereotactic delivery of radiation therapy has been considered for many decades, but only over the last 20 years has there been a marked increase in use of this approach thanks to advances in treatment technology. Stereotactic radiosurgery (SRS), used to treat select benign and malignant brain tumors and some functional disorders, is generally delivered as a single, large dose of approximately 20 Gy or more [55]. The term radiosurgery was first coined by neurosurgeon Lars Leskel in 1951 [56]. Stereotactic body radiation therapy (SBRT), sometimes called stereotactic ablative radiotherapy (SABR), is used in select cases for small, extracranial tumors and is typically delivered in 1–5 fractions of 7–20 Gy each [57]. Both of these approaches necessarily involve "extreme" hypofractionation. The reader should be aware, however, that there are other radiotherapy treatment regimens more reminiscent of conventional radiotherapy that involve "milder" forms of hypofractionation using doses per fraction in the 2–4 Gy range [58]. The UK START [59, 60], FAST [61], and FAST-Forward [62] clinical trials are excellent examples of stepwise, carefully designed and biologically informed trials that have led to widespread implementation of moderate hypofractionation for the treatment of early breast cancer. However, these moderately hypofractionated regimens are not necessarily intended to be ablative, involve larger treatment volumes than used in SRS and SBRT, and for some, overall treatment times extend several weeks.

In the simplest sense, the radiobiological rationale for using extreme hypofractionation seems clear, namely that the biological potency of the treatment should increase and that this increase would be selective for the tumor to the extent that the highly precise and conformal treatment planning characteristic of SRS and SBRT would minimize the exposure to normal tissues at risk of complication [63].

Time, dose, and fractionation schedules used in conventional radiotherapy evolved over many decades, developed by trial and error and the invoking of educated guesses. By successively building on previous work, sufficient clinical data accrued with respect to normal tissue tolerance and tumor control doses to deem a particular schedule generally safe and effective. Seminal publications that comprehensively reviewed the then-current understanding of dose-volume-outcome constraints for late normal tissue complications included those by Rubin and Casarett in the late 1960s [64] and later, in the early 1990s, by Emami et al. [65]. Then, in 2010, the Quantitative Analysis of Normal Tissue Effects in the Clinic (QUANTEC) compilation was published [66], with the goal of further refining Emami's earlier work by providing up-to-date dose-response and dose-volume relationships for clinically relevant normal tissue complications, and in so doing, offer practical guidance to radiation oncologists on what would constitute an optimal, or at least minimally acceptable, treatment plan based on 3D dose distributions [67]. Each successive compilation—at approximately 20 year intervals—of these dose constraints not only took into account changes in technology and practice patterns and the growing understanding of cancer biology, but also included additional clinical data collected since the previous compilation.

In much the same way as with conventional radiotherapy, the time, dose, and fractionation schedules used for extreme hypofractionation evolved "organically," [68, 69] albeit over a much shorter period of time; some of the pioneering clinical trial results for the treatment of small, inoperable lung cancers with SBRT were published as recently as 15 years ago, e.g., Chang and Timmerman [70], Martin and Gaya [57], Mehta et al. [71]. Since that time, clinical experience with treating numerous other sites has grown substantially [72].

Early on, the use of SBRT was considered revolutionary by some but foolhardy and potentially dangerous by others, due in part to institutional memory of disastrous results with hypofractionation dating back to the early twentieth century, but mainly because all the carefully vetted dose constraints based on conventional fractionation were not applicable for extreme hypofractionation, leaving no frame of reference for its safe and effective use. Even so, the prospect of being able to treat and sometimes even cure otherwise inoperable primary tumors in a non-invasive, convenient, and time- and cost-saving manner was alluring, as was the possibility of treating oligometastatic disease in a similar fashion [73–77].

A consensus guideline that provided a frame of reference for the use extreme hypofractionation became available in 2021, after an arduous undertaking over a comparatively short period of time by dedicated radiation oncologists, medical physicists, radiation biologists, and biostatisticians. In keeping with the earlier QUANTEC study, the High Dose per Fraction, Hypofractionated Treatment Effects in the Clinic (HyTEC) project [78] sought to provide radiation oncologists with guidelines to reasonably assess the risk of normal tissue complications based on dose-response and dose-volume parameters, and to do so in the era of intensity-modulated dose distributions, a technology that had not yet been widely available at the time of QUANTEC. HyTEC data sets were obtained from peer-reviewed publications of hypofractionation used to treat cancers in the lung, brain, spinal cord, head and neck, abdomen, and pelvis. Unlike QUANTEC, the HyTEC project also compiled dose-response data for tumor control probabilities. The promise of improved tumor control with higher, more biologically potent radiation doses was the original driving force for the adoption of extreme hypofractionation.

Even with HyTEC to help guide clinical practice, beyond the presumption that the ablation of small tumors using extreme hypofractionation was possible due to greater biological effectiveness (discussed above), what accounts, mechanistically speaking, for that greater biological effectiveness is not that well defined. It is also the subject of considerable controversy, with some defending the continued use of "classical" radiation biology concepts and the LQ model [79], and others claiming that "new biology" uniquely associated with the high doses used in SRS and SBRT isn't explained sufficiently by classical concepts and therefore invalidates the use of the LQ model [80–84].

Part of the problem is that the *clinical* rationale for the use of SRS or SBRT/SABR is different from that of conventional and hyperfractionation. The goal of the former is to completely ablate small lesions, with the likelihood of producing normal tissue complications of lesser concern—with certain caveats—due to the more precise tumor targeting and small volumes of normal tissue incidentally irradiated. In contrast, both conventional and hyperfractionated radiation therapy are driven principally by the *avoidance* of normal tissue complications, particularly late complications, and within those constraints, a hopefully sufficient total dose to achieve good tumor control.

What isn't controversial is that SRS and SBRT have been surprisingly successful for the treatment of small brain, lung, breast, liver, prostate, and spine tumors, yielding high local control rates for tumors and usually, no worse normal tissue complications [71, 85–88]. This is the case regardless of any assumed, inferred, or proposed biological underpinnings.

Below, some of the biological effects of hypofractionation are discussed in a general way, with most of the emphasis on whether such effects would or would not be consistent with the continued use of the LQ model for isoeffect analysis. Readers interested in a more in-depth discussion of the molecular biology of radiation-induced effects, including cell death, vascular injury, immunomodulation of the tumor microenvironment, and others not discussed herein, are referred to Chap. 2.

1.3 The Validity of the LQ Model

For more than 30 years, the LQ model has demonstrated its usefulness—for the relatively small dose fractions used in more conventional radiotherapy—for the calculation of isoeffective treatment schedules and to assess qualitatively how a change in fractionation pattern would affect both tumor control and normal tissue complication probabilities (i.e., comparison of BEDs). However, with the return of hypofractionation in the form of SRS or SBRT using high or very high doses per fraction, many radiation oncologists have continued to use the LQ model and BEDs despite such schedules being, in many cases, outside the range of the data sets used to formulate and validate the model in the first place [78]. Are they justified in doing so, even in the face of BEDs often greater than 150 Gy_3's, suggesting an unacceptable risk for late complications [71]? Or, are these high BEDs overestimates of the actual biological effectiveness of hypofractionation? If so, is it possible that the LQ model is simply incorrect?

A number of radiobiological concepts are discussed below, some that would argue against the continued use of the LQ model for hypofractionated radiotherapy, and others that would argue for the model's continued use. It is hoped that the reader can use this information to make better informed decisions about the use of hypofractionation.

1.3.1 Shapes of Dose Response Curves

Cell survival curves fitted to the LQ model are characterized by non-zero initial slopes represented by the α-component and, as the β-component becomes more prominent at increasing doses, a continuously bending curve. Could the continuously bending curve account for the LQ model's apparent overestimation of the biological effectiveness of hypofractionation? In theory, yes, if only because this is assumed to be the case in order to justify the use of the LQ model for measuring fractionation sensitivity in vivo. But what if the "real" dose response curve has a different shape?

Park and colleagues [89] proposed that the LQ model be modified in order to better align it with clinical results and expectations and to aid in determining isoeffective treatments using hypofractionation, by replacing the continuously bending portion of the dose response curve with an exponential function. Fowler [90] maintained that the modification of the LQ formula to create such a "Universal Survival Curve" [89] was not necessary, when simply assigning a higher α/β ratio to the tissue would accomplish nearly the same thing, a "straightening" of the dose response curve at high doses. Both approaches—mixing and matching survival curve models and adjusting α/β ratios—seem rather arbitrary, although the latter does have some biological justification.

According to the LQ model, α/β ratios for different tissues can be used as a metric to describe the tissue's fractionation sensitivity which—to a first approximation at least—is a reflection of the inherent radiosensitivity and repair capacity of the tissue's cells. However, the other R's, repopulation and reoxygenation in particular, could very well be ongoing during treatment, and influence the measured α/β ratios. Accordingly, how might α/β ratios change?

In rodent tumors, Williams et al. [91] determined the effect on the measured α/β ratio with and without the influence of each R. For example, the persistence of tumor hypoxia during treatment decreased the α/β ratio, whereas allowing reoxygenation to occur increased it. Repopulation had the net effect of decreasing the measured α/β ratio, suggesting that assigning a higher ratio for a tissue known to proliferate rapidly might better represent its "true" fractionation sensitivity. Redistribution or reassortment of tumor cells into more radiosensitive phases of the cell cycle during the course of radiotherapy also increased the α/β ratio.

1.3.2 Modes of Cell Death

The mechanism of radiation-induced death for most mammalian cells is mitotic catastrophe, which occurs secondary to chromosome aberrations and/or spindle defects that physically interfere with the cell division process [92, 93]. This type of cell death occurs during or soon after the cell next attempts to divide after irradiation. Cells killed in this manner initially appear intact, if multinucleated and/or containing cytoplasmic micronuclei, but over several days are removed from the tumor.

Apoptosis, or programmed cell death, is a type of interphase death associated with embryonic development and normal tissue remodeling and homeostasis [94], and is an active and carefully regulated process responsive to various stimuli. A modest subset of normal tissue and tumor cells undergo apoptosis after irradiation [95]. Cells undergoing apoptosis fragment into self-contained apoptotic bodies which ultimately are consumed by phagocytes and typically do not elicit an immune response [93].

Senescence refers to a type of genetically controlled cellular growth arrest that, while cells may persist physically for extended periods, halts permanently their continued movement through the cell cycle [96]. It is a natural process associated with the shortening of DNA telomeres with each subsequent cell division as normal cells age. Radiation-induced senescence is similar, but to distinguish it from the natural process, it is more properly termed "radiation-induced permanent growth arrest" [97].

Necrosis is another form of cell death characterized by cell swelling followed by membrane rupture and the release of cellular contents into the extracellular space, eliciting inflammation and an immune response. Historically, necrosis was considered a relatively passive process that occurred secondary to prolonged nutrient deprivation or hypoxia; however, under certain circumstances, it also can follow a molecular program akin to apoptosis. "Programmed" necrosis is more properly termed necroptosis [98].

Immunogenic cell death is a more recently identified mode of cell death observed after exposure to certain chemotherapy agents and ionizing radiation [99–101]. It is somewhat apoptosis-like, but due to some unique features, it *does* elicit an immune response to released tumor antigens, unlike apoptosis [100]. Of particular interest is that the immune response can act systemically as well as locally, and in theory, could elicit distant, abscopal effects.

There is a complicated interplay between the different modes of cell death, with several having biochemical features in common, some seeming to substitute for one another in cases where one pathway is downregulated or inhibited, and at other times some seeming to compete with each other [93]. These complex relationships make it difficult to predict which type or types of cell death might predominate in response to the high doses characteristic of SRS and SBRT, and whether the dose response for such would or would not be linear-quadratic.

1.4 The Role of the Tumor Vasculature

That vascular injury is responsible, at least in part, for radiation-induced complications in some normal tissues has long been appreciated [64], but the role vascular injury plays in tumors remains less well understood. Nevertheless, the targeting of tumor vasculature using radiation or other agents remains an attractive goal because the loss of a single microvessel has the potential to kill hundreds, if not thousands, of clonogenic tumor cells [102].

A loss or reduction in tumor vasculature could act as a radiosensitizer causing secondary ischemic death of tumor cells, reducing the tumor's overall growth rate, or leading to so-called vascular normalization [103, 104], the regression of small, inefficient vessels and the retention and promotion of more mature, larger vessels that would permit better access of chemotherapeutics. In addition, vascular normalization could lead to reoxygenation of hypoxic regions of the tumor. On the other hand, loss of small vasculature could also increase tumor hypoxia, which in turn could increase radioresistance as well as facilitate tumor progression [105, 106]. Reoxygenation secondary to vascular normalization might also stimulate proliferation of tumor cells. To complicate matters further, there is also evidence that radiation can *protect* tumor vasculature by causing the upregulation of proangiogenic factors [107].

Nearly 20 years ago, Fuks, Kolesnick, and colleagues [108, 109] suggested that the radiation sensitivity of tumors, especially after large dose fractions such as those used in SRS/SBRT, was mediated by the apoptotic death of vascular endothelial cells. The proposed mechanism for this was that radiation activated the acid sphingomyelinase pathway—highly enriched in endothelial cells—which lead to the generation of ceramide, a potent mediator of apoptosis. In support of this idea was the finding that vascular endothelial cells in animal models lacking the acid sphingomyelinase pathway were resistant to radiation-induced apoptosis after large, single doses, but those with the pathway intact experienced a rapid wave of endothelial

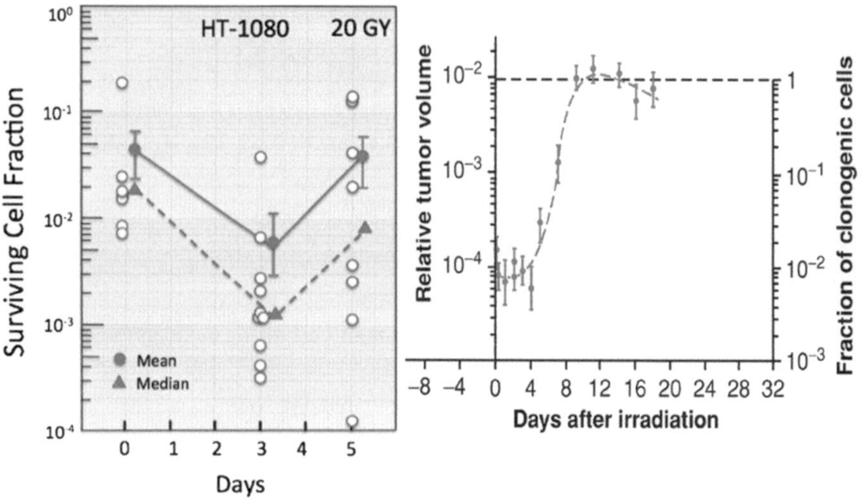

Fig. 1.7 Response of tumor clonogens as a function of time after a large, single dose of 20 Gy. *Left panel*: Mean and median surviving fractions of clonogens from a human HT-1080 fibrosarcoma xenograft assayed using an in vivo-to-in vitro excision assay. The surviving fraction of clonogens from tumors left in situ for the times indicated significantly decreased at 3 days after irradiation and then began to rebound. (From Song et al. [113].) *Right panel*: Fraction of clonogenic rat rhabdomyosarcoma cells, expressed as tumor volume relative to size-matched unirradiated tumors and assayed as above. Regrowth delay is evident for the first 4 days after irradiation before accelerated repopulation begins, but no significant decrease in surviving fraction is noted. (Adapted from Hermens and Barendsen [114])

cell apoptosis within hours of irradiation, yet with little evidence of damage to the tumor cells themselves for 2–3 additional days [108], yet others (e.g., Moding et al. [110]) found no influence of the presence or absence of endothelial cell apoptosis on overall radiation response in a genetically engineered murine sarcoma model.

Further, albeit less direct, evidence supporting a role for vascular injury in tumor cell death was the finding that in select rodent tumors and human tumor xenografts irradiated with single doses of 10 or 20 Gy, the clonogenic cell survival (assessed using an in vivo-to-in vitro assay) decreased for 2–3 days after irradiation [111–113] (left panel of Fig. 1.7).

The time scale for this additional tumor cell death was consistent with that observed for the loss of endothelial cells. Song and colleagues further suggested that the presence of indirect tumor cell death secondary to vascular injury could change the shape of the dose response curve for the tumor, and in so doing, potentially invalidate the LQ model [115]. That said, there are also reports in the literature that do *not* demonstrate a further reduction in tumor clonogens in the days immediately following irradiation with a single dose of 20 Gy, a notable example being the work of Hermens and Barendsen [114] showing a steady *increase* in tumor clonogen number after irradiation of a rat rhabdomyosarcoma (right panel of Fig. 1.7).

The LQ model does not specifically address vascular injury as a distinct mechanism of radiation-induced cell killing, although in cases where it does play a role, use of the model might not be appropriate. However, the fact is that there are multiple examples in the literature both supporting and refuting the role of the microvasculature in influencing tumor response to hypofractionation, and that it also remains unclear whether loss of vasculature would result in tumor radiosensitization or radioprotection. Thus, it is perhaps premature to conclude one way or the other about the applicability of the LQ model for hypofractionation.

1.5 The Role of the Immune System

Much contemporary radiobiology research focuses on the potential of radiation therapy to act as an immune system stimulant [116–121]. Generally speaking, most human tumors are not particularly immunogenic either before, during, or after conventional radiation therapy [116], presumably because of an immunosuppressive tumor microenvironment. Immuno-stimulatory effects after the high radiation doses characteristic of SRS or SBRT could be different and potentially greater; although, admittedly, there is still much to be learned about the time-dose-fractionation dependencies of these effects [117, 120, 122, 123].

Some of the ways irradiated cells die (necrosis and immunogenic cell death especially) have the potential to release subcellular materials into the tumor microenvironment, liberating large quantities of tumor-associated antigens, eliciting a local inflammatory response and causing the release of inflammatory cytokines that in turn could enhance antigen presentation and processing by dendritic cells and macrophages. Further, irradiated tumor cells in the process of dying by mitotic catastrophe that contain micronuclei stimulate the cytosolic DNA sensing system, the cyclic GMP–AMP synthase (cGAS)-stimulator of interferon genes (STING) pathway, which likewise triggers an immune response [124, 125]. Taken together, these radiation-induced effects could convert the tumor milieu into an in situ vaccine, paving the way for non-local effector T cells bearing immune memory to be recruited to the tumor site [126, 127].

The use of immune checkpoint inhibitors in combination with hypofractionated radiotherapy has been proposed as a means of further overcoming the immunosuppressive tumor microenvironment locally, and therefore augmenting the in situ vaccine. In addition, although still relatively rare events and of questionable clinical significance [128–133], abscopal effects have also been noted. These have been observed in preclinical mouse models, small subsets of patients with metastatic melanoma and non-small cell lung cancer, and anecdotally for other cancers treated with combinations of radiotherapy and immunotherapy [122, 134–138]. Such intriguing observations have spawned dozens of clinical trials of combined radiotherapy and ipilimumab for patients with melanoma, lung, cervix, and head and neck cancers [139]. Expanding indications for immune checkpoint inhibitors including ipilimumab and other next generation, FDA-approved drugs (e.g., nivolumab, pembrolizumab, avelumab, durvalumab, and atezolizumab) [140], along with a pipeline of new immunotherapeutics targeting different immunosuppressive pathways used by tumors, guarantee more trials of these drugs with radiation therapy in the future [141–143].

The existence of immune system effects unique to hypofractionation are not accommodated currently in the LQ isoeffect model, to the extent that increased tumor immunogenicity actually affects clinical outcome. If it does, the expectation would be that enhanced immunity would behave as a radiosensitizer, although it remains to be seen whether this radiosensitization would manifest as a change in dose response curve shape away from linear-quadratic.

1.6 The Role of Treatment Volume and Normal Tissue Organization

SRS and SBRT are critically dependent on very precise dose localization and delivery to the tumor, with as small a volume of surrounding normal tissue irradiated as currently feasible. Under such irradiation conditions, the likelihood of a clinically significant normal tissue complication should be quite low, provided the tissue at risk is not especially critical or in very close proximity to one that is [144–147]. The tissue's structural and functional organization could also play a role.

A simplistic model for describing the structural/functional organization of normal tissues was proposed by Withers and colleagues [148], who envisioned tissues as being composed of functional subunits (FSUs), minimum anatomic entities capable of carrying out the function of the tissue or maintaining its structural integrity. By analogy with electrical circuits, the arrangement of FSUs in different tissues could be either "parallel" or "serial" (or some combination), and that this arrangement would dictate to a first approximation the tissue's radiation tolerance as a function of treatment volume. The spinal cord, the skin, and many tubular or sack-like organs behave as if their FSUs are arranged in series, that is, that an injury to even a small volume of tissue potentially could inactivate it and produce a major functional loss. Conversely, for tissues such as the lung, liver, and kidney, FSU's are arranged in parallel, meaning that provided the treatment volume is small, little, or no functional loss would occur even for high or very high doses. As such, SRS and SBRT may be better suited for, and less likely to produce complications in, parallel tissues than serial ones.

At present, the LQ model does not make provisions for the volume of normal tissue irradiated nor the tissue's structural/functional organization, but given that much of the advantage of SRS and SBRT lies in the small volumes irradiated overall and the exclusion of nearly all surrounding normal tissue, the LQ model should not be rejected on this basis alone.

1.7 The Role of the Five R's

Proponents of the continued used of the LQ model and the calculation of BEDs for SRS and SBRT [79, 149–152] claim that the five R's of radiotherapy still apply for hypofractionation and can explain the excellent outcomes, even though the R's were initially proposed to describe the radiobiological underpinnings of conventional fractionation [30]. In the case of hypofractionation, however, the roles and relative importance of the R's are likely to be different.

For example, when cells are irradiated with low-to-moderate doses of radiation, cell cycle arrest is temporary, so eventually survivors would resume proliferating and redistribute themselves around the cell cycle. However, after exposure to high-to-very-high doses characteristic of SRS or SBRT, cells are more likely to become permanently growth-arrested and undergo senescence, apoptosis, or necrosis. This would effectively eliminate the possibility of cells either repopulating or redistributing, although the short overall treatment times characteristic of SRS and SBRT would limit their influence regardless.

These short overall treatment times could be problematic when it comes to reoxygenation. In hypoxic tumors, short overall times could lead to incomplete reoxygenation which would have the net effect of making tumors more resistant, even to such high, ablative doses. Based on sample calculations of the effectiveness of commonly used SBRT regimens in either the presence or absence of tumor hypoxia (20% hypoxic fraction and an OER of 2.8 assumed), Brown et al. [153] recommend therefore that hypoxic cell radiosensitizers be used in conjunction with SBRT, particularly single-dose SBRT.

In spite of presumed differences in the influence of the R's when hypofractionation is used, Brenner, Brown, and colleagues [79, 150, 151, 154] have argued that use of the LQ model is not only still relevant, but relevant even for the high or very high doses used for SRS and SBRT. They cite two lines of evidence in support of this. First, reciprocal dose isoeffect curves for different normal tissue endpoints generated from multifraction experiments in rodents are linear, and remain so up to doses of nearly 25 Gy, suggesting adherence to the LQ model (left panel of Fig. 1.8) [79, 151]. Second, using human data on the control of non-small cell lung cancers treated with either single fraction SBRT, 3–8 fraction SBRT or 3D conformal radiotherapy using greater than 10 fractions, these authors found a monotonic relationship between the tumor control probability (TCP) and the BED calculated using the LQ model (right panel of Fig. 1.8). In other words, a given TCP was achieved for a given BED *regardless* of whether the treatment was single or multi-fraction SBRT or more conventional 3D conformal therapy. This suggests that there is nothing unique about SBRT in terms of its biological effectiveness compared to more conventional treatment, and that its efficacy lies simply in the higher BED it delivers and not any new or unique biology.

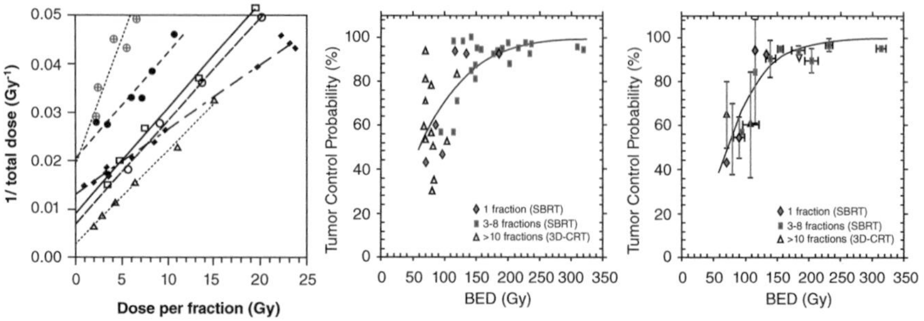

Fig. 1.8 Evidence for adherence of SBRT fractionation schemes to the LQ isoeffect model. *Left panel*: Reciprocal dose plot isoeffect curves for different normal tissue complications in rodents, including late effects in rat spinal cord, early reactions in mouse skin, and early and late murine intestinal injury. Isoeffect data that fall on a straight line on a reciprocal dose plot conform to the LQ model [79, 151]. (From Brenner [79].) *Right panels*: Mean tumor control probability (TCP) as a function of BED (Gy_{10}) for Stage I non-small cell lung cancer in patients treated with either single fraction SBRT, 3–8 fraction SBRT or 3D conformal radiotherapy using greater than 10 fractions, weighted for the number of patients in each treatment group. A given TCP was achieved for a given BED regardless of how the dose was delivered, suggesting that SBRT was not different from more conventional treatment in terms of biological effectiveness [150, 151]. (From Brown et al. [151])

1.8 Conclusions

Thanks to technological advances in recent years allowing highly conformal treatment of small tumors, hypofractionation has made an impressive comeback compared to its use during the early days of radiotherapy at the turn of the twentieth century. In terms of the biology of hypofractionation, there are conflicting findings and still much to be learned, although, in general, it appears that “old school” radiobiology in the form of the five R’s of radiotherapy still applies, with the proviso that the R’s may exert different influences in the case of hypofractionation than for conventionally fractionated radiotherapy. These influences could explain the impressive success of ablative radiotherapy in some settings, yet it is also clear that biological effects unique to hypofractionation also exist and could play a role, and, as some suggest, invalidate the use of the LQ model for the calculation of isoeffects.

References

1. Roentgen WC. Uber eine neue Art von Strahlen. Sitzgsber Physik-Med Ges Wuerzburg. 1895;137:132–41.
2. Becquerel H. Emission of the new radiations by metallic uranium. CR Acad Sci. 1896;122:1086–8.
3. Curie P, Curie MS. Sur une substance nouvelle radioactive, contenue dans la pechblende. CR Acad Sci. 1898;127:175–8.

4. Stenbeck T. Ein Fall von Hautkrebs geheilt durch Rontgenbestrahlung. Mitteil Grenzgeb Med Chir. 1900;6:347–9.
5. Kogelnik HD. The history and evolution of radiotherapy and radiation oncology in Austria. Int J Radiat Oncol Biol Phys. 1996;35:219–26.
6. Leszczynski K, Boyko S. On the controversies surrounding the origins of radiation therapy. Radiother Oncol. 1997;42:213–7.
7. Bernier J, Hall EJ, Giaccia A. Radiation oncology: a century of achievements. Nat Rev Cancer. 2004;4:737–47.
8. Kaplan HS. Present status of radiation therapy of cancer: an overview. In: Becker FF, editor. Cancer 6: a comprehensive treatise. New York: Plenum Press; 1977. p. 1–34.
9. Thames HD, Hendry JH. Fractionation in radiotherapy. Philadelphia: Taylor and Francis; 1987.
10. Bergonie J, Tribondeau L. Interpretation de quelques resultats de la radiotherapie. CR Acad Sci. 1906;143:983–8.
11. Regaud C. The influence of the duration of irradiation on the changes produced in the testicle by radium. Int J Radiat Oncol Biol Phys. 1977;2:565–7.
12. Regaud C, Ferroux R. Discordance des effets de rayons X, d'une part dans le testicule, par le peau, d'autre part dans la fractionnement de la dose. CR Societe de Biologie. 1927;97:431–4.
13. Coutard H. Roentgen therapy of epitheliomas of the tonsillar region, hypopharynx and larynx from 1920 to 1926. Am J Roentgenol. 1932;28:313–31.
14. Coutard H. Present conception of treatment of cancer of the larynx. Radiology. 1940;34:136–45.
15. Reisner A. Untersuchungen uber die veranderungen der Hauttoleranz bei verschiedener Unterterlung. Strahlentherapie. 1930;37:779–87.
16. Quimby E, MacComb WS. Further studies on the rate of recovery of human skin from the effects of roentgen or gamma rays. Radiology. 1937;29:305–12.
17. Paterson R. The value of assessing and prescribing dosage in radiation therapy in simple terms. Radiology. 1939;32:221–7.
18. Ellis F. Tolerance dose in radiotherapy with 200 keV X-rays. Br J Radiol. 1942;15:348–50.
19. Strandqvist M. Studien uber die kumulative wirkung der roentgenstrahlen bei fraktionierung. Acta Radiol Suppl. 1944;55:1–300.
20. Fletcher GH. Keynote address: the scientific basis of the present and future practice of clinical radiotherapy. Int J Radiat Oncol Biol Phys. 1983;9:1073–82.
21. Ellis F. Relationship of biological effect to dose-time-fractionation factors in radiotherapy. In: Ebert M, Howard M, editors. Current topics in radiation research. Amsterdam: North Holland Publishing; 1968. p. 357–97.
22. Ellis F. Dose, time and fractionation: a clinical hypothesis. Clin Radiol. 1969;20:1–8.
23. Fowler JF, Stern BE. Dose-time relationships in radiotherapy and the validity of cell survival curve models. Br J Radiol. 1963;36:163–73.
24. Fowler JF, Morgan RL, Silvester JA, Bewley DK, Turner BA. Experiments with fractionated x-ray treatment of the skin of pigs. I. Fractionation up to 28 days. Br J Radiol. 1963;36:188–96.
25. Orton CG, Ellis F. A simplification in the use of the NSD concept in practical radiotherapy. Br J Radiol. 1973;46:529–37.
26. Bentzen SM. Estimation of radiobiological parameters from clinical data. In: Hagen U, Jung H, Streffer C, editors. Radiation research 1895–1995: volume 2, congress lectures. Wurzburg: Universitatsdruckerei H. Sturtz AG; 1995. p. 833–8.
27. Thomlinson RH, Gray LH. The histological structure of some human lung cancers and the possible implications for radiotherapy. Br J Cancer. 1955;9:539–49.
28. Palcic B, Skarsgard LD. Reduced oxygen enhancement ratio at low doses of ionizing radiation. Radiat Res. 1984;100:328–39.
29. Fowler JF, Morgan RL, Wood CAP. Pretherapeutic experiments with the fast neutron beam from the Medical Research Council cyclotron. I. The biological and physical advantages and problems of neutron therapy. Br J Radiol. 1963;36:163–73.

30. Withers HR. The four R's of radiotherapy. In: Adler H, Lett JT, Zelle M, editors. Advances in radiation biology, vol. 5. New York: Academic Press; 1975. p. 241–71.
31. Steel GG, McMillan TJ, Peacock JH. The 5Rs of radiobiology. Int J Radiat Biol. 1989;56:1045–8.
32. Elkind MM, Sutton H. X-ray damage and recovery in mammalian cells. Nature. 1959;184:1293–11295.
33. Bedford JS, Mitchell JB, Fox MH. Variations in responses of several mammalian cell lines to low dose-rate irradiation. In: Meyn RE, Withers HR, editors. Radiation biology in cancer research. New York: Raven Press; 1980. p. 251–62.
34. Zeman EM, Bedford JS. Dose-rate effects in mammalian cells: V. Dose fractionation effects in noncycling C3H 10T1/2 cells. Int J Radiat Oncol Biol Phys. 1984;10:2089–98.
35. Denekamp J. Changes in the rate of proliferation in normal tissues after irradiation. In: Nygaard O, Adler HI, Sinclair WK, editors. Radiation research: biomedical, chemical and physical perspectives. New York: Academic Press, Inc.; 1975. p. 810–25.
36. Steel GG. The heyday of cell population kinetics: insights from the 1960's and 1970's. Semin Radiat Oncol. 1993;3:78–83.
37. Alper T, Howard-Flanders P. The role of oxygen in modifying the radiosensitivity of *E. coli B*. Nature. 1956;178:978–9.
38. Kallman RF. The phenomenon of reoxygenation and its implications for fractionated radiotherapy. Radiology. 1972;105:135–42.
39. Brown JM. Evidence for acutely hypoxic cells in mouse tumours, and a possible mechanism of reoxygenation. Br J Radiol. 1979;52:650–6.
40. Chaplin DJ, Durand RE, Olive PL. Acute hypoxia in tumors: implication for modifiers of radiation effects. Int J Radiat Oncol Biol Phys. 1986;12:1279–82.
41. Dewhirst MW. Relationships between cycling hypoxia, HIF-1, angiogenesis and oxidative stress. Radiat Res. 2009;172:653–65.
42. Douglas BG, Fowler JF. The effect of multiple small doses of X-rays on skin reactions in the mouse and a basic interpretation. Radiat Res. 1976;66:401–26.
43. Joiner M, Van der Kogel A. Basic clinical radiobiology. 5th ed. London: Hodder Arnold; 2019.
44. Thames HD, Withers HR, Peters LJ, Fletcher G. Changes in early and late radiation responses with altered dose fractionation: implications for dose-survival relationships. Int J Radiat Oncol Biol Phys. 1982;8:219–26.
45. Withers HR, Thames HD, Peters LJ. Differences in the fractionation response of acutely and late-responding tissues. In: Karcher KH, Kogelnik HD, Reinartz G, editors. Progress in radio oncology II. New York: Raven Press; 1982. p. 287–96.
46. Withers HR, Thames HD, Peters LJ. A new isoeffect curve for change in dose per fraction. Radiother Oncol. 1983;1:187–91.
47. Zeman EM, Schreiber EC, Tepper JE. Basics of radiation therapy. In: Abeloff MD, Armitage JO, Niederhuber JE, Kastan MB, McKenna WG, editors. Abeloff's clinical oncology. 6th ed. Philadelphia: Churchill Livingstone; 2019. p. 431–60.
48. Fowler JF. Non-standard fractionation in radiotherapy. Int J Radiat Oncol Biol Phys. 1984;10:755–9.
49. Fowler JF. The James Kirk Memorial Lecture. What next in fractionated radiotherapy? Br J Cancer Suppl. 1984;46:285–300.
50. Fowler JF. The linear-quadratic formula and progress in fractionated radiotherapy. Br J Radiol. 1989;62:679–94.
51. Fowler JF. 21 years of biologically effective dose. Br J Radiol. 2010;83:554–68.
52. Barendsen GW. Differences among tissues with respect to iso-effect relations for fractionated irradiation. Strahlentherapie. 1984;160:667–9.
53. Lee AW, Sze WM, Fowler JF, Chappell R, Leung SF, Teo P. Caution on the use of altered fractionation for nasopharyngeal carcinoma. Radiother Oncol. 1999;52:201–11.

54. Fowler JF, Harari PM, Leborgne F, Leborgne JH. Acute radiation reactions in oral and pharyngeal mucosa: tolerable levels in altered fractionation schedules. Radiother Oncol. 2003;69:161–8.
55. Phillips MH, Stelzer KJ, Griffin TW, Mayberg MR, Winn HR. Stereotactic radiosurgery: a review and comparison of methods. J Clin Oncol. 1994;12:1085–99.
56. Leskel L. The stereotactic method and radiosurgery of the brain. Acta Chir Scand. 1951;102:316–9.
57. Martin A, Gaya A. Stereotactic body radiotherapy: a review. Clin Oncol (R Coll Radiol). 2010;22:157–72.
58. Hickey BE, James ML, Lehman M, Hider PN, Jeffery M, Francis DP, et al. Fraction size in radiation therapy for breast conservation in early breast cancer. Cochrane Database Syst Rev. 2016;7:CD003860.
59. Whelan TJ, Pignol JP, Levine MN, Julian JA, MacKenzie R, Parpia S, et al. Long-term results of hypofractionated radiation therapy for breast cancer. N Engl J Med. 2010;362:513–20.
60. Haviland JS, Owen JR, Dewar JA, Agrawal RK, Barrett J, Barrett-Lee PJ, et al. The UK Standardisation of Breast Radiotherapy (START) trials of radiotherapy hypofractionation for treatment of early breast cancer: 10-year follow-up results of two randomised controlled trials. Lancet Oncol. 2013;14:1086–94.
61. Agrawal RK, Alhasso A, Barrett-Lee PJ, Bliss JM, Bliss P, Bloomfield D, et al. First results of the randomised UK FAST Trial of radiotherapy hypofractionation for treatment of early breast cancer (CRUKE/04/015). Radiother Oncol. 2011;100:93–100.
62. Murray Brunt A, Haviland JS, Wheatley DA, Sydenham MA, Alhasso A, Bloomfield DJ, et al. Hypofractionated breast radiotherapy for 1 week versus 3 weeks (FAST-Forward): 5-year efficacy and late normal tissue effects results from a multicentre, non-inferiority, randomised, phase 3 trial. Lancet. 2020;395:1613–26.
63. Benedict SH, Yenice KM, Followill D, Galvin JM, Hinson W, Kavanagh B, et al. Stereotactic body radiation therapy: the report of AAPM Task Group 101. Med Phys. 2010;37:4078–101.
64. Rubin P, Constine LS, Marks LB, editors. ALERT—adverse late effects of cancer treatment. Heidelberg: Springer; 2014.
65. Emami B, Lyman J, Brown A, Cola L, Goitein M, Munzenrider JE, et al. Tolerance of normal tissue to therapeutic irradiation. Int J Radiat Oncol Biol Phys. 1991;21:109–22.
66. Marks LB, Ten Haken RK, Martel MK. Guest editor's introduction to QUANTEC: a users guide. Int J Radiat Oncol Biol Phys. 2010;76:S1–2.
67. Bentzen SM, Constine LS, Deasy JO, Eisbruch A, Jackson A, Marks LB, et al. Quantitative analyses of normal tissue effects in the clinic (QUANTEC): an introduction to the scientific issues. Int J Radiat Oncol Biol Phys. 2010;76:S3–9.
68. Timmerman R. An overview of hypofractionation and introduction to this issue of seminars in radiation oncology. Semin Radiat Oncol. 2008;18:215–22.
69. Timmerman R. A story of hypofractionation and the table on the wall. Int J Radiat Oncol Biol Phys. 2022;112:4–21.
70. Chang BK, Timmerman RD. Stereotactic body radiation therapy: a comprehensive review. Am J Clin Oncol. 2007;30:637–44.
71. Mehta N, King CR, Agazaryan N, Steinberg M, Hua A, Lee P. Stereotactic body radiation therapy and 3-dimensional conformal radiotherapy for stage I non-small cell lung cancer: a pooled analysis of biological equivalent dose and local control. Pract Radiat Oncol. 2012;2:288–95.
72. Gerhard SG, Palma DA, Arifin AJ, Louie AV, Li GJ, Al-Shafa F, et al. Organ at risk dose constraints in SABR: a systematic review of active clinical trials. Pract Radiat Oncol. 2021;11(4):e355.
73. Corbin KS, Hellman S, Weichselbaum RR. Extracranial oligometastases: a subset of metastases curable with stereotactic radiotherapy. J Clin Oncol. 2013;31:1384–90.
74. Tree AC, Khoo VS, Eeles RA, Ahmed M, Dearnaley DP, Hawkins MA, et al. Stereotactic body radiotherapy for oligometastases. Lancet Oncol. 2013;14:e28–37.

75. Ahmed KA, Torres-Roca JF. Stereotactic body radiotherapy in the management of oligometastatic disease. Cancer Control. 2016;23:21–9.
76. Palma DA, Olson R, Harrow S, Gaede S, Louie AV, Haasbeek C, et al. Stereotactic ablative radiotherapy versus standard of care palliative treatment in patients with oligometastatic cancers (SABR-COMET): a randomised, phase 2, open-label trial. Lancet. 2019;393:2051–8.
77. Palma DA, Olson R, Harrow S, Gaede S, Louie AV, Haasbeek C, et al. Stereotactic ablative radiotherapy for the comprehensive treatment of oligometastatic cancers: long-term results of the SABR-COMET phase II randomized trial. J Clin Oncol. 2020;38:2830–8.
78. Grimm J, Marks LB, Jackson A, Kavanagh BD, Xue J, Yorke E. High dose per fraction, hypofractionated treatment effects in the clinic (HyTEC): an overview. Int J Radiat Oncol Biol Phys. 2021;110:1–10.
79. Brenner DJ. The linear-quadratic model is an appropriate methodology for determining isoeffective doses at large doses per fraction. Semin Radiat Oncol. 2008;18:234–9.
80. Astrahan M. Some implications of linear-quadratic-linear radiation dose-response with regard to hypofractionation. Med Phys. 2008;35:4161–72.
81. Kirkpatrick JP, Meyer JJ, Marks LB. The linear-quadratic model is inappropriate to model high dose per fraction effects in radiosurgery. Semin Radiat Oncol. 2008;18:240–3.
82. Kirkpatrick JP, Brenner DJ, Orton CG. Point/counterpoint. The linear-quadratic model is inappropriate to model high dose per fraction effects in radiosurgery. Med Phys. 2009;36:3381–4.
83. Wang JZ, Huang Z, Lo SS, Yuh WT, Mayr NA. A generalized linear-quadratic model for radiosurgery, stereotactic body radiation therapy, and high-dose rate brachytherapy. Sci Transl Med. 2010;2:39ra48.
84. Sheu T, Molkentine J, Transtrum MK, Buchholz TA, Withers HR, Thames HD, et al. Use of the LQ model with large fraction sizes results in underestimation of isoeffect doses. Radiother Oncol. 2013;109:21–5.
85. Ritter M. Rationale, conduct, and outcome using hypofractionated radiotherapy in prostate cancer. Semin Radiat Oncol. 2008;18:249–56.
86. Timmerman R, Paulus R, Galvin J, Michalski J, Straube W, Bradley J, et al. Stereotactic body radiation therapy for inoperable early stage lung cancer. JAMA. 2010;303:1070–6.
87. Shuryak I, Carlson DJ, Brown JM, Brenner DJ. High-dose and fractionation effects in stereotactic radiation therapy: analysis of tumor control data from 2965 patients. Radiother Oncol. 2015;115:327–34.
88. Katsoulakis E, Laufer I, Bilsky M, Agaram NP, Lovelock M, Yamada Y. Pathological characteristics of spine metastases treated with high-dose single-fraction stereotactic radiosurgery. Neurosurg Focus. 2017;42:E7.
89. Park C, Papiez L, Zhang S, Story M, Timmerman RD. Universal survival curve and single fraction equivalent dose: useful tools in understanding potency of ablative radiotherapy. Int J Radiat Oncol Biol Phys. 2008;70:847–52.
90. Fowler JF. Linear quadratics is alive and well: in regard to Park et al. (Int J Radiat Oncol Biol Phys 2008;70:847–852). Int J Radiat Oncol Biol Phys. 2008;72:957–8.
91. Williams MV, Denekamp J, Fowler JF. A review of alpha/beta ratios for experimental tumors: implications for clinical studies of altered fractionation. Int J Radiat Oncol Biol Phys. 1985;11:87–96.
92. Vitale I, Galluzzi L, Castedo M, Kroemer G. Mitotic catastrophe: a mechanism for avoiding genomic instability. Nat Rev Mol Cell Biol. 2011;12:385–92.
93. Galluzzi L, Vitale I, Abrams JM, Alnemri ES, Baehrecke EH, Blagosklonny MV, et al. Molecular definitions of cell death subroutines: recommendations of the Nomenclature Committee on Cell Death 2012. Cell Death Differ. 2012;19:107–20.
94. Kerr JFR, Wyllie AH, Currie AR. Apoptosis: a basic biological phenomenon with wide ranging implications in tissue kinetics. Br J Cancer. 1972;26:239–57.
95. Meyn R. Apoptosis and response to radiation: implications for radiation therapy. Oncology. 1997;11:349–56.
96. Campisi J. Aging, cellular senescence, and cancer. Annu Rev Physiol. 2013;75:685–705.

97. Gewirtz DA, Holt SE, Elmore LW. Accelerated senescence: an emerging role in tumor cell response to chemotherapy and radiation. Biochem Pharmacol. 2008;76:947–57.
98. Cho YS, Park SY, Shin HS, Chan FK. Physiological consequences of programmed necrosis, an alternative form of cell demise. Mol Cells. 2010;29:327–32.
99. Golden EB, Pellicciotta I, Demaria S, Barcellos-Hoff MH, Formenti SC. The convergence of radiation and immunogenic cell death signaling pathways. Front Oncol. 2012;2:88.
100. Galluzzi L, Kepp O, Kroemer G. Immunogenic cell death in radiation therapy. Onco Targets Ther. 2013;2:e26536.
101. D'Souza NM, Fang P, Logan J, Yang J, Jiang W, Li J. Combining radiation therapy with immune checkpoint blockade for central nervous system malignancies. Front Oncol. 2016;6:212.
102. Denekamp J. Vascular endothelium as the vulnerable element in tumours. Acta Radiol Oncol. 1984;23:217–25.
103. Goel S, Duda DG, Xu L, Munn LL, Boucher Y, Fukumura D, et al. Normalization of the vasculature for treatment of cancer and other diseases. Physiol Rev. 2011;91:1071–121.
104. Lan J, Wan XL, Deng L, Xue JX, Wang LS, Meng MB, et al. Ablative hypofractionated radiotherapy normalizes tumor vasculature in Lewis lung carcinoma mice model. Radiat Res. 2013;179:458–64.
105. Semenza GL. Hypoxia, clonal selection, and the role of HIF-1 in tumor progression. Crit Rev Biochem Mol Biol. 2000;35:71–103.
106. Semenza GL. Defining the role of hypoxia-inducible factor 1 in cancer biology and therapeutics. Oncogene. 2010;29:625–34.
107. Moeller BJ, Dreher MR, Rabbani ZN, Schroeder T, Cao Y, Li CY, et al. Pleiotropic effects of HIF-1 blockade on tumor radiosensitivity. Cancer Cell. 2005;8:99–110.
108. Garcia-Barros M, Paris F, Cordon-Cardo C, Lyden D, Rafii S, Haimovitz-Friedman A, et al. Tumor response to radiotherapy regulated by endothelial cell apoptosis. Science. 2003;300:1155–9.
109. Fuks Z, Kolesnick R. Engaging the vascular component of the tumor response. Cancer Cell. 2005;8:89–91.
110. Moding EJ, Castle KD, Perez BA, Oh P, Min HD, Norris H, et al. Tumor cells, but not endothelial cells, mediate eradication of primary sarcomas by stereotactic body radiation therapy. Sci Transl Med. 2015;7:278ra34.
111. Song CW, Kim MS, Cho LC, Dusenbery K, Sperduto PW. Radiobiological basis of SBRT and SRS. Int J Clin Oncol. 2014;19:570–8.
112. Kim MS, Kim W, Park IH, Kim HJ, Lee E, Jung JH, et al. Radiobiological mechanisms of stereotactic body radiation therapy and stereotactic radiation surgery. Radiat Oncol J. 2015;33:265–75.
113. Song CW, Lee YJ, Griffin RJ, Park I, Koonce NA, Hui S, et al. Indirect tumor cell death after high-dose hypofractionated irradiation: implications for stereotactic body radiation therapy and stereotactic radiation surgery. Int J Radiat Oncol Biol Phys. 2015;93:166–72.
114. Hermens AF, Barendsen GW. Changes of cell proliferation characteristics in a rat rhabdomyosarcoma before and after X-irradiation. Eur J Cancer. 1969;5:173–89.
115. Song CW, Terezakis S, Emami B, Griffin RJ, Sperduto PW, Kim MS, et al. Indirect cell death and the LQ model in SBRT and SRS. J Radiosurg SBRT. 2020;7:1–4.
116. Formenti SC, Demaria S. Systemic effects of local radiotherapy. Lancet Oncol. 2009;10:718–26.
117. Demaria S, Formenti SC. Radiation as an immunological adjuvant: current evidence on dose and fractionation. Front Oncol. 2012;2:153.
118. Demaria S, Formenti SC. Radiotherapy effects on anti-tumor immunity: implications for cancer treatment. Front Oncol. 2013;3:128.
119. Burnette B, Weichselbaum RR. The immunology of ablative radiation. Semin Radiat Oncol. 2015;25:40–5.

120. Demaria S, Golden EB, Formenti SC. Role of local radiation therapy in cancer immunotherapy. JAMA Oncol. 2015;1:1325–32.
121. Golden EB, Marciscano AE, Formenti SC. Radiation therapy and the in situ vaccination approach. Int J Radiat Oncol Biol Phys. 2020;108:891–8.
122. Ko EC, Formenti SC. Radiotherapy and checkpoint inhibitors: a winning new combination. Ther Adv Med Oncol. 2018;10:1758835918768240.
123. Walle T, Martinez Monge R, Cerwenka A, Ajona D, Melero I, Lecanda F. Radiation effects on antitumor immune responses: current perspectives and challenges. Ther Adv Med Oncol. 2018;10:1758834017742575.
124. Vanpouille-Box C, Demaria S, Formenti SC, Galluzzi L. Cytosolic DNA sensing in organismal tumor control. Cancer Cell. 2018;34:361–78.
125. Decout A, Katz JD, Venkatraman S, Ablasser A. The cGAS-STING pathway as a therapeutic target in inflammatory diseases. Nat Rev Immunol. 2021;21:548–69.
126. Demaria S, Pilones KA, Vanpouille-Box C, Golden EB, Formenti SC. The optimal partnership of radiation and immunotherapy: from preclinical studies to clinical translation. Radiat Res. 2014;182:170–81.
127. Ishihara D, Pop L, Takeshima T, Iyengar P, Hannan R. Rationale and evidence to combine radiation therapy and immunotherapy for cancer treatment. Cancer Immunol Immunother. 2016;66:281–98.
128. Xing D, Siva S, Hanna GG. The abscopal effect of stereotactic radiotherapy and immunotherapy: Fool's Gold or El Dorado? Clin Oncol (R Coll Radiol). 2019;31:432–43.
129. Yilmaz MT, Elmali A, Yazici G. Abscopal effect, from myth to reality: from radiation oncologists' perspective. Cureus. 2019;11:e3860.
130. Romesser PB, Crane CH. Pursuit of the abscopal effect. Digest Dis Interv. 2020;04:369–72.
131. Tubin S, Yan W, Mourad WF, Fossati P, Khan MK. The future of radiation-induced abscopal response: beyond conventional radiotherapy approaches. Future Oncol. 2020;16:1137–51.
132. Seiwert TY, Kiess AP. Time to debunk an urban myth? The "abscopal effect" with radiation and anti-PD-1. J Clin Oncol. 2021;39:1–3.
133. Mirjolet C, Truc G. Abscopal effect: myth or reality? Cancer Radiother. 2021;25:533.
134. Postow MA, Callahan MK, Barker CA, Yamada Y, Yuan J, Kitano S, et al. Immunologic correlates of the abscopal effect in a patient with melanoma. N Engl J Med. 2012;366:925–31.
135. Golden EB, Demaria S, Schiff PB, Chachoua A, Formenti SC. An abscopal response to radiation and ipilimumab in a patient with metastatic non-small cell lung cancer. Immunol Res. 2013;1:365–72.
136. Chicas-Sett R, Morales-Orue I, Castilla-Martinez J, Zafra-Martin J, Kannemann A, Blanco J, et al. Stereotactic ablative radiotherapy combined with immune checkpoint inhibitors reboots the immune response assisted by immunotherapy in metastatic lung cancer: a systematic review. Int J Mol Sci. 2019;20:2173.
137. Takahashi J, Nagasawa S. Immunostimulatory effects of radiotherapy for local and systemic control of melanoma: a review. Int J Mol Sci. 2020;21:9324.
138. Donlon NE, Power R, Hayes C, Reynolds JV, Lysaght J. Radiotherapy, immunotherapy, and the tumour microenvironment: turning an immunosuppressive milieu into a therapeutic opportunity. Cancer Lett. 2021;502:84–96.
139. Vatner RE, Cooper BT, Vanpouille-Box C, Demaria S, Formenti SC. Combinations of immunotherapy and radiation in cancer therapy. Front Oncol. 2014;4:325.
140. Vaddepally RK, Kharel P, Pandey R, Garje R, Chandra AB. Review of indications of FDA-approved immune checkpoint inhibitors per NCCN guidelines with the level of evidence. Cancers (Basel). 2020;12:738.
141. Kon E, Benhar I. Immune checkpoint inhibitor combinations: current efforts and important aspects for success. Drug Resist Updates. 2019;45:13–29.
142. Bagchi S, Yuan R, Engleman EG. Immune checkpoint inhibitors for the treatment of cancer: clinical impact and mechanisms of response and resistance. Annu Rev Pathol. 2021;16:223–49.

143. Sharma P, Siddiqui BA, Anandhan S, Yadav SS, Subudhi SK, Gao J, et al. The next decade of immune checkpoint therapy. Cancer Discov. 2021;11:838–57.
144. Timmerman R, McGarry R, Yiannoutsos C, Papiez L, Tudor K, DeLuca J, et al. Excessive toxicity when treating central tumors in a phase II study of stereotactic body radiation therapy for medically inoperable early-stage lung cancer. J Clin Oncol. 2006;24:4833–9.
145. Lo SS, Sahgal A, Chang EL, Mayr NA, Teh BS, Huang Z, et al. Serious complications associated with stereotactic ablative radiotherapy and strategies to mitigate the risk. Clin Oncol (R Coll Radiol). 2013;25:378–87.
146. Cozzarini C, Fiorino C, Deantoni C, Briganti A, Fodor A, La Macchia M, et al. Higher-than-expected severe (Grade 3–4) late urinary toxicity after postprostatectomy hypofractionated radiotherapy: a single-institution analysis of 1176 patients. Eur Urol. 2014;66:1024–30.
147. Modh A, Rimner A, Williams E, Foster A, Shah M, Shi W, et al. Local control and toxicity in a large cohort of central lung tumors treated with stereotactic body radiation therapy. Int J Radiat Oncol Biol Phys. 2014;90:1168–76.
148. Withers HR, Taylor JMG, Maciejewski B. Treatment volume and tissue tolerance. Int J Radiat Oncol Biol Phys. 1988;14:751–9.
149. Chapman JD, Gillespie CJ. The power of radiation biophysics—let's use it. Int J Radiat Oncol Biol Phys. 2012;84:309–11.
150. Brown JM, Brenner DJ, Carlson DJ. Dose escalation, not "new biology," can account for the efficacy of stereotactic body radiation therapy with non-small cell lung cancer. Int J Radiat Oncol Biol Phys. 2013;85:1159.
151. Brown JM, Carlson DJ, Brenner DJ. The tumor radiobiology of SRS and SBRT: are more than the 5 Rs involved. Int J Radiat Oncol Biol Phys. 2014;88:254–62.
152. Nahum AE. The radiobiology of hypofractionation. Clin Oncol (R Coll Radiol). 2015;27:260–9.
153. Brown JM, Diehn M, Loo BW. Stereotactic ablative radiotherapy should be combined with a hypoxic cell radiosensitizer. Int J Radiat Oncol Biol Phys. 2010;78:323–7.
154. Brenner DJ, Hlatky LR, Hahnfeldt PJ, Huang Y, Sachs RK. The linear-quadratic model and most other common radiobiological models result in similar predictions of time-dose relationships. Radiat Res. 1998;150:83–91.

Chapter 2
Simplifying the Biology: Stem, Stroma and Beyond

Subhrajit Saha and Bruce F. Kimler

2.1 Introduction

Hypofractionated radiation therapy (RT) was first used in the early twentieth century. Since then technological improvements have made dose delivery more precise, reducing concern about deleterious effects of large single doses to critical organs. In parallel, a better understanding is required of the biological aspects of large dose radiation effects in both normal and malignant tissue. Tissue responses to radiation are regulated by multiple factors starting from stem progenitor cell populations, the tissue microenvironment including the stromal niche, and major signaling cross-talk between the stem cell compartment, stroma, and the immune microenvironment, not only locally but also systemically via abscopal effects. Recent studies indicated that the gut microbiome also plays a significant role in malignancy, not only its natural history but also its response to therapeutic interventions. This chapter will cover these new biological factors and mechanisms, and their involvement in the overall consequences of hypofractionated RT.

S. Saha (✉) · B. F. Kimler
Department of Radiation Oncology, University of Kansas Medical Center, Kansas City, Kansas, USA
e-mail: ssaha@kumc.edu

O. Kaidar-Person, R. Chen (eds.), *Hypofractionated and Stereotactic Radiation Therapy*, https://doi.org/10.1007/978-3-031-47701-0_2

2.2 Acute and Late Effects of Hypofractionated Radiation

Radiation-induced normal tissue toxicity is a major limiting factor for effective therapy. The linear-quadratic model has been used traditionally to model isoeffect doses for loss of tissue function following conventional RT as well as hypofractionated RT. In Chap. 1, the utilization of this model is described in detail. Chap. 2 covers biological functions influencing radiation-induced acute and delayed toxicity. Radiation-induced acute toxicity often results in premature suspension or discontinuation of treatment, with the reduced dose allowing continued tumor growth or subsequent increased probability of tumor recurrence. Radiation-induced chronic or late effects may not interfere with treatment completion but significantly reduces post-treatment quality of life for some patients. Radiation-induced toxicity depends on the tissue type. Organs such as the intestine or bone marrow enriched with rapidly self-renewing cells are more radiosensitive and often develop acute toxicity. However, organs such as the liver or lung with predominantly slow cycling cells are prone to develop late effects of radiation such as fibrosis.

Radiation-induced intestinal toxicity is a major limiting factor for effective radiotherapy against abdominal malignancies. Even with precise dose delivery using SBRT to such tumors, the small bowel epithelium will still be exposed to radiation. Patients undergoing abdominal radiotherapy can experience anorexia, vomiting, diarrhea, and weight loss. These patients are at risk of developing acute intestinal inflammation and loss of mucosal integrity which also introduces the risk of bacterial influx and sepsis. Similarly, patients undergoing pelvic radiotherapy are also at increased risk for rectal epithelial damage, hemorrhage, and inflammation. A detailed understanding of normal tissue homeostasis and injury processes is necessary to develop therapeutic strategies against radiation-induced toxicity.

In a rapidly self-renewing tissue such as the intestine, both homeostasis and regeneration processes primarily depend on the presence of tissue stem cells. Stem cells in the intestine are located within the base of the crypts. These cells divide and differentiate into mature cell types including absorptive enterocytes, goblet cells, enteroendocrine cells, and tuft cells. Multiple studies have shown that the intestine has an active reserve stem cell pool [1]. Rapidly dividing crypt base columnar cells (CBCs) are primarily involved in epithelial self-renewal. However, due to their rapid self-renewal rate, CBCs are highly sensitive to radiation or chemotherapy. CBCs are enriched with multiple cell surface proteins including LGR5, ASCL2, OLFM4, SMOC2, PROM1, and SOX9^{lo}. Over the past decade, LGR5 has been used extensively to identify and characterize the intestinal stem cells [2–5]. The importance of LGR5 positive CBCs in the regenerative process and their high sensitivity to genotoxic insult make them a major therapeutic target to rescue the intestinal epithelium against radiation-induced toxicity. Reserve stem cell pools consist of long-lived, mostly quiescent stem cells present at the +4 position of the crypt base [1, 6, 7]. These cells can interconvert with more rapidly proliferating LGR5-positive CBCs, while quiescent these cells express BMI1, MTERT, HOPX, LRIG1, SOX9^{hi}, DCLK1, and KRT19 [6, 8–10] as surface proteins which are distinct from CBCs. Compared to LGR5-positive CBCs, +4 position cells are relatively radio-resistant. Multiple signaling pathways are involved in radiation-induced DNA damage and apoptosis, as well as in repair and regenerative processes in intestinal stem cells. Clinical/preclinical efforts to ameliorate radiation-induced toxicity in the intestine epithelium have focused on (1) of intestinal stem cell regeneration, (2) induction of cell cycle arrest to minimize radiation-induced DNA damage, and (3) modulation of stromal signals. Several radioprotectors, ranging from physiological growth factors to small molecule agents, have been tested in preclinical settings. So far there are no FDA-approved therapies available to protect/mitigate radiation-induced intestinal injury.

Radiation-induced chronic or long-term effects often consist of fibrosis which may occur not only in the intestine but also in the skin and subcutaneous tissue, lung, and genitourinary tract, as well as any other organs in the treatment field. Radiation-induced chronic inflammation often leads to accumulation of inflammatory immune cells which along with endogenous pro-fibrotic cells then undergo differentiation to acquire a fibrotic phenotype. In addition, myofibroblasts produce excess collagen and other extracellular matrix (ECM) components, the consequence of which is compounded by a reduction in remodeling enzymes. The majority of anti-fibrotic therapy is focused on reducing fibrosis once developed, which may be helpful to avoid immediate mortality but has thus far failed to improve a patient's quality of life. The use of SBRT in treating gastrointestinal (GI) malignancies is growing [11]. Currently, for SBRT involving GI organs-at-risk (OARs), there is wide variation in fractionation schedules, contouring of organs, and methodologies used to describe toxicities. However dose tolerance for conventionally fractionated RT and hypofractionated RT in some OARs is not well-described even with the QUANTEC (Quantitative Analysis of Normal Tissue Effects in the Clinic) system [12]. A recent publication of the HyTEC (High Dose per Fraction, Hypofractionated Treatment Effect in the Clinic) initiative [13] summarizes published peer-reviewed clinical data to further refine dose, volume, and outcome estimates for both normal tissue complication probability (NTCP) and tumor control probability (TCP) for SRS/SBRT. The HyTEC reports include organ/tumor-specific papers addressing TCP and NTCP for six anatomic regions: cranial [14] head and neck [15] thoracic [16, 17], abdominal [18–20], pelvic [21, 22], and spinal [23, 24] (a total of nine articles for TCP and seven for NTCP). A clear understanding of dose, volume, and outcome data for both tumors and normal tissues is essential to optimize the therapeutic ratio and maximize the value of care to the patient when hypofractionated RT is utilized.

2.3 Cancer Stem Cells: A Major Target for Hypofractionated RT

Cells with self-renewal ability followed by capacity to differentiate into multiple lineages are known as stem cells [1, 2]. In many tumors, a subpopulation of malignant cells with similar properties exhibits significant resistance to radiation therapy and chemotherapy. Over the years these cells have been identified as cancer stem cells (CSCs) as they show significant involvement in recurrence and tumor growth even after therapy. High free radical scavenger levels and low proteasome activity further promote CSC survival following cytotoxic therapy. Although many researchers disagree over various aspects of cancer stem cell biology and nomenclature, there clearly exists a population of tumor cells that exhibit an exclusive ability for self-renewal and differentiation into the heterogeneous lineages that promote tumor maintenance [25, 26]. Results of studies indicate that targeting cancer stem cells may improve therapeutic outcomes. In response to fractionated radiation, cell populations become enriched for cells expressing putative markers of "stemness." Specific phenotypes vary based on tumor type and methodology, but common features of these cells after radiation often include increased survival, reduced apoptosis, and rapid resolution of H2AX foci (i.e., fast repair of DNA double strand breaks). For example, one study demonstrated an enrichment of glial cancer stem cells after radiation, and that these cells exhibited preferential activation of the DNA damage checkpoint responses and increases in DNA repair capacity [27]. Compared to conventional fractionation, the effect of hypofractionation on CSCs differs among different cancer types [28]. In glioblastoma, hypofractionation led to a worse outcome. In contrast, for other tumors such as non-small cell lung cancer, hypofractionation demonstrated a better result than conventional fractionation. From these studies it has been postulated that radiosensitivity and overall survival of CSCs primarily depend on compartmental equilibrium between CSCs and differentiated cancer cells (DCCs) [29].

The therapeutic resistance of tumors is therefore multifactorial and complex but the fact that CSCs may differ in the way they handle radiation-induced DNA damage should be considered as a potential parameter determining the outcome of fractionated radiotherapy. In essence, if the dose per fraction of radiation is inadequate to cause sufficient cell death in the CSC population, the frequency of CSCs in a tumor may even increase during treatment, although clinically the tumor may shrink macroscopically.

Identification of signaling pathways in favor of or against CSC survival is crucial. Some of these pathways may be modulated by hypofractionated or ablative RT. Signaling pathways (Fig. 2.1), such as SHH, Notch, and Oct4, can be potential CSC targets to treat cancers as they promote stem cell proliferation. Targeting SHH signaling also demonstrates the involvement of the autophagy regulator BMI1 in the self-renewal of stem cells [30]. Autophagy can be pro or anti-tumorigenic. Autophagy functions as a tumor suppressor by degrading potentially oncogenic molecules. Autophagy can also play a role as a tumor enhancer by improving stress tolerance which facilitates cell survival by sustaining energy production that can lead to tumor growth and therapeutic resistance [31]. Blocking autophagy therefore may also be therapeutically advantageous. Some radioresistant tumors continue or accelerate their autophagic flux when exposed to conventional fractionation, whereas hypofractionation may block the autophagic flux and at least partially overcome radioresistance. However, pretreatment of some tumors with autophagy inducers, followed by hypofractionated radiotherapy, could enhance antineoplastic efficacy by leading to non-functional autophagic death.

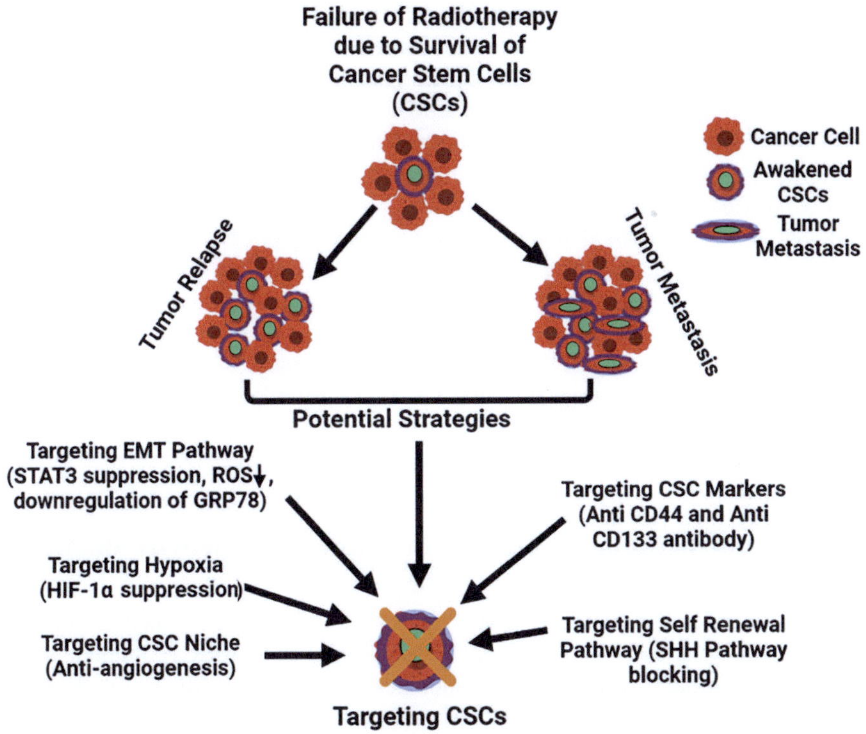

Fig. 2.1 Potential therapeutic targets to radiosensitize CSCs. Treatments targeting CSC markers, CSC self-renewal pathways, CSC niche, CSC-associated EMT, and hypoxia may radiosensitize CSCs. [Modified from Fig. 3, Liu et al., International Journal of Oral Science (2020) 12:19]

Radiation-induced transition from an epithelial to a mesenchymal state (EMT) may be another potential target to minimize the CSC population (Fig. 2.1). EMT promotes the CSC phenotype and may contribute to the development of therapeutic resistance. In response to EMT, signal transducer and activator of transcription 3 (STAT3) has been found to promote CSCs in pancreatic cancer. Inhibition of the DNA binding activity of STAT3 reduces CSCs and enhances the radiosensitivity of pancreatic cancer cells [32]. Pharmacological targeting of EMT has shown success against multiple cancers with improvement in efficacy of radiotherapy. Metformin has been shown to inhibit EMT with increase in radiosensitivity of prostate cancer cells, colorectal cancer cells, and breast cancer cells [29, 33–37].

The CSC niche itself is another potential target to radiosensitize CSCs (Fig. 2.1). In solid organ cancers such as glioblastoma, bone marrow-derived cells provide signals that promote tumor recurrence [38]. These bone marrow-derived cells contribute to a CSC niche consisting of multiple cell types such as myeloid derived suppressor cells, macrophages, fibrocytes, mesenchymal cells, and endothelial progenitor cells [39]. Non-ablative fractionated or low dose hypofractionated RT promotes recruitment of bone marrow-derived cells by inducing the expression of

HIF-1-dependent stromal derived factor-1 (SDF-1) [40, 41]. SDF-1 interacts with CXCR4-positive bone marrow-derived cells and promotes their recruitment to the irradiated tumor. Therefore, CXCR4 can be a potential target to inhibit tumor recurrence [41]. Targeted elimination of the CSC vascular niche may enhance effectiveness of RT by reducing nutrient support and the secretion of signaling molecules required by CSCs. Targeting tumor angiogenesis by an antiangiogenic agent significantly reduces CSC numbers as well as tumor growth in mice [42, 43]. Moreover, elimination of tumor blood vessels promotes sensitivity of CSCs to cytotoxic drugs [44]. Thus, the application of anti-angiogenesis drugs targeting CSC niches in combination with radiotherapy may be a promising therapeutic strategy in cancer; but further studies are needed.

A better understanding of the potential therapeutic targets for CSC sensitization for hypofractionated RT may lead to safer and more efficient combination strategies, which in turn will improve curability of cancer patients.

2.4 Hypofractionated RT and the Tumor Microenvironment

The tumor microenvironment (TME) consists of cancer-associated fibroblasts (CAFs), epithelial cells (ECs), mesenchymal stromal cells (MSCs), immune cells, and their paracrine signals such as chemokines and cytokines. All are key determinants of tumor growth and treatment resistance [45–48]. The immune cell compartment of the TME includes tumor-associated macrophages, tumor-associated neutrophils, myeloid-derived suppressor cells, natural killer cells (NKs), T cells, B cells, dendritic cells, and mast cells. Variation in radiosensitivity among different TME cell types provides a significant impact on treatment outcome and may be further modulated by different dose fractionations and schedules of radiotherapy.

RT can stimulate innate and adaptive immunity to promote an anti-tumor immune response. The enhancement effect of hypofractionated RT on the immune response has been widely investigated as it is considered an approach to expand the benefit of immunotherapy. Recent evidence suggests that hypofractionated RT may either promote or suppress the immune microenvironment [41, 49]. However, the specific doses and fractionation schedules required to either activate or suppress the anti-tumor immune response are still not clear. A combination with immunotherapy could possibly improve the curative potential of hypofractionated RT [49].

The immunoreactive effect of radiation therapy is dose-dependent and preclinical studies revealed that doses of 8–10 Gy or more per fraction are more effective in enhancing the anti-tumor immune response [50–52]. In addition to the activation of DNA damage-mediated cell death, hypofractionated RT can induce immunogenic death of tumor cells and promote anti-tumor immune response [53]. Immunogenic cell death is also associated with expression of damage-associated molecular patterns (DAMP) signals and pro-inflammatory cytokines to activate a cytotoxic T cell response [54]. DAMPs activate dendritic cells via toll-like receptors (TLRs) and facilitate the uptake of tumor antigens and their presentation on major histocompatibility complex class 1 (MHC-1) to activate tumor-specific cytotoxic T lymphocytes [55, 56]. Many preclinical studies have demonstrated that hypofractionated RT can increase presentation of tumor antigens to CD8+ T cells and enhance the antitumor T-cell-mediated immune response [41].

One of the major immune evasion mechanisms for cancer cells is surface expression of immune suppressive molecules (e.g., CD47), known as "don't eat me" signals. However, tumor cells exposed to hypofractionated RT often demonstrate surface expression of many immunogenic molecules, such as adhesion molecules, death receptors, stress-induced ligands, heat shock proteins, and stimulatory molecules (such as MHC-I and CD80), HMG®-CoA, Careticulin, collectively known as "eat me" signals [57, 58] (Fig. 2.2). The balance between eat me and don't eat me signals is key for tumor antigen recognition by the immune system and T cell-mediated local and systemic tumor cell eradication [59–62]. Based on their immunogenicity and treatment responsiveness, tumors can be classified as either hot or cold tumors. The TME associated with a hot tumor primarily demonstrates an inflammatory phenotype of myeloid cells, high level of T cell infiltration, high number of other effector cells such as NK cells, and antigen presenting cells. A TME

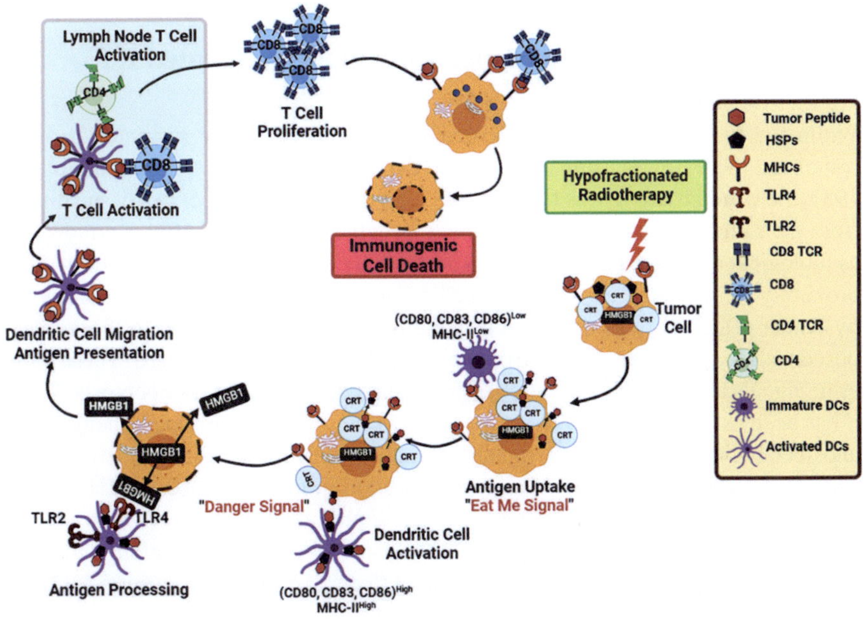

Fig. 2.2 Hypofractionated RT in modulation of tumor microenvironment. Large dose irradiation often demonstrates surface expression of many immunogenic molecules, such as adhesion molecules, death receptors, stress-induced ligands, heat shock proteins, and stimulatory molecules (such as MHC-I and CD80), HMG®-CoA, Careticulin collectively known as eat me signals. These signals along with DAMPs activate dendritic cells and their presentation on major histocompatibility complex class 1 (MHC-1) to activate the tumor-specific cytotoxic T lymphocytes. Activated T cells then recognize both local and systemic tumor cells expressing those antigens and induces cancer cell death

consisting of very low T cell infiltrates and other effector cells with a high number of Tregs and myeloid-derived suppressor cells lead to a cold tumor.

While large radiation doses may be optimal for activation of immune responses, there is also the potential that they induce damage to the tumor vasculature, limiting infiltration of cytotoxic T lymphocytes into the tumor and promoting hypoxia [63–66]. Moreover, radiation doses >6 Gy upregulate the expression and activity of endothelial nitric oxide synthase (eNOS), which promotes endothelial cell activity and tumor neo-angiogenesis [67]. Formation of dysregulated vasculature leads to the recruitment of radioresistant suppressor cells, including myeloid-derived suppressor cells, Tregs, and tissue associated macrophages with the M2 phenotype [68, 69]. Radioresistant CAFs favor an immunosuppressive TME by releasing pro-tumorigenic paracrine signals consisting of growth factors, proteolytic enzymes, and cytokines [70–72]. However, the immunosuppressive role of CAFs depends on the dose and fraction of radiotherapy and the specific tumor types [73].

In conclusion, it is evident that immunomodulatory effects of hypofractionated RT are bi-directional and further mechanistic insight is needed before optimization of doses and fractionation schedules can be realized.

2.5 Abscopal/Bystander Effects of Hypofractionated RT

While the focus on the tumor microenvironment is primarily restricted to local responses, there is increasing appreciation that abscopal effects are also possible. In 1953, the word abscopal was first referred to as the radiation effect to a tissue distant from the radiation exposure field. Radiation-induced bystander effects are defined as biological effects expressed in cells not directly exposed to radiation but in close proximity to irradiated cells. Cell-to-cell communications are key in mediating the bystander effect. Effects of ionizing radiation were communicated to these unexposed cells by paracrine signals from nearby cells which were exposed. These paracrine signals modulate proliferation, differentiation, quiescence, or apoptosis. So far it has been established that secretory factors in the form of cytokines, chemokines, and metabolites carry critical signals to induce both local bystander effects and distant abscopal effects. For example, radiation-induced release of TNF-α and TRAIL function as major paracrine signals and promotes apoptosis [74–78].

The bystander effect has numerous associated phenomena, including adaptive response, genomic instability, and abscopal effects. Additionally, genetic variation between individuals may further influence both normal tissue collateral damage and beneficial bystander/abscopal effects.

In 1992, Hatsumi Nagasawa and John B. Little first reported about radiation-induced bystander effect [79]. In subsequent multiple reports, it has been demonstrated that cells that are not directly hit by an alpha particle, but are in the vicinity of one that is hit, also contribute to the genotoxic response of the cell population [80–82]. Similarly, when cells are irradiated, and the culture medium is transferred to un-irradiated cells, these un-irradiated cells show bystander responses when assayed for clonogenic survival and oncogenic transformation [83, 84]. These observations are also attributed to the bystander effect.

The bystander effect is nicely illustrated by spatially fractionated grid radiation therapy (SFGRT)—where only parts of the tumor/target region receive high-dose hypofractionated irradiation, while the rest of the target region receives much lower doses. A preclinical study further demonstrated bystander and abscopal effects in mice bearing bilateral A549 lung adenocarcinoma xenograft tumors [85]. In this study maximal abscopal effect was observed in unirradiated right tumor when mice was exposed to 15 Gy SFGRT followed by 5 fractions of 2 Gy to the left tumor suggesting that the abscopal effect can be amplified by sequential combination of SFGRT with conventional fractionation [60]. Similar results were obtained using LATTICE therapy in mice bearing bilateral Lewis Lung Carcinoma (LLC) tumors. SFGRT was compared to the effects of high-dose RT directed to the total tumor volume versus RT directed to partial tumor volumes (10, 20 and 50%). Maximal regression was seen in tumors treated with RT (20 Gy) directed to 10% of tumor volume and in non-irradiated tumors with the highest levels of cytokine response and infiltration of CD3+ T cells. These results clearly suggest that high-dose RT directed to partial tumor volumes elicits more robust immune stimulation than RT to total tumor volume. Therefore, SFGRT can be considered as one of the most potent approaches to promote bystander and abscopal effects [85].

Antitumor immunity observed in lesions distant from the irradiated field is a prime example of the abscopal effect. Radiation-induced modification of immune cell infiltration and alteration in immune cell phenotypes such as macrophages and lymphocytes produces a systemic effect to inhibit non-irradiated tumors and metastases [86]. Preclinical studies demonstrated that radiation has a local anti-tumor effect with initial immune priming and subsequent immune-effector functions. However, this local immune response can carry a memory and exhibit a systemic response for tumor rechallenge in the same animal. This local anti-tumor immune response also has been extended to out-of-field lesions at local or distant sites [87]. This systemic anti-tumoral humoral response can be used as an in situ autologous tumor vaccine and can be considered a combinatorial strategy with immunotherapy. The use of SBRT to enhance antitumor immunity is being tested in pre-clinical studies and clinical trials. Clinical studies utilizing hypofractionation with regimens of 60 Gy in 8 fractions or 50 Gy in 4 fractions have demonstrated increases in immunoactive CD8+ cytotoxic T-cells in the peripheral blood samples of patients [88, 89]. Impressively, these changes were evident as early as 72 h following completion of SBRT, and they persisted for up to 6 months [89]. Some studies also demonstrated that renal cell carcinoma patients treated with SBRT ranging from 30 Gy in 2 fractions or 32 Gy in 4 fractions exhibited complete regression of non-irradiated lesions [90]. A preclinical study with 8 Gy in 1 fraction in murine MC38 adenocarcinoma lines demonstrated increase in immune recognition by upregulation of MHC1 antigen presenting molecules [91]. These studies suggested that hypofractionation may induce the recruitment of dendritic cells which then enhance the visibility of tumor antigens for immune cell signaling and thereby promote antitumor immunity even in non-irradiated lesions. Although these observations are encouraging, there are also reports showing immunosuppressive effects of SBRT—thus warranting further studies to improve our understanding of the influence of dose and timing of treatment. Moreover, the biological mechanisms of the immunomodulatory effect of SBRT are still not clear. Therefore, in parallel to clinical studies, additional mechanistic pre-clinical studies need to be performed.

The interval between individual fractions is now considered as one of the key factors preserving innate immune function and modulating overall tumor control. Mice receiving a combination of anti-PDL1 and radiation treatment showed better tumor control with prolonged spacing of radiation fractions of 10 days apart compared to daily or 4-day intervals [92]. This Personalized Ultrafractionated Stereotactic Adaptive Radiation Therapy (PULSAR) has now been tested in several early phase clinical trials with an expectation that longer treatment intervals will work better synergistically with checkpoint inhibitor therapy, minimize acute toxicity, and finally provide a better control over metastatic cancer. Patients with metastatic renal cancer [93] or prostate cancer [94] demonstrated better tumor control in response to PULSAR without any side effects. Although further study is needed, available evidence suggests that prolonged spacing of radiation fractionation may provide a better local and systemic effect.

2.6 Microbiome: Implications for Hypofractionated Radiotherapy

A better understanding of the interaction between the host microbiome, tumor, and radiation therapy that will influence clinical outcomes is emerging. Studies to date mostly utilized standard fractionation to demonstrate that gut flora may be altered to an inflammatory activation pattern which may help with the recruitment of immune cells and reduce immunosuppressive nature of tumor. Recent evidence also suggests that the gut microbiota composition may in turn impact the response to radiation. Preclinical studies demonstrate that microbiota can be altered to improve hypofractionated RT efficacy. Oral supplementation in mice of Vancomycin, a glycopeptide antibiotic that acts mainly on gram-positive bacteria, elicited antitumor effect of hypofractionated RT against melanoma, lung, and cervical cancer [95]. A functioning immune system was required for this effect which could also be eliminated by treatment with sodium butyrate, known to be a critical metabolite for gram-positive bacteria. This implicates the gram-positive gut microbiome as mediating remodeling of the tumor microenvironment, increasing antigen presentation in adjacent lymph nodes, and ultimately improving the effectiveness of radiation therapy against the primary tumor. A more practical means of achieving a similar response might be to employ the widely used and safe antibiotic vancomycin so as to improve the efficacy of hypofractionated RT. Recent reports have suggested that the intestinal microbiome also modulates radiation-induced toxicity [96, 97]. Patients with good clinical outcomes may benefit more from pronounced changes in the abundance of particular flora.

The microbiome is becoming a potential therapeutic target to improve the therapeutic ratio of radiotherapy. Several clinical and pre-clinical studies over the past decade established that microbiome composition is one of the major determining factors for radiosensitivity of both normal and malignant tissue. However, there are numerous outstanding questions that need to be answered before the development of a comprehensive approach for microbiome-targeted or microbiome-based treatment can become reality. It is likely that dose and dose fractionation effects on microbiome composition will be crucial to improve the therapeutic ratio. Thus, it is critical that ongoing research includes use of hypofractionated RT in addition to conventional fractionation in efforts to determine the involvement of the microbiome in local and systemic effects of radiation, as well as key signaling crosstalk between irradiated tissue and microbiome.

2.7 Summary

Success of new applications of hypofractionated RT will depend on multiple biological or physiological factors such as cancer stem cell niche, tumor microenvironment, immune responses, and acute and late effects of treatment. Therefore, continued advances in the use of hypofractionation and SBRT to improve patient care and outcomes will rely heavily on continued elucidation of the biological mechanisms associated with hypofractionated RT.

References

1. Barker N. Adult intestinal stem cells: critical drivers of epithelial homeostasis and regeneration. Nat Rev Mol Cell Biol. 2014;15(1):19–33. Epub 2013/12/12. https://doi.org/10.1038/nrm3721.
2. Barker N, van Es JH, Kuipers J, Kujala P, van den Born M, Cozijnsen M, Haegebarth A, Korving J, Begthel H, Peters PJ, Clevers H. Identification of stem cells in small intestine and colon by marker gene Lgr5. Nature. 2007;449(7165):1003–7. Epub 2007/10/16. https://doi.org/10.1038/nature06196.
3. van der Flier LG, van Gijn ME, Hatzis P, Kujala P, Haegebarth A, Stange DE, Begthel H, van den Born M, Guryev V, Oving I, van Es JH, Barker N, Peters PJ, van de Wetering M, Clevers H. Transcription factor achaete scute-like 2 controls intestinal stem cell fate. Cell. 2009;136(5):903–12. Epub 2009/03/10. https://doi.org/10.1016/j.cell.2009.01.031.
4. van der Flier LG, Haegebarth A, Stange DE, van de Wetering M, Clevers H. OLFM4 is a robust marker for stem cells in human intestine and marks a subset of colorectal cancer cells. Gastroenterology. 2009;137(1):15–7. Epub 2009/05/20. https://doi.org/10.1053/j.gastro.2009.05.035.
5. Munoz J, Stange DE, Schepers AG, van de Wetering M, Koo BK, Itzkovitz S, Volckmann R, Kung KS, Koster J, Radulescu S, Myant K, Versteeg R, Sansom OJ, van Es JH, Barker N, van Oudenaarden A, Mohammed S, Heck AJ, Clevers H. The Lgr5 intestinal stem cell signature: robust expression of proposed quiescent '+4' cell markers. EMBO J. 2012;31(14):3079–91. https://doi.org/10.1038/emboj.2012.166. PubMed PMID: 22692129; PMCID: PMC3400017.

6. Asfaha S, Hayakawa Y, Muley A, Stokes S, Graham TA, Ericksen RE, Westphalen CB, von Burstin J, Mastracci TL, Worthley DL, Guha C, Quante M, Rustgi AK, Wang TC. Krt19(+)/Lgr5(−) cells are radioresistant cancer-initiating stem cells in the colon and intestine. Cell Stem Cell. 2015;16(6):627–38. https://doi.org/10.1016/j.stem.2015.04.013. Epub 2015/06/06. PubMed PMID: 26046762; PMCID: PMC4457942.
7. Yan KS, Chia LA, Li X, Ootani A, Su J, Lee JY, Su N, Luo Y, Heilshorn SC, Amieva MR, Sangiorgi E, Capecchi MR, Kuo CJ. The intestinal stem cell markers Bmi1 and Lgr5 identify two functionally distinct populations. Proc Natl Acad Sci U S A. 2012;109(2):466–71. https://doi.org/10.1073/pnas.1118857109. Epub 2011/12/23. PubMed PMID: 22190486; PMCID: PMC3258636.
8. Fre S, Hannezo E, Sale S, Huyghe M, Lafkas D, Kissel H, Louvi A, Greve J, Louvard D, Artavanis-Tsakonas S. Notch lineages and activity in intestinal stem cells determined by a new set of knock-in mice. PLoS One. 2011;6(10):e25785. https://doi.org/10.1371/journal.pone.0025785. Epub 2011/10/13. PubMed PMID: 21991352; PMCID: PMC3185035.
9. Furuyama K, Kawaguchi Y, Akiyama H, Horiguchi M, Kodama S, Kuhara T, Hosokawa S, Elbahrawy A, Soeda T, Koizumi M, Masui T, Kawaguchi M, Takaori K, Doi R, Nishi E, Kakinoki R, Deng JM, Behringer RR, Nakamura T, Uemoto S. Continuous cell supply from a Sox9-expressing progenitor zone in adult liver, exocrine pancreas and intestine. Nat Genet. 2011;43(1):34–41. Epub 2010/11/30. https://doi.org/10.1038/ng.722.
10. Montgomery RK, Carlone DL, Richmond CA, Farilla L, Kranendonk ME, Henderson DE, Baffour-Awuah NY, Ambruzs DM, Fogli LK, Algra S, Breault DT. Mouse telomerase reverse transcriptase (mTert) expression marks slowly cycling intestinal stem cells. Proc Natl Acad Sci U S A. 2011;108(1):179–84. https://doi.org/10.1073/pnas.1013004108. Epub 2010/12/22. PubMed PMID: 21173232; PMCID: PMC3017192.
11. Tchelebi L, Zaorsky N, Mackley H. Stereotactic body radiation therapy in the management of upper GI malignancies. Biomedicines. 2018;6(1):6010007. https://doi.org/10.3390/biomedicines6010007. Epub 2018/01/06. PubMed PMID: 29301352; PMCID: PMC5874664.
12. Marks LB, Yorke ED, Jackson A, Ten Haken RK, Constine LS, Eisbruch A, Bentzen SM, Nam J, Deasy JO. Use of normal tissue complication probability models in the clinic. Int J Radiat Oncol Biol Phys. 2010;76(3 Suppl):S10–9. Epub 2010/03/05. https://doi.org/10.1016/j.ijrobp.2009.07.1754.
13. Grimm J, Marks LB, Jackson A, Kavanagh BD, Xue J, Yorke E. High dose per fraction, hypofractionated treatment effects in the clinic (HyTEC): an overview. Int J Radiat Oncol Biol Phys. 2021;110(1):1–10. https://doi.org/10.1016/j.ijrobp.2020.10.039. Epub 2021/04/18. PubMed PMID: 33864823; PMCID: PMC9447432.
14. Milano MT, Grimm J, Soltys SG, Yorke E, Moiseenko V, Tome WA, Sahgal A, Xue J, Ma L, Solberg TD, Kirkpatrick JP, Constine LS, Flickinger JC, Marks LB, El Naqa I. Single- and multi-fraction stereotactic radiosurgery dose tolerances of the optic pathways. Int J Radiat Oncol Biol Phys. 2021;110(1):87–99. https://doi.org/10.1016/j.ijrobp.2018.01.053. Epub 2018/03/15. PubMed PMID: 29534899; PMCID: PMC9479557.
15. Grimm J, Vargo JA, Mavroidis P, Moiseenko V, Emami B, Jain S, Caudell JJ, Clump DA, Ling DC, Das S, Moros EG, Vinogradskiy Y, Xue J, Heron DE. Initial data pooling for radiation dose-volume tolerance for carotid artery blowout and other bleeding events in hypofractionated head and neck retreatments. Int J Radiat Oncol Biol Phys. 2021;110(1):147–59. Epub 2021/02/16. https://doi.org/10.1016/j.ijrobp.2020.12.037.
16. Kong FS, Moiseenko V, Zhao J, Milano MT, Li L, Rimner A, Das S, Li XA, Miften M, Liao Z, Martel M, Bentzen SM, Jackson A, Grimm J, Marks LB, Yorke E. Organs at risk considerations for thoracic stereotactic body radiation therapy: what is safe for lung parenchyma? Int J Radiat Oncol Biol Phys. 2021;110(1):172–87. https://doi.org/10.1016/j.ijrobp.2018.11.028. Epub 2018/11/30. PubMed PMID: 30496880; PMCID: PMC9454379.
17. Lee P, Loo BW Jr, Biswas T, Ding GX, El Naqa IM, Jackson A, Kong FM, LaCouture T, Miften M, Solberg T, Tome WA, Tai A, Yorke E, Li XA. Local control after stereotactic body radiation therapy for stage I non-small cell lung cancer. Int J Radiat Oncol Biol Phys.

2021;110(1):160–71. https://doi.org/10.1016/j.ijrobp.2019.03.045. Epub 2019/04/08. PubMed PMID: 30954520; PMCID: PMC9446070.

18. Ohri N, Tome WA, Mendez Romero A, Miften M, Ten Haken RK, Dawson LA, Grimm J, Yorke E, Jackson A. Local control after stereotactic body radiation therapy for liver tumors. Int J Radiat Oncol Biol Phys. 2021;110(1):188–95. https://doi.org/10.1016/j.ijrobp.2017.12.288. Epub 2018/02/06. PubMed PMID: 29395629; PMCID: PMC6102100.
19. Miften M, Vinogradskiy Y, Moiseenko V, Grimm J, Yorke E, Jackson A, Tome WA, Ten Haken RK, Ohri N, Mendez Romero A, Goodman KA, Marks LB, Kavanagh B, Dawson LA. Radiation dose-volume effects for liver SBRT. Int J Radiat Oncol Biol Phys. 2021;110(1):196–205. https://doi.org/10.1016/j.ijrobp.2017.12.290. Epub 2018/02/28. PubMed PMID: 29482870; PMCID: PMC6095822.
20. Mahadevan A, Moningi S, Grimm J, Li XA, Forster KM, Palta M, Prior P, Goodman KA, Narang A, Heron DE, Lo SS, Urbanic J, Herman JM. Maximizing tumor control and limiting complications with stereotactic body radiation therapy for pancreatic cancer. Int J Radiat Oncol Biol Phys. 2021;110(1):206–16. Epub 2020/12/29. https://doi.org/10.1016/j.ijrobp.2020.11.017.
21. Wang K, Mavroidis P, Royce TJ, Falchook AD, Collins SP, Sapareto S, Sheets NC, Fuller DB, El Naqa I, Yorke E, Grimm J, Jackson A, Chen RC. Prostate stereotactic body radiation therapy: an overview of toxicity and dose response. Int J Radiat Oncol Biol Phys. 2021;110(1):237–48. https://doi.org/10.1016/j.ijrobp.2020.09.054. Epub 2020/12/29. PubMed PMID: 33358229; PMCID: PMC8053668.
22. Royce TJ, Mavroidis P, Wang K, Falchook AD, Sheets NC, Fuller DB, Collins SP, El Naqa I, Song DY, Ding GX, Nahum AE, Jackson A, Grimm J, Yorke E, Chen RC. Tumor control probability modeling and systematic review of the literature of stereotactic body radiation therapy for prostate cancer. Int J Radiat Oncol Biol Phys. 2021;110(1):227–36. https://doi.org/10.1016/j.ijrobp.2020.08.014. Epub 2020/09/10. PubMed PMID: 32900561; PMCID: PMC9445430.
23. Soltys SG, Grimm J, Milano MT, Xue J, Sahgal A, Yorke E, Yamada Y, Ding GX, Li XA, Lovelock DM, Jackson A, Ma L, El Naqa I, Gibbs IC, Marks LB, Benedict S. Stereotactic body radiation therapy for spinal metastases: tumor control probability analyses and recommended reporting standards. Int J Radiat Oncol Biol Phys. 2021;110(1):112–23. Epub 2021/02/01. https://doi.org/10.1016/j.ijrobp.2020.11.021.
24. Sahgal A, Chang JH, Ma L, Marks LB, Milano MT, Medin P, Niemierko A, Soltys SG, Tome WA, Wong CS, Yorke E, Grimm J, Jackson A. Spinal cord dose tolerance to stereotactic body radiation therapy. Int J Radiat Oncol Biol Phys. 2021;110(1):124–36. Epub 2019/10/14. https://doi.org/10.1016/j.ijrobp.2019.09.038.
25. Chen J, Li Y, Yu TS, McKay RM, Burns DK, Kernie SG, Parada LF. A restricted cell population propagates glioblastoma growth after chemotherapy. Nature. 2012;488(7412):522–6. Epub 2012/08/03. https://doi.org/10.1038/nature11287.
26. Schepers AG, Snippert HJ, Stange DE, van den Born M, van Es JH, van de Wetering M, Clevers H. Lineage tracing reveals Lgr5+ stem cell activity in mouse intestinal adenomas. Science. 2012;337(6095):730–5. Epub 2012/08/03. https://doi.org/10.1126/science.1224676.
27. Bao S, Wu Q, McLendon RE, Hao Y, Shi Q, Hjelmeland AB, Dewhirst MW, Bigner DD, Rich JN. Glioma stem cells promote radioresistance by preferential activation of the DNA damage response. Nature. 2006;444(7120):756–60. Epub 2006/10/20. https://doi.org/10.1038/nature05236.
28. Yu VY, Nguyen D, Pajonk F, Kupelian P, Kaprealian T, Selch M, Low DA, Sheng K. Incorporating cancer stem cells in radiation therapy treatment response modeling and the implication in glioblastoma multiforme treatment resistance. Int J Radiat Oncol Biol Phys. 2015;91(4):866–75. Epub 2015/03/11. https://doi.org/10.1016/j.ijrobp.2014.12.004.
29. Zannella VE, Dal Pra A, Muaddi H, McKee TD, Stapleton S, Sykes J, Glicksman R, Chaib S, Zamiara P, Milosevic M, Wouters BG, Bristow RG, Koritzinsky M. Reprogramming metabolism with metformin improves tumor oxygenation and radiotherapy response. Clin Cancer Res. 2013;19(24):6741–50. Epub 2013/10/22. https://doi.org/10.1158/1078-0432.CCR-13-1787.

30. Leung C, Lingbeek M, Shakhova O, Liu J, Tanger E, Saremaslani P, Van Lohuizen M, Marino S. Bmi1 is essential for cerebellar development and is overexpressed in human medulloblastomas. Nature. 2004;428(6980):337–41. Epub 2004/03/19. https://doi.org/10.1038/nature02385.
31. Nagelkerke A, Sweep FC, Geurts-Moespot A, Bussink J, Span PN. Therapeutic targeting of autophagy in cancer. Part I: molecular pathways controlling autophagy. Semin Cancer Biol. 2015;31:89–98. Epub 2014/06/01. https://doi.org/10.1016/j.semcancer.2014.05.004.
32. Wu X, Tang W, Marquez RT, Li K, Highfill CA, He F, Lian J, Lin J, Fuchs JR, Ji M, Li L, Xu L. Overcoming chemo/radio-resistance of pancreatic cancer by inhibiting STAT3 signaling. Oncotarget. 2016;7(10):11708–23. https://doi.org/10.18632/oncotarget.7336. Epub 2016/02/18. PubMed PMID: 26887043; PMCID: PMC4905505.
33. Zhao Z, Cheng X, Wang Y, Han R, Li L, Xiang T, He L, Long H, Zhu B, He Y. Metformin inhibits the IL-6-induced epithelial-mesenchymal transition and lung adenocarcinoma growth and metastasis. PLoS One. 2014;9(4):e95884. https://doi.org/10.1371/journal.pone.0095884. Epub 2014/05/03. PubMed PMID: 24789104; PMCID: PMC4005743.
34. Vazquez-Martin A, Oliveras-Ferraros C, Cufi S, Del Barco S, Martin-Castillo B, Menendez JA. Metformin regulates breast cancer stem cell ontogeny by transcriptional regulation of the epithelial-mesenchymal transition (EMT) status. Cell Cycle. 2010;9(18):3807–14. Epub 2010/10/05. PubMed PMID: 20890129.
35. Qu C, Zhang W, Zheng G, Zhang Z, Yin J, He Z. Metformin reverses multidrug resistance and epithelial-mesenchymal transition (EMT) via activating AMP-activated protein kinase (AMPK) in human breast cancer cells. Mol Cell Biochem. 2014;386(1–2):63–71. Epub 2013/10/08. https://doi.org/10.1007/s11010-013-1845-x.
36. Ferro A, Goyal S, Kim S, Wu H, Taunk NK, Schiff D, Pirlamarla A, Haffty BG. Evaluation of diabetic patients with breast cancer treated with metformin during adjuvant radiotherapy. Int J Breast Cancer. 2013;2013:659723. https://doi.org/10.1155/2013/659723. Epub 2014/01/15. PubMed PMID: 24416595; PMCID: PMC3876696.
37. Spratt DE, Zhang C, Zumsteg ZS, Pei X, Zhang Z, Zelefsky MJ. Metformin and prostate cancer: reduced development of castration-resistant disease and prostate cancer mortality. Eur Urol. 2013;63(4):709–16. https://doi.org/10.1016/j.eururo.2012.12.004. Epub 2013/01/05. PubMed PMID: 23287698; PMCID: PMC4034673.
38. Thomas JG, Parker Kerrigan BC, Hossain A, Gumin J, Shinojima N, Nwajei F, Ezhilarasan R, Love P, Sulman EP, Lang FF. Ionizing radiation augments glioma tropism of mesenchymal stem cells. J Neurosurg. 2018;128(1):287–95. https://doi.org/10.3171/2016.9.JNS16278. Epub 2017/04/01. PubMed PMID: 28362237; PMCID: PMC6008155.
39. Quante M, Tu SP, Tomita H, Gonda T, Wang SS, Takashi S, Baik GH, Shibata W, Diprete B, Betz KS, Friedman R, Varro A, Tycko B, Wang TC. Bone marrow-derived myofibroblasts contribute to the mesenchymal stem cell niche and promote tumor growth. Cancer Cell. 2011;19(2):257–72. https://doi.org/10.1016/j.ccr.2011.01.020. Epub 2011/02/15. PubMed PMID: 21316604; PMCID: PMC3060401.
40. Barker HE, Paget JT, Khan AA, Harrington KJ. The tumour microenvironment after radiotherapy: mechanisms of resistance and recurrence. Nat Rev Cancer. 2015;15(7):409–25. https://doi.org/10.1038/nrc3958. Epub 2015/06/25. PubMed PMID: 26105538; PMCID: PMC4896389.
41. Arnold KM, Flynn NJ, Raben A, Romak L, Yu Y, Dicker AP, Mourtada F, Sims-Mourtada J. The impact of radiation on the tumor microenvironment: effect of dose and fractionation schedules. Cancer Growth Metastasis. 2018;11:1179064418761639. https://doi.org/10.1177/1179064418761639. Epub 2018/03/20. PubMed PMID: 29551910; PMCID: PMC5846913.
42. Calabrese C, Poppleton H, Kocak M, Hogg TL, Fuller C, Hamner B, Oh EY, Gaber MW, Finklestein D, Allen M, Frank A, Bayazitov IT, Zakharenko SS, Gajjar A, Davidoff A, Gilbertson RJ. A perivascular niche for brain tumor stem cells. Cancer Cell. 2007;11(1):69–82. Epub 2007/01/16. https://doi.org/10.1016/j.ccr.2006.11.020.

43. Yang ZJ, Wechsler-Reya RJ. Hit 'em where they live: targeting the cancer stem cell niche. Cancer Cell. 2007;11(1):3–5. Epub 2007/01/16. https://doi.org/10.1016/j.ccr.2006.12.007.
44. Brabletz T, Jung A, Spaderna S, Hlubek F, Kirchner T. Opinion: migrating cancer stem cells—an integrated concept of malignant tumour progression. Nat Rev Cancer. 2005;5(9):744–9. Epub 2005/09/09. https://doi.org/10.1038/nrc1694.
45. Portella L, Scala S. Ionizing radiation effects on the tumor microenvironment. Semin Oncol. 2019;46(3):254–60. Epub 2019/08/07. https://doi.org/10.1053/j.seminoncol.2019.07.003.
46. Junttila MR, de Sauvage FJ. Influence of tumour micro-environment heterogeneity on therapeutic response. Nature. 2013;501(7467):346–54. Epub 2013/09/21. https://doi.org/10.1038/nature12626.
47. Wu T, Dai Y. Tumor microenvironment and therapeutic response. Cancer Lett. 2017;387:61–8. Epub 2016/02/05. https://doi.org/10.1016/j.canlet.2016.01.043.
48. Ansems M, Span PN. The tumor microenvironment and radiotherapy response; a central role for cancer-associated fibroblasts. Clin Transl Radiat Oncol. 2020;22:90–7. https://doi.org/10.1016/j.ctro.2020.04.001. Epub 2020/04/28. PubMed PMID: 32337377; PMCID: PMC7177030.
49. Wang Y. Advances in hypofractionated irradiation-induced immunosuppression of tumor microenvironment. Front Immunol. 2020;11:612072. https://doi.org/10.3389/fimmu.2020.612072. Epub 2021/02/12. PubMed PMID: 33569059; PMCID: PMC7868375.
50. Popp I, Grosu AL, Niedermann G, Duda DG. Immune modulation by hypofractionated stereotactic radiation therapy: therapeutic implications. Radiother Oncol. 2016;120(2):185–94. Epub 2016/08/09. https://doi.org/10.1016/j.radonc.2016.07.013.
51. Garg AD, Nowis D, Golab J, Vandenabeele P, Krysko DV, Agostinis P. Immunogenic cell death, DAMPs and anticancer therapeutics: an emerging amalgamation. Biochim Biophys Acta. 2010;1805(1):53–71. Epub 2009/09/02. https://doi.org/10.1016/j.bbcan.2009.08.003.
52. Golden EB, Demaria S, Schiff PB, Chachoua A, Formenti SC. An abscopal response to radiation and ipilimumab in a patient with metastatic non-small cell lung cancer. Cancer Immunol Res. 2013;1(6):365–72. https://doi.org/10.1158/2326-6066.CIR-13-0115. Epub 2014/02/25. PubMed PMID: 24563870; PMCID: PMC3930458.
53. Menon H, Ramapriyan R, Cushman TR, Verma V, Kim HH, Schoenhals JE, Atalar C, Selek U, Chun SG, Chang JY, Barsoumian HB, Nguyen QN, Altan M, Cortez MA, Hahn SM, Welsh JW. Role of radiation therapy in modulation of the tumor stroma and microenvironment. Front Immunol. 2019;10:193. https://doi.org/10.3389/fimmu.2019.00193. Epub 2019/03/05. PubMed PMID: 30828330; PMCID: PMC6384252.
54. Tesniere A, Panaretakis T, Kepp O, Apetoh L, Ghiringhelli F, Zitvogel L, Kroemer G. Molecular characteristics of immunogenic cancer cell death. Cell Death Differ. 2008;15(1):3–12. Epub 2007/11/17. https://doi.org/10.1038/sj.cdd.4402269.
55. Tharmalingam H, Hoskin PJ. The optimism surrounding stereotactic body radiation therapy and immunomodulation. Chin Clin Oncol. 2017;6(Suppl 2):S9. Epub 2017/09/18. https://doi.org/10.21037/cco.2017.05.01.
56. Yang Y, Liu B, Dai J, Srivastava PK, Zammit DJ, Lefrancois L, Li Z. Heat shock protein gp96 is a master chaperone for toll-like receptors and is important in the innate function of macrophages. Immunity. 2007;26(2):215–26. https://doi.org/10.1016/j.immuni.2006.12.005. Epub 2007/02/06. PubMed PMID: 17275357; PMCID: PMC2847270.
57. Moding EJ, Mowery YM, Kirsch DG. Opportunities for radiosensitization in the stereotactic body radiation therapy (SBRT) era. Cancer J. 2016;22(4):267–73. https://doi.org/10.1097/PPO.0000000000000203. Epub 2016/07/22. PubMed PMID: 27441746; PMCID: PMC4957656.
58. Schaue D, McBride WH. Opportunities and challenges of radiotherapy for treating cancer. Nat Rev Clin Oncol. 2015;12(9):527–40. https://doi.org/10.1038/nrclinonc.2015.120. Epub 2015/07/01. PubMed PMID: 26122185; PMCID: PMC8396062.
59. Diegeler S, Hellweg CE. Intercellular communication of tumor cells and immune cells after exposure to different ionizing radiation qualities. Front Immunol. 2017;8:664. https://doi.

org/10.3389/fimmu.2017.00664. Epub 2017/06/24. PubMed PMID: 28638385; PMCID: PMC5461334.
60. Wattenberg MM, Fahim A, Ahmed MM, Hodge JW. Unlocking the combination: potentiation of radiation-induced antitumor responses with immunotherapy. Radiat Res. 2014;182(2):126–38. https://doi.org/10.1667/RR13374.1. Epub 2014/06/25. PubMed PMID: 24960415; PMCID: PMC4128341.
61. Frey B, Rubner Y, Kulzer L, Werthmoller N, Weiss EM, Fietkau R, Gaipl US. Antitumor immune responses induced by ionizing irradiation and further immune stimulation. Cancer Immunol Immunother. 2014;63(1):29–36. Epub 2013/09/21. https://doi.org/10.1007/s00262-013-1474-y.
62. Deng L, Liang H, Burnette B, Weicheslbaum RR, Fu YX. Radiation and anti-PD-L1 antibody combinatorial therapy induces T cell-mediated depletion of myeloid-derived suppressor cells and tumor regression. Oncoimmunology. 2014;3:e28499. https://doi.org/10.4161/onci.28499. Epub 2014/07/23. PubMed PMID: 25050217; PMCID: PMC4063144.
63. Hellevik T, Martinez-Zubiaurre I. Radiotherapy and the tumor stroma: the importance of dose and fractionation. Front Oncol. 2014;4:1. https://doi.org/10.3389/fonc.2014.00001. Epub 2014/01/31. PubMed PMID: 24478982; PMCID: PMC3896881.
64. Begg K, Tavassoli M. Inside the hypoxic tumour: reprogramming of the DDR and radioresistance. Cell Death Discov. 2020;6:77. https://doi.org/10.1038/s41420-020-00311-0. Epub 2020/08/31. PubMed PMID: 32864165; PMCID: PMC7434912.
65. Wang Y, Liu ZG, Yuan H, Deng W, Li J, Huang Y, Kim BYS, Story MD, Jiang W. The reciprocity between radiotherapy and cancer immunotherapy. Clin Cancer Res. 2019;25(6):1709–17. https://doi.org/10.1158/1078-0432.CCR-18-2581. Epub 2018/11/11. PubMed PMID: 30413527; PMCID: PMC6420874.
66. Sun X, Lv X, Yan Y, Zhao Y, Ma R, He M, Wei M. Hypoxia-mediated cancer stem cell resistance and targeted therapy. Biomed Pharmacother. 2020;130:110623. Epub 2020/08/14. https://doi.org/10.1016/j.biopha.2020.110623.
67. Grabham P, Hu B, Sharma P, Geard C. Effects of ionizing radiation on three-dimensional human vessel models: differential effects according to radiation quality and cellular development. Radiat Res. 2011;175(1):21–8. Epub 2010/12/24. https://doi.org/10.1667/RR2289.1.
68. Park HJ, Griffin RJ, Hui S, Levitt SH, Song CW. Radiation-induced vascular damage in tumors: implications of vascular damage in ablative hypofractionated radiotherapy (SBRT and SRS). Radiat Res. 2012;177(3):311–27. Epub 2012/01/11. https://doi.org/10.1667/rr2773.1.
69. Sun X, Deng L, Lu Y. Challenges and opportunities of using stereotactic body radiotherapy with anti-angiogenesis agents in tumor therapy. Chin J Cancer Res. 2018;30(1):147–56. https://doi.org/10.21147/j.issn.1000-9604.2018.01.15. Epub 2018/03/17. PubMed PMID: 29545728; PMCID: PMC5842229.
70. Piper M, Mueller AC, Karam SD. The interplay between cancer associated fibroblasts and immune cells in the context of radiation therapy. Mol Carcinog. 2020;59(7):754–65. https://doi.org/10.1002/mc.23205. Epub 2020/05/05. PubMed PMID: 32363633; PMCID: PMC8011858.
71. Rodier F, Coppe JP, Patil CK, Hoeijmakers WA, Munoz DP, Raza SR, Freund A, Campeau E, Davalos AR, Campisi J. Persistent DNA damage signalling triggers senescence-associated inflammatory cytokine secretion. Nat Cell Biol. 2009;11(8):973–9. Epub 2009/07/15. https://doi.org/10.1038/ncb1909.
72. Nguyen HQ, To NH, Zadigue P, Kerbrat S, De La Taille A, Le Gouvello S, Belkacemi Y. Ionizing radiation-induced cellular senescence promotes tissue fibrosis after radiotherapy. A review. Crit Rev Oncol Hematol. 2018;129:13–26. Epub 2018/08/12. https://doi.org/10.1016/j.critrevonc.2018.06.012.
73. Hellevik T, Pettersen I, Berg V, Winberg JO, Moe BT, Bartnes K, Paulssen RH, Busund LT, Bremnes R, Chalmers A, Martinez-Zubiaurre I. Cancer-associated fibroblasts from human NSCLC survive ablative doses of radiation but their invasive capacity is reduced. Radiat Oncol. 2012;7:59. https://doi.org/10.1186/1748-717X-7-59. Epub 2012/04/17. PubMed PMID: 22500976; PMCID: PMC3359264.

74. Ahmed MM, Sells SF, Venkatasubbarao K, Fruitwala SM, Muthukkumar S, Harp C, Mohiuddin M, Rangnekar VM. Ionizing radiation-inducible apoptosis in the absence of p53 linked to transcription factor EGR-1. J Biol Chem. 1997;272(52):33056–61. Epub 1998/01/31. https://doi.org/10.1074/jbc.272.52.33056.
75. Hallahan DE, Spriggs DR, Beckett MA, Kufe DW, Weichselbaum RR. Increased tumor necrosis factor alpha mRNA after cellular exposure to ionizing radiation. Proc Natl Acad Sci U S A. 1989;86(24):10104–7. https://doi.org/10.1073/pnas.86.24.10104. Epub 1989/12/01. PubMed PMID: 2602359; PMCID: PMC298653.
76. Hallahan DE, Haimovitz-Friedman A, Kufe DW, Fuks Z, Weichselbaum RR. The role of cytokines in radiation oncology. Important Adv Oncol. 1993:71–80. Epub 1993/01/01. PubMed PMID: 8505057.
77. Hallahan DE, Virudachalam S, Sherman ML, Huberman E, Kufe DW, Weichselbaum RR. Tumor necrosis factor gene expression is mediated by protein kinase C following activation by ionizing radiation. Cancer Res. 1991;51(17):4565–9. Epub 1991/09/01. PubMed PMID: 1873801.
78. Unnithan J, Macklis RM. TRAIL induction by radiation in lymphoma patients. Cancer Investig. 2004;22(4):522–5. Epub 2004/11/30. https://doi.org/10.1081/cnv-200026397.
79. Nagasawa H, Little JB. Induction of sister chromatid exchanges by extremely low doses of alpha-particles. Cancer Res. 1992;52(22):6394–6. Epub 1992/11/15. PubMed PMID: 1423287.
80. Wu LJ, Randers-Pehrson G, Xu A, Waldren CA, Geard CR, Yu Z, Hei TK. Targeted cytoplasmic irradiation with alpha particles induces mutations in mammalian cells. Proc Natl Acad Sci U S A. 1999;96(9):4959–64. https://doi.org/10.1073/pnas.96.9.4959. Epub 1999/04/29. PubMed PMID: 10220401; PMCID: PMC21799.
81. Zhou H, Randers-Pehrson G, Waldren CA, Vannais D, Hall EJ, Hei TK. Induction of a bystander mutagenic effect of alpha particles in mammalian cells. Proc Natl Acad Sci U S A. 2000;97(5):2099–104. https://doi.org/10.1073/pnas.030420797. Epub 2000/02/19. PubMed PMID: 10681418; PMCID: PMC15760.
82. Prise KM, Belyakov OV, Folkard M, Michael BD. Studies of bystander effects in human fibroblasts using a charged particle microbeam. Int J Radiat Biol. 1998;74(6):793–8. Epub 1999/01/09. https://doi.org/10.1080/095530098141087.
83. Mitchell SA, Randers-Pehrson G, Brenner DJ, Hall EJ. The bystander response in C3H 10T1/2 cells: the influence of cell-to-cell contact. Radiat Res. 2004;161(4):397–401. Epub 2004/03/25. https://doi.org/10.1667/rr3137.
84. Mitchell SA, Marino SA, Brenner DJ, Hall EJ. Bystander effect and adaptive response in C3H 10T(1/2) cells. Int J Radiat Biol. 2004;80(7):465–72. Epub 2004/09/14. https://doi.org/10.1080/09553000410001725116.
85. Prasanna A, Ahmed MM, Mohiuddin M, Coleman CN. Exploiting sensitization windows of opportunity in hyper and hypo-fractionated radiation therapy. J Thorac Dis. 2014;6(4):287–302. https://doi.org/10.3978/j.issn.2072-1439.2014.01.14. Epub 2014/04/02. PubMed PMID: 24688774; PMCID: PMC3968552.
86. Ngwa W, Irabor OC, Schoenfeld JD, Hesser J, Demaria S, Formenti SC. Using immunotherapy to boost the abscopal effect. Nat Rev Cancer. 2018;18(5):313–22. https://doi.org/10.1038/nrc.2018.6. Epub 2018/02/17. PubMed PMID: 29449659; PMCID: PMC5912991.
87. Brix N, Tiefenthaller A, Anders H, Belka C, Lauber K. Abscopal, immunological effects of radiotherapy: narrowing the gap between clinical and preclinical experiences. Immunol Rev. 2017;280(1):249–79. Epub 2017/10/14. https://doi.org/10.1111/imr.12573.
88. Siva S, MacManus MP, Martin RF, Martin OA. Abscopal effects of radiation therapy: a clinical review for the radiobiologist. Cancer Lett. 2015;356(1):82–90. Epub 2013/10/16. https://doi.org/10.1016/j.canlet.2013.09.018.
89. Jayaraman P, Parikh F, Newton JM, Hanoteau A, Rivas C, Krupar R, Rajapakshe K, Pathak R, Kanthaswamy K, MacLaren C, Huang S, Coarfa C, Spanos C, Edwards DP, Parihar R, Sikora AG. TGF-beta1 programmed myeloid-derived suppressor cells (MDSC) acquire immune-stimulating and tumor killing activity capable of rejecting established tumors in

combination with radiotherapy. Oncoimmunology. 2018;7(10):e1490853. https://doi.org/10.1080/2162402X.2018.1490853. Epub 2018/10/06. PubMed PMID: 30288358; PMCID: PMC6169570.

90. Wersall PJ, Blomgren H, Pisa P, Lax I, Kalkner KM, Svedman C. Regression of non-irradiated metastases after extracranial stereotactic radiotherapy in metastatic renal cell carcinoma. Acta Oncol. 2006;45(4):493–7. Epub 2006/06/09. https://doi.org/10.1080/02841860600604611.
91. Reits EA, Hodge JW, Herberts CA, Groothuis TA, Chakraborty M, Wansley EK, Camphausen K, Luiten RM, de Ru AH, Neijssen J, Griekspoor A, Mesman E, Verreck FA, Spits H, Schlom J, van Veelen P, Neefjes JJ. Radiation modulates the peptide repertoire, enhances MHC class I expression, and induces successful antitumor immunotherapy. J Exp Med. 2006;203(5):1259–71. https://doi.org/10.1084/jem.20052494. Epub 2006/04/26. PubMed PMID: 16636135; PMCID: PMC3212727.
92. Moore C, Hsu CC, Chen WM, Chen BPC, Han C, Story M, Aguilera T, Pop LM, Hannan R, Fu YX, Saha D, Timmerman R. Personalized ultrafractionated stereotactic adaptive radiotherapy (PULSAR) in preclinical models enhances single-agent immune checkpoint blockade. Int J Radiat Oncol Biol Phys. 2021;110(5):1306–16. https://doi.org/10.1016/j.ijrobp.2021.03.047. Epub 2021/04/02. PubMed PMID: 33794306; PMCID: PMC8286324.
93. Morris Z, Dohopolski M, Rahimi A, Timmerman R. Future directions in the use of SAbR for the treatment of oligometastatic cancers. Semin Radiat Oncol. 2021;31(3):253–62. Epub 2021/06/07. https://doi.org/10.1016/j.semradonc.2021.03.004.
94. Alayed Y, Quon H, Ong A, Cheung P, Chu W, Chung H, Vesprini D, Chowdhury A, Panjwani D, Pang G, Korol R, Davidson M, Ravi A, McCurdy B, Zhang L, Mamedov A, Deabreu A, Loblaw A. Accelerating prostate stereotactic ablative body radiotherapy: efficacy and toxicity of a randomized phase II study of 11 versus 29 days overall treatment time (PATRIOT). Radiother Oncol. 2020;149:8–13. Epub 2020/05/18. https://doi.org/10.1016/j.radonc.2020.04.039.
95. Uribe-Herranz M, Rafail S, Beghi S, Gil-de-Gomez L, Verginadis I, Bittinger K, Pustylnikov S, Pierini S, Perales-Linares R, Blair IA, Mesaros CA, Snyder NW, Bushman F, Koumenis C, Facciabene A. Gut microbiota modulate dendritic cell antigen presentation and radiotherapy-induced antitumor immune response. J Clin Invest. 2020;130(1):466–79. https://doi.org/10.1172/JCI124332. Epub 2019/12/10. PubMed PMID: 31815742; PMCID: PMC6934221.
96. Liu J, Liu C, Yue J. Radiotherapy and the gut microbiome: facts and fiction. Radiat Oncol. 2021;16(1):9. https://doi.org/10.1186/s13014-020-01735-9. Epub 2021/01/14. PubMed PMID: 33436010; PMCID: PMC7805150.
97. Kumagai T, Rahman F, Smith AM. The microbiome and radiation induced-bowel injury: evidence for potential mechanistic role in disease pathogenesis. Nutrients. 2018;10(10):101405. https://doi.org/10.3390/nu10101405. Epub 2018/10/04. PubMed PMID: 30279338; PMCID: PMC6213333.

Chapter 3
The Physics of Hypofractionation and SRS/SBRT

Jason Matney and Leith Rankine

3.1 Introduction

The practice of SRS/SBRT and other hypofractionated RT relies on the accurate delivery of large doses in a limited number of fractions. To minimize normal tissue toxicities, RT is typically required to be highly conformal with rapid falloff of dose outside of the target volume. In SRS/SBRT cases, this requirement is achieved through a combination of specialized simulation, treatment planning, imaging, positional setup, motion management, and delivery technologies. Since SRS/SBRT requires a hypofractionated regimen with little tolerance for error, establishing and following guidelines for rigorous quality assurance (QA) and quality control is extremely important. The quality of the SRS/SBRT program depends on the coordinated interactions of a team of skilled health care professionals.

This chapter outlines the physics of hypofractionation by starting with definitions, basic premise, and reviewing some currently available delivery systems. This chapter includes a discussion of the basic SRS/SBRT strategy for simulation, motion management, treatment planning, and treatment delivery. Finally, the chapter concludes with a discussion of physics considerations for commissioning a clinical program and developing a comprehensive quality assurance program.

- In the mid-twentieth century, stereotactic radiosurgery (SRS) was developed to treat intracranial sites [1].

J. Matney (✉)
Department of Radiation Oncology, University of California at Davis Cancer Center, Sacramento, CA, USA
e-mail: jematney@ucdavis.edu

L. Rankine
Department of Radiation Oncology, University of North Carolina School of Medicine, Chapel Hill, NC, USA
e-mail: Leith_Rankine@med.unc.edu

O. Kaidar-Person, R. Chen (eds.), *Hypofractionated and Stereotactic Radiation Therapy*, https://doi.org/10.1007/978-3-031-47701-0_3

- Stereotaxis is a method in neurosurgery for locating points within the brain using an external, three-dimensional frame of reference usually based on the Cartesian coordinate system.
- The earliest use of the term "stereotactic radiosurgery" was reported by Lars Leksell in 1951 [2]. Typically, SRS is used to describe single fraction radiotherapy to intracranial targets, initially used as an alternative to neurosurgery.
- Stereotactic radiotherapy (SRT) is a term for fractionated SRS to localized sites within the brain or spine.
- The first combined use of X-rays with a stereotactic device (or frame) for immobilization and localization occurred in 1950 [2].
- SRS was first developed using orthovoltage X-rays, followed by protons, heavy charged particles, and gamma rays from Cobalt-60 treatment machines.
- Two broad categories have been used to immobilize and localize intracranial targets: Invasive and non-invasive systems [3].
  - Historically, skull fixation frames were used to immobilize and localize the head prior to simulation and treatment planning. These devices would remain in place until completion of treatment. These systems often used a physical frame affixed to the patient's skull, commonly using pins or screws.
  - Recently, frameless systems have been developed that use radiographic imaging and non-radiographic tracking to verify and monitor patient alignment. These systems can utilize a customized mask to immobilize the patient for simulation and treatment.
- The combination of clinical experience of SRS combined with developments in technology led to similar techniques over the past two decades in extracranial sites: stereotactic ablative radiation therapy (SABR) or stereotactic body radiation therapy (SBRT) [4].
- Both techniques (SRS/SBRT) differ from traditional radiotherapy in that large doses are delivered in 1–5 fractions.
- The goal of SRS/SBRT is to deliver a high biologically effective dose while minimizing dose to normal tissues using highly conformal treatment beams to achieve rapid dose fall-off outside the target.
- To achieve such highly conformal dose deliveries, it is imperative that the entire treatment process achieves accuracy and precision beyond that of conventional radiation therapy.
- Clinical patient outcomes of SBRT were first published in 1995, initially focusing on lung, liver, and retroperitoneal disease sites [5].
- In 2020, the NRG Oncology Medical Physics Subcommittee distributed a survey and received responses from 568 institutions on general policies and procedures for delivery of SRS/SBRT. Among responding clinics, 97.5% treat lung SBRT patients, 77.0% perform brain SRT, and 29.1% deliver prostate SBRT [6].
- The clinical implementation recommendations including protocols, equipment, resources, and QA procedures have been outlined in AAPM Task Group 101 publication [7]. Major features of SRS/SBRT adapted from AAPM TG-101 are summarized in Table 3.1.

Table 3.1 General comparison of conventional (3D/IMRT) to stereotactic (SRS/SBRT) radiotherapy

Treatment	Conventional 3D/IMRT	SRS/SBRT
Dose/fx	1.8–3 Gy	5–30 Gy
Fractions	10–30	1–5
Target definition	CTV/PTV (gross disease + subclinical extent). Tumor might not have sharp boundary	GTV/CTV/ITV/PTV Well defined tumors: GTV = CTV
Prescription isodose line	~90–95%	~50–90%
Dose gradient outside PTV	Moderate falloff	Very steep falloff
Margin	~Centimeter	Millimeters
Beam arrangement	Typically coplanar beams	Typically include non-coplanar beams
Physics/dosimetry involvement and monitoring	Indirect	Direct
Primary imaging modality	Multi-modality: CT/MR/PET	Multi-modality: CT/MR/PET
Redundancy in geometric verification	No	Yes, imaging prior to each treatment, possibly during
Maintenance of target accuracy throughout treatment	Moderate patient positioning control and monitoring	High; strict immobilization and high frequency position monitoring
Need for respiratory motion management?	Potentially	Necessary in sites with potential for respiratory motion
Staff training requirements	High	High + additional SBRT training

3.2 Treatment Systems for SRS/SBRT

3.2.1 GammaKnife

- The GammaKnife® Perfexion [8] and Icon system (Elekta, Crowley, UK) treats cranial sites with 192 Cobalt-60 sources in a conical configuration. Older models used over 200 sources that were arranged in a hemispherical pattern and a helmet-type collimation system.
- Primary and secondary collimation in the GammaKnife Perfexion® system is achieved by a single 12-cm thick tungsten collimator array, in which collimators are arranged in a series of five concentric rings around the patient, divided into independently moving 8 regions called "sectors".
- The collimation device produces individual beams of 4, 8 and 16 mm converging at the isocenter. Beam diameters are changed by moving the source tray over the selected collimator set.
  - Due to the pattern of source placements, the source to focus distance ranges from 374 to 433 mm.

- Each exposure is referred to as a "shot" of radiation where the circular beams intersect to produce a roughly spherical dose distribution.
  - Multiple spherical shots can be combined to "pack" a volume, leading to the term "sphere packing" to describe the method of treatment planning in GammaKnife.
- The patient is moved into the treatment unit using the couch. The only other main moving part on the GammaKnife unit is the drive which moves the source tray into position over the desired beam collimator holes.
- Patients are affixed in a head frame which is attached to the patient's skull with screws. This remains in place during imaging, planning and treatment.
  - This provides a rigid frame around the patient, but traditionally limits the GammaKnife to a single fraction, to avoid repeated placement of the head frame onto the patient.
- The GammaKnife® Icon (shown in Fig. 3.1) was introduced in 2016 and expands on the Perfexion by adding a gantry mounted with an X-ray tube and imaging detector for CBCT acquisition. GammaKnife Icon enables on-board CBCT and thus allows for frameless radiosurgery using a thermoplastic mask.
  - The Icon also has the "Intra-Fraction Motion Management" (IFMM) system that uses an infrared camera system to monitor a reflector dot placed on the patient's nose. This allows the system to monitor for patient shifting or motion during the duration of treatment. The system allows for a treatment interruption when the patient infrared dot moves outside of a set value.
- Plans on the GammaKnife system were traditionally prescribed to the 50% isodose line. Thus, the maximum dose point is twice the prescription value. Now the GammaPlan® system allows the user to define the prescription line.
- Advantages of GammaKnife include sharp penumbra and treatment planning with the ability to easily place multiple isocenters.
- Disadvantages of GammaKnife include the need for source replacement approximately every 7 years due to the 5.26 year half-life of Cobalt-60, the ability to treat only intracranial lesions, and the limited field size/shaping available.

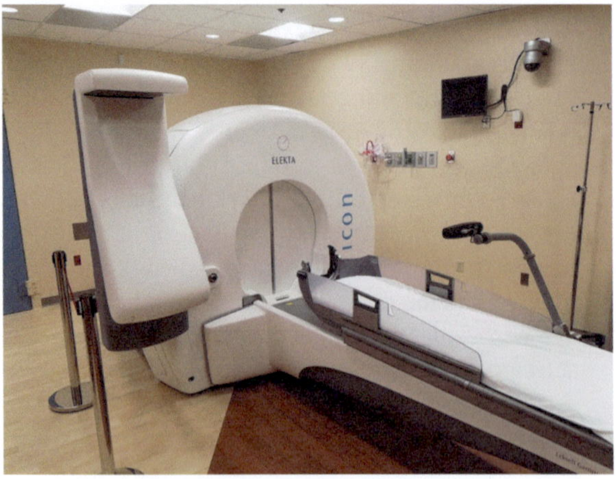

Fig. 3.1 Elekta GammaKnife® Icon unit, which collimates 192 Cobalt-60 sources to deliver multiple beams simultaneously to the focal point. The gantry-mounted CBCT system is seen to the left of the treatment unit

3.2.2 CyberKnife

- The CyberKnife® system (Accuray, Sunnyvale, CA) shown in Fig. 3.2 consists of a 6 MV flattening filter free linear (FFF) accelerator mounted on a robotic arm and a robotic couch [9].
- The robotic arm can manipulate the accelerator into hundreds of predefined positions, called nodes. From each node, the system can produce non-coplanar, non-isocentric beams.
- Radiographic image guidance is performed with two planar X-ray systems for patient alignment and intrafractional tracking.
- Initial CyberKnife treatments used fixed circular stereotactic cones with sizes 5–60 mm as measured at a reference source-to-axis distance (SAD) of 800 mm.
- The Iris™ variable aperture device can reproduce each of the fixed cones [10]. This allows for more field sizes to be used in a plan without the therapist needing to enter the room to physically exchange cones.
- The CyberKnife InCise multileaf collimator system allows for MLC-defined step-and-shoot field shapes to be used.
  - This compact MLC is designed to achieve a maximum field size of 120×102.5 mm^2, using 41 leaf pairs with a width of 2.5 mm at the reference source-axis-distance of 800 mm [11].
- Depending on the type/location of tumor, the CyberKnife allows for multiple, frameless patient setup and tracking methods.
  - 6D skull tracking system: A frameless system using orthogonal X-rays to determine translation and rotation to align bony skull anatomy to planned position using a series of digitally reconstructed radiographs (DRR).
  - Xsight Spine Alignment system: Similar to 6D skull tracking, spine tracking aligns the spine to the planned position using the X-ray imaging system and a series of DRRs from the treatment plan.

    Options exist to treat patients in both prone and supine positions.

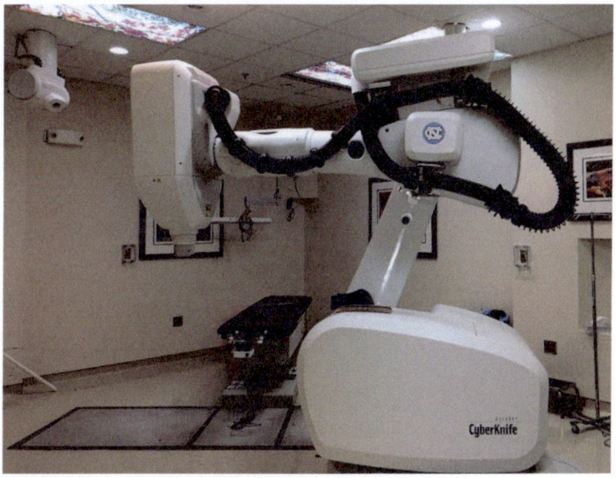

Fig. 3.2 Accuray CyberKnife system with a linear accelerator mounted on a robotic arm. Also shown are the ceiling and in-floor X-ray imaging system and robotic treatment couch

- Synchrony Tracking System: The system synchronizes the beam delivery with the motion of internal fiducials.
  The system continuously monitors external markers placed on the patient's chest/abdomen.
  By observing the fiducials through intermittent stereoscopic X-ray imaging, the system correlates the motion of the external markers with the internal fiducials.
  The CyberKnife system adjusts the treatment beam to track the position of the moving target in real time using the correlation model between the external markers and internal fiducials.

3.2.3 *Linear Accelerators*

- Two of the largest manufacturers, Varian and Elekta, have similar system configurations for their linear accelerators (Table 3.2).
  - Both offer 6 and 10 MV beam energies with flattening filter free mode, which are common for SRS/SBRT.
- Varian (Palo Alto, CA) accelerators that may be used for SRS/SBRT include the TrueBeam and older Trilogy and Clinac platforms when used with the Varian On-Board Imaging (OBI) kV imaging system.

Table 3.2 Comparison of two recent accelerator models from Varian and Elekta

Machine	Varian TrueBeam	Elekta VersaHD
Years of manufacture	2010-current	2013-current
Photon energy available	6 and 10/15/18	6 and 10/15/18
RF power source	Klystron	Magnetron
Maximum dose rate	6 MV FFF: 1400 MU/min 10 MV FFF: 2400 MU/min	6 MV FFF: 1400 MU/min 10 MV FFF: 2400 MU/min
Maximum field size	40×40 cm^2	40×40 cm^2
MLC	120 MLC 5 mm leaf width at isocenter 10 mm width on outside leaves at isocenter	160 MLC 5 mm leaf thickness at isocenter
Portal imager	Amorphous silicon: aS1000	Amorphous silicon: iViewGT
Treatment delivery	3D/IMRT/SRS/SBRT/arc	3D/IMRT/SRS/SBRT/arc
Arc therapy	Yes: RapidArc	Yes: VMAT
IGRT	OBI system with CBCT: 3D-CBCT kV planar Fluoroscopy Fiducial tracking algorithms	XVI system with CBCT: 3D-CBCT kV planar Fluoroscopy Online 4D-CBCT
Couch	3D: Exact IGRT table or 6D: PerfectPitch	3D: Precise table or 6D: HexaPOD

- Elekta (Crowley, UK) accelerators that may be used for SRS/SBRT include the VersaHD and older Infinity and Synergy platforms when used with the Elekta X-ray Volumetric Imaging (XVI) kV imaging system.
- A few design differences between Varian and Elekta linear accelerators shown for comparison in Fig. 3.3:
  - Elekta uses a magnetron to produce microwaves and a traveling wave guide in contrast to Varian addition of a klystron to amplify microwaves and a standing wave guide to accelerate electrons.
  - Varian features a gridded triode electron gun. This grid allows the user to rapidly start or terminate the injection of electrons to the waveguide, which allows faster gating of the beam. This is an important feature for gated treatment deliveries.
  - Recent Elekta machines are designed without *x*-direction jaws, instead using the MLC carriage with backup diaphragm to replace the jaws.
  - Varian machines are designed with tertiary MLCs. Two sets of *x*-direction and *y*-direction jaws are still used.
- Both manufacturers offer high dose rate flattening filter free (FFF) modes. These modes remove the flattening filter from the beam. A cross-profile comparison of a flattened and FFF beam is shown in Fig. 3.4.
- For SRS and SBRT planning, the target dose is not meant to be uniform, thus FFF modes lend well to such treatments.

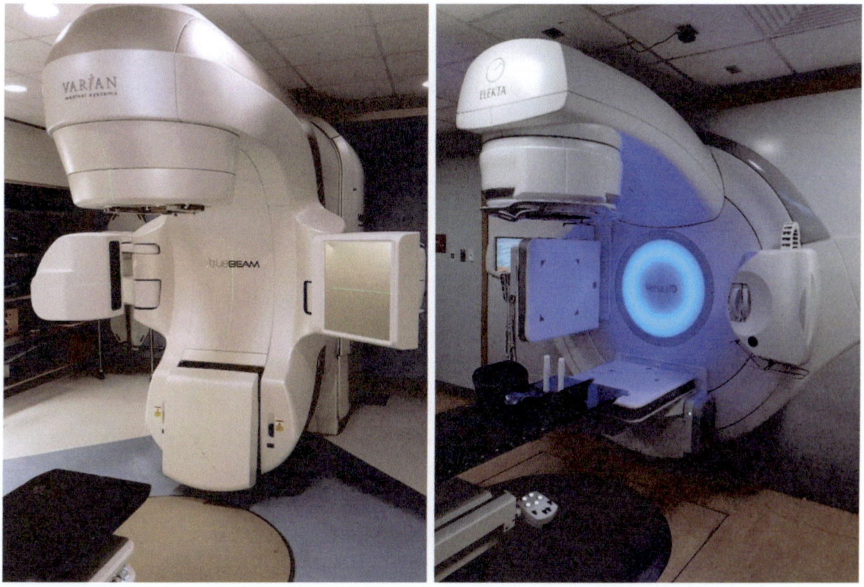

Fig. 3.3 Images of two standard modern linear accelerators with IGRT capabilities: Varian TrueBeam® and Elekta VersaHD® which show the kV imaging source and panels, and carbon fiber couches on both systems

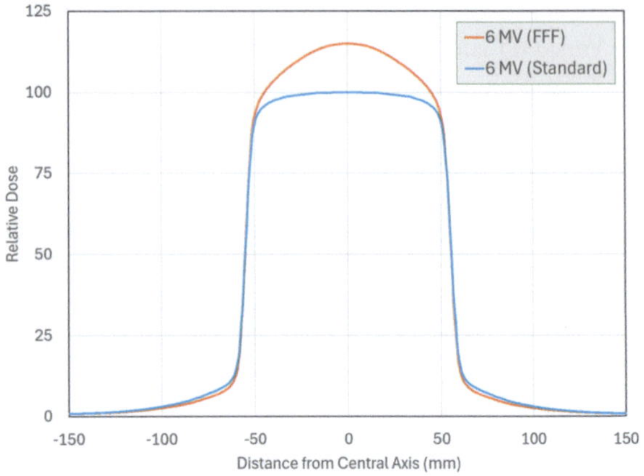

Fig. 3.4 Profile comparison of a 6 MV flattened beam (blue) with a flattening filter free (red) beam for a 10 × 10 cm² field at a depth of 10 cm in water. The peaked profile is advantageous for planning SBRT/SRS treatments where uniformity in target dose is not a goal

- The removal of the flattening filter for FFF mode results in a peaked profile, lower average photon energy (no beam hardening from the flattening filter), faster dose rate, lower head leakage, reduced scatter and less neutron production for 10+ MV beams.
- Both manufacturers include IGRT systems that incorporate both MV and kV energies. This includes the ability to acquire fluoroscopic studies for motion assessment and volumetric imaging which includes both CBCT and 4D CBCT capabilities.
  - Typical imaging kV energies range from 70–150 kVp.
- BrainLab Novalis™ Radiosurgery system features a high-definition MLC with 2.5 mm central leaves on a Varian linear accelerator with a 6D robotic couch and the ExacTrac® system that incorporates an infrared guidance with a stereoscopic X-ray system.
  - The combined kV/optical system allows for continuous monitoring of optical markers on the patient with X-ray verification of internal positioning.
- The Varian Edge™ radiosurgery system has 6, 6 FFF and 10 FFF MV energies only, and 120 MLCs with 2.5 mm leaf width at isocenter with a maximum field size of 40 × 22 cm². This system also incorporates an optical surface monitoring system.
- Magnetic resonance guided radiation therapy combines MR imaging into patient setup and treatment delivery.
  - The inclusion of MR imaging allows for continuous, non-ionizing imaging during treatment with superior soft tissue contrast. Such imaging may be useful, for example, in monitoring tumors moving with respiration such as liver SBRT.
  - Cobalt therapy can be combined with MR guidance during treatment. One example is the ViewRay MRIdian® system (ViewRay, Oakwood Village, Ohio) that incorporates three independent, high activity cobalt sources mounted on a ring gantry with 120° separation with a 0.35 Tesla MR system [12]. Each source has an independent MLC. The MR and MV systems share

a common isocenter, enabling simultaneous and continuous MRI during treatment delivery.
  - Disadvantages include the currently low MR field strength. Also with Cobalt-60 therapies, there is increased penumbra due to the source size and a limited dose rate: maximum 600 cGy/min which decays over time.
- Several vendors currently offer linear accelerators with MR imaging capabilities.
  - Elekta Unity MR-linac combines a 1.5 T Philips MRI with a ring based gantry system that houses a 7 MV FFF accelerator. The system uses a 160 leaf MLC similar to the Agility MLC found on standard Elekta linear accelerators [13]. The maximum field size in the isocenter plane is 57.4 × 22.0 cm^2. The Unity has a source to isocenter distance of 143.5 cm and an inner-bore diameter of 70 cm.
  - MRIdian Linac is a single source MR-linac with 6MV FFF energy with a 0.35 Tesla MR system. The system uses 138 MLC leaves arranged in a dual stack configuration to minimize leakage radiation. Since the dual MLC stacks are shifted against each other by one half of a leaf width, the resulting effective leaf width is 4.15 mm. Maximum field size by the MRIdian linac is 27.4 × 27.4 cm^2 in the current system.

3.2.4 *Helical Delivery Systems*

- Helical treatment delivery can also be used for SBRT (Fig. 3.5). This differs from traditional linear accelerators by mounting the gantry on a ring and enclosing the ring. This allows for a much-faster rotation time of the gantry compared to traditional linear accelerators which are limited to one rotation per minute. By rotating the beam around the patient quickly and translating the couch through the rotating beam, arc therapy can be delivered in a helical pattern. This helical treatment method can be used for SBRT delivery.

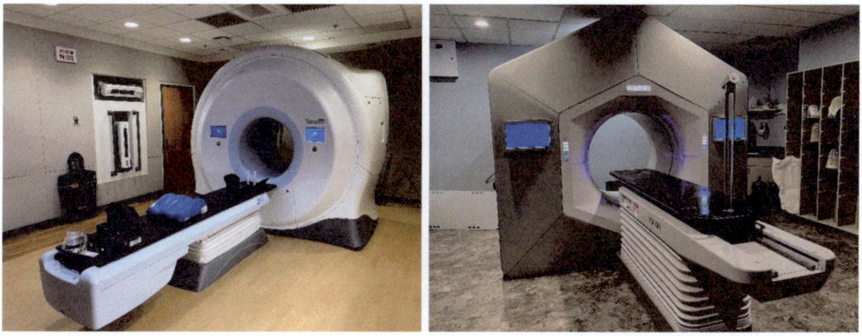

Fig. 3.5 Images of two helical delivery systems with IGRT capabilities: Accuray TomoTherapy (left) and the Varian Halcyon (right) accelerators. Both units feature an enclosed-ring mounted gantry which safely allows for faster gantry rotation compared to C-arm linear accelerators

- The TomoTherapy Hi-ART (Accuray Inc., Sunnyvale, CA) features a compact 6 MV FFF linear accelerator mounted on a rotating ring. TomoTherapy allows the combination of a continuously rotating linear accelerator with a continuously translating couch for both imaging and treatment delivery [14].
  - The beam is collimated into a fan-shaped beam that is collimated by longitudinal jaws to a width of 1–5 cm. The fan can extend 40 cm wide at isocenter, which is 80 cm from the source. The TomoTherapy machine jaw width can also be adjusted during the treatment, referred to as "dynamic jaws."
  - Beam modulation and collimation of the fan beam is achieved with a "binary" multileaf collimator. In the lateral direction, a 64 leaf collimator is used with a leaf width of 0.625 cm at isocenter. There are 51 gantry positions (or projections) per gantry rotation used to define the delivery by changing the leaf pattern to modulate the beam. The leaves are binary; hence, each leaf is either completely open or closed across the beam.
  - The TomoTherapy system is capable of using the linear accelerator to create a 3.5 MV fan beam for CT imaging (MVCT). The MVCT allows for daily patient setup and imaging.
  - TomoTherapy Radixact® is the latest model from Accuray that includes a ring-mounted kilovoltage CT system for improved image quality and imaging speed compared to MVCT. The Radixact system can achieve a dose rate of 1000 MU/min compared to the older system limitation of 850 MU/min. Additionally, the Synchrony tracking system from CyberKnife has been added to the Radixact system to allow for tumor tracking in real time.
- The Varian Halcyon™ delivers with 6 MV FFF only with a 15-s rotation time and uses a unique dual-layer stacked MLC design with maximum field size of 28 × 28 cm^2. The stacked design enables faster dynamic leaf motion (5 cm/s) and an "effective" size of 0.5 cm at isocenter (individual MLCs are each 1 cm thick, but the two layers are offset by 0.5 cm). The on-board imaging uses an orthogonal kV system with an offset detector panel allowing for large field-of-view CBCT acquisition for image-guidance [15].
- Helical fan-beam delivery and motion-induced interplay may be of concern in moving targets, especially lung and liver targets [16]. As the helical delivery focuses on one region or slice of the patient, the target could be moving into and out of the treated slice.
  - In the context of targets potentially affected by respiratory motion and SBRT, the interplay effect is a concern with helical fan-beam delivery.
  - Kissick et al. concluded the interplay effect was likely small in the presence of a sinusoidal motion; however, even a small amount of randomness in motion trace can alter the delivery dramatically [17].
  - Price, et al. concluded that narrow jaw (1 cm) Tomotherapy delivery interplay with respiratory motion could greatly compromise the target coverage. In comparison, larger jaw sizes (2.5 cm) were less sensitive to interplay effects.

3.3 Other Hypofractionation Systems

3.3.1 Brachytherapy

- High dose rate brachytherapy is a short course of radiation, usually $\leq$10 fractions where a high-activity Iridium-192 (typically 5–10 Curies in source strength) source is placed into or near the tumor site using a remote afterloader to place the source.
- High dose rate is usually quantified as greater than 12 Gy/h [18].
- Remote HDR afterloaders are an application of the "As Low as Reasonably Achievable" (ALARA) principle in radiation protection. By removing the need to hand place sources, remote afterloaders reduce exposure to all staff. Remote afterloading also allows for optimization of source dwell time to optimize the dose distribution.
- Two common remote afterloaders are shown in Fig. 3.6. Newer remote afterloader units include the Varian GammaMedplus™, Varian Bravos™, and Elekta Flexitron™.
- Various applicators are used to direct and separate the source from the patient. Different applicators exist for lung/bronchial, skin, gynecological, and breast treatments.

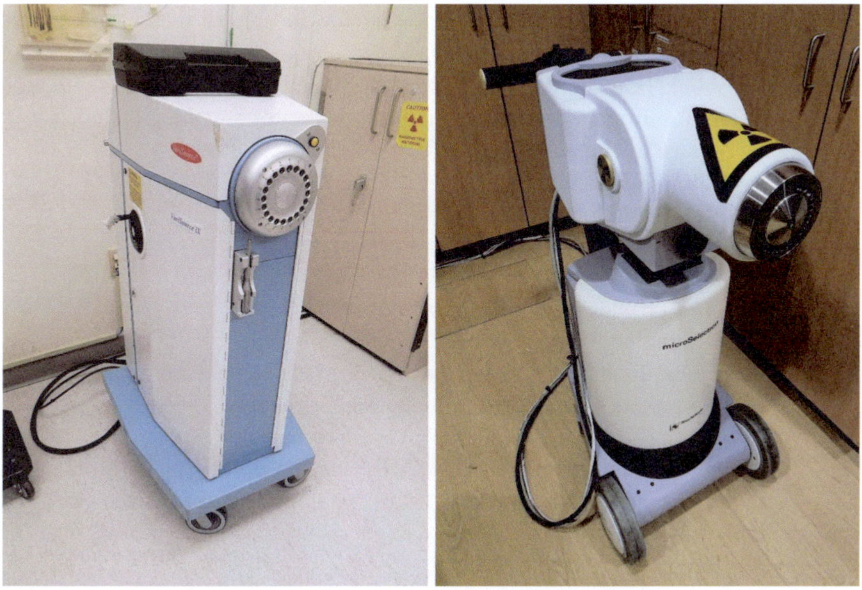

Fig. 3.6 Images of two common remote afterloaders for HDR brachytherapy: Varian Varisource® iX (left) and Elekta MicroSelectron® (right). Both allow for the controlled placement of a sealed Iridium-192 source into a variety of applicators placed inside/on a patient

3.3.2 *Patient Simulation*

- Computed tomography (CT) is typically used for treatment planning.
- Task Group 101 Recommendations:
  - Scan extent should include target and all relevant OARs.
  - Scan at least 5–10 cm in the superior-inferior direction beyond the OARs.
  - When using non-coplanar beams, scan upwards to 15 cm in the superior–inferior direction to accurately model dose within the patient.
  - Slice thickness should be 1–3 mm.
  - Deep inspiration breath-hold CT scans help reduce normal tissue dose [19].
- Simulation for Respiratory Motion:
  - Tumors in the thorax (lung, rib) or abdomen (liver, pancreas, kidney) can be affected by respiratory motion.
  - Respiratory motion can induce artifacts in free-breathing planning CT, leading to target/normal-tissue delineation errors.
  - Breath hold CT scans can be used to limit motion during a simulation/treatment.
  - 4DCTs take advantage of time-resolved information of couch position and breathing motion to reconstruct a 4DCT.
  - Breath hold CTs may overestimate tumor motion compared to 4DCTs as the patients may breathe more than normal tidal breathing.
  - 4DCTs are imperative when treating free breathing treatment sites because it will demonstrate the extent of tumor motion to help in creating treatment margins [20].
  - 4DCT should be acquired in addition to the planning CT at time of simulation

    External surrogates that are often used to monitor breathing include.
    - Surface tracking (e.g., AlignRT®, Catalyst® systems)
    - Bellows device
    - Infra-red/optical reflective marker tracking
    - Spirometry

    Breathing wave consistency and tag placement should be checked for errors by physics prior to reconstruction.

    4DCT imaging typically sorts CT images into ten different phases.

    Amplitude-binning is generally less artifact-prone than phase-binning [21], but is only supported on modern CT scanners. Typically, amplitude values range from full-exhale (0%) to full-inhale (100%).

    Maximum intensity projections (MIP) can be useful for lung planning; minimum intensity projections (MinIP) can be useful for liver planning; both projection images can cause target delineation errors if used near the diaphragm.

    Most robust planning information is obtained by using all reconstructed 4DCT phases. Using only end-inhale and end-inhale imaging may underestimate respiratory motion due to hysteresis.

  - Inhale breath-hold and exhale breath-hold CT scans can be additionally attained to estimate extent of tumor motion, may overestimate tumor motion compared to free-breathing motion 4DCT.
  - Some systems permit treatment during breath hold. However, variation between breath holds should be quantified and included in margins.
- Immobilization devices.
  - Minimize inter-fraction and intra-fraction motion.
  - Currently available commercial immobilization systems include:

    Vacuum bag immobilization devices: (e.g., Vac-Lok Bag, Alpha Cradle)
    - Vacuum sealed bag with plastic beads or foam that conform to the patient
    - Patient in bag which hardens around patient to immobilize

    Thermo-plastic masks and molds
    - Plastic that is pliable when heated and formed to the patient where it is locked into anchors and hardens around the patient

    Compression belt/paddles
    - Abdominal compression is used for lower lobe lung lesions or liver lesions to help reduce respiratory motion

    Body frames: (e.g., Elekta BodyFIX system)
    - Similar to a vacuum bag system but also has a plastic wrap that suctions around the patient to help decrease motion of body areas not in contact with the bag

    Full Body SBRT Frames
    - Several vendors offer a complete body immobilization system that attaches to the simulation CT couch and accelerator couch that includes an immobilization bag, wingboard, head sponge, handles, abdominal compression device, knee sponge, and leg specific immobilization

3.3.3 Image Registration

- Image registration has an important role in target delineation. Many different imaging modalities have been used in SRS/SBRT planning.
  - MRI has better soft tissue and cerebral tissue delineation compared to CT. Task Group 101 considered MRI to be the gold standard for brain imaging.
  - When registering MRI and CT, one should be careful about:

    The two scans are not always a complete match due to different patient positions between MR scan and simulation scan.

    MRI does not provide electron density needed for the calculation of dose as is the case for CT.

    One must be aware that MRI is prone to geometric distortions, especially at the periphery of a scan, which could cause limitations in the quality of a registration [22].

MRI can also have "ghost" artifacts which are the representation of more than one of the same object due to motion [22].

- Positron Emission Tomography (PET) scans are used in conjunction with CT scans to add biological information provided in the PET scan.
  PET has attenuation corrections utilizing the CT taken concurrently and the attenuation corrected PET scan should be used for registration.
  Fuse CT from PET/CT to planning CT to limit error since the PET/CT should already be registered. One must verify that the patient did not move between the CT and PET acquisitions.
  Some disadvantages of a PET scan include [23]:
  - PET is quantified in terms of standard uptake value (SUV) of the PET radionuclide. One must work with standard update value cautiously as visual appearance can change greatly from window and level, and SUV may not be reproducible from one scan to the next.
  - Since PET scans take a longer time compared to CT, the PET scan is more prone to motion blurring and other artifacts.

3.3.4 Patient Setup and Treatment Delivery

- Current SBRT systems rely on image guidance for patient setup before every fraction. The details of the IGRT available depend on the treatment machine.
- Typically simulation CT images or DRR are transferred to the treatment console to perform registration with kV and/or MV images acquired with the in-room imaging systems.
- It is important to consider the potential imaging dose to the patient over the course of SRS/SBRT. The management of imaging dose during IGRT is discussed in AAPM Task Group 75 [24].
  - The dose is dependent on the technique of imaging. Overall kV imaging dose depends on many factors, such as energy.
    Planar imaging will deposit the high dose at the imaged entrance skin surface.
    Volumetric imaging (e.g., CBCT) will deliver roughly uniform dose throughout the imaged volume.
  - To ALARA, collimate radiographic imaging studies to the areas of interest to reduce imaging dose to the patient.
  - The imaging dose for a given imaging technique should be quantified by a qualified medical physicist.
- Resulting IGRT offsets in the co-registration signify setup shifts required to bring the patient into the planned position.
  - All SRS/SBRT systems have methods to align the patient after image guidance, typically by moving the treatment couch.
- In our clinic, after any patient shift, we repeat the imaging study to ensure that the patient positioning system performed as intended.

  - While all patient positioning systems should undergo daily quality assurance procedures, the high dose and limited number of fractions in SBRT/SRS warrant additional imaging to ensure proper patient alignment.
- Prior to the first treatment, our clinic's policies state that the in-room images must be reviewed by a physician.
- Additional delivery considerations to account for tumor motion.
  - Magnitude and frequency of tumor motion can vary [25]:
    - Between simulation and treatment
    - Day-to-day between treatments
    - During a treatment fraction
  - For all approaches (ITV, Mid-Position, gating, breath-hold) daily pre-treatment dynamic imaging is vital to confirm estimated tumor motion and correlation with any external surrogates [26].
  - Examples of pre-treatment respiratory motion assessment include:
    - 4D-CBCT
    - CBCT or on-board fluoroscopy fiducial tracking
    - MRI (e.g., MRgRT real-target imaging)
  - For extended treatment times encountered in SBRT, periodic monitoring of internal motion is recommended as patient respiration can vary during treatment.

3.3.5 Patient-Specific Physics Quality Assurance

- In our clinic, several additional tasks are performed for SBRT/SRS beyond that of conventional radiotherapy treatments.
- A physician and physicist are present throughout the simulation to assist with selection and usage of immobilization devices. The immobilization devices for SRS/SBRT are often more complex than conventional radiotherapy.
- A pretreatment physics chart check is performed to check relevant parameters such as treatment intent, simulation images, contouring, image registration, isocenter location (if applicable), and overall plan quality. An important check is the comparison of parameters in the patient's electronic chart against the TPS.
- A secondary monitor unit (MU) calculation is performed for every patient. Typically the second check and TPS MU are within 5% agreement per beam and 3% overall calculation point dose.
- Any patient treated with arc therapy will have a measurement-based QA performed. Often, this is similar to QA measurements performed for standard fractionation arc plans. This also serves to verify that the leaf position/sequencing from the TPS was correctly transferred to the record and verify system and the treatment machine control station.
- For cone defined fields (such as CyberKnife), our clinic does not perform patient-specific beam measurements. Each cone has been thoroughly measured and quantified during linear accelerator commissioning.

  - Beam data for a selection of cones is verified during annual QA.
- For SBRT/SRS treated with MLC-based 3D conformal radiotherapy, the combination of irregular treatment field shapes and small treatment field areas (e.g., usually less than 4 cm × 4 cm) are an indication for individual field ion chamber output measurements. An ion chamber with small collecting volume dimensions must be used, so as not to succumb to partial volume effects. Additionally, we check the MLC transfer from planning system to the linear accelerator and MLC positioning accuracy by way of diode array measurements or EPID-based films of each field.
- Similarly, for VMAT/IMRT, with many irregular and small segments, the dose output is measured using a small ion chamber, and the relative dose distributions of each field/arc are measured through one plane of the treatment field, using either film or diode array.
  - Note: ion chamber and diode array measurements seldom test the accuracy of the dose calculation algorithm in heterogeneous media; this test should be performed during commissioning, and validated by way of a third-party heterogeneous phantom measurement (e.g., Imaging and Radiation Oncology Core [IROC], MD Anderson Cancer Center, Houston, TX).
- AAPM Task Group 101 [7] recommends that:
  - At least one qualified medical physicist is present from beginning to end of the first fraction and is available for therapists to consult for any subsequent fractions.
  - A radiation oncologist approves the results of image guidance and verifies portal imaging before every fraction.
  - All systems to align the patient must be checked with specific quality assurance procedures. Daily imaging isocenter checks and simple localization checks are performed as part of routine morning QA in our clinic.

3.3.6 Machine-Specific Physics Quality Assurance

- Quality assurance programs for SRS/SBRT should be an extension of already existing tests.
  - The same format of daily, monthly, and annual testing procedures is recommended.
  - These procedures should be designed to detect any deviations from the baseline performance determined at acceptance and commissioning.

    Daily QA should be designed to verify the basic functionality and safe usage of all delivery and IGRT systems.

    Monthly QA should be designed to detect trends in performance away from the baseline and focus on tests most likely to affect patient treatment.

    Annual QA should be a thorough retesting of all individual and combined systems used and sets a baseline for monthly comparisons.

- Our departmental linear accelerator quality assurance policies and procedures have been developed based on the following AAPM Task Group Reports:
  - TG-40—Comprehensive QA for Radiation Oncology: This older report provides a comprehensive list of tests, testing frequencies, and tolerance for linear accelerator-based quality assurance [27].
  - TG-142—Quality assurance of medical accelerators: This report is an update to TG-40 with increased testing recommendations for accelerators used for IGRT and SRS/SBRT techniques [28].
  - TG-104—The Role of In-Room kV X-Ray Imaging for Patient Setup and Target Localization: This report outlines the different types of planar X-ray imaging systems available and recommends quality assurance tests for these systems [29].
  - TG-179—Quality assurance for image-guided radiation therapy utilizing CT-based technologies: This report outlines available technology and general quality assurance testing and frequency of tests for kV CBCT and MV CBCT, and CT-on-rails units used for patient positioning [30].
  - TG-147—Quality Assurance for non-radiographic localization and positioning systems: This report summarizes various systems and outlines quality assurance test and testing frequencies for non-radiographic systems used to align patients [31].
  - QA of robotic radiosurgery devices is covered by AAPM Task Group 135 [32].
  - AAPM Task Group 142 recommends daily, monthly, and annual quality assurance tests that should be performed for all linear accelerators and additional tests for SRS/SBRT units.
  - In addition, an ASTRO executive summary recommended additional tests not mentioned in the earlier report [33].
  - Table 3.3 summarizes recommendations from ASTRO and Task Group 142.
  - Additional tests or more frequent testing may be appropriate depending on the treatment machine and technologies used.
- The Winston–Lutz test is an important test of a linear accelerator used for SRS/SBRT.
  - This test was developed by Lutz et al. where a metal sphere is placed at isocenter. A film was acquired of the treatment beam, and the center of the sphere is compared to the center of the treatment field [34].
  - This test checks the gantry, table, and collimator isocenter alignments in various angles.

    Mechanical flex in the system as the gantry angles changes or variation in the center of the couch or collimator rotation can all be detected using this test.
  - Winston–Lutz films can now be acquired using the EPID imagers of most linear accelerators.
  - Typically, this test is performed daily to verify the imaging isocenter aligns to the treatment (MV) isocenter.
  - Figure 3.7 demonstrates typical Winston–Lutz images.

Table 3.3 Combined AAPM Task Group 142 and ASTRO recommended minimum quality assurance testing specifically for SRS/SBRT linear accelerators

Test type	Procedure	Tolerance for SRS/ SBRT accelerator
Daily tests (in addition to TG 142 guidelines)		
Dosimetric	X-ray output constancy	3%
Mechanical	Laser localization	1 mm
	Optical distance indicator at isocenter	2 mm
	Collimator/jaw size indicator	1 mm
	Winston–Lutz MV–kV isocenter coincidence (single angle)	≤1 mm, <0.75 mm average
	IGRT system couch positioning/repositioning	1 mm
Safety	Stereotactic interlocks/lockouts	Functional
	Collisional interlocks of kV/MV systems	Functional
	Imaging system interlocks	Functional
Monthly tests (in addition to TG 142 guidelines)		
Dosimetric	X-ray output	2%
	Dose rate output constancy	2%
Mechanical	Treatment couch positioning indicators	1 mm and 0.5°
	MV–kV isocenter coincidence (cardinal angles)	1 mm
Imaging	Hidden target test using frame or IGRT system	≤1 mm
	Planar kV and MV geometrical scaling	≤1 mm kV ≤2 mm MV
	CBCT contrast, spatial resolution, HU constancy, uniformity and noise	Baseline
	CBCT geometrical accuracy	≤1 mm
Annual tests (in addition to TG 142 guidelines)		
Dosimetric	SRS arc rotation	1 MU or 2%
	MU linearity	≤5% or 2–4 MU
	Spot check of small field beam data including output factors, depth dose and off-axis factors	≤1% from baseline
Mechanical	MV–kV isocenter coincidence	1 mm
Imaging	CBCT imaging dose	Baseline
	Planar kV or MV imaging dose	Baseline
	KV beam quality and energy	Baseline
	Imager position of full range of travel	±5 mm
	End-to-end localization assessment	≤1 mm
	End-to-end dosimetric measurement	≤2%

- One recommended monthly QA addition is use of "hidden target" end-to-end test of the IGRT systems, in which the user aligns a phantom with an internal spherical target to the machine isocenter using the IGRT capabilities, and then verifies the target position using kV and MV imaging.
  – Intentionally misaligning the phantom initially by a known off-set, and then testing the IGRT system's ability to adequately correct the position, is a more thorough version of this recommended test.

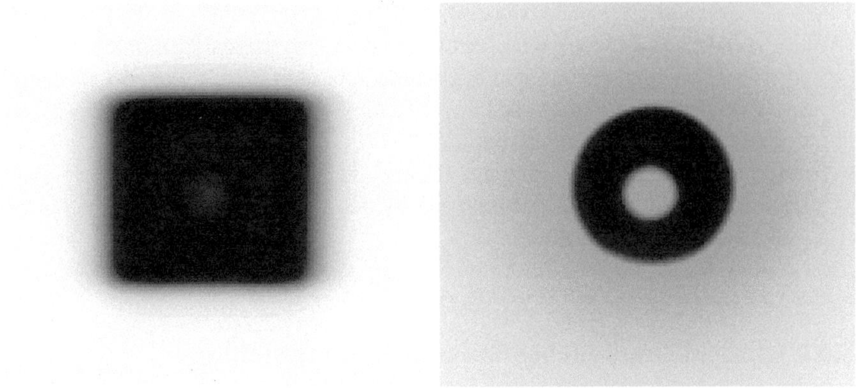

Fig. 3.7 Examples of Winston–Lutz tests for a MLC-defined field (left) and a cone-defined field (right) on a linear accelerator. The test compares the center of the radiation field to the center of a metal sphere placed at isocenter. In the image on the right, a small variation in the radiation field relative to the sphere is easily detected by the human eye

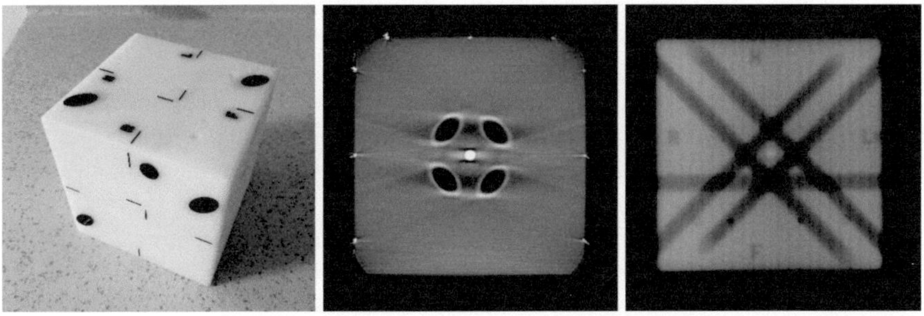

Fig. 3.8 A "hidden object" end-to-end test can be performed with commercial phantoms. Shown here are the MIMI phantom (left) and its resulting CBCT (center), which is used to align its central Winston–Lutz-style metal sphere to the kV isocenter. Finally, an MV portal image (right) can be taken to verify alignment of the metal sphere with the MV isocenter

- Several vendors have designed phantoms to facilitate this test for a variety of systems. These phantoms are able to test alignment of the laser, kV, and MV isocenters.
- In our clinic, the "hidden target" test is performed using the "Multiple Imaging Modality Isocentricity" (MIMI) phantom (Fig. 3.8) from Standard Imaging (Middleton, WI).

    The phantom has a hidden, metal sphere embedded at the center for Winston–Lutz testing and multiple open air columns assist with image registration.

    Marked on the outside of the phantom are off-center lines to align the phantom with a known offset from the central sphere.

    A CBCT of the phantom is acquired. The IGRT system automated registration algorithm aligns the phantom's center to isocenter and performs the

couch shift. This tests the couch alignment capabilities of the system and should equal the known offset from sphere to external laser marking.
The previous step aligned the central sphere to the kV imaging isocenter. MV portal imaging is used to verify the central sphere aligns with the central axis of the radiation field.
- Any ancillary imaging system isocenter, such as an optical surface tracking system, can also be tested with the hidden target test once the phantom is aligned to the MV isocenter.

3.4 Clinical Implementation and Commissioning

- AAPM Task Group 101 outlines the critical steps for initiating a clinical SBRT program:
  - Establish the scope of the program including goals for each treatment site.
  - Determine the treatment modality, dose, fractionation scheme, and treatment planning goals that support the clinical goals for each treatment site.
  - Determine the equipment requirements for patient positioning, treatment delivery, and positional verification.
  - Determine the personnel needs for implementation, including additional requirements for therapists, dosimetrists, physicists, and physicians.
  - Establish and perform acceptance testing and commissioning test procedures for all SBRT equipment.
  - Establish quality assurance procedures for simulation, treatment planning, treatment delivery, and IGRT verification guidelines. Include reporting methodologies and action levels for these guidelines.
  - Conduct personnel training for all new equipment, procedures, and guidelines.
- Acceptance testing is not the same as commissioning but is only the first step of the process for physics.
  - Acceptance testing is generally performed with the vendor's personnel to ensure that the system is functional, operates within intended specifications, and in compliance with all regulatory requirements.
- Commissioning testing should be developed by the institution's physics team to establish a comprehensive baseline characterization of the SRS/SBRT system's performance. A time consuming but crucial portion of the commissioning process is the measurement and characterization of the radiation from the machine.
  - AAPM Task Group 106 provides guidelines and recommendations on standard linear accelerator beam data commissioning [35].
  - SBRT/SRS commonly uses small treatment fields to achieve the necessary conformality. Accurate dosimetric measurement of small fields is complicated by several issues:
    Detector volume averaging
    Loss of lateral electronic equilibrium
    Collimator effects (e.g., MLC leakage, leaf end transmission)
    Detector position uncertainty

  - AAPM TG 101 recommends that the active diameter of the detector should be less than half of the full-width half maximum of the smallest beam measured.
- The TPS must be commissioned using beam data to ensure accurate calculation of dose and monitor units. This includes a systematic comparison of calculation and measurement ranging from simple configurations such as a single beam to sophisticated arrangements of beams replicating all potential SRS/SBRT clinical scenarios [33].
- There are large potential clinical consequences for incorrect beam data and machine calibration, especially in SRS/SBRT.
  - Due to the increased potential for errors, commissioning data should be compared to published data (often termed "golden data") and any inconsistencies should be investigated.
- Acceptance testing and commissioning should characterize each step of the SRS/SBRT process. Once the individual components of the SRS/SBRT planning and treatment technique are commissioned, it is recommended to perform an all-encompassing "end-to-end" test of the entire system [20].
  - The testing should mimic actual patient treatment and should use all of the same equipment used for treating the patient.
  - "End-to-end" testing using anthropomorphic phantoms is a recommended procedure prior to final commissioning and as part of on-going quality assurance.
- Prior to releasing the machine for clinical usage, it is recommended to independently verify the absolute machine calibration utilizing a remote dosimetry monitoring service.
  - One example is the MD Anderson IROC Houston Quality Assurance Center which provides dosimeters and phantoms via mail order service [36].
- Table 3.4 outlines recommendations of comprehensive quality control measures from ASTRO [33].

Table 3.4 ASTRO recommendations of comprehensive quality control measures

Recommendations to guard against catastrophic failures in SRS and SBRT			
Procedure and tests	Principal	Primary review	Secondary review
1. Commissioning treatment devices and planning systems			
Machine output calibrations and factors in accordance with relevant guidelines (TG-51, TG-101, TG-142)	Physicist	2nd physicist	Independent assessment (RPC, etc.)
Treatment planning system commissioning should include test cases similar to those encountered in SBRT (TG-53)	Physicist	2nd physicist	Physicists and dosimetrists
2. Patient selection			
Patient selection should be in accordance with an approved clinical protocol	Physician	Physicians and physicists	ALL

(continued)

Table 3.4 (continued)

Recommendations to guard against catastrophic failures in SRS and SBRT			
Procedure and tests	Principal	Primary review	Secondary review
3. Patient simulation			
Patient simulated in accordance with approved protocol (immobilization and respiratory management) and supervised by physician	Simulation therapist	Physician	Physicists and dosimetrists
4. Patient treatment planning			
Verify the patient information, treatment site, and prescription	Dosimetrist	Physician	All
Verify correct positioning of the high dose and intermediate regions of isodose plan relative to targets	Dosimetrist	Physician	Physicist
Verify the reference images and any shift information—physician determines IGRT technique	Dosimetrist	Physicist	ALL
5. Pre-treatment quality assurance			
Verify that the correct version of the patient's treatment plan is approved, sent to treatment management system, and used for patient-specific QA	Dosimetrist	Physicist	ALL
Perform a thorough chart review	Therapist	Physicist	ALL
Perform a complete chart check including review of information in treatment management system, field apertures in treatment management system, and check of dose to verify TPS calculation	Dosimetrist	Physicist	ALL
Before the first treatment or for any change in treatment, perform patient-specific QA to guarantee that data transfer between systems is correct before patient treatment begins	Physicist	Physicist	ALL
6. Treatment delivery			
Halt a procedure if the operator is unclear about what is being done	ALL	ALL	ALL
Perform a check of treatment parameters before start of each treatment against a fixed version of the treatment plan	Therapist	2nd therapist	ALL
Perform a time out prior to treatment delivery	Therapist	2nd therapist	ALL
Assess patient clinically during course of SBRT to identify any acute effects	Physician, therapist, and nurse	Physician, therapist, and nurse	
7. Quality performance and improvement			
Perform end-to-end testing to guarantee transfer of data among all systems involved in imaging, planning and dose delivery (annually and after any software or hardware changes)	Physicist	Second physicist	Physicists and dosimetrists

References

1. Leksell L. Stereotactic radiosurgery. J Neurol Neurosurg Psychiatry. 1983;46(9):797–803.
2. Leksell L. The stereotaxic method and radiosurgery of the brain. Acta Chir Scand. 1951;102(4):316–9.
3. Lightstone AW, Benedict SH, Bova FJ, Solberg TD, Stern RL. Intracranial stereotactic positioning systems: Report of the American Association of Physicists in Medicine radiation therapy committee task group no. 68. Med Phys. 2005;32(7):2380–98.
4. Potters L, Steinberg M, Rose C, et al. American Society for Therapeutic Radiology and Oncology and American College of Radiology Practice Guideline for the performance of stereotactic body radiation therapy. Int J Radiat Oncol Biol Phys. 2004;60(4):1026–32.
5. Blomgren H, Lax I, Näslund I, Svanström R. Stereotactic high dose fraction radiation therapy of extracranial tumors using an accelerator: clinical experience of the first thirty-one patients. Acta Oncol. 1995;34(6):861–70.
6. Chetvertkov M, Monroe JI, Boparai J, Solberg TD, Pafundi DH, Ruo RL, Gladstone DJ, Yin FF, Chetty IJ, Benedict S, Followill DS, Xiao Y, Sohn JW. NRG oncology survey on practice and technology use in SRT and SBRT delivery. Front Oncol. 2020;10:602–7.
7. Benedict SH, Yenice KM, Followill D, et al. Stereotactic body radiation therapy: the report of AAPM task group 101. Med Phys. 2010;37(8):4078–101.
8. Lindquist C, Paddick I. The Leksell Gamma Knife Perfexion and comparisons with its predecessors. Neurosurgery. 2007;61(3 Suppl):ONS-130–40.
9. Adler JR Jr, Chang SD, Murphy MJ, Doty J, Geis P, Hancock SL. The Cyberknife: a frameless robotic system for radiosurgery. Stereotact Funct Neurosurg. 1997;69(1–4):124–8.
10. Van De Water S, Hoogeman MS, Breedveld S, Nuyttens JJME, Schaart DR, Heijmen BJM. Variable circular collimator in robotic radiosurgery: a time-efficient alternative to a mini-multileaf collimator? Int J Radiat Oncol Biol Phys. 2011;81(3):863–70.
11. Fürweger C, Prins P, Coskan H, Heijmen BJM. Characteristics and performance of the first commercial multileaf collimator for a robotic radiosurgery system. Med Phys. 2016;43(5):2063–71.
12. Mutic S, Dempsey JF. The ViewRay system: magnetic resonance-guided and controlled radiotherapy. Semin Radiat Oncol. 2014;24(3):196–9.
13. Raaymakers BW, Lagendijk JJW, Overweg J, et al. Integrating a 1.5 T MRI scanner with a 6 MV accelerator: proof of concept. Phys Med Biol. 2009;54(12):N229–37.
14. Langen KM, Papanikolaou N, Balog J, et al. QA for helical tomotherapy: report of the AAPM task group 148. Med Phys. 2010;37(9):4817–53.
15. Netherton T, Li Y, Gao S, et al. Experience in commissioning the halcyon linac. Med Phys. 2019;46(10):4304–13.
16. Price A, Chen J, Chao E, et al. Compensation of intrafractional motion for lung stereotactic body radiotherapy (SBRT) on helical TomoTherapy. Biomed Phys Eng Express. 2019;5(2):025043.
17. Kissick MW, Mo X, McCall KC, Schubert LK, Westerly DC, MacKie TR. A phantom model demonstration of tomotherapy dose painting delivery, including managed respiratory motion without motion management. Phys Med Biol. 2010;55(10):2983–95.
18. ICRU. Dose and volume specification for reporting intracavitary therapy in gynecology. Bethesda: International Commission on Radiation Units and Measurements; 1991. p. 38.
19. Mageras GS, Yorke E. Deep inspiration breath hold and respiratory gating strategies for reducing organ motion in radiation treatment. Semin Radiat Oncol. 2004;14(1):65–75.
20. Potters L, Kavanagh B, Galvin JM, et al. American Society for Therapeutic Radiology and Oncology (ASTRO) and American College of Radiology (ACR) practice guideline for the performance of stereotactic body radiation therapy. Int J Radiat Oncol Biol Phys. 2010;76(2):326–32.
21. Olsen JR, Lu W, Hubenschmidt JP, et al. Effect of novel amplitude/phase binning algorithm on commercial four-dimensional computed tomography quality. Int J Radiat Oncol Biol Phys. 2008;70(1):243–52.

22. Hill DLG, Batchelor PG, Holden M, Hawkes DJ. Medical image registration. Phys Med Biol. 2001;46(3):R1–R45.
23. Prince JL. Medical imaging signals and systems. Upper Saddle River: Pearson Prentice Hall; 2006.
24. Murphy MJ, Balter J, Balter S, et al. The management of imaging dose during image-guided radiotherapy: report of the AAPM task group 75. Med Phys. 2007;34(10):4041–63.
25. Ge J, Santanam L, Noel C, Parikh PJ. Planning 4-dimensional computed tomography (4DCT) cannot adequately represent daily intrafractional motion of abdominal tumors. Int J Radiat Oncol Biol Phys. 2013;85(4):999–1005.
26. Rankine L, Wan H, Parikh P, et al. Cone-beam computed tomography internal motion tracking should be used to validate 4-dimensional computed tomography for abdominal radiation therapy patients. Int J Radiat Oncol Biol Phys. 2016;95(2):818–26.
27. Kutcher GJ, Coia L, Gillin M, et al. Comprehensive Qa for radiation oncology: report of AAPM radiation therapy committee task group 40. Med Phys. 1994;21(4):581–618.
28. Klein EE, Hanley J, Bayouth J, et al. Task group 142 report: quality assurance of medical accelerators. Med Phys. 2009;36(9):4197–212.
29. Yin FF, Wong J, Balter J, et al. The role of in-room kV X-ray imaging for patient setup and target localization: report of AAPM task group 104. AAPM Rep. 2009:62.
30. Bissonnette JP, Balter PA, Dong L, et al. Quality assurance for image-guided radiation therapy utilizing CT-based technologies: a report of the AAPM TG-179. Med Phys. 2012;39(4):1946–63.
31. Willoughby T, Lehmann J, Bencomo JA, et al. Quality assurance for nonradiographic radiotherapy localization and positioning systems: report of task group 147. Med Phys. 2012;39(4):1728–47.
32. Dieterich S, Cavedon C, Chuang CF, et al. Report of AAPM TG 135: quality assurance for robotic radiosurgery. Med Phys. 2011;38(6):2914–36.
33. Solberg TD, Balter JM, Benedict SH, et al. Quality and safety considerations in stereotactic radiosurgery and stereotactic body radiation therapy: executive summary. Pract Radiat Oncol. 2012;2(1):2–9.
34. Lutz W, Winston KR, Maleki N. A system for stereotactic radiosurgery with a linear accelerator. Int J Radiat Oncol Biol Phys. 1988;14(2):373–81.
35. Das IJ, Cheng CW, Watts RJ, et al. Accelerator beam data commissioning equipment and procedures: report of the TG-106 of the therapy physics committee of the AAPM. Med Phys. 2008;35(9):4186–215.
36. Ibbott GS. QA in radiation therapy: the RPC perspective. J Phys Conf Ser. 2010;250:1–7.

Chapter 4
Treatment Planning for Hypofractionated RT and SRS/SBRT

Kenny Guida, Dima Soultan, and Harold Li

4.1 Introduction

Treatment planning for SRS and SBRT relies on designing a highly precise plan that delivers a large, concentrated dose of radiation to the intended target in a single treatment, or over the course of a few treatments, while ensuring optimal sparing of surrounding organs at risk (OARs). While similar to conventional planning in many aspects, the stakes are much higher in hypofractionation; higher daily doses, smaller margins, and exponential increase of the potential toxicity for nearby organs pose serious challenges. When planning these difficult scenarios, the Radiation Oncology team investigates all the potential options to ensure the best possible outcome for the patient.

This chapter serves as a comprehensive guide for SRS, SBRT, and hypofractionated treatment planning for various disease sites. The process of treatment planning, from simulation and image registration, through contouring and beam selection, and finally culminating in dose calculation and plan analysis, will be explored in this chapter. Treatment modalities and techniques will be explored for different body sites, including brain, spine, thorax, abdomen, and pelvis, giving the reader insight on planning strategies.

K. Guida (✉) · D. Soultan · H. Li
Department of Radiation Oncology, University of Kansas Medical Center, Kansas City, KS, USA
e-mail: kguida@kumc.edu; dsoultan@kumc.edu; hli5@kumc.edu

O. Kaidar-Person, R. Chen (eds.), *Hypofractionated and Stereotactic Radiation Therapy*, https://doi.org/10.1007/978-3-031-47701-0_4

4.2 Simulation and Image Registration

4.2.1 Imaging and Simulation

- For most SRS and SBRT plans, CT is the primary imaging modality for dose calculation. With many planning systems relying on HU values and electron density for dose calculations, CT data sets are crucial in the treatment planning process [1].
- MRI is the gold standard for delineating lesions within the brain. Over the last two decades, MRI has proven useful in visualizing extracranial disease as well, as many employ this modality to identify lesions within the prostate, spine, and abdomen.
- PET imaging, with the use of ^{18}F-Fluorodeocyglucose (FDG), has been utilized for cancer staging and identifying sites of disease. Due to limitations of spatial resolution, PET typically is not as useful as CT and MRI in stereotactic planning. Trimodality planning using PET/MRI and CT is currently evaluated in clinical practice.
- In treatment simulation, the patient should be immobilized in a reproducible manner over the entire treatment course.
  - Immobilization techniques should be developed at Radiation Oncology centers for each body site treated via stereotactic radiotherapy, as each site may necessitate a different setup.
  - For example, cranial cases generally require immobilization via head frames or thermoplastic masks. New methods using frameless/open masks and SGRT are currently available for cranial RT, whereas SBRT cases may need some combination of stereotactic cradle and breathing motion management devices [2].
- CT simulation scans should envelop the tumor site and extend at least 5–10 cm in the superior and inferior directions. If non-coplanar beams are to be used, scans should be lengthened in both superior and inferior directions by an additional 5 cm to adequately capture the patient anatomy for planning and dose calculation purposes.
  - Typically, for SRS, the entire head is scanned for treatment planning purposes, while a lung SBRT plan will generally require the entirety of the lungs to be scanned, for calculation and dose tracking purposes.
- Treatment simulation scans should not truncate portions of the patient. Scans should capture sufficient patient data superiorly and inferiorly of the target.
  - Wide bore scanners and extended field of view mode help ensure capturing the entire width of the patient by the CT scan.
  - Since noncoplanar beams are needed for many of these treatments, sufficient scan data around the target is needed to account for beam attenuation in any direction.
- For SRS, CT slice thickness should be no more than 1.5 mm. For SBRT, CT slice thickness should be 1–3 mm [1].

- AAPM TG 76 put forth a process of implementing respiratory motion management (RMM) in the clinical setting.
  - If tumor motion exceeds 5 mm or if normal tissue could be significantly spared, the task group recommends using RMM techniques.
  - When using RMM techniques in the simulation process, it is important to review all scans and account for possible artifacts due to respiratory motion; there could be variations in the breathing cycle that could impact the generation of 4D CT images [3].

4.2.2 Image Registration

- Image registration is defined as the transformations performed on one or more image data sets with respect to a primary reference image in order to map identical anatomic points in the imaging studies into a Common Coordinate System (CCS), while fusion is combining the inputs of the registered imaging data sets in a single representation.
- Registration can be classified by the following criteria [4, 5]:
  - Dimensionality: spatial dimensions 2D/2D, 2D/3D, 3D/3D, and time series (4D).
  - Nature of registration basis:

    Extrinsic:

    (a) Invasive: stereotactic frame;

    (b) Non-invasive: frame, dental adapter, and skin markers.

    Intrinsic:

    (a) Geometry or feature-based metric using point or surface matching;

    (b) Intensity-based metric which exploits voxel data directly to extract similarity metrics. Common algorithms in clinical use are Sum of Squared Differences (SSD), Cross Correlation (CC), and Mutual Information (MI).
  - Nature of transformation:

    Geometric:

    (a) Rigid: rotation and translation transformations where every pixel-to-pixel relationship is unchanged by the transformation.

    (b) Affine: adds scaling, shearing, and plane reflection to rigid transformations.

    (c) Deformable: adds non-linear transformations such as shrinkage and stretching to the affine transformations, e.g., global spline-based or local spline-based methods.

    Physical: applies local Deformation Vector Fields (DVFs), such as viscous, elastic, and optical flow, or finite element analysis using biomechanical tissue properties.
  - Domain of transformation:

    Local

    Global

  - Interaction: user's manual adjustment must be limited to rigid registration:
    Interactive
    Semi-automatic
    Automatic
  - Optimization: to converge to an optimal solution:
    Gradient-based methods: parameters computed
    Stochastic-based methods: parameters searched for
- Image registration and fusion for SRS/SBRT involve registration between the same or multiple imaging modalities, e.g., CT-CT, MRI-CT, PET/CT-CT, CT Angio-CT, CBCT-CT, KV-CT, and MV-CT [6].
  - The spatial resolution of the anatomical imaging modalities (≤1 mm for CT and 1–2 mm for MRI) provides details about lesion site, size, morphology, and structural changes to bordering tissues. MRI has a superior contrast resolution; as a result, MRI enhances soft tissue visualization. The AAPM Task Group 101 considers MRI to be the gold standard for brain neoplasm in addition to the increased presence in SBRT for prostate, spinal, chest, and solid abdominal tumors [1].
  - Functional imaging modalities, such as SPECT and PET, display thc targeted molecular structure of the lesion via radio-labeled tracers, providing biological function information of the lesion and surrounding tissues [7]. Hybrid modalities, like PET/CT (as seen in Fig. 4.1), SPECT/CT, and PET/MRI, combine anatomical imaging with functional imaging, which integrate their

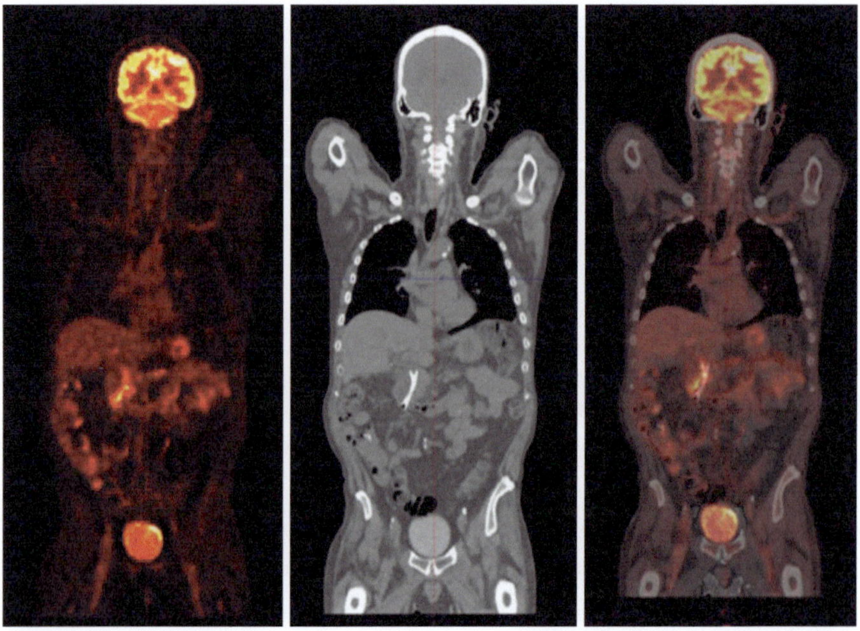

Fig. 4.1 Functional PET image and anatomical CT image registered and fused

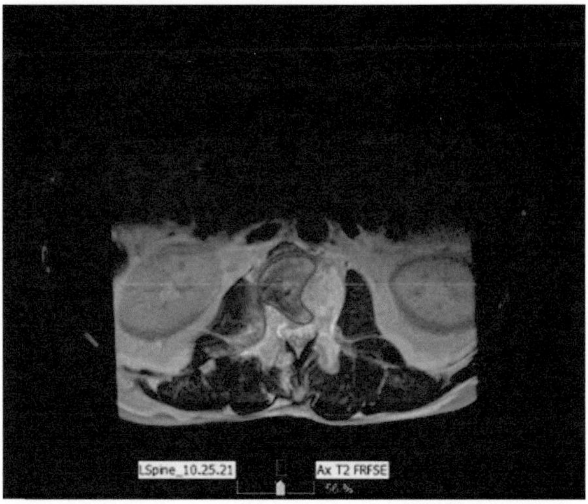

Fig. 4.2 An MRI is fused with a CT to delineate an L-spine spine lesion (red contour) during the SBRT planning process

individual strengths and provide the tumor's physiological and biological process on a detailed anatomical and structural visualization [8].

- Image registration and fusion are extensively utilized in SRS and SBRT.
  - Target volume and normal tissue segmentation for treatment planning may require registration and fusion to allow for mapping relevant information from one image set to the treatment planning CT, as seen in Fig. 4.2.
- Image registration plays an essential role in Adaptive Radiation Therapy, which provides clinicians the opportunity to improve clinical outcomes by refining the treatment plan throughout the course of treatment by accounting for treatment response and changes in anatomy [9].

  Deformable Image Registration (DIR) deforms the target and OAR volumes and then propagates the dose from the planning CT to recently obtained CT or in-room 3D imaging sets; estimates of dose accumulation and toxicity predictions can be performed after DIR.
- IGRT for target localization

  Registration between in-room and planning images reveals the possible physiological changes to the patient such as bladder filling, peristalsis, or weight loss, and determines the necessary translational and rotational shifts to match treatment planning CT; however, shifts are limited by the system capabilities. Six-degrees-of-freedom (6DOF) couches in modern LINACs account for pitch and roll rotational shifts in addition to the standard couch capabilities. 6DOF couches are becoming increasingly crucial for LINAC based SRS/SBRT.
- Evaluation of treatment response and follow-up

  Due to the complex and heterogeneous tumor and normal tissue response to radiation therapy, DIR and fusion of functional and anatomical images allow for both qualitative and quantitative assessment of the treatment response.

  Radiomics is based on extracting a sizable number of tumor features from multimodality images at different phases using data classification algorithms in order to uncover tumor characteristics and response patterns. DIR is crucial to the accuracy and integrity of the radiomics assessment, and thus the accuracy and integrity of the radiomics derived predictive models [10].

- Sources of errors and uncertainties in image registration:
  - Issues with registration inputs, such as image acquisition errors (incorrect scan parameters), image quality (noise), susceptibility to distortion and motion artifacts, or high-density artifacts (dental fillings), can lead to errors in image registration [5].

    Verifying geometric fidelity and creating scan protocols dedicated for radiation therapy application are advised.

    Oblique MRI scans suffer from rectangular voxel shapes; hence, these images require resampling which jeopardizes the geometric integrity. Axial 3D MRI acquisitions are advised for stereotactic applications.

    MRI's geometric fidelity is affected by water-fat shift of 0.5–1 mm, as displayed in Fig. 4.3 [11].

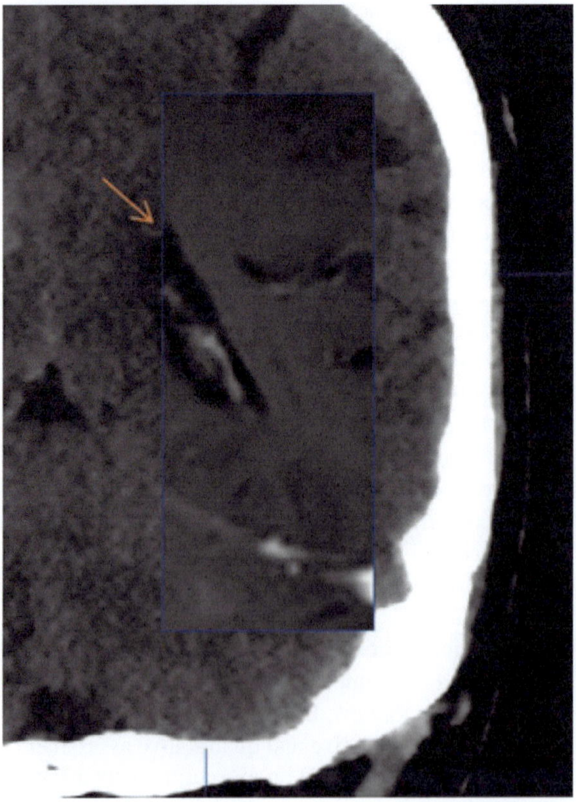

Fig. 4.3 The arrow (orange) points at a water-fat shift involving the ventricle in the MRI relative to the treatment planning CT, as seen through the spy glass

MRI distortion, which is more pronounced at the periphery, limits the registration accuracy. For stereotactic applications, geometrical distortion should be less than 1 mm.

Motion induces ghost artifacts in MRI where the same object appears to be repeated multiple times in the same image.

PET has an inherent lower spatial resolution of about 3 mm compared to CT and MRI.

PET/CT reduces registration and fusion uncertainties to less than 2 mm due to the combined PET-CT hardware and acquisition of both images during the same session.

Transmission CT that is used in attenuation correction for PET in PET/CT should be used to register with the planning CT.

- Algorithms using too few or too many degrees of freedom can result in larger numbers of errors than what the optimizer can mitigate. It is important for the user to understand the limitations of the registration algorithms and the goal of registration.
- Uncertainties greater than a voxel size should be accounted for by incorporating them in margin expansion.
- Caution should be exercised when applying a registration transformation result to a third image data set by understanding the properties of each image; for example, registration of PET/CT to CT-MRI results with PET-MRI registration. It is an indication of a misregistration if the FDG-avid areas from the PET image aligns to the bones on the MRI image.
- ASTRO and ACR recommend that IGRT image registration is approved by the clinician prior to SRS or SBRT treatment delivery [12].

• Registration Quality Assurance (QA):
  - Qualitative validation and verification of image registration accuracy are usually done by visual inspection using available tools such as split screen or spy glass at every step that involves registration. Important anatomical landmarks should be carefully checked for a match [5].

    Brain: orbits, optic nerves, ventricles, nose, external auditory canal (to correct for the roll), and clivus (to correct for yaw), and sagittal suture, as seen in Fig. 4.4.

    Neck: cervical spine that is one vertebral body above and one below the treatment site.

    Chest: T spine or L spine.

    Abdomen, liver, spleen, and kidney boundaries, and axial alignment of abdominal aorta.
  - Quantitative analysis of registration accuracy can be done by computing one of the following matrices

    Target Registration Error (TRE) $\leq$1 mm

    Mean Distance to Agreement (MDA) $\leq$1 mm

    Dice Similarity Coefficient (DSC): 0.8–0.9

    Jacobian determinant $\leq$1 mm

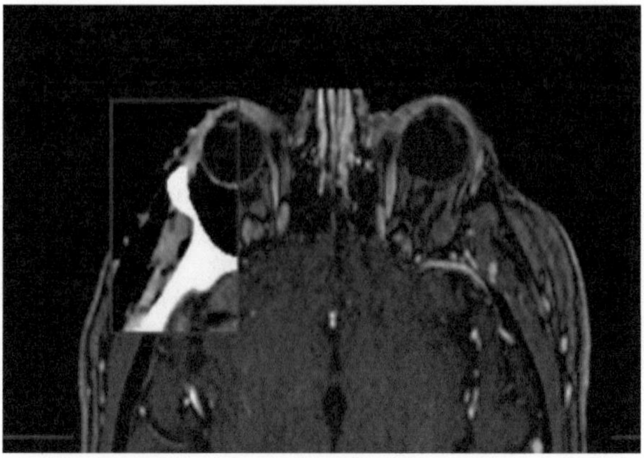

Fig. 4.4 A spy glass tool is used to check alignment of the right orbit between MRI and CT data sets to validate the image registration

Consistency should be less than 1 mm, which suggests the independence of the registration from the direction of the registration.

- Registration software commissioning and end-to-end testing
  - Most commercially available treatment planning software systems offer image registration solutions.
  - The AAPM Task Group 132 recommends performing end-to-end testing to image registration software annually, as well as after major upgrades and imager repair or replacement; physical or digital phantoms can aid in these quality assurance tasks [5].
  - A set of digital phantoms is supplied by ImSimQA software and DIR-Lab 4DCT with descriptions of each dataset and instructions for test type, tolerances, and registration uncertainty assessment level by rejection and acceptance criteria.
  - If the software algorithm does not meet commissioning tolerances, the projected uncertainties should be included in treatment protocols, and performance status of the algorithm should be communicated with the clinical team.

4.3 Contouring

- Contouring in modern treatment planning for SRS, SBRT, and hypofractionated treatments includes target volumes, organs at risk (OARs), planning organ at risk volumes (PRVs), and optimization structures to maximize target coverage.
- Image registration of planning images to imaging studies obtained from different imaging modalities, such as MRI, contrast CT, and PET/CT, is helpful in visualizing and delineating target structures and OARs that may not be apparent on treatment planning CT data sets.
- Like conventional planning, Gross Tumor (GTV), Clinical Target (CTV), Internal Target (ITV), and Planning Target (PTV) volumes are utilized in SRS and SBRT planning.

  - Target volumes, OARs, and PRVs should follow the concepts outlined by the ICRU 50 and 62 publications [13, 14].
- Internal Target Volumes, or ITVs, are contoured by the physician. The ITV accounts for a moving tumor's trajectory, which can be visualized on 4DCT data sets.
  - Obtaining ITVs from 4DCT data set is becoming the standard practice in modern radiation therapy. The PTV can be generated by adding margin to the ITV.
  - Maximum Intensity Projection (MIP) data sets should be used for contouring hyperdense tumors, in comparison to surrounding tissues (e.g., lung tumors). Figure 4.5 shows an average CT (left) vs a MIP; the ITV was contoured from the MIP scan and transferred to the average scan for planning and dose calculation.
  - Minimum Intensity Projection (minIP) data sets should be used for delineating hypodense tumors in comparison to surrounding tissues (e.g., liver lesions).
  - Extent of tumor motion should be measured throughout the breathing cycle.
    For cases with excursion above 5 mm, the use of VMAT should be cautioned due to the interplay effect.
    If excursion is above 1 cm, another method of breathing motion management should be investigated, as the ITV volume will have increased and thus normal tissue sparing will be compromised; gating, such as breath hold or amplitude-based techniques, should be investigated when tumor motion can compromise normal tissue sparing.
- In SRS treatment planning, the GTV equals the CTV [13, 14] and most cases are planned to the GTV rather than expanding to a PTV. Expanding the GTV by 1 mm to a PTV can ensure GTV coverage but will also increase normal brain dose, thereby increasing the risk of radionecrosis.
- For SBRT, margins are typically added to the GTV or ITV yielding a PTV. The PTV should account for geometric variations of the GTV location throughout the duration of the patient's treatment due to intrafraction tumor motion and delivery limitations.
- OAR structures are typically contoured by physicians or dosimetrists and are reviewed by the physician [13, 14]. Contouring of these structures is of paramount importance in treatment planning since the advent of inverse planning.
  - IMRT enables the user to set dose constraints to OARs to ensure clinical tolerances are met during the planning process.
  - For critical structures near a target, especially serial structures like the spinal cord, brainstem, and optics, it is important to generate a PRV by adding margin. Optimizing to the PRV can aid in bending the isodose curves away from a specific OAR, ensuring normal tissue tolerance is met.
- Optimization structures can be used to enhance the coverage of a PTV structure, increase conformity, and drive rapid dose falloff. Concentric rings have been used to drive conformity and generate steep dose gradients for SRS and SBRT cases [15].

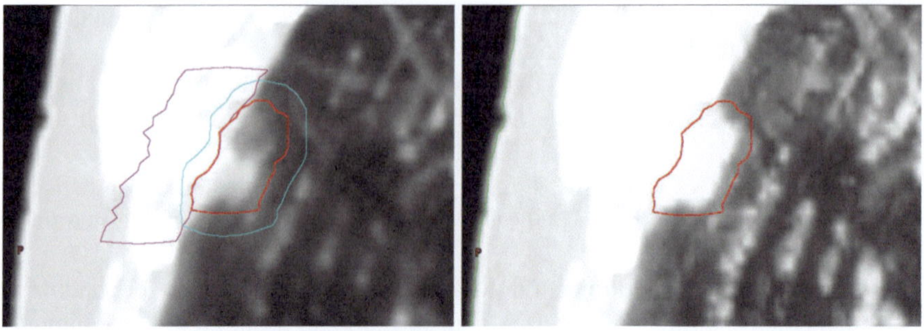

Fig. 4.5 A right lower lobe lesion is shown on both the average CT (left) and MIP CT. The MIP captures the trajectory of the tumor during the breathing cycle, allowing the radiation oncology team to generate a plan on a free breathing scan

  - Such structures can reduce the R50%, the ratio of the 50% isodose volume to the PTV volume. Ring structures are often used to measure dose falloff in SBRT cases. D_{2cm} was popularized by the RTOG 0813 and 0915 trials as a dose metric measuring the maximum isodose at 2 cm from the PTV structure [15].
- Support structures should be considered during the treatment planning and dose calculation processes. Structures that attenuate the beam should be included in dose calculations, including the treatment couch, mask, headrest, and immobilization devices. Neglecting attenuation by these structures could lead to surface dose calculations errors, resulting in skin dose underestimation.

4.4 Beam Energy

- For SRS and SBRT, lower beam energies are preferred since penumbra increases with increasing beam energy. Increased penumbra counteracts the generation of sharp dose falloff, which is crucial in SRS and SBRT cases.
  - 6 MV is widely available for linear accelerators and CyberKnife (Accuray, Madison, WI) units. GammaKnife (Elekta, Crawley, UK) utilizes Cobalt-60, which has an average energy of 1.25 MeV. 6–10 MV photon beams are often employed for SBRT cases, depending on location and tumor depth.
  - 6 MV beams should be used for most thoracic cases due to increased lateral scattering of higher energy beams.
  - 10 MV photon fields can be employed in pelvic or abdominal cases in an effort to reduce intermediate dose and achieve a high level of conformality.

Many linear accelerators have been equipped with Flattening Filter Free (FFF) Mode, which increases the dose rate and allows for sharper falloff due to the center-peaked nature of these beams.

- In SRS/SBRT dose prescription is defined at 50–90% IDL to achieve high dose gradient, eliminating the need for penumbra margins. SRS and SBRT isodose line prescriptions assume the acceptance of hotspots within the target volume.
  - Linac-based brain SRS and SRT prescriptions are typically specified at 80% IDL.
  - GammaKnife SRS treatments are specified at 50% IDL.
  - Spine, lung, and liver prescriptions are specified at 60–80% IDL.

4.5 Planning Modalities and Techniques

4.5.1 Photons

From dedicated radiosurgery units to linear accelerators, photon beams can provide precise beamlets of radiation to targets within the brain and body. Below, we cover different devices and techniques of employing photon beams to deliver hypofractionated doses of radiation.

- Cones:
  - Linear accelerators can deliver radiosurgery dose distributions akin to Gamma Knife by using cone-based techniques. SRS cones can be utilized in cranial cases for lesions smaller than 3 cm.
  - SRS cones come in a variety of sizes, ranging from 4 to 30 mm in diameter. SRS cones are mounted on an applicator that fits on the gantry head.
  - Field sizes should be fixed to vendor standards, to limit fluence through the applicator, usually no greater than 5 × 5 cm^2.
  - Visualizing the target in the BEV window during planning aids the planner to select the appropriate cone size. It is important to fit the target within the cone, and possibly via using multiple cone sizes; nevertheless, it is imperative to tailor the cone selection to create a sharp dose gradient reducing the volume of brain receiving high and intermediate dose; all attempts should be carefully made for each beam or arc to decrease margins between the target and the cone edges.
  - Cone-based SRS typically yields a spherical high dose region like GammaKnife, making it a perfect solution for small, spherical lesions in the brain.
- MLCs:
  - MLCs are often used for SRS and SBRT cases. Most linear accelerators generally come with standard MLCs with leaf widths of about 5–10 mm, while stereotactic linear accelerators employ high-definition MLCs (HD-MLCs) as small as 2.5 mm. Studies have shown that plans using high-definition MLCs achieved greater dose conformity for SRS cases [16]. HD-MLCs can be implemented for extracranial cases as well; improvements in PTV coverage and OAR sparing have been realized in these cases, especially those with irregular targets such as spine SBRT [17]. For SRS, SRT, and SBRT, HD-

MLC and standard MLC can be used for treating targets with the largest dimension greater than 1 cm.

For targets smaller than 1 cm, HD-MLC is superior in terms of conformity. For irregular lesions, HD-MLC plans can generate more conformal plans than standard MLC plans [18].

- Upgrading from standard MLCs to HD-MLCs has shown slight improvements in SBRT treatments, with minor reduction in spinal cord dose for spine SBRT treatments at the expense of plan complexity [19].

- Static fields:
  - Despite being the most basic linear accelerator-based treatment option, static field delivery is a viable option for SRS, SBRT, and hypofractionated treatments. From APBI to SRS, static field delivery can be utilized to adequately cover the PTV while creating sharp gradients to spare nearby normal tissue.

    Field-in-field planning can help increase the homogeneity within the PTV if desired.

    Static fields can also be added to arcs to create a hybrid plan; static fields can be used in this case to enhance PTV coverage and steer isodose lines away from OARs in order to meet normal tissue tolerances.
- Conformal Arcs:
  - Conformal arcs can be employed to deliver a highly conformal dose distribution with sharp falloff. This conformity is achieved by continuously refitting the MLCs to target, i.e., MLC shape matches the beam's eye view of the target along the entire arc trajectory.
  - Conformal arcs can be employed in cranial and extracranial cases and for a variety of target shapes and sizes; however, concave shapes are better suited for IMRT and VMAT.
  - One caveat in utilizing conformal arc therapy for moving targets is the interplay effect. Conformal arcs avoid the interplay effect, whereas modulated techniques have more dose delivery uncertainty for lung and abdominal lesions. Figure 4.6 shows an SBRT lung plan with conformal arcs (left) and VMAT (right). The VMAT plan blocks the PTV and ITV during the delivery, whereas the MLCs will hug the PTV throughout the delivery, reducing any chance of blocking the tumor during delivery.
- IMRT
  - IMRT can be employed for any shape target; however it excels in treating irregular targets. Using multiple beam arrangements can be helpful for cranial and extracranial cases to attain high dose conformity and OAR sparing.
  - Beams should be spaced apart enough to spread the low dose around the surrounding tissue and reduce streaks of high dose outside the target. Static IMRT fields can be generated to avoid entering or exiting certain regions; for example, avoiding entrance through the contralateral lung in lung cases should be a priority.

    For cases that require the reduction of low dose spray, such as retreatment or patients with implantable electronic devices such as pacemakers and defibrillators, IMRT provides a better solution than VMAT.

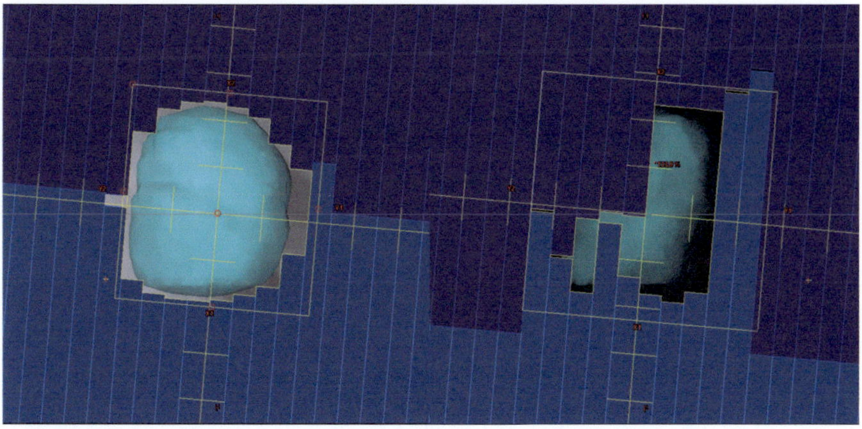

Fig. 4.6 Conformal (left) and VMAT SBRT lung plans, showcasing the possibility of interplay effect due to MLCs blocking the PTV during VMAT delivery

- VMAT
  - VMAT can be used for cranial and extracranial stereotactic treatments and is considered a potent technique combining arc delivery and inverse optimization.
  - VMAT can achieve a highly conformal dose distribution with steep gradient, as MLCs constantly move to modulate the dose distribution for complex targets.

    Because of the dynamic nature of the MLCs, tumor motion within the field could cause discrepancies between predicted and delivered dose.
  - VMAT can be used for a multitude of target shapes and sizes. Whereas conformal arc therapy is ideal for round targets, VMAT can conquer even the most complex shapes, including spinal lesions.
  - VMAT tends to spray low dose around the patient along the arc direction; organs at risk on the level of the target volumes will tend to have higher volumes of low dose with VMAT as compared to IMRT. However, VMAT reduces skin dose at entry points more effectively than static field delivery methods.

    Arc creation techniques and avoidance sectors can help prevent entrance dose in designated portions of the patient, helping to further shape the dose distribution.
  - Simultaneous-integrated boost (SIB) is feasible with VMAT; when some hypofractionation treatments necessitate multiple prescription dose levels, like SRS for multiple brain metastases and prostate SBRT with urethra sparing, VMAT is an ideal solution.

    At our institution, an SIB optimization is often utilized in SBRT lung planning; lower limits of 110–120% of the PTV prescription are placed on the ITV to generate a hotspot within the tumor and sharp falloff outside the target volumes.

- Grid and Lattice Therapy:
  - Studies have shown that SBRT for large lesions (greater than 5 cm) have caused unacceptable toxicities in patients. GRID therapy has successfully been used for large sarcomas, where creating high-dose peaks and low-dose valleys within the target has yielded excellent local control while maintaining low toxicity.
  - GRID therapy utilizes a fabricated block made of high Z material with holes spaced throughout.
    A single field is typically utilized in 2D GRID therapy [20].
  - Tumors deeper than 8 cm may necessitate the switch from a 2D GRID plan to Tomotherapy or VMAT-based GRID techniques.
  - Spatially Fractionated Radiation Therapy (SFRT) is a 3D technique that creates a lattice of small, high dose islands of dose within a lower prescription isodose line and can be used to treat lesions too deep for standard GRID Therapy.
    SFRT can be delivered via VMAT; planning requires contouring SIB spheres within the tumor volume to create the lattice of high dose.
    SFRT can be used to treat large, radioresistant diseases that traditionally would not be considered for SBRT [21].

4.5.2 Protons

The proton therapy market is projected to grow worldwide and the use of proton beams in SRS and SBRT is expected to continue gaining more steam.

- Proton SBRT has been used to treat lung, liver, kidney, prostate, and head and neck cancers at various centers.
- Proton beams exhibit sharp dose falloff beyond the Bragg Peak, allowing for increased OAR sparing beyond the treated volume.
- Compared to photon planning and the use of PTVs to enhance plan robustness to the GTV or ITV, proton planning typically does not rely on PTV structures. Conventional margins used in photon planning can be ineffective in proton planning.
  - Some commercial planning systems, like RayStation (RaySearch Laboratories, Stockholm, Sweden), employ a robust optimization mechanism to ensure adequate dose is delivered by each field, taking uncertainties in tissue density, range, organ motion, and patient setup into account [22].
- Proton treatments can reduce the dose to nearby OARs more effectively than photon plans for many cases.
  - For lung SBRT, proton therapy shows lower OAR dose compared to photon VMAT and CyberKnife [22].

- New technology, such as FLASH Proton Therapy, could reduce treatment time to a few seconds per beam, making proton therapy a useful tool in treating targets with motion.

4.6 Inverse Planning

- In inverse planning, the dose distribution is obtained by finding a global optimal solution and then translating the reached numerical solution into deliverable intensity patterns, where the objective cost function is the mathematical formalism of the clinical requirements. Objective cost functions can be dose based, dose-volume based, or dose-response based. The cost (score) is the numeric value returned by the objective function. The cost quantifies the treatment plan quality and indicates the need to re-run the optimization until the clinical objectives are met.
- Optimization techniques of inverse planning are mainly categorized into the following [23–25]:
  - Deterministic methods: Linear, Non-linear programming, and Iterative methods.

    Iterative methods start with an initially estimated solution that converges through a multi-layered approach that leverages optimization efficiency, adequacy, and speed to reach an optimal solution.

    - Gradient Search algorithms are based on a multi-variable, differentiable, and convex function. When the function descends in the negative gradient direction, it reaches a global minimum.
      - A known limitation of gradient search algorithms is reaching multiple local minima, which can act as a false solution.
      - Eclipse Treatment Planning Software's (Varian, Palo Alto, CA) PO, DVO, and PRO optimizers are examples of commercially available gradient search algorithms.
    - Filtered back projection algorithms (akin to those used in image reconstruction) have been proposed for its simplicity and straightforwardness.
  - Stochastic methods: the change of the objective cost function's score is controlled by a probability function:
    (a) If $\Delta C_n < 0$, where C_n is the cost function value at the nth iteration, then change of variables is accepted.
    (b) If $\Delta C_n > 0$, the change is accepted with an acceptance probability.
    (c) The acceptance probability decreases exponentially as the optimization proceeds, driving the system to an optimal global solution.

      Simulated Annealing (SA) is the most widely used stochastic algorithm. SA simulates the cooling process of heated metal where the atoms attempt to place themselves in global energy minimum of a perfect lattice.

- Pareto Optimization
  - Long used by engineers and economists to obtain balanced, optimal solutions, Pareto Optimization has found its way into Radiation Oncology over recent years, as Multi-Criteria Optimization (MCO) has been implemented by several vendors.
  - Pareto Optimality is a state for an allocation of resources in which it is impossible to make any one individual resource better without making at least another individual worse. Planners using MCO can make tradeoffs within a set, rather than considering the full range of each parameter.
  - MCO requires the creation of a large database of plans based on a set of planning goals. From this database, optimal solutions along the Pareto front are identified and the user can balance planning goals to yield a desired solution.
  - MCO allows better selection of treatment plans and reduces the duration and number of iterations to achieve a quality plan using forward and other inverse optimization methods [26].
  - Several Treatment Planning Systems, such as RayStation and Eclipse, have made MCO available.

    At our institution, the use of MCO has been examined. Physicians have increased input in dosimetric trade offs during the planning process, as the relationship between two objectives is more visible due to sliders associated with these optimizers. Moving a slider to improve one objective will worsen another objective to some degree, and a DVH calculation can quantify these changes in real time.
- Knowledge-Based Planning
  - Knowledge-Based Planning (KBP) is an automated process that relies on a model formed from similar, previously devised treatment plans. KBP can generate high quality IMRT or VMAT plans for various disease sites. Varian RapidPlan and RayStation Machine Learning are two examples of commercial KBP platforms.
  - To build a model, high quality plans are identified for the training set; previously treated patients in concordance with certain protocols or with in-house standards are often utilized in building successful models.

    Data are extracted from a planning set, including prescription dose levels, structure dose volume histograms, PTV and OAR volumes, and structure overlap.

    Principal component analysis is employed to build a DVH estimation model and help identify potential outliers within the group.

    Dosimetric and geometrical outliers may degrade the model and users will have to navigate these outliers during model generation.

    Once completed, models are tested amongst a verification cohort prior to clinical implementation.
  - KBP models can be used to predict DVH data for OARs based on anatomy, prescription dose, and beam geometry. Line optimization can be used to pull the OAR dose closer to the lower limit of these predictions. In Fig. 4.7, a prostate SBRT case is optimized using RapidPlan; the model provides predic-

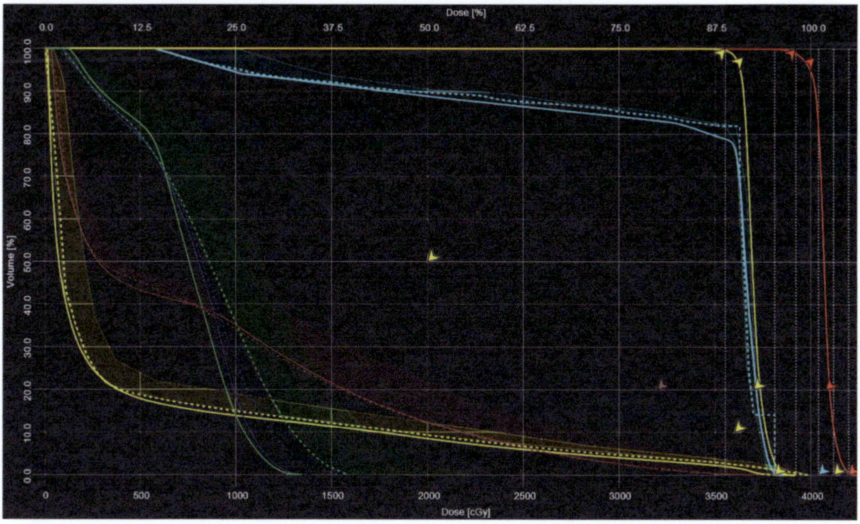

Fig. 4.7 A prostate SBRT is optimized using RapidPlan. Bladder (yellow), rectum (brown), urethra (cyan), and femoral heads (dark green and navy) are optimized with clinical constraints (arrows) and line objectives, with model predictions in the shaded regions. The predictions help planners assess what is possible during the optimization, allowing for improvements to OARs

tions for the rectum, bladder, femoral heads, and urethra, helping the user reduce dose to these OARs and meet clinical tolerances.

- Studies have shown that KBP reduces planning time and standardizes the quality of treatment plans across a cohort [27]. KBP models can also help inexperienced planners attain clinically feasible plans for difficult cases, such as SBRT Spine [28].
- KBP models have been created for SRS and SRT cases for single and multiple lesions, as well as SBRT cases for various extracranial sites.

  Publications have shown KBP models' capability of generating clinically viable plans for difficult cases, such as multi-lesion SRS, liver, lung, and spine SBRT [27–30].
- At our institution, models have been developed for SRT and lung, prostate, and spine SBRT. These models have enhanced our treatment planning, conformity, and dose reduction, especially intermediate dose, to nearby OARs.

  KBP models provide a blueprint for planners, viewing OAR dose predictions early in the optimization process, hence allowing users to push objectives accordingly in order to produce ideal plans in a short amount of time.

4.7 Dose Calculation

- Convolution-Superposition, Linear Boltzmann Transport Equation Solver, and Monte Carlo are the favorable dose calculations algorithms for stereotactic and hypofractionated planning.

- Monte Carlo has been established as the Gold Standard of treatment plan dose calculations and is available on several commercial platforms.
- Convolution-Superposition algorithms like Varian's Analytical Anisotropic Algorithm (AAA) and Pinnacle's Collapsed Cone Convolution have been utilized successfully in the clinical setting for over a decade.
- Linear Boltzmann Transport Equation Solvers, like Acuros XB, have seen increased clinical use over the last decade. The deterministic approach used by this algorithm achieves results similar to Monte Carlo while greatly improving calculation time for VMAT plans over AAA.

  Acuros XB calculations tend to be more accurate than AAA in heterogeneous media, especially in air cavities, making this algorithm essential for SBRT Lung planning [31]. Acuros XB can perform dose calculations to medium or water, depending on clinical preference.

- AAPM TG 101 recommends an isotropic calculation grid size of 2 mm or finer for stereotactic treatment planning [1].

4.8 Plan Analysis

- Stereotactic protocols specify a PTV $D_{95\%}$ of 100%, with the entire GTV receiving the prescription dose. Depending on the case, reducing the coverage may be acceptable in order to meet clinical tolerances for normal tissue; however, all avenues should be explored in order to prevent cold spots within the GTV and PTV if possible.
- CI100 is the conformity index defined as the ratio of the prescription isodose volume (PIV) to the volume of the PTV. CI100 measures how closely the prescription isodose line conforms to the target.
  - For SRS and SBRT, the ideal CI100 is unity; clinically, CI100 values should at least fall within 1.2–1.5.
  - For lesions over 0.7 cc in volume, values over 1.5 indicate non-conformality, resulting in the surrounding normal tissues receiving an unnecessary amount of the prescribed dose.
  - CI100 values up to 2.0 may be acceptable for lesions smaller than 0.7 cc, especially if planned with MLCs.
- HI is the Homogeneity Index proposed by RTOG to assess the homogeneity of the dose distribution within the target volume. HI is defined in the most used formula in the literature as $(D_{2\%} - D_{98\%})/D_p \times 100$, where $D_{2\%}$ is the minimum dose to 2% of the target, representing "maximum dose;" $D_{98\%}$ is the minimum dose to 98% of the target, representing the "minimum dose;" and D_p is the prescription dose [32].
  - SRS and SBRT planning should not pursue homogeneous target dose coverage in most cases. Hotspots within the PTV are desirable and allow delivering higher doses to radioresistant hypoxic sub-volumes of the PTV.

- R50% is a metric that measures the intermediate dose spill. R50% is the ratio of volume receiving 50% of the prescribed dose to the volume of the PTV. RTOG 0813 and RTOG 0915 popularized this metric and provided a table on ideal and acceptable R50% values based on PTV volume for Lung SBRT. Even though steep dose fall off is more difficult to achieve for larger lesions, R50% tends to decrease with increasing PTV volume. When planning SRS and SRT cases, the 50% isodose line should be nearly isotropic around the target [15].
- Gradient index (GI) is a metric resembling R50% in that it evaluates intermediate dose fall off outside the target. GI, which is typically used in SRS, is defined as the ratio of the volume receiving 50% of the prescribed dose to the PIV volume. GI is a complementary metric to CI100 in analyzing radiosurgery plans and can be a predictive tool of brain radionecrosis [33].
- Gradient measure (GM) is a metric used to assess the high dose fall off. GM is defined as the difference in centimeters between the equivalent spheres' radii of the 50% and 100% of prescription isodose volumes. Published literature identified the dependence of clinically achievable GM on PTV size, especially in Lung SBRT [33].
- D_{2cm} is the maximum dose at 2 cm from the PTV. This metric was included in RTOG 0813 and 0915 to assess Lung SBRT plans. These two protocols included a table dictating ideal and acceptable values for D_{2cm} based on PTV volume [15]. The greater the PTV volume, the higher the allowed dose is at 2 cm away from the PTV. To determine the D_{2cm}, a ring structure at 2 cm from the PTV is created. This structure can also aid in plan optimization to drive down the intermediate dose and create a sharper gradient, as seen in Fig. 4.8.

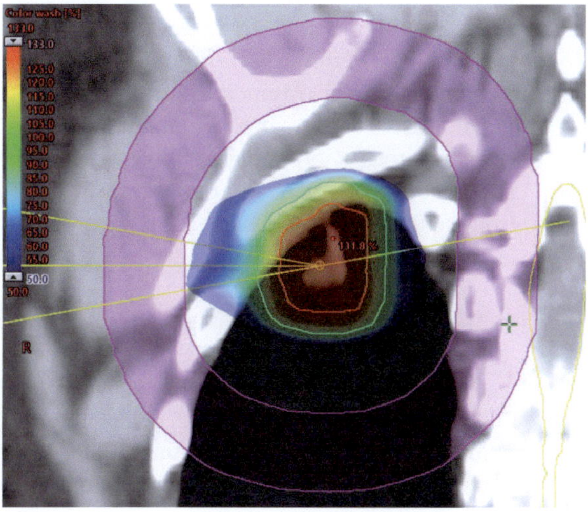

Fig. 4.8 The D_{2cm} ring (pink) can be used to measure the maximum dose at 2 cm away from the PTV and drive dose falloff in the optimization process. Using non-coplanar arcs can help spread out low and intermediate doses and help create sharper dose falloff, as the 50% isoshade does not touch the ring structure seen above

4.9 Treatment Planning Strategies Per Body Site

4.9.1 Brain

- SRS and SRT can be delivered using Linear Accelerators by using multiple fixed beams or arcs. SRS treatments, in particular, are often delivered with multiple coplanar and non-coplanar static fields and arcs in order to achieve a highly conformal dose distribution.
- Cranial treatments generally have greater clearance than extracranial treatments, allowing for a greater range of couch and gantry angles.
- The use of non-coplanar arrangements tends to increase target conformity, reduce integral dose, and improve R50%.
- When planning SRS and SRT, plans should use at least 350° arc degrees in total to spread out the low dose within the brain and reduce maximum entry dose at the skin level.
- Software has been developed to predict collisions and can be implemented into treatment planning to determine feasible isocenter placements and non-coplanar arrangements. The use of non-coplanar beams does increase the treatment duration. Dry runs should be performed for all SRS and SRT cases prior to treating the first fraction to ensure clearance.
- For lesions of diameter less than 2 cm, cones or high-definition MLCs are often needed to generate a steep dose gradient
  - Stereotactic cones are helpful in achieving high conformity for spherical lesions in the brain.
  - MLCs can achieve high levels of conformity for spherical and irregularly shaped tumors in both cranial and extracranial cases through conformal dynamic arcs delivery, static IMRT fields, and VMAT arcs. IMRT and VMAT are employed to generate conformal plans for larger lesions, especially in SRT and SBRT cases.
- Single Isocenter, Multiple Metastases
  - Elements (Brainlab, Munich, Germany) software is a proprietary Pi algorithm by BrainLab's SRS treatment planning platform. The software automates the planning process, grouping multiple brain metastases for a single isocenter and creating volumetrically optimized dynamic conformal arcs to treat each group to the prescribed dose.

    Elements can generate a single-fraction SRS or multi-fraction SRT plans for multiple brain lesions.

    The software platform can generate plans using up to five table positions and ten total arcs.

    During the optimization process, MLCs and collimator angles will be selected by the system to generate highly conformal apertures for the lesions within the selected group.

    For cases where the distribution of metastases is too widespread, multiple groups with separate isocenters may be necessary to maintain delivery precision, accuracy, and dose conformity, while reducing whole brain dose to within clinical tolerance [34].

- HyperArc is Varian's VMAT solution for SRS for single isocenter planning delivery of one or more brain metastases.
  - In addition to VMAT inverse planning feature, HyperArc automates isocenter placement, arc creation, and collimator angle selection.
  - HyperArc plans have four 180° arcs, with one coplanar arc and three non-coplanar arcs at couch kicks of 45°, 315°, and 270°.
  - SRS-NTO, which is the normal tissue optimizer for HyperArc SRS cases, generates sharper dose gradients than the original version, thus sparing greater volumes of normal brain receiving intermediate and low isodose levels.
  - The streamlined planning process reduces the planning time for difficult SRS cases, often yielding superior results to manual VMAT planning [35].
  - HyperArc integrates a virtual collision system into the treatment planning realm, allowing for planners to perform a dry run virtually to mitigate the chances of collision.
- Elements and HyperArc utilize jaw tracking to reduce low dose to surrounding normal tissue. The combination of these techniques helps reduce dose bridging between lesions, which is commonly seen in single isocenter plans for multiple lesions.
- A multi-institutional comparison study was performed analyzing plans for multiple brain metastases generated by VMAT, Varian HyperArc, BrainLab Elements, and GammaKnife.
  - For lesions less than 1 cm in diameter, GammaKnife plans achieved the best conformity and reduced whole brain dose better compared to the other modalities.
  - HyperArc compared favorably for small targets but excels at larger targets; for targets greater than 1 cm in diameter, HyperArc and manual VMAT achieved superior conformity while reducing treatment time as compared to GammaKnife [35].

4.9.2 *Head and Neck*

- For patients experiencing recurrent head and neck cancer, the options for further treatment include surgery and reirradiation.
  - Due to risks of fistula, carotid blowout, and ulceration, reirradiation poses serious risks. SBRT has been employed to target the recurrent tumor to deliver a high dose per fraction with a sharp gradient to minimize dose to the surrounding normal tissue.
  - One to five fractions of SBRT are prescribed to recurrent disease in the head and neck of the body.
- CT imaging is utilized for treatment planning and dose calculation; MRI imaging helps in identifying the extent of the recurrence.
  - Typically, SBRT plans for recurrent Head and Neck cancers will target the GTV.

   - Small margins of 2–3 mm have been used to reduce the risk of missing the target; nevertheless, caution should be exercised when the recurrence site borders a critical structure.
- The use of coplanar and non-coplanar beams is of a paramount importance in the cases of Head and Neck SBRT:
   - CyberKnife plans typically have 80–120 nodes, giving users the ability to target the lesion from many angles [36].
   - On linear accelerators, users can create IMRT plans with multiple coplanar and non-coplanar arrangements to avoid entry or exit dose through critical structures.

     A mix of coplanar and non-coplanar arcs could function like SRS, creating a sharp dose gradient beyond the lesion and spreading the low dose around the head and neck region. Figure 4.9 shows the use of IMRT in creating a highly conformal dose distribution for a recurrent head and neck lesion.
- Proton therapy poses an effective solution in treating head and neck cancer with SBRT. For primary and recurrent tumors near OARs, proton therapy can reduce dose to adjacent tissues allowing for target dose escalation.

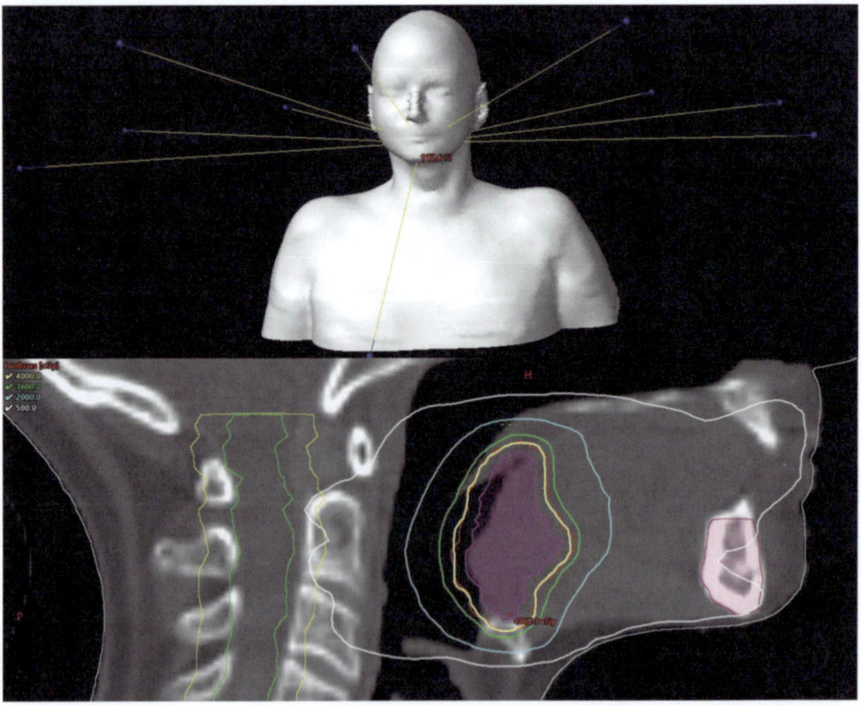

Fig. 4.9 (Top) A mix of coplanar and non-coplanar IMRT fields were utilized in retreating a recurrent floor of mouth lesion. The use of 6FFF and Jaw Tracking helped drive the high and intermediate dose conformity (bottom), sparing nearby mandible and the spinal cord

4.9.3 Lung

- Lung SBRT can be delivered by multiple treatment systems. MR-guided systems, CyberKnife, Linear Accelerators, Tomotherapy, and Proton units have all been utilized in Lung SBRT treatments.
- For LINACs, 3D planning technique utilizes 5–8 unique coplanar and non-coplanar beam arrangements that can deliver conformal plans with sharp dose gradients. MLCs are fitted to the PTV, minimizing the margin to create the sharp gradients needed to deliver SBRT.
  – Field-in-field techniques can be utilized for further dose shaping. It is important not to oppose 3D static fields, as this will increase the intermediate dose spray along the field direction.
- Conformal arcs are utilized on linear accelerators to spread entry dose around the patient.
  – A combination of static beams and conformal arcs can be used to enhance conformity for lung lesions.
- IMRT and VMAT can improve high dose conformity, reduce OAR dose, and generate an SIB.
  – IMRT plans, using 5–8 coplanar and non-coplanar beams, can deliver conformal plans.
  – VMAT plans utilizing multiple full or partial arcs deliver effective SBRT treatments, while reducing delivery times as compared to IMRT and 3D conformal plans.
  – VMAT plans typically use multiple partial arcs. Stylistically, arc lengths are selected to avoid entry through the contralateral (unaffected) lung.

    For cases involving lateral lesions, full arcs would present possibilities of gantry-patient collisions.

    Partial arcs with small table kicks of 5°–20° can be helpful in spreading the entry dose and increasing high dose conformity. Care should be taken when introducing non-coplanar field arrangements for extracranial SBRT cases.

    Short arcs (40°–60°) with table kicks of 90° can increase the dose delivered in the sagittal plane, thus reducing lateral dose spread. This technique can help reduce dose to nearby organs at risk, especially for medial lesions, as evidenced in Fig. 4.10.
- Recent studies have shown that in addition to PTV volume, dose heterogeneity and surface volume also play a role in R50%.
  – Heterogeneous plans with a higher HI value and mean dose tend to yield a lower R50% compared to homogenous plans.
  – Tumors that have a higher surface area will also exhibit higher R50% values than PTVs of the same volume that are more spherical in nature [37].
- Studies have shown that the use of FFF beams can provide similar target coverage to flattened beams, while displaying better dose conformity and reducing

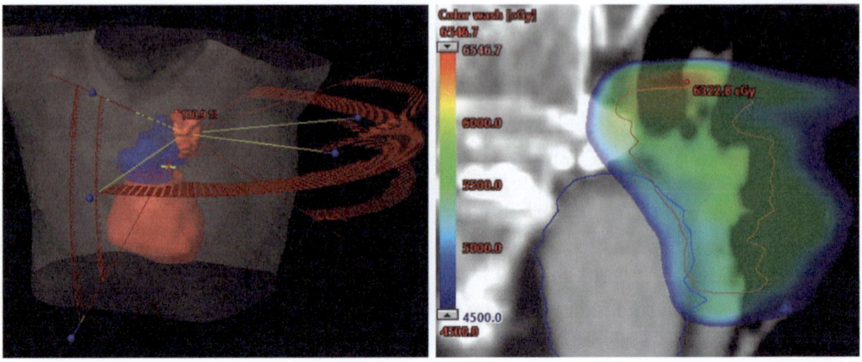

Fig. 4.10 The use of short arcs with 90° table kicks helped spread out dose along the sagittal direction (left) to reduce dose to the great vessels (blue contour, right) in this case. This technique can be applied to reduce dose to the spinal cord, esophagus, and major airways

intermediate dose spillage. 6FFF arcs also have shown the capability of reducing OAR dose, including nearby lung and chest wall [38].

- Jaw tracking is a feature enabled on most modern linear accelerators that reduces the field size to the largest MLC opening at any given time, reducing interleaf leakage, low and intermediate dose to surrounding tissues.
  - Jaw tracking has been successfully utilized in single-isocenter SBRT lung cases treating multiple lesions [39].
  - For small, single lesion cases, jaw tracking should be thoroughly investigated.
    If a plan is highly modulated, the jaws will reduce in size to match the field opening. If the MLC opening is very small, the field size will reduce as well, opening the risk of having field sizes smaller than data used to commission the linear accelerator.
    Care should be taken to ensure that no beamlets are smaller than the smallest field size in the TPS output factor tables.
- Proton therapy is suitable for lung SBRT as well. Tumors with largest dimension over 5 cm are often excluded from photon SBRT protocols due to the increase in intermediate and low dose spray; however, proton beams can reduce the dose to normal tissue for these cases.
  - Due to potential increased sparing of OARs posed by proton therapy, this modality could be used to maximize the dose to central lesions while minimizing toxicity to the esophagus, major airways, heart, and great vessels.
  - The Particle Therapy Co-operative Group (PTCOG) suggests that protons or carbon ions be utilized for large lesions (greater than 5 cm) and centrally located lesions, as protons can be stopped by soft tissue in the mediastinum; even patients with multiple or recurrent lesions could be ideal candidates for proton therapy [40, 41].

4.9.4 Breast

- Hypofractionation has become increasingly popular in breast cancer treatments. Accelerated Partial Breast Irradiation (APBI) has been treated via HDR brachytherapy and external beam treatments [42].
  - Per the B39/RTOG 0413 protocol, APBI can be delivered in ten fractions via external beam or HDR over the course of 5 days.
  - 3D conformal radiotherapy was typically utilized for the external beam option, while interstitial applicators such as Mammosite, Contura, or SAVI were allowed for HDR treatments.

    From our experience, SAVI provides the best quality treatment plans of the HDR applicators, as the catheters are closest to the lumpectomy cavity, thus providing the most conformal treatment.
- Another option to treat breast cancer via hypofractionation is Intraoperative Radiotherapy (IORT). At the time of surgery, a dose of about 20 Gy can be delivered to the lumpectomy cavity via low-energy X-ray units, such as the Zeiss Intrabeam (Carl Zeiss Surgical, Oberkochen, Germany) or Xoft Axxent (iCAD, Nashua, NH), or high energy electron beams. Pre-configured treatment plans can be loaded at the time of surgery based on tumor cavity size.
- Advances in treatment planning and delivery have enabled treating the tumor bed to higher doses in fewer fractions.
  - A study from Florence, Italy, utilized IMRT to deliver a conformal dose of 30 Gy in 5 fractions to the lumpectomy bed plus margin [43]. A mix of coplanar and non-coplanar IMRT beams can deliver a homogenous dose to the PTV while sparing the ipsilateral lung, heart, and contralateral breast and lung. Flash can be applied to the IMRT fields to ensure adequate coverage of shallow lesions.
  - Care should be taken when setting up fields; avoid exit dose through the heart and contralateral breast [44]. Figure 4.11 shows an IMRT setup for a breast lumpectomy cavity receiving 30 Gy in 5 fractions.
- CyberKnife has also been utilized for hypofractionated breast treatments. Multiple centers across the US have employed CyberKnife to deliver highly conformal dose to the lumpectomy bed while sparing nearby OARs.
  - Using the Synchrony Respiratory Tracking System, CyberKnife units can deliver APBI without breath hold or amplitude-based techniques. This proprietary gating system can help reduce heart and skin toxicity seen in some IMRT approaches [45, 46].
- IMRT does come with the inherent disadvantage of increased integral dose, as compared to brachytherapy and IORT. IMRT poses a greater secondary cancer risk compared to these other techniques [43].
- MR-IGRT has been explored over the last few years in treating breast cancer. Using MR-IGRT during treatments, it is possible to view the tumor cavity during treatment and use this system for gating and adaptive planning.

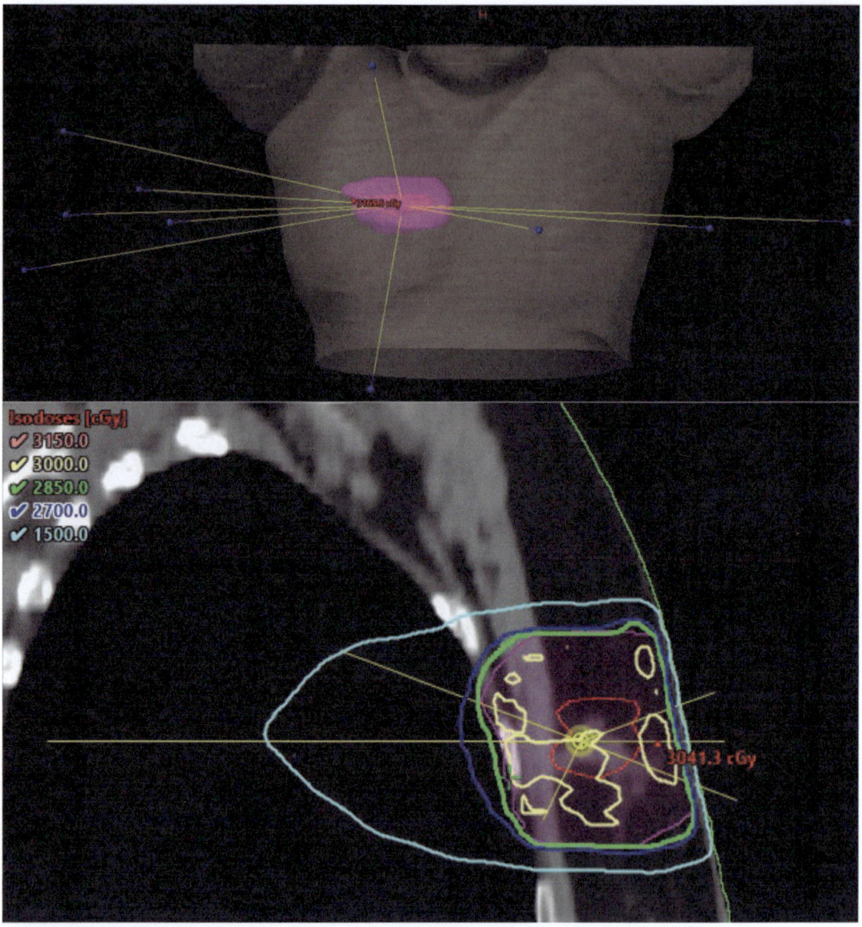

Fig. 4.11 A mix of coplanar and non-coplanar IMRT fields (top) can be used to treat the lumpectomy bed to 30 Gy, ensuring a highly conformal dose distribution with excellent coverage (bottom), per the Florence Protocol

- Studies have shown that mean cavity displacement during treatment was about 0.6 mm in the AP and SI directions [47]. Due to small cavity displacements and ability to perform MR cine imaging, it is possible to perform APBI as well as dose escalation treatments such as SBRT (Florence Trial) and Single-Fraction, High-Gradient Partial-Breast Irradiation (SFHGPBI).
- A recent phase 1/2 multi-institutional trial allowed for a single treatment, similar to single dose targeted intraoperative radiotherapy during lumpectomy (TARGIT) using external beam radiation.

  A dose of 15–22 Gy to the tumor bed, with a minimum dose of 5 Gy to a 1 cm expansion, is prescribed on the SFHGPBI trial. Both kV and MR-guided linear accelerators can be utilized for these treatments, granted the tumor bed can be visualized using these imaging techniques.

Utilizing beam geometry and IMRT, a high dose of at least 15 Gy is delivered to the lumpectomy bed for these cases. Using MR-IGRT for these cases allows for smaller PTV expansions than conventional radiotherapy, allowing for dose escalation and greater OAR dose reduction than previous APBI trials using 2–2.5 cm margins [48].

4.9.5 Abdomen

- Abdominal SBRT is achievable with 3D conformal radiation therapy, IMRT/VMAT, CyberKnife, and Tomotherapy. Studies have identified dosimetric discrepancies between the different techniques and modalities [49].
- Patients are simulated in the supine position with minor differences with respect to arms position between CyberKnife and Linacs [50].
  - Simulation utilizes different immobilization techniques and devices to mitigate respiratory induced motion, intra-fraction and inter-fraction motion, such as Vac-Lok cushions, thermoplastic body mask, and abdominal compression blocks.
  - MRI with contrast is the standard imaging modality for GTV delineation.
    - Image registration and fusion of MRI images to planning CT is recommended to focus on the lesion location due to diaphragm motion induced deformations.
  - 4DCT is the standard simulation approach to quantify tumor motion and determine the ITV [49].
    - Intravenous contrast is usually administered for better visualization and delineation of the tumor and OARs [51].
    - minIP CT aids with hypodense liver lesion excursion assessment and delineation.
    - Slice thickness is recommended to be 1 mm.
    - Average CT is used for treatment planning.
  - PTV margins are governed by the capability of tumor tracking via internal or external surrogate, and gating technology: free breathing, active breathing, or breathhold.
    - Residual uncertainties resulting from motion magnitude greater than 5 mm or suboptimal MRI fusion should be accounted for in the PTV margin expansion; typical PTV margins are 5–10 mm.
    - Due to larger respiratory induced motion magnitude in the sup-inf direction, the sup-inf PTV expansion can be greater by a few millimeters than radial PTV expansion to account for motion.
    - Fiducial markers can be implanted in the liver parenchyma within the tumor perimeter by Interventional Radiology at least a week before simulation [52].

  - Fiducial markers serve as internal landmarks for IGRT and tumor tracking.
  - Implanting fiducials supports reducing margins expansion, hence reducing radiation toxicity.
- Daily CBCT is the standard IGRT for abdominal SBRT cases.
- VMAT is preferred over other approaches. Usually, two to three partial arcs are used with the possibility of using avoidance sectors and ring optimization structures to avoid OARs and unjustified dose spillage, as seen in Fig. 4.12.

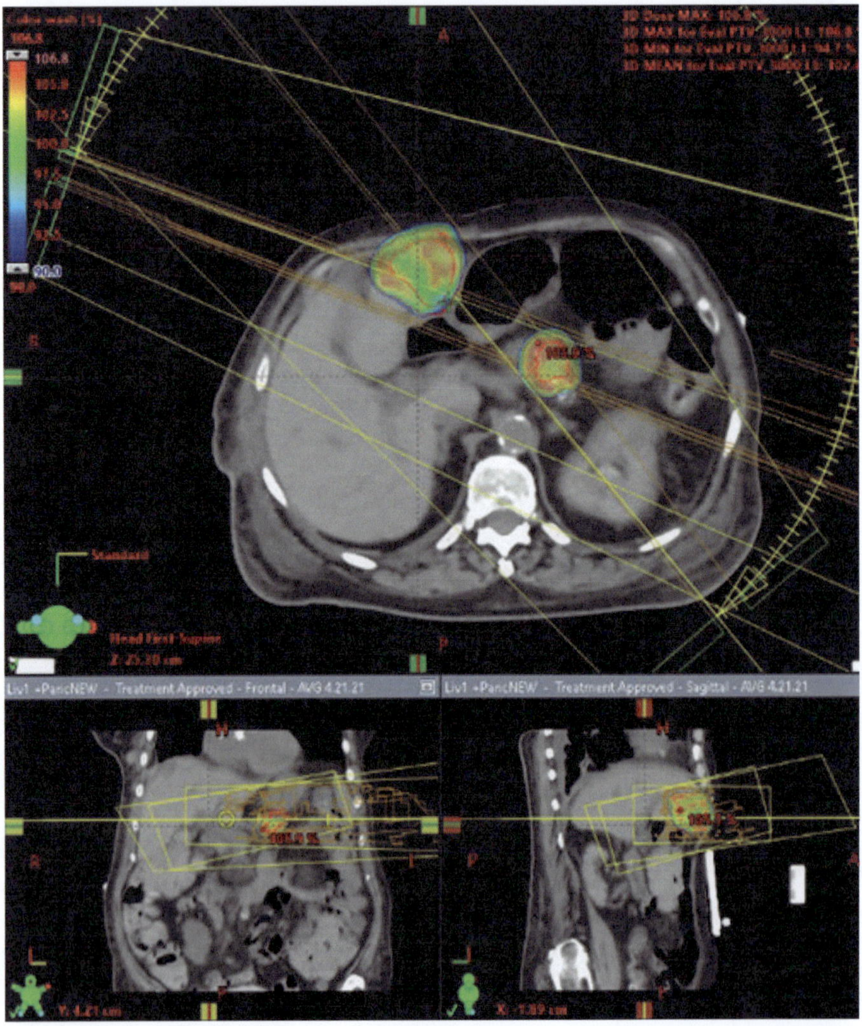

Fig. 4.12 Liver and pancreas SBRT 30 Gy in 3 fx treated simultaneously on Novalis TX, HD MLCs. The VMAT plan utilizes three partial arcs in this case. An abdominal compression plate was used for respiratory induced motion management

- FFF VMAT achieves significantly shorter beam on time, hence reducing adverse intrafraction motion effects, and allows for shorter overall treatment time and higher beam duty cycle if gating is utilized [50].
- One of the benefits of VMAT for liver SBRT is high conformity level and sharp dose falloff.

  Nearby OARs include the healthy liver (Liver-GTV), spinal cord, kidneys, stomach, duodenum, and small bowel [50, 51, 53].

  The ideal target coverage is $V_{100\%}$ of 95%; inverse planning optimization objectives are geared towards avoiding radiation induced liver disease (RILD) and other GI toxicities by meeting the dose constraints of the healthy liver and critical structures.
- Reducing PTV margins to decrease dose to healthy liver and/or OARs should be carefully assessed with respect to the immobilization and motion management techniques utilized.

• Stereotactic Magnetic Resonance-Guided Radiation Therapy (SMART) provides clinicians the ability to deliver high doses of radiation safely to pancreatic tumors [54].
  - Using MR-IGRT, adaptive planning can be utilized in the clinical setting for abdominal lesions.
  - Studies have shown that using MR-guidance can improve visualization and delineation of surrounding OARs within the abdomen, allowing for the target dose-escalation and sparing of nearby critical structures. Tumors in the head of the pancreas often border the duodenum, one of the critical OARs for these treatments. Because of proximity of the duodenum, clinicians are often limited in dose prescriptions when relying on kV imaging for image guidance [55].

4.9.6 *Prostate*

• Prostate SBRT can be delivered via CyberKnife or IMRT/VMAT, which has seen increasing use over the last decade. Most of the long-term patient data have been captured from CyberKnife centers
  - Treatment plans are typically performed using a CT data set. MRI sequences can be registered to planning CT enabling the physician to delineate the prostate gland from normal tissue.
  - Typical prostate SBRT margins are 5 mm in all directions, except posteriorly, where a 3 mm margin should suffice to reduce rectal dose.
  - Rectal spacers, can be utilized to reduce rectal toxicity.

    Endorectal balloons can spread the posterior wall of the rectum further from the PTV volume, whereas hydrogel such as SpaceOAR (Augmenix, Inc, Watertown, MA) can push a segment of the organ further from the PTV.

    Endorectal balloons need to be placed for each treatment, whereas SpaceOAR will remain in place for up to 6 months post-injection.

    SpaceOAR can be visualized on MRI and CT and can be contoured for visualization of the target and nearby OARs.

  - The urethra can be contoured from CT data sets; this organ can be visualized if a catheter is placed prior to simulation. To reduce urethra dose, a 1–2 mm PRV expansion can be made.

    A more heterogeneous dose distribution within the PTV can help spare the urethra [56]. Optimizing to the PRV should force hot spots away from the urethra, similar to the modified-peripheral approach in prostate brachytherapy. The figure below (Fig. 4.13) shows a sagittal view of current SBRT prostate planning; SpaceOAR creates separation between the rectum and prostate to reduce toxicity, an SIB of 40 Gy is delivered to high risk regions, and a urethra PRV is used in optimization to reduce urethra dose to about 38 Gy.

- Fiducials are often implanted within the prostate for match-and-review during setup, or fiducial tracking at the treatment unit. To assist with this process, these fiducials should be contoured.
  - If using Calypso to track the prostate in real time, each beacon should be contoured and reference points need to be placed to locate each beacon for treatment.
- CyberKnife treatments consist of about 100–120 nodes and treatments are delivered in about 40 min. Because CyberKnife plans do not typically enter through the posterior, bladder dose tends to be higher than plans delivered via linear accelerator [57].
- VMAT can be delivered by linear accelerators or Tomotherapy units. VMAT techniques tend to produce more homogenous dose distributions within the PTV than CyberKnife [58]. VMAT can also allow for dose painting techniques; simul-

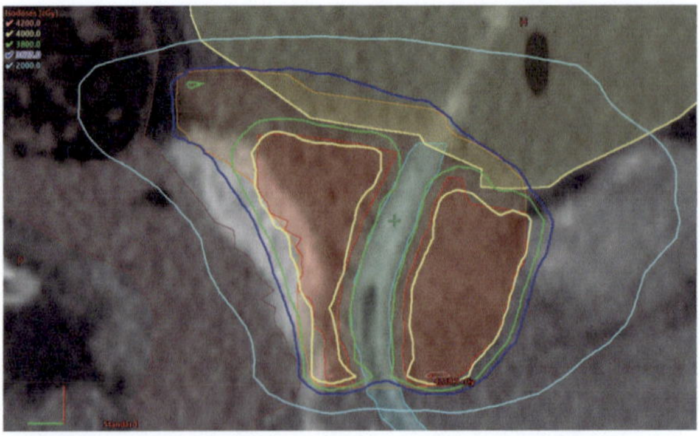

Fig. 4.13 Prostate SBRT is planned with VMAT to deliver 36 Gy to the whole gland (orange) plus 40 Gy to high-risk regions (red) of the prostate, while meeting bladder, rectum, and urethra tolerances

taneous-integrated boost of intraprostatic lesions and urethra sparing can be achieved with this technique.
  - At our institution, a typical prostate SBRT will be delivered in five fractions with VMAT. Our plans strive to deliver a homogenous dose within the prostate PTV for patients receiving 3625 cGy over five treatments; however, for plans with PTVs receiving simultaneous-integrated boosts to 4000 cGy, a urethra PRV will be used in the optimization to reduce the urethra dose to clinical tolerance.
- Studies have shown that, while CyberKnife and IMRT-based techniques achieve similar dosimetric outcomes, IMRT and VMAT plans are able to reduce the Rectal *V*50% and *V*90% greater than CyberKnife plans. IMRT and VMAT typically reduce the amount of intermediate to high dose to the rectum and bladder [59].

4.9.7 Spine

The spinal cord is a serial organ; when planning for spine SBRT cases, extreme caution should be taken in reducing the maximum dose to the spinal cord. D_{max} as well as the $D_{0.35cc}$ and $D_{1.2cc}$, are dosimetric constraints often employed when analyzing spine SBRT plans.

- Contouring is performed on CT scans with the aid of MRI and Myelogram data sets to delineate the GTV, spinal cord, and cauda equina. Tumor volumes should follow the International Spine Radiosurgery Consortium (ISRC) guidelines.
- IMRT and VMAT are popular linear accelerator techniques in treating spine SBRT.
  - Typically, IMRT beams are spaced 15°–20° along the posterior portion of the patient to avoid entry through the lungs, per TG 101 [1]. This technique has shown to generate a sharp dose gradient between the target and spinal cord upwards of 12% per mm. Coplanar VMAT arcs are efficient in delivering quality SBRT plans. It is rather difficult to utilize non-coplanar arcs due to the location of the spine lesions and patient anatomy. Two to three arcs should be sufficient to create a conformal SBRT plan with sharp gradients to spare the spinal cord.

    Like IMRT, it is important to assign more weight to arcs posteriorly in the thoracic and abdominal regions; this can be achieved with avoidance sectors, avoidance structures, posterior arcs, or optimization structures.
  - Compared with step and shoot IMRT, coplanar VMAT arcs have been shown to reduce $D_{0.03cc}$ and $V_{10\ Gy}$, as well as improve the CI_{100}, for single fraction SBRT spine cases. Two coplanar arcs were sufficient to deliver a prescription dose of 18 Gy to over 90% of the PTV volume while meeting RTOG 0631 normal tissue standards [60].

- A recent study showed that spine SBRT could be feasibly delivered via MR-LINAC. While conformity and heterogeneity worsened, the study showed reduced dose to the spinal cord and cord PRV. With real-time MR imaging, it is possible that PTV margins could be reduced, allowing for possible dose escalation [61].
- $V_{105\%}$ is the volume of tissue outside of the PTV receiving 105% of the prescription volume. With SBRT spine cases, the volume should be restricted as much as possible.
  - RTOG 0631 recommended that the volume outside of the PTV receiving 105% should be less than 2 cc and that the 105% isodose line should be within 1 cm of the PTV [15].
- Hot spots within the PTV are allowed for SBRT cases. Because sharp gradients are needed to attain target coverage while sparing the spinal cord to clinical tolerances, hot spots of over 150% are allowed in many studies.
- Since the spinal cord is a serial organ, a PRV can be utilized to reduce the maximum dose to the cord for planning purposes.
  - A 2–3 mm margin can be added to the spinal cord or cauda equina. When optimizing, a hard constraint can be placed on the maximum dose to the PRV structure in order to drive a sharp gradient and maintain normal tissue tolerance to the spinal cord.
  - In some cases, the GTV or PTV overlaps the cord. Meeting cord tolerance typically trumps PTV coverage, and some protocols will accept a $V_{100\%}$ of 90% if the spinal cord meets specifications.
- Retreatment of the spine presents a challenge. Patients returning for spinal irradiation after receiving a previous course of radiation in the same region, as in the case of bone metastases at the same level as prior breast or lung treatment, could be candidates for SBRT.
  - The challenge is determining previous spinal cord dose and determining a feasible dose to the cord for new treatment planning. Biologically Effective Dose (BED) calculation is essential in retreat spine cases, as the possibility of developing myelitis increases as dose to the spinal cord increases beyond a cumulative dose of 70 Gy at 2 Gy equivalent fractions [61].

    Varian's Velocity software has a biological dose calculation mechanic that allows the user to translate plan dose to equivalent dose at 2 Gy fractions; isoshades and DVH data can be displayed (Fig. 4.14) in equivalent dose using this module in velocity for comparisons, cumulative dose summation, and guiding planning process.

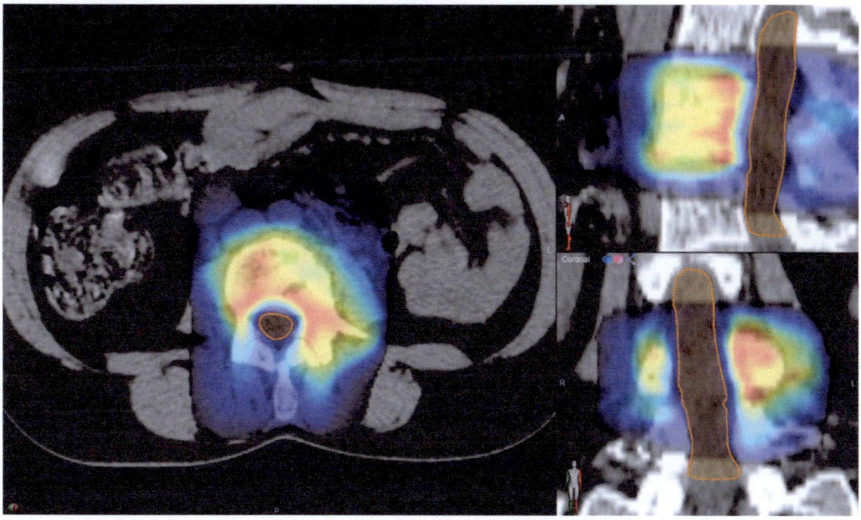

Fig. 4.14 A $EQD_{2\,Gy}$ dose summation in Velocity between a previous palliative spine plan using AP/PA fields and spine SBRT using VMAT. The isoshades show a minimum dose of 60 Gy; the goal was to reduce the canal to a cumulative dose of 70 Gy at 2 Gy-equivalent fractions

References

1. Benedict SH, Yenice KM, Followill D, et al. Stereotactic body radiation therapy: the report of AAPM task group 101. Med Phys. 2010;37(8):4078–101.
2. Halvorsen PH, Cirino E, Das IJ, Garrett JA, Yang J, Yin FF, Fairobent LA. AAPM-RSS medical physics practice guideline 9. A. For SRS-SBRT. J Appl Clin Med Phys. 2017;18(5):10–21.
3. Keall PJ, Mageras GS, Balter JM, Emery RS, Forster KM, Jiang SB, Kapatoes JM, Kubo HD, Low DA, Murphy MJ, Murray BR, Ramsey CR, van Herk MB, Vedam SS, Wong JW, Yorke E. The management of respiratory motion in radiation oncology: report of AAPM task group 76. AAPM report no. 91. Med Phys. 2006;33(10):3874–900.
4. Maintz JBA, Viergever MA. A survey of medical image registration. Med Image Anal. 1998;2(1):1–36.
5. Brock KK, Mutic S, McNutt TR, Li H, Kessler ML. Use of image registration and fusion algorithms and techniques in radiotherapy: report of the AAPM radiation therapy committee task group no. 132. Med Phys. 2017;44(7):e43–76.
6. Dasarathy BV. Medical image fusion: a survey of the state of the art. Inf Fusion. 2014;19(9):4–19.
7. Buck AK, et al. SPECT/CT. J Nucl Med. 2008;49(8):1305–19.
8. Histed SN, Lindenberg ML, Mena E, Turkbey B, Choyke PL, Kurdziel KA. Review of functional/anatomic imaging in oncology. Nucl Med Commun. 2012;33(4):349–61.
9. Brock KK. Adaptive radiotherapy: moving into the future. Semin Radiat Oncol. 2019;29(3):181–4.
10. Shiri I, et al. Repeatability of radiomic features in magnetic resonance imaging of glioblastoma: test–retest and image registration analyses. Med Phys. 2020;47(9):4265–80.
11. van der Heide UA, Frantzen-Steneker M, Astreinidou E, Nowee ME, van Houdt PJ. MRI basics for radiation oncologists. Clin Transl Radiat Oncol. 2019;18:74–9.
12. Potters L, et al. American Society for Therapeutic Radiology and Oncology (ASTRO) and American College of Radiology (ACR) practice guideline for the performance of stereotactic body radiation therapy. Int J Radiat Oncol Biol Phys. 2010;76(2):326–32.

13. ICRU. Prescribing, recording and reporting photon beam therapy. ICRU Report 50; 1993.
14. ICRU. Prescribing, recording and reporting photon beam therapy (Supplement to ICRU Report 50). ICRU Report 62; 1999.
15. Desai D, Narayanasamy G, Bimali M, Cordrey I, Elasmar H, Srinivasan S, Johnson EL. Cleaning the dose falloff in lung SBRT plan. J Appl Clin Med Phys. 2021;22(1):100–8.
16. Tanyi JA, Kato CM, Chen Y, Chen Z, Fuss M. Impact of the high-definition multileaf collimator on linear accelerator-based intracranial stereotactic radiosurgery. Br J Radiol. 2011;84:629–38.
17. Wu QJ, Wang Z, Kirkpatrick JP, Chang Z, Meyer JJ, Lu M, Huntzinger C, Yin FF. Radiat Oncol. 2009;4:3.
18. Jalbout W, Abou Zahr J, Youssef B, Shahine B. On the feasibility of stereotactic radiosurgery with 5.0 and 10.0 mm MLC leaves as a function of target size and shape. Front Oncol. 2019;9:741.
19. Younge KC, Kuchta JR, Mikell JK, Rosen B, Bredfeldt JS, Matuszak MM. The impact of a high-definition multileaf collimator for spine SBRT. J Appl Clin Med Phys. 2017;18(6):97–103.
20. Yan W, Khan MK, Wu X, Simone CB, Fan J, Gressen E, Zhang X, Limoli CL, Bahig H, Tubin S, Mourad WF. Spatially fractionated radiation therapy: history, present and the future. Clin Transl Radiat Oncol. 2020;20:30–8.
21. Duriseti S, Kavanaugh J, Goddu S, Price A, Knutson N, Reynoso F, Michalski J, Mutic S, Robinson C, Spraker MB. Spatially fractionated stereotactic body radiation therapy (lattice) for large tumors. Adv Radiat Oncol. 2021;6:1–6.
22. Stuschke M, Kaiser A, Abu-Jawad J, Pottgen C, Levengrun S, Farr J. Multi-scenario based robust intensity-modulated proton therapy (IMPT) plans can account for set-up errors more effectively in terms of normal tissue sparing than planning target volume (PTV) based intensity-modulated photon plans in the head and neck region. Radiat Oncol. 2013;8:145.
23. Ehrgott M, Güler Ç, Hamacher HW, Shao L. Mathematical optimization in intensity modulated radiation therapy. Ann Oper Res. 2010;175(1):309–65.
24. Mundt AJ, Roenke JC. Intensity modulated radiation therapy: a clinical perspective. USA: PMPH USA; 2005.
25. Purdy JA. Intensity-modulated radiotherapy: current status and issues of interest. Int J Radiat Oncol Biol Phys. 2001;51(4):880–914.
26. Fiege J, McCurdy B, Potrebko P, Champion H, Cull A. PARETO: a novel evolutionary optimization approach to multiobjective IMRT planning. Med Phys. 2011;38(9):5217–29.
27. Snyder KC, Kim J, Reding A, Fraser C, Gordon J, Ajlouni M, Movsas B, Chetty IJ. Development and evaluation of a clinical model for lung cancer patients using stereotactic body radiotherapy (SBRT) within a knowledge-based algorithm for treatment planning. J Appl Clin Med Phys. 2016;17(6):263–75.
28. Jeong C, Park JW, Kwak J, Song SY, Cho B. Volumetric-modulated arc radiotherapy using knowledge-based planning: application to spine stereotactic body radiotherapy. Progr Med Phys. 2019;30(4):94–103.
29. Gits HC, Dow J, Feng M, Matuszak MM. Using a knowledge-based planning model for quality assurance of liver stereotactic body radiation therapy plans. Int J Radiat Oncol Biol Phys. 2016;96(2S):E645–6.
30. Dumane VA, Tseng TC, Sheu RD, Lo YC, Gupta V, Saitta A, Rosenzweig KE, Green S. Training and evaluation of a knowledge-based model for automated treatment planning of multiple brain metastases. J Cancer Metastasis. 2019;5:42–51.
31. Yan C, Combine AG, Bednarz G, Lalonde RJ, Hu B, Dickens K, Wynn R, Pavord DC, Hug MS. Clinical implementation and evaluation of the Acuros dose calculation algorithm. J Appl Clin Med Phys. 2017;18(5):195–209.
32. Kataria T, Sharma K, Subramani V, Karrthick KP, Bisht SS. Homogeneity index: an objective tool for assessment of conformal radiation treatments. J Med Phys. 2012;37(4):207–13.
33. Hoffman D, Dragojević I, Hoisak J, Hoopes D, Manger R. Lung stereotactic body radiation therapy (SBRT) dose gradient and PTV volume: a retrospective multi-center analysis. Radiat Oncol. 2019;14(1):1–7.

34. Meeks SL, Mercado CE, Popple RA, Agazaryan N, Kaprealian T, Fiveash JB, Tenn S. Practical considerations for single Isocenter LINAC radiosurgery of multiple brain metastases. Pract Radiat Oncol. 2021;12:195–9.
35. Vergalasova I, Liu H, Alonso-Basanta M, Dong L, Li J, Nie K, Shi W, Teo BKK, Yu Y, Yue NJ, Zou W, Li T. Multi-institutional dosimetric evaluation of modern day stereotactic radiosurgery (SRS) treatment options for multiple brain metastases. Front Oncol. 2019;9:483.
36. Lim CM, Clump DA, Heron DE, Ferris RL. Stereotactic body radiotherapy (SBRT) for primary and recurrent head and neck tumors. Oral Oncol. 2013;49:401–6.
37. Desai DD, Cordrey IL, Johnson EL. A physically meaningful relationship between R50% and PTV surface area in lung SBRT. J Appl Clin Med Phys. 2020;21(9):47–56.
38. Pokhrel D, Halfman M, Sanford L. FFF-VMAT for SBRT of lung lesions: improves dose coverage at tumor-lung interface compared to flattened beams. J Appl Clin Med Phys. 2020;21(1):26–35.
39. Pokhrel D, Sanfard L, Halfman M, Molloy J. Potential reduction of lung dose via VMAT with jaw tracking in the treatment of single-isocenter/two-lesion lung SBRT. J Appl Clin Med Phys. 2019;20(5):55–63.
40. Wink KJC, Roelofs E, Simone CB 2nd, et al. Photons, protons, or carbon ions for stage I non-small cell lung cancer: results of multicentric ROCOCO in silico study. Radiother Oncol. 2018;128(1):139–46.
41. Chang YJ, Jabbour SK, De Ruysscher D, Schild SE, Simone CB, Rengan R, Feigenberg S, Khan AJ, Choi NC, Bradley JD, Zhue XR, Lomax AJ, Hoppe BS. Consensus statement on proton therapy in early-stage and locally advanced non-small cell lung cancer. Int J Radiat Oncol Biol Phys. 2016;95(1):505–16.
42. Radiation Therapy Oncology Group (RTOG). NSABP Protocol B-39, RTOG Protocol 0413: a randomized phase III study of conventional whole breast irradiation (WBI) versus partial breast irradiation (PBI) for women with Stage 0, I, or II breast cancer. 2005.
43. Livi L, Buonamici FB, Simontacchi G, Scotti V, Fambrini M, Compagnucci A, Paiar F, Scoccianti S, Pallotta S, Detti B, Agresti B, Talamonti C, Mangoni M, Bianchi S, Cataliotti L, Marrazzo L, Bucciolini M, Biti G. Accelerated partial breast irradiation with IMRT: new technical approach and interim analysis of acute toxicity in a phase III randomized clinical trial. Int J Radiat Oncol Biol Phys. 2010;77(2):509–15.
44. Lewin AA, Derhagopian R, Saigal K, Panoff JE, Abitbol A, Wieczorek DJ, Mishra V, Reis I, Ferrell A, Moreno L, Takita C. Accelerated partial breast irradiation is safe and effective using intensity-modulated radiation therapy in selected early-stage breast cancer. Int J Radiat Oncol Biol Phys. 2012;82(5):2104–10.
45. Rahimi A, Thomas K, Spangler A, Rao R, Leitch M, Wooldridge R, Rivers A, Seiler S, Albuquerque K, Stevenson S, Goudreau S, Garwood D, Haley B, Euhus D, Heinzerling J, Ding C, Gao A, Ahn C, Timmerman R. Preliminary results of a phase 1 dose-escalation trial for early-stage breast cancer using 5-fraction stereotactic body radiation therapy for partial breast irradiation. Int J Radiat Oncol Biol Phys. 2017;98(1):196–205 e2.
46. Jagsi R, Ben-David MA, Moran JM, Marsh RB, Griffith KA, Hayman JA, Pierce LJ. Unacceptable cosmesis in a protocol investigating intensity-modulated radiotherapy with active breathing control for accelerated partial-breast irradiation. Int J Radiat Oncol Biol Phys. 2010;76:71–8.
47. Acharya S, Fischer-Valuck BW, Mazur TR, Curcuru A, Sona K, Kashani R, Green O, Ochoa L, Mutic S, Zoberi I, Li HH, Thomas MA. Magnetic resonance image guided radiation therapy for external beam accelerated partial-breast irradiation: evaluation of delivered dose and intrafractional cavity motion. Int J Radiat Biol Phys. 2016;96(4):785–92.
48. Kennedy WR, Thomas MA, Stanley JA, Luo J, Ochoa LL, Clifton KK, Cyr AE, Margenthaler JA, DeWees TA, Price A, Kashani R, Green O, Zoberi I. Single-institution phase 1/2 clinical trial of single-fraction, high-gradient adjuvant partial-breast irradiation for hormone sensitive stage 0–1 breast cancer. Int J Radiat Biol Phys. 2020;107(2):344–52.

49. Schefter TE, Kavanagh BD. Radiation therapy for liver metastases. Semin Radiat Oncol. 2011;21(4):264–70.
50. Esposito M, et al. Multicentre treatment planning inter-comparison in a national context: the liver stereotactic ablative radiotherapy case. Phys Med. 2016;32(1):277–83.
51. Miften M, et al. Radiation dose-volume effects for liver SBRT. Int J Radiat Oncol Biol Phys. 2021;110(1):196–205.
52. Llacer-Moscardo C, et al. Imaged-guided liver stereotactic body radiotherapy using VMAT and real-time adaptive tumor gating: concerns about technique and preliminary clinical results. Pract Oncol Radiother. 2017;22(2):141–9.
53. Huang WY, et al. Stereotactic body radiation therapy in recurrent hepatocellular carcinoma. Int J Radiat Oncol Biol Phys. 2012;84(2):355–61.
54. Hassanzadeh C, Rudra S, Bommireddy A, Hawkins WG, Wang-Gillam A, Fields RC, Cai B, Park J, Green O, Roach M, Henke L, Kim H. Ablative five-fraction stereotactic body radiation therapy for inoperable pancreatic cancer using online MR-guided adaptation. Adv Radiat Oncol. 2021;6:1–8.
55. Krishnan S, Chadha AS, Suh Y, Chen HC, Rao A, Das P, Minsky BD, Mahmood U, Delclos ME, Sawakuchi GO, Beddar S, Katz MH, Fleming JB, Javle MM, Varadhachary GR, Wolff RA, Crane CH. Focal radiation therapy dose escalation improves overall survival in locally advanced pancreatic cancer patients receiving induction chemotherapy and consolidative chemoradiation. Int J Radiat Oncol Biol Phys. 2016;94(4):755–65.
56. Scobiola S, Kittel C, Elsayad K, Kroeger K, Oertal M, Samhouri L, Haverkamp U, Eich HT. A treatment planning study comparing IMRT techniques and cyber knife for stereotactic body radiotherapy of low-risk prostate carcinoma. Radiat Oncol. 2019;14:143–53.
57. Pawlicki T, Kim GY, Hsu A, Cotrutz C, Boyer AL, Xing L, King CR, Luxton G. Investigation of Linac-based image-guided hypofractionated prostate radiotherapy. Med Dosim. 2007;32(2):71–9.
58. Lin YW, Lin KH, Ho HW, et al. Treatment plan comparison between stereotactic body radiation therapy techniques for prostate cancer: non-isocentric Cyberknife versus isocentric RapidArc. Phys Med. 2014;30(6):654–61.
59. Ouyang Z, Lahurd DV, Balagamwala EH, Chao ST, Suh JH, Xia P. Treatment planning of VMAT and step-and-shoot IMRT delivery techniques for single fraction spine SBRT: an intercomparative dosimetric analysis and phantom-based quality assurance measurements. J Appl Clin Med Phys. 2020;21(1):62–8.
60. Redler G, Stevens T, Cammin J, et al. Dosimetric feasibility of utilizing the ViewRay magnetic resonance guided Linac system for image-guided spine stereotactic body radiation therapy. Cureus. 2019;11:12.
61. Sahgal A, Chang JH, Ma L, Marks LB, Milano MT, Medin P, Niermierko A, Soltys SG, Tome WA, Wong CS, Yorke E, Grimm J, Jackson A. Spinal cord dose tolerance to stereotactic body radiation therapy. Int J Radiat Oncol Biol Phys. 2021;110(1):124–36.

Chapter 5
Grid and Lattice Radiation

Orit Kaidar-Person, Maoz Ben-Ayun, and Yaccov R. Lawrence

5.1 Introduction

- Grid-RT is based on an old 2D radiation technique often referred to as mini-beam-RT, or spatially fractionated radiation therapy (SFGRT).
- Grid-RT was applied clinically with kV X-ray delivery systems to treat initially superficial targets and later deep-seated tumors [1, 2].
- Grid-RT was designed to achieve a very high-dose of radiation concentrated in small regions while not exceeding the tolerance dose of nearby healthy tissue.
- In the past decades, the use of megavoltage LINAC and advances in RT such as imaging for defining the target volume, improvement in RT planning and delivery, allowing for steep-gradient and volumetric modulated arc, led to a revival of the concept of 2D grid-RT and extending it to a 3D configuration (i.e., Lattice RT [LRT]).
- The high-radiation dose regions are referred to as vertices. They are located inside the tumor in a way that allows a dosimetric distribution to maintain a conventional dose at the tumor edge, thus not affecting the tolerance dose of the OARs [3–5].

O. Kaidar-Person (✉)
Breast Cancer Radiation Unit, Radiation Department, Sheba Tel Hashomer, Ramat Gan, Israel

School of Medicine, Tel-Aviv University (TAU), Tel Aviv, Israel
e-mail: Orit.kaidarperson@sheba.health.gov.il

M. Ben-Ayun
Radiation Department, Sheba Tel Hashomer, Ramat Gan, Israel
e-mail: maoz.Ben-Ayun@sheba.health.gov.il

Y. R. Lawrence
Radiation Department, Sheba Tel Hashomer, Ramat Gan, Israel

School of Medicine, Tel-Aviv University (TAU), Tel Aviv, Israel
e-mail: Yaacov.Lawrence@sheba.health.gov.il

O. Kaidar-Person, R. Chen (eds.), *Hypofractionated and Stereotactic Radiation Therapy*, https://doi.org/10.1007/978-3-031-47701-0_5

- Therefore, it was an attractive technique to manage patients with bulky tumors, which are often refractory to conventional RT and the size of the target does not allow for safe delivery of SBRT [6].
- In large bulky tumors, grid-RT or LRT is thought to have less radiation toxicity than other RT techniques without compromising tumor control due to its unique radiobiological effect [4, 7].
- Grid-RT or LRT is somewhat similar to high-dose-rate interstitial brachytherapy, based on the objectives of delivering a high RT dose to areas of the tumor forming peak-to-valley dose distribution within the tumor volume, with minimized toxicity.
- Additionally, grid-RT or LRT can be used as a RT boost to facilitate tumor response in bulky tumors [8].
- In 2020, the Radiosurgery Society (RSS) GRID/LATTICE, Microbeam and FLASH Radiotherapy Working Group published a white paper about grid-RT which provided a clinical physics consensus and guidelines for technology selection, commissioning, QA, dose prescription, treatment planning, and reporting [9].
- Grid-RT is being applied to proton-RT by employing pencil beam scanning [9].
- LRT or proton grid-RT are not discussed in the RSS publication and are currently evaluated in clinical trials [9].
- As data are scarce and there is a wide variety in its clinical application, this chapter provides a short introduction to the topic and not as a guide for clinical application of grid-RT/LRT.
- For the purpose of this section, SFRT will relate to both grid-RT or LRT.

5.2 Radiobiology of Grid/LRT

- SFRT appears to induce rapid tumor cell apoptosis in bulky and hypoxic tumors despite parts of the tumor receiving only low dose "valley" radiation (see also Chap. 2) [10, 11].
- Potential explanations for SFGRT's effectiveness include vascular damage, bystander effects, and immune effects.
- Bystander effects refer to the ability of irradiated cells to induce the death of non-irradiated neighboring cells. The bystander effect may be due to molecules such as TNF-a, TRAIL, and ceramide being released from irradiated cells and acting upon non-irradiated cells, initiating a cell death cascade [10, 11].
- It has been hypothesized that SFRT induces a more effective immunostimulatory effect than conventional radiation therapy [12, 13], possibly due to the former sparing immune effector cells.

5.3 Techniques in Creating a GRID/Lattice Pattern

- The original technique was to place a physical grid block or grid collimator that contains arrays of apertures within a cerrobend or brass block [14] (Fig. 5.1).

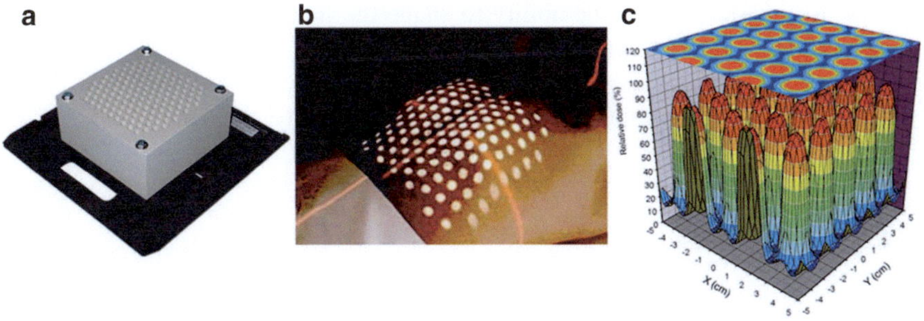

Fig. 5.1 The GRID block (**a**). Commercially available GRID collimator (High Dose Radiation Grid; Radiation Products Design). (**b**) Light field on patient's body using GRID block. (**c**) Spatial dosimetric distribution of the GRID block. [Reproduced with permission from Zhang H, Wu X, Zhang X, et al. Photon GRID Radiation Therapy: A Physics and Dosimetry White Paper from the Radiosurgery Society (RSS) GRID/LATTICE, Microbeam and FLASH Radiotherapy Working Group. Radiat Res. 2020;194: 665–677. "© 2021 Radiation Research Society"]

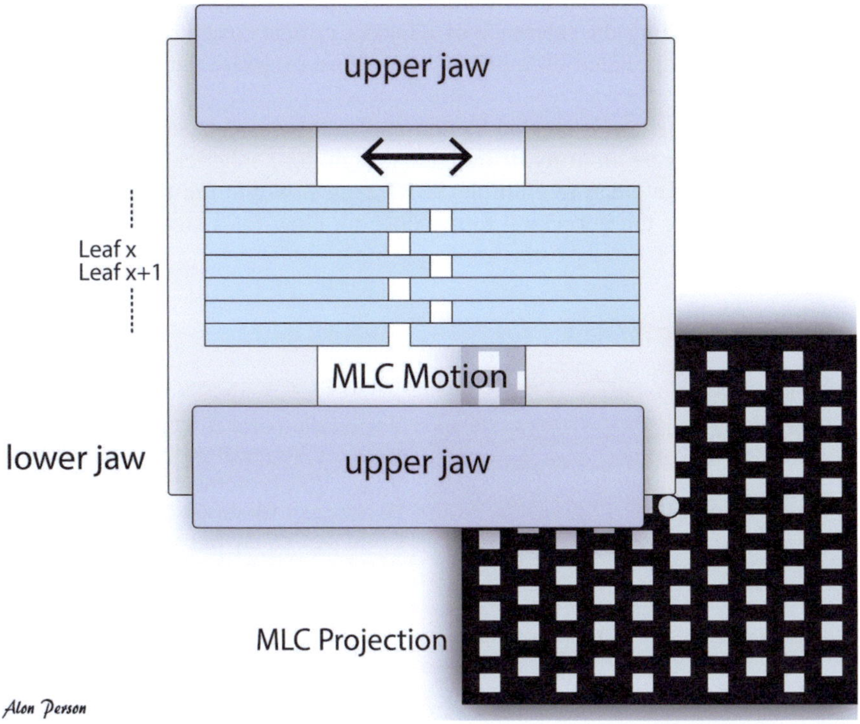

Fig. 5.2 MLC based LRT. The MLC-created GRID pattern radiation field (checkerboard). MLCs could be used with static beams or dynamic planning

- The circular apertures in a grid cerrobend block are typically arranged in a hexagonal pattern, with a diameter of around 1–1.4 cm mm and center-to-center spacing of approximately 2 cm, in the plane of the isocenter [14].
- New RT techniques allow the creation of a virtual block entirely using MLC modulation, resulting in a grid or a 3D lattice pattern [1] (Fig. 5.2).

- The use of MLC added the ability to shape the field to conform to the tumor volume and thereby spare OARs [9, 15].
- The most commonly used diameters of peak dose regions are about 1–1.25 cm wide with spacing (center-to-center distance) of about 1.5–2 cm [13].

5.4 RT Planning

- The dosimetric features of SFRT are defined by the ratio of the valley dose (areas of lower doses) and the peak doses (vertices = higher doses), or the valley-to-peak dose ratio, and are dependent on tumor size/volume (Fig. 5.3).
- Treatment prescription is non-uniform and should include a specification for peak and valley dose, ratio, and equivalent uniform dose [9].
- This ratio quantifies the degree of spatial fractionation, and its spatial location is within the gross tumor as seen on imaging for RT planning (Fig. 5.3).
- SFRT dosimetric planning is committed to deliver high doses of radiation without exceeding the tolerance of adjacent critical structures, and the total volume is encapsulated by a rim of valley dose to assure the safety of OARs (Fig. 5.4).
- The 3D LRT pattern is created by non-coplanar focused beams or volumetric IMRT to generate an array of individual high-dose spherical vertices within the tumor—like creating multiple SBRT targets within the tumor volume—while reducing the peripheral tumor dose to allow for a steep gradient near the OARs.

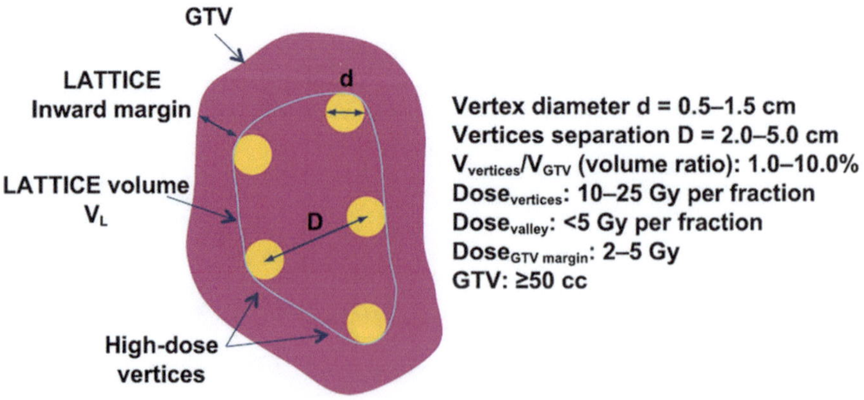

Fig. 5.3 Parameters and ranges of a typical LRT plan. [Reproduced with permission from Wu X, Perez NC, Zheng Y, et al. The Technical and Clinical Implementation of LATTICE Radiation Therapy (LRT). Radiat Res. 2020;194: 737–746. "© 2021 Radiation Research Society"]

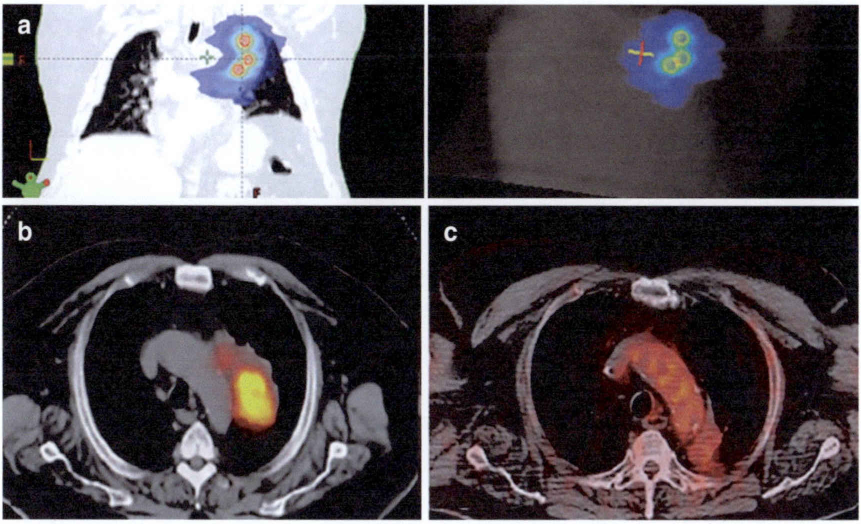

Fig. 5.4 LRT for a stage IIIA lung tumor as upfront boost: 18 Gy to the vertices, 3 Gy to the periphery of the PTV. (**a**) (Top row): dose distribution. (**b**) Tumor prior to treatment. (**c**) Follow-up PET-CT 15 months after LRT followed by additional 29 fractions of 2 Gy per fraction using VMAT. [Reproduced with permission from Wu X, Perez NC, Zheng Y, et al. The Technical and Clinical Implementation of LATTICE Radiation Therapy (LRT). Radiat Res. 2020;194: 737–746. "© 2021 Radiation Research Society"]

5.5 RT Delivery

- SFRT delivery techniques may include 3DCRT, conformal arc, IMRT, TomoTherapy, VMAT, and proton therapy [9].
- Similar to conventional RT planning, selection of beam energy is based on considerations of target coverage and sparing of critical OARs.
- Similar to conventional RT planning, the RT team should consider neutron and electron contamination, treatment delivery time, and other factors that might interfere with a safe delivery of treatment. Immobilization and intrafraction movement are also important considerations.
- Tumor response and shrinkage can lead to significant dosimetric changes. Thus, a limited number of fractions and overall treatment time may be important for SFRT.

5.6 Clinical Application

- Currently it is estimated that over 2000 patients with late-stage bulky tumors have received SFRT [9, 16] including lung, gynecological, renal cell, head and neck, sarcoma, breast, thymoma, liver, upper and lower gastrointestinal, chordoma, lymphoma, skin, and other cancers [16].
- Table 5.1 summarizes clinical applications of SFRT.

Table 5.1 Summary of experiences with lattice radiotherapy

First author (publication year)	Treated sites	Median volume (cc) (range)	Vertices (*n*)	Patients (*n*)	Follow-up median (range) (month)	Histology	Lattice RT dose/fx (Gy) (total dose, Gy)	Further EBRT	Volume reduction (tumor response) (range, %)	Side effects
Amendola [19] (2010)	Pelvis	915	15	1	1	Cervix squamous cell carcinoma	2.4 (48 Gy)	Yes (prior)	70%	Diarrhea (G1)
Suarez [5] (2015)	Pelvis	1495	12	1	20	Ovarian carcinosarcoma	9 (27 Gy)	Yes (post)	70%	None
Amendola [4] (2018)	Thorax	175 (46–487)	3	10	6 (1–71)	NSCLC	18 (18 Gy)	Yes (post)	64% (15–83)	Radiation pneumonitis (G1)
Amendola [18] (2020)	Pelvis	200.35 (74.1–412.4)	2–11	10	28.5 (4–77)	NSCLC	8 (24 Gy)	Yes (post)	48% (6–91)	Diarrhea G1, G2 cystitis
Pollack [21] (2020)	Prostate	NA	1–3 (cylinders)	25	66 (21–7)	High-risk prostate cancer	12–14 (12–14 Gy)	Yes (post)	–	No acute G3 GU/GI Late GU toxicity: G1 (15), G2 (4) and G4 (1) = sepsis after a post-treatment transurethral resection Late GI toxicity: G1 (11) and G2 (4)
Jiang [17] (2021)	Posterior chest wall	63.2	6	1	7	NSCLC	20 Gy at 69% isodose line	NA	–	None

Toxicity outcomes reported according to RTOG scale. Modified with permission from Ferini G, Valenti V, Tripoli A, et al. Lattice or Oxygen-Guided Radiotherapy: What If They Converge? Possible Future Directions in the Era of Immunotherapy. Cancers. 2021;13: 3290.
Abbreviations: *GI* gastrointestinal, *GU* genitourinary, *NSCLC* non-small cell lung cancer, *EBRT* external beam radiation therapy

- SFRT has been used under diverse clinical regimens, as monotherapy, as a boost to conventionally fractionated radiotherapy, and as re-irradiation.
- The tumor volume (GTV) ranged in various reports from 40.5 to 1494.9 cc.
- SFRT has been given as a single fraction or multiple fractions, with vertex dose ranging from 2.4 to 20 Gy per fraction, planned with/without concomitant systemic therapy, including chemotherapy, small molecular inhibitors, and immunotherapy [4, 5, 16–22].

5.7 Future Directions

In conventional LRT the position of the peaks and valleys is somewhat arbitrary. New imaging modalities can differentiate areas within the tumor based upon biological characteristics, such as increased glucose uptake and hypoxia—therefore, future research should explore placement of peak and valley doses based on such characteristics, especially as a single fraction boost in residual viable disease after RT.

5.8 Summary

SFRT has evolved from technically simple 2D grid treatments to complex 3D-LRT. Such treatments require vigorous treatment planning and delivery. Although SFRT promises to provide an effective and safe treatment to large tumors, clinical data are scarce. A number of clinical trials are in progress.

References

1. Ha JK, Zhang G, Naqvi SA, Regine WF, Yu CX. Feasibility of delivering grid therapy using a multileaf collimator. Med Phys. 2006;33:76–82.
2. Marks H. Clinical experience with irradiation through a grid. Radiology. 1952;58:338–42.
3. Neuner G, Mohiuddin MM, Vander Walde N, et al. High-dose spatially fractionated GRID radiation therapy (SFGRT): a comparison of treatment outcomes with Cerrobend vs. MLC SFGRT. Int J Radiat Oncol Biol Phys. 2012;82:1642–9.
4. Amendola BE, Perez NC, Wu X, Blanco Suarez JM, Lu JJ, Amendola M. Improved outcome of treating locally advanced lung cancer with the use of lattice radiotherapy (LRT): a case report. Clin Transl Radiat Oncol. 2018;9:68–71.
5. Blanco Suarez JM, Amendola BE, Perez N, Amendola M, Wu X. The use of lattice radiation therapy (LRT) in the treatment of bulky tumors: a case report of a large metastatic mixed Mullerian ovarian tumor. Cureus. 2015;7:e389.
6. Mohiuddin M, Curtis DL, Grizos WT, Komarnicky L. Palliative treatment of advanced cancer using multiple nonconfluent pencil beam radiation. A pilot study. Cancer. 1990;66:114–8.
7. Haring W. Twenty-five years of grid irradiation. Z Gesamte Inn Med. 1958;13:752–5.

8. Mohiuddin M, Fujita M, Regine WF, Megooni AS, Ibbott GS, Ahmed MM. High-dose spatially-fractionated radiation (GRID): a new paradigm in the management of advanced cancers. Int J Radiat Oncol Biol Phys. 1999;45:721–7.
9. Zhang H, Wu X, Zhang X, et al. Photon GRID radiation therapy: a physics and dosimetry white paper from the radiosurgery society (RSS) GRID/LATTICE, microbeam and FLASH radiotherapy working group. Radiat Res. 2020;194:665–77.
10. Sathishkumar S, Boyanovsky B, Karakashian AA, et al. Elevated sphingomyelinase activity and ceramide concentration in serum of patients undergoing high dose spatially fractionated radiation treatment: implications for endothelial apoptosis. Cancer Biol Ther. 2005;4:979–86.
11. Sathishkumar S, Dey S, Meigooni AS, et al. The impact of TNF-alpha induction on therapeutic efficacy following high dose spatially fractionated (GRID) radiation. Technol Cancer Res Treat. 2002;1:141–7.
12. Kanagavelu S, Gupta S, Wu X, et al. In vivo effects of lattice radiation therapy on local and distant lung cancer: potential role of immunomodulation. Radiat Res. 2014;182:149–62.
13. Ferini G, Valenti V, Tripoli A, et al. Lattice or oxygen-guided radiotherapy: what if they converge? Possible future directions in the era of immunotherapy. Cancers. 2021;13:3290.
14. Meigooni AS, Dou K, Meigooni NJ, et al. Dosimetric characteristics of a newly designed grid block for megavoltage photon radiation and its therapeutic advantage using a linear quadratic model. Med Phys. 2006;33:3165–73.
15. Pokhrel D, Halfman M, Sanford L, Chen Q, Kudrimoti M. A novel, yet simple MLC-based 3D-crossfire technique for spatially fractionated GRID therapy treatment of deep-seated bulky tumors. J Appl Clin Med Phys. 2020;21:68–74.
16. Wu X, Perez NC, Zheng Y, et al. The technical and clinical implementation of LATTICE radiation therapy (LRT). Radiat Res. 2020;194:737–46.
17. Jiang L, Li X, Zhang J, et al. Combined high-dose LATTICE radiation therapy and immune checkpoint blockade for advanced bulky tumors: the concept and a case report. Front Oncol. 2020;10:548132.
18. Amendola BE, Perez NC, Mayr NA, Wu X, Amendola M. Spatially fractionated radiation therapy using lattice radiation in far-advanced bulky cervical cancer: a clinical and molecular imaging and outcome study. Radiat Res. 2020;194:724–36.
19. Amendola B, Perez N, Amendola MA, et al. Lattice radiotherapy with RapidArc for treatment of gynecological tumors: dosimetric and early clinical evaluations. Cureus. 2010;2(9):e15. https://doi.org/10.7759/cureus.15.
20. Duriseti S, Kavanaugh J, Goddu S, Price A, Knutson N, Reynoso F, Michalski J, Mutic S, Robinson C, Spraker MB. Spatially fractionated stereotactic body radiation therapy (lattice) for large tumors. Adv Radiat Oncol. 2021;6:100639.
21. Pollack A, Chinea FM, Bossart E, Kwon D, Abramowitz MC, Lynne C, Jorda M, Marples B, Patel VN, Wu X, et al. Phase I trial of MRI-guided prostate cancer lattice extreme ablative dose (LEAD) boost radiation therapy. Int J Radiat Oncol. 2020;107:305–15.
22. Kopchick B, Xu H, Niu Y, Becker S, Qiu X, Yu C. Technical note: Dosimetric feasibility of lattice radiotherapy for breast cancer using GammaPod. Med Phys. 2020;47:3928–34.

Part I
Benign Central Nervous System Tumors

Chapter 6
Arteriovenous Malformation

Felix Ehret, Katelyn M. Atkins, Marc Bussière, and Helen A. Shih

6.1 Introduction

Neurosurgeon Lars Leksell first described radiosurgery in 1951 and the first clinical application involved GammaKnife-based treatment of benign conditions such as trigeminal neuralgia and arteriovenous malformations (AVM). The principles of stereotactic radiosurgery (SRS) have been applied to fractionated stereotactic radiotherapy (FSRT) techniques for treatment of a variety of commonly treated benign tumors and functional disorders of the CNS. This chapter summarizes hypofractionated radiotherapy techniques, including SRS and FSRT, for AVM.

6.2 Pearls

- Cerebral AVMs are abnormal vascular lesions that bypass the capillary network by shunting blood from feeding arteries to draining veins via a tortuous nidus of vascular connections.

F. Ehret (✉)
Department of Radiation Oncology, Charité - Universitätsmedizin Berlin, Berlin, Germany
e-mail: felix.ehret@charite.de

K. M. Atkins
Department of Radiation Oncology, Cedars-Sinai Medical Center, Los Angeles, CA, USA
e-mail: katelyn.atkins@cshs.org

M. Bussière · H. A. Shih (✉)
Department of Radiation Oncology, Massachusetts General Hospital, Francis H. Burr Proton Therapy Center, Boston, MA, USA
e-mail: bussiere.marc@mgh.harvard.edu; hshih@mgh.harvard.edu

O. Kaidar-Person, R. Chen (eds.), *Hypofractionated and Stereotactic Radiation Therapy*, https://doi.org/10.1007/978-3-031-47701-0_6

- The point prevalence is 18 in 100,000, accounting for 1–2% of all strokes and 9% of subarachnoid hemorrhages.
- The majority (80–90%) are supratentorial and isolated in nature, while up to 9% occur in multiple.
- While generally considered sporadic congenital malformations, the presence of multiple AVMs is associated with hereditary hemorrhagic telangiectasia (also termed Osler–Weber–Rendu syndrome).
- Brain AVMs most often present between the ages of 10 and 40 years.
- The most common presenting symptoms are:
  - Intracranial hemorrhage (usually intraparenchymal).
  - Seizure (more likely with large, cortical AVMs with superficial drainage).
  - Headaches.
  - Focal neurologic deficits (secondary to mass effect, hemorrhage, or vascular steal).
- AVMs carry an estimated risk of hemorrhage of 1–4% per year:
  - The strongest predictors of hemorrhage include prior hemorrhage (at presentation, or clinically silent), deep location, exclusively deep drainage, and associated aneurysms.
- Medical workup: H&P, including assessment of performance status, with emphasis on preceding neurological symptoms (headaches, seizures, focal neurologic deficits) and thorough neurologic examination.
- Imaging workup:
  - CT: Arterial malformations are typically identified on CT, which demonstrate strong contrast enhancement and appear as isodense or hyperdense tortuous vessels. There may be areas of hemorrhage surrounding the nidus. More sensitive imaging is usually required.
  - MRI/MRA: Increased sensitivity for evaluating the nidus, which demonstrate strong contrast enhancement and appear as hypointense flow voids on both T1- and T2-weighted series. Depending on the AVM location, functional MRI could be considered.
  - Angiography: The gold standard modality for AVM diagnosis and nidus delineation.
- Given the morbidity and mortality of hemorrhage, treatment is often considered for asymptomatic and symptomatic patients.
- Management strategies include observation, surgical resection, SRS, and embolization.
- For resectable lesions, surgery is the treatment of choice—as the risk of hemorrhage is immediately removed.
- For unresectable lesions or those with high-associated surgical risk, SRS is a well-established alternative.
  - High-dose RT is presumed to result in a fibrointimal reaction with associated thrombosis and eventual obliteration of the AVM nidus often between 2 and 4 years post-treatment (typical single-fraction SRS dose of 15–24 Gy with higher doses more effective but also with higher risk of morbidity).

Table 6.1 Spetzler–Martin grading scale

Size		Brain location		Venous drainage	
0–3 cm	1	Non-eloquent	0	Superficial	0
3.1–6.0 cm	2	Eloquent[a]	1	Deep	1
>6 cm	3				

Grade IV is considered as inoperable
Modified from Spetzler et al. [1]
[a]Involving or directly adjacent to primary motor or somatosensory cortex, primary visual cortex, Broca'a area, Wernicke's area, hypothalamus, thalamus, deep nuclei, brainstem, or cerebellar nuclei

- Endovascular treatment or embolization (while rarely curative as an isolated intervention) can be a useful adjuvant technique prior to surgery or SRS.

6.3 Staging, Grading, and Other Classifications

Classically, the surgical risk associated with AVMs has been classified based on the 1986 Spetzler–Martin grading scale, which accounts for multiple or large lesions, those in eloquent brain regions, and superficial versus deep drainage, to predict surgical outcomes (Table 6.1, [1]). The total score is the sum in all categories (e.g., grade I = 1 point, grade V = 5 points), where the higher the score, the higher the risk of operative morbidity and mortality [2].

More recently, several radiosurgery-based AVM-scoring systems have been developed to more effectively predict outcomes following AVM radiosurgery. One of the most commonly used is the modified radiosurgery-based AVM score that incorporates AVM nidus volume, patient age, and AVM location by the following equation: AVM score = (0.1) (volume, mL) + (0.02) (age, year) + (0.5) (location; hemispheric/corpus callosum/cerebellar = 0, basal ganglia/thalamus/brainstem = 1) [3]. The score predicts the probability of complete AVM obliteration without any new neurological deficits after treatment [3]. Other AVM score systems are available, but a recent analysis showed continuous scores to outperform integer-based scoring systems at predicting AVM obliteration after SRS without functional decline [4].

6.4 Patient Selection

- Factors influencing treatment recommendations include patient age, medical comorbidities, cranial nerve deficits, AVM size and/or growth rate, presenting symptoms, competing symptoms (i.e., contralateral hearing or vision loss), and proximity to critical organs at risk (OAR, such as brainstem, cochlea, optic apparatus, and eloquent brain).
- Single-fraction SRS for low-grade or small-volume AVMs (SM Grade I–II, low AVM score, nidus volume <10–15 cc), including those in eloquent or deep locations not amenable to surgical resection.

- For single-fraction SRS, targets should generally be:
  - <3 cm.
  - Not directly abutting critical OAR.
  - >3–5 mm from the optic apparatus (optic chiasm, optic nerves) to achieve adequate dose fall-off between the prescription dose and OAR tolerance (<8–10 Gy for single-fraction SRS).
- For FSRT, AVM may be larger (>3–4 cm), in closer proximity to or involving OAR.
- For high-risk AVMs (e.g., large size, deep or eloquent location, close to or involving OAR), the optimal treatment approach remains controversial, but includes FSRT versus volume-staged SRS:
  - FSRT: Total dose is divided into ≥2 equal fractions delivered approximately weekly [5].
  - Volume-staged SRS: The AVM nidus is divided into several regions based upon branches of vascular flow (typically 2–4), each of which is treated to an effective single-fraction dose, commonly with a 3–9-month break interval [6, 7].

6.5 Treatment Planning Considerations

Treatment planning considerations, including critical components of simulation, target delineation, coverage considerations, and planning strategies are described in (Table 6.2) and depicted in (Fig. 6.2).

Table 6.2 Treatment planning considerations

Simulation instructions	**Position**: Supine, arms at sides, head and neck neutral **Immobilization**: A rigid (frame or frameless) stereotactic immobilization system[a] • GammaKnife: Head frame in conjunction with a metal collimator helmet • Linac based: Various, including rigid frame with external skull fixation, noninvasive modified GTC frame (noninvasive fixation by use of a dental plate), or a three-point thermoplastic mask with a modified stereotactic frame (Fig. 6.1) **CT**: Thin-cut CT images (1.0–1.5 mm slice thickness) ideally with IV contrast spanning from vertex to mid-cervical spine **Diagnostic imaging**: Co-registration of planning CT with the appropriate diagnostic imaging (contrast-enhanced MRI or CT) for target and OAR delineation • MRI sequences should include pre- and post-contrast T1-weighted, pre-contrast T2-weighted and FLAIR, and multi-planar (axial, sagittal, and coronal) post-contrast T1-weighted images. Post-contrast T1-weighted images with thin (1 mm) sectioning ideally should be obtained
Image guidance	Imaging options include CBCT, orthogonal kV X-rays; misalignment corrections via positional systems with four or six rotational axes of the patient couch/platform

Table 6.2 (continued)

Target delineation	Target is the entire nidus (see Fig. 6.2a), delineated by co-registration with brain MRI/MRA and/or CT angiography. Draining veins best visualized during arterial phase of angiogram are not part of the target
Margins	The target is the nidus (GTV = CTV) PTV = CTV plus 0–2 mm uniform expansion (depending on institutional setup error, including accuracy and reproducibility of immobilization). For standard thermoplastic mask, generally CTV plus 0–2 mm uniform expansion. For stereotactic frame, generally CTV plus 0–1 mm uniform expansion
Target coverage considerations	≥95% of the AVM (GTV) should receive the prescription dose
Treatment modality	Linac, GammaKnife, CyberKnife, or proton beam
Planning strategies/ assessment	Steep PTV to OAR dose gradients are generated using multiple beam arrangements or non-coplanar arcs together with dose prescription to the steepest portion of the beam profile (often the 50% IDL for GammaKnife or the 70–90% IDL for Linac-based). For Linac-based SRS, the standard beam profile is shaped by collimation with cones or MLCs. An example treatment plan is depicted in Fig. 6.2b Notably, as target size increases, the dosimetric advantages of SRS tend to decline—as the sharp dose fall-off becomes shallower and the higher doses to adjacent normal tissue become prohibitive, thereby generally precluding safe and effective SRS delivery to targets >3 cm in diameter The following indices should be generated [8]: **Conformality index**: Prescription isodose volume/target volume (ideally ≤1.5) **Homogeneity index**: Maximum dose to target volume/prescription dose (ideally ≤2) **Gradient index**: Volume receiving half the prescription isodose/volume receiving the full prescription isodose (ideally ≤4)

Abbreviations: *GTC* Gill–Thomas–Cosman, *FLAIR* fluid-attenuated inversion recovery, *CBCT* cone beam CT, *Linac* linear accelerator

[a]Based on delivery system and institutional protocol

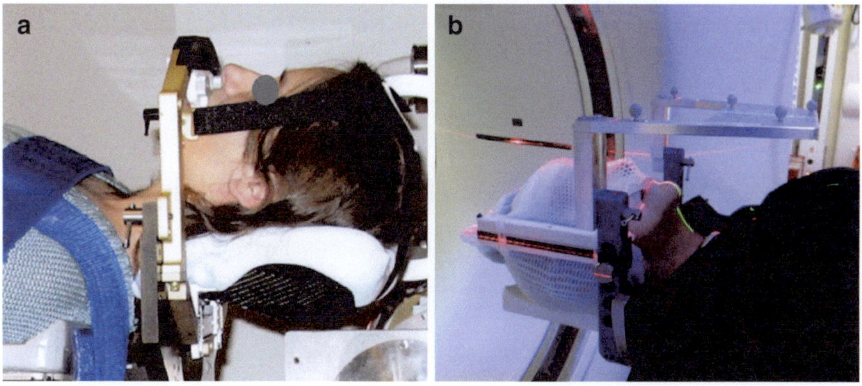

Fig. 6.1 Immobilization depicted using (**a**) a modified Gill–Thomas–Cosman (mGTC) frame (Integra NeuroSciences, USA) and (**b**) a thermoplastic mask (Brainlab, Germany)

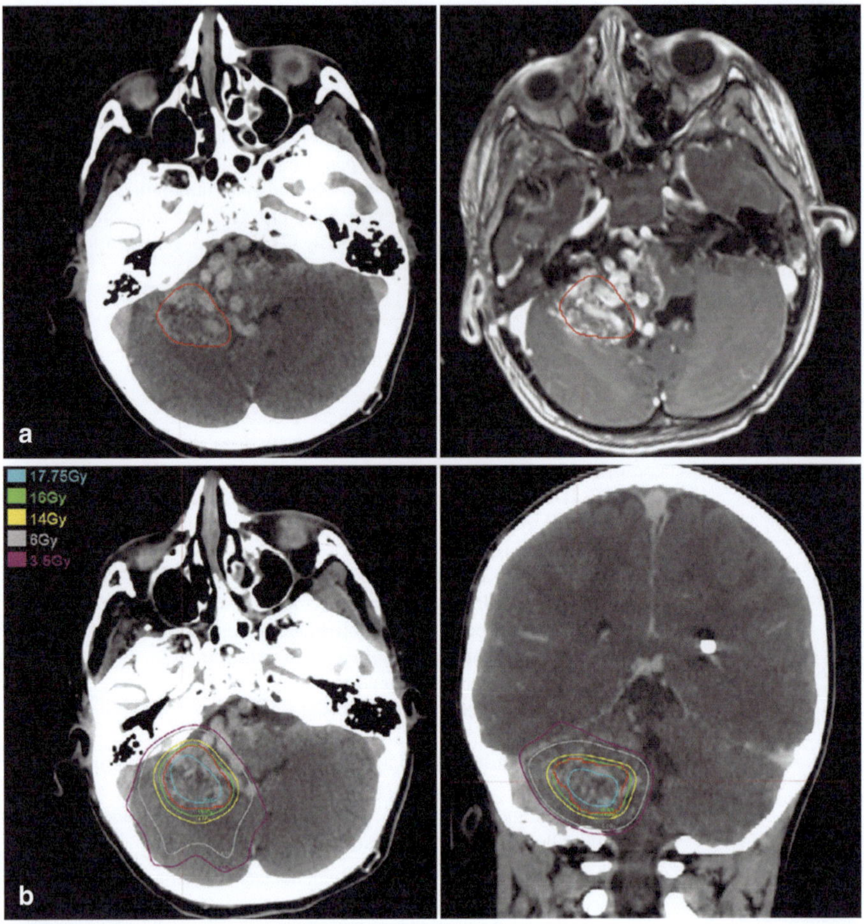

Fig. 6.2 A 6.5 cc right cerebellar AVM in a 12-year-old child; GTV target delineation in red. (**a**) Simulation CT (left), 3D FSPGR MRI sequence (right). (**b**) Treatment plans with prescription IDL in green, effective normalization 90%. SRS, 8 GyRBE protons × 2 fx (16 Gy RBE total). Simulation CT axial (left) and coronal (right). *IDL* isodose line

6.6 Commonly Used Dose/Fractionation Schemes

Commonly utilized dose/fractionation schemes for SRS and FSRT are described in Table 6.3.

Table 6.3 Commonly used dose/fractionation schemes

Commonly used dose/fractionation schemes		
	Patient selection considerations	Dose/fx
SRS	SM grade I–II, low risk	15–24 Gy × 1 fx, prescribed to the 50%, 70–85%, 90%, and 80% prescription isodose lines for GammaKnife, CyberKnife, proton beam, and Linac [9–12]
FSRT	Large lesion, high risk	16–28 Gy, in 2–4 fx (e.g., 8 Gy × 3 fx or 7 Gy × 3 fx), ≥7 days apart or treatment of the entire nidus in separate SRS treatments [5, 13]
Volume staged	Large lesion, high risk	13–18 Gy each, with 2–4 fx, 3–9 months apart [6, 7]

Abbreviations: *SM* Spetzler–Martin, *fx* fraction(s), *Linac* linear accelerator

6.7 Normal Tissue Tolerances

Normal tissue tolerances for SRS and FSRT are described in Table 6.4. In particular, the estimated rates of radiation-induced optic neuropathy are very rare at <8–10 Gy but reach >10% at single-SRS doses between 12 and 15 Gy [18, 19]. In a study by Kano et al. patients with vestibular schwannomas treated with GammaKnife SRS who received a median central cochlea dose <4.2 Gy had better hearing preservation [17].

Table 6.4 Normal tissue tolerances for SRS and FSRT

*D*max[a] (Gy) in critical structures for SRS and FSRT				
Organ	Authors' recommendations	TG101 [14]	QUANTEC [15]	HyTEC [16]
Brainstem				
1 fx	≤12 Gy	15 Gy	<12.5 Gy	–
3 fx	≤21 Gy	23.1 Gy	–	–
5 fx	≤30 Gy	31 Gy	–	–
Cochlea				
1 fx	≤11 Gy, median <4.2 Gy [17]	9 Gy	≤14 Gy	–
3 fx	–	17.1 Gy	–	–
5 fx	–	25 Gy	–	–
Optic apparatus				
1 fx	≤8 Gy	10 Gy	–	<10 Gy
3 fx	≤16.5 Gy	17.4 Gy	–	<20 Gy
5 fx	≤25 Gy	25 Gy	–	<25 Gy
Optic chiasm				
1 fx	≤8 Gy	–	<12 Gy	–
3 fx	–	–	–	–
5 fx	–	–	–	–
Optic nerve				
1 fx	≤8 Gy	–	<12 Gy	–
3 fx	–	–	–	–
5 fx	–	–	–	–

[a]Maximum point dose

6.8 Patient Management Considerations

- Premedication/prophylactic medication:
  - There is no standard premedication regimen.
  - Consideration of steroids, benzodiazepines, and/or anticonvulsants is dependent on severity and tempo of symptoms or neurologic deficit(s), treatment volume/location and number of fractions, if known prior seizures, as well as patient age and/or medical comorbidities.
- Acute toxicity:
  - Generally well tolerated; expected higher risk of toxicity with high-grade AVMs requiring FSRT or volume-staged radiotherapy.
  - Headaches (<5–15%), transient neurologic changes (<1–10%) [9, 10, 20]:
    Consider short-course dexamethasone 2–4 mg QD (can increase to BID), taper, and/or discontinue as soon as feasible.
    Second line: Referral to neurology.
  - Seizures (<10–15%) [9, 10, 20]: Referral to neurology.

- Late toxicity:
  - Headaches (<10–15%), seizures (<5–10%), neurologic changes (<10%), cyst development (1–3%, occurrence mostly >5 years after treament) [5, 6, 9, 10, 13, 21–24].
  - To note, there remains an inherent risk of hemorrhage until obliteration occurs, including any hemorrhage (low-grade lesion 0–6%, high grade lesion 2–22%) and fatal hemorrhage (low-grade lesion 0–3%, high-grade lesion 0–15%) [5, 6, 9, 10, 13, 21, 22].

6.9 Follow-Up

- H&P every 6–12 months, or as needed.
- MRI with contrast every 6 months for 2 years, then annually (CT with contrast if non-tolerant or MRI contraindicated).
  - At the time of apparent radiographic resolution, perform angiography to confirm obliteration.
- For AVM close to the optic system, monitor eyesight.
- For base of skull locations, monitor for hypopituitarism with regular serum analyses annually.
  - Recommend endocrinologist for long-term management and monitoring of endocrine dysfunction.

6.10 Relevant Literature

- Low-grade AVMs (SM Grade I–II, low AVM score, nidus volume <10–15 cc) are effectively treated with single-fraction SRS (general dose 15–24 Gy) [25]. Typical reported obliteration rates are 70–90%, including those in eloquent or deep locations not amenable to surgical resection ([9, 10, 20, 25] and see Table 6.5).
- For large or high-risk AVMs, the optimal treatment approach remains controversial, as delivery of effective single-fraction SRS doses is limited by increasing treatment volumes and associated risk of treatment-related toxicity. To mitigate this, there are two main strategies, FSRT or volume-staged SRS.
  - In FSRT, the total dose is divided into ≥2 equal fractions delivered weekly, with the rationale of improving tolerance of adjacent normal brain tissue to higher doses, however at the expense of obliteration rates (15–27%) [5, 13, 21].
  - For volume-staged SRS, the AVM nidus is divided into several regions (typically 2–4), for which each section is treated to an effective single-fraction dose, typically with a 3–9-month interval to allow for normal brain tissue recovery [6, 7, 32].

Table 6.5 Relevant literature

Study	Patients (*n*)	Median follow-up (months)	Median AVM vol (cm^3)	Modality, dose, fractionation	Obliteration rate (%)
Pan (2000) [26]	240 (60% SM I–III, 40% SM IV–VI)	26	32% >10	GammaKnife, 15–18 Gy × 1 fx	• Vol 10–15 cm^3: 77% at 40 months • Vol >15 cm^3: 25% at 40 months • 58% at 50 months
Flores (2011) [27]	213 (69% SM I–II, 31% SM III)	48	2.1 (mean)	Linac, 14 Gy × 1 fx	• 66% at 3 years • 82% at 5 years
Kano (2012) [20]	217 (SM I–II)	64	2.3	GammaKnife, 22 Gy × 1 fx	• 58% at 3 years • 87% at 4 years • 90% at 5 years • 93% at 10 years
Stark (2013) [28]	1012 (52% SM I–II, 48% SM III–IV)	96	3.5 (mean)	GammaKnife, mean 21.1 Gy × 1 fx	69% overall
Hattangadi-Gluth (2014) [10]	248	35	3.5	Proton beam, 15 Gy (RBE) × 1 fx	• 65% at 2.9 years • 70% at 5 years
Ding (2014) [9]	502 (SM I–II)	48 (radiographic) 62 (clinical)	2.4	GammaKnife, 23 Gy × 1 fx	• 66% at 5 years • 80% at 10 years
Silander (2004) [21]	26 (65% SM I–III, 35% SM IV–V)	NA	13	Proton beam, 20–25 Gy (RBE) total in 2–4 fx	• Vol <25 cm^3: 70% • Vol ≥25 cm^3: 30%
Vernimmen (2005) [29]	64 (50% SM I–III, 50% SM IV–V)	62	41% <14 59% ≥14	Proton beam, 2–3 fx • Volume <14 cm^3: Minimum target vol total dose 15 Gy (RBE) • Volume ≥14 cm^3: Minimum target vol total dose 10.4 Gy (RBE)	• Vol <14 cm^3: 75% • Vol ≥14 cm^3: 43%

Table 6.5 (continued)

Study	Patients (n)	Median follow-up (months)	Median AVM vol (cm^3)	Modality, dose, fractionation	Obliteration rate (%)
Hattangadi (2012) [13]	59	56	22.9	Proton beam, 16 Gy (RBE) total in 2 fx	Total 15%, partial 34%, stable 51%
Blamek (2013) [5]	49 (67% SM II–III, 33% SM IV–V)	29	18	Linac, 19.9 Gy (mean)/21 Gy (median) total dose in 2–4 fx	• 7% at 1 year • 11% at 2 years • 21% at 3 years
Pollock (2017) [30]	34 (71% SM IV–V)	98	22.2	GammaKnife, 16 × 2 fx	• 14% at 3 years • 54% at 5 years • 75% at 7 years
Graffeo (2019) [31]	173 (SM I–II)	68	2.1 (diameter in cm)	GammaKnife, 20 Gy × 1 fx	• 61% at 4 years • 78% at 8 years • 83% at last follow-up
Greve (2021) [11]	215 (54% SM I–III, 46% SM IV–VI)	40	2.4	CyberKnife, 18 Gy × 1 fx	• 47% at 3 years • 67% at last follow-up

Abbreviations: *SM* Spetzler–Martin, *fx* fraction(s), *vol* volume, *Linac* linear accelerator

- Notably, a literature review by Moosa et al. suggests that the higher delivered BED in volume-staged SRS may result in higher obliteration rates compared to FSRT (47 vs. 22%), with the noted disadvantage that partial obliteration may result in altered blood flow patterns and an uncertain impact on the risk of hemorrhage, although rates of hemorrhage do not appear to be increased [22].

References

1. Spetzler RF, Martin NA. A proposed grading system for arteriovenous malformations. J Neurosurg. 1986;65(4):476–83.
2. Hamilton MG, Spetzler RF. The prospective application of a grading system for arteriovenous malformations. Neurosurgery. 1994;34(1):2–6. discussion-7.
3. Pollock BE, Flickinger JC. Modification of the radiosurgery-based arteriovenous malformation grading system. Neurosurgery. 2008;63(2):239–43. discussion 43.
4. Pollock BE, Storlie CB, Link MJ, Stafford SL, Garces YI, Foote RL. Comparative analysis of arteriovenous malformation grading scales in predicting outcomes after stereotactic radiosurgery. J Neurosurg. 2015;126(3):852–8.
5. Blamek S, Larysz D, Miszczyk L, Idasiak A, Rudnik A, Tarnawski R. Hypofractionated stereotactic radiotherapy for large or involving critical organs cerebral arteriovenous malformations. Radiol Oncol. 2013;47(1):50–6.

6. Kano H, Kondziolka D, Flickinger JC, Park KJ, Parry PV, Yang HC, et al. Stereotactic radiosurgery for arteriovenous malformations, part 6: multistaged volumetric management of large arteriovenous malformations. J Neurosurg. 2012;116(1):54–65.
7. Seymour ZA, Sneed PK, Gupta N, Lawton MT, Molinaro AM, Young W, et al. Volume-staged radiosurgery for large arteriovenous malformations: an evolving paradigm. J Neurosurg. 2016;124(1):163–74.
8. Balagamwala EH, Suh JH, Barnett GH, Khan MK, Neyman G, Cai RS, et al. The importance of the conformality, heterogeneity, and gradient indices in evaluating Gamma Knife radiosurgery treatment plans for intracranial meningiomas. Int J Radiat Oncol Biol Phys. 2012;83(5):1406–13.
9. Ding D, Yen CP, Xu Z, Starke RM, Sheehan JP. Radiosurgery for low-grade intracranial arteriovenous malformations. J Neurosurg. 2014;121(2):457–67.
10. Hattangadi-Gluth JA, Chapman PH, Kim D, Niemierko A, Bussiere MR, Stringham A, et al. Single-fraction proton beam stereotactic radiosurgery for cerebral arteriovenous malformations. Int J Radiat Oncol Biol Phys. 2014;89(2):338–46.
11. Greve T, Ehret F, Hofmann T, Thorsteinsdottir J, Dorn F, Švigelj V, Resman-Gašperšič A, Tonn JC, Schichor C, Muacevic A. Magnetic resonance imaging-based robotic radiosurgery of arteriovenous malformations. Front Oncol. 2021;10:608750.
12. Zabel-du Bois A, Milker-Zabel S, Huber P, Schlegel W, Debus J. Stereotactic linac-based radiosurgery in the treatment of cerebral arteriovenous malformations located deep involving corpus callosum motor cortex or brainstem. Int J Radiat Oncol Biol Phys. 2006;64(4):1044–8.
13. Hattangadi JA, Chapman PH, Bussiere MR, Niemierko A, Ogilvy CS, Rowell A, et al. Planned two-fraction proton beam stereotactic radiosurgery for high-risk inoperable cerebral arteriovenous malformations. Int J Radiat Oncol Biol Phys. 2012;83(2):533–41.
14. Benedict SH, Yenice KM, Followill D, Galvin JM, Hinson W, Kavanagh B, et al. Stereotactic body radiation therapy: the report of AAPM task group 101. Med Phys. 2010;37(8):4078–101.
15. Marks LB, Yorke ED, Jackson A, Ten Haken RK, Constine LS, Eisbruch A, et al. Use of normal tissue complication probability models in the clinic. Int J Radiat Oncol Biol Phys. 2010;76(3 Suppl):S10–9.
16. Milano MT, Grimm J, Soltys SG, Yorke E, Moiseenko V, Tomé WA, Sahgal A, Xue J, Ma L, Solberg TD, Kirkpatrick JP, Constine LS, Flickinger JC, Marks LB, El Naqa I. Single- and multi-fraction stereotactic radiosurgery dose tolerances of the optic pathways. Int J Radiat Oncol Biol Phys. 2018;110(1):87–99.
17. Kano H, Kondziolka D, Khan A, Flickinger JC, Lunsford LD. Predictors of hearing preservation after stereotactic radiosurgery for acoustic neuroma. J Neurosurg. 2009;111(4):863–73.
18. Mayo C, Martel MK, Marks LB, Flickinger J, Nam J, Kirkpatrick J. Radiation dose-volume effects of optic nerves and chiasm. Int J Radiat Oncol Biol Phys. 2010;76(3 Suppl):S28–35.
19. Tishler RB, Loeffler JS, Lunsford LD, Duma C, Alexander E 3rd, Kooy HM, et al. Tolerance of cranial nerves of the cavernous sinus to radiosurgery. Int J Radiat Oncol Biol Phys. 1993;27(2):215–21.
20. Kano H, Lunsford LD, Flickinger JC, Yang HC, Flannery TJ, Awan NR, et al. Stereotactic radiosurgery for arteriovenous malformations, part 1: management of Spetzler–Martin Grade I and II arteriovenous malformations. J Neurosurg. 2012;116(1):11–20.
21. Silander H, Pellettieri L, Enblad P, Montelius A, Grusell E, Vallhagen-Dahlgren C, et al. Fractionated, stereotactic proton beam treatment of cerebral arteriovenous malformations. Acta Neurol Scand. 2004;109(2):85–90.
22. Moosa S, Chen CJ, Ding D, Lee CC, Chivukula S, Starke RM, et al. Volume-staged versus dose-staged radiosurgery outcomes for large intracranial arteriovenous malformations. Neurosurg Focus. 2014;37(3):E18.
23. Chen CJ, Ding D, Derdeyn CP, Lanzino G, Friedlander RM, Southerland AM, Lawton MT, Sheehan JP. Brain arteriovenous malformations. Neurology. 2020;95(20):917–27.

24. Ilyas A, Chen CJ, Ding D, Mastorakos P, Taylor DG, Pomeraniec IJ, Lee CC, Sheehan JP. Cyst formation after stereotactic radiosurgery for brain arteriovenous malformations: a systematic review. J Neurosurg. 2017;128(5):1354–63.
25. Musa C, Amisha V, Scott HC, Cornel T, Grover Patrick J. Gamma Knife radiosurgery for cerebral arteriovenous malformations: a systematic review and meta-analysis. Neurosurg Rev. 2022;45(3):1987–2004.
26. Pan DH, Guo WY, Chung WY, Shiau CY, Chang YC, Wang LW. Gamma knife radiosurgery as a single treatment modality for large cerebral arteriovenous malformations. J Neurosurg. 2000;93(Suppl 3):113–9.
27. Flores GL, Sallabanda K, dos Santos MA, Gutiérrez J, Salcedo JCBP, Beltrán C, et al. Linac stereotactic radiosurgery for the treatment of small arteriovenous malformations: lower doses can be equally effective. Stereotact Funct Neurosurg. 2011;89(6):338–45.
28. Starke RM, Yen CP, Ding D, Sheehan JP. A practical grading scale for predicting outcome after radiosurgery for arteriovenous malformations: analysis of 1012 treated patients. J Neurosurg. 2013;119(4):981–7.
29. Vernimmen FJ, Slabbert JP, Wilson JA, Fredericks S, Melvill R. Stereotactic proton beam therapy for intracranial arteriovenous malformations. Int J Radiat Oncol Biol Phys. 2005;62(1):44–52.
30. Pollock BE, Link MJ, Stafford SL, Lanzino G, Garces YI, Foote RL. Volume-staged stereotactic radiosurgery for intracranial arteriovenous malformations: outcomes based on an 18-year experience. Neurosurgery. 2017;80(4):543–50.
31. Graffeo CS, Link MJ, Stafford SL, Garces YI, Foote RL, Pollock BE. More II It than Meets the Eye: outcomes after single-fraction stereotactic radiosurgery in a case series of low-grade arteriovenous malformations. Oper Neurosurg (Hagerstown). 2019;18:136–44. https://doi.org/10.1093/ons/opz153.
32. Pollock BE, Kline RW, Stafford SL, Foote RL, Schomberg PJ. The rationale and technique of staged-volume arteriovenous malformation radiosurgery. Int J Radiat Oncol Biol Phys. 2000;48(3):817–24.

Chapter 7
Trigeminal Neuralgia

Felix Ehret, Katelyn M. Atkins, Marc Bussière, and Helen A. Shih

7.1 Introduction

The GammaKnife-based treatment of trigeminal neuralgia is well-established and was firstly reported by Lars Leksell in 1971. Recent advances in linac-based stereotactic radiosurgery (SRS) approaches have shown efficacy as an acceptable alternative modality. This chapter summarizes the SRS treatment for trigeminal neuralgia.

7.2 Pearls

- Trigeminal neuralgia (also known as tic douloureux) is a rare condition characterized Trigeminal neuralgia by paroxysmal facial pain with an annual incidence of 4–13 per 100,000 people.
- The incidence gradually increases with age, with most idiopathic cases occurring beyond age 50 and occurring more frequently in women than men (1.5–1.7:1).
- The vast majority is sporadic, while rare familial cases have been reported and hypertension may be a risk factor.

F. Ehret
Department of Radiation Oncology, Charité - Universitätsmedizin Berlin, Berlin, Germany
e-mail: felix.ehret@charite.de

K. M. Atkins
Department of Radiation Oncology, Cedars-Sinai Medical Center, Los Angeles, CA, USA
e-mail: katelyn.atkins@cshs.org

M. Bussière · H. A. Shih (✉)
Department of Radiation Oncology, Massachusetts General Hospital, Francis H. Burr Proton Therapy Center, Boston, MA, USA
e-mail: bussiere.marc@mgh.harvard.edu; hshih@mgh.harvard.edu

O. Kaidar-Person, R. Chen (eds.), *Hypofractionated and Stereotactic Radiation Therapy*, https://doi.org/10.1007/978-3-031-47701-0_7

- While the precise cause is not well understood, the majority of classic cases are thought to result from aberrant vascular compression of the trigeminal nerve root at the entry to the pons (dorsal root entry zone, DREZ).
  - Secondary, or non-classic, causes of trigeminal neuralgia may result from tumors (e.g., vestibular schwannoma or meningioma), multiple sclerosis, acute herpes zoster, postherpetic neuralgia, or trauma.
- Patients often present with brief, paroxysmal episodes of unilateral, shock-like pains that are abrupt in onset and termination, typically triggered by otherwise innocuous stimuli, and occur within the distribution of one or more divisions of the trigeminal nerve (CN V).
- Local anatomy:
  - The trigeminal nerve has three major divisions, ophthalmic (V_1), maxillary (V_2), and mandibular (V_3), which together supply sensory innervation to the face (V_1–V_3) and sensory and motor innervation to the muscles of mastication (V_3). The DREZ is at the mid-lateral surface of the pons and the sensory ganglion (gasserian ganglion) resides in Meckel's cave within the floor of the middle cranial fossa.
- Medical workup:
  - Detailed H&P, including assessment of pain characteristics and performance status:
    Many secondary causes of trigeminal neuralgia, such as trauma, postherpetic neuralgia, acute herpes zoster, and multiple sclerosis, can be revealed by thorough history and physical examination.
- Imaging workup: MRI or CT is often obtained to rule out secondary or structural causes of trigeminal neuralgia symptoms.
  - MRI: The trigeminal nerve can be visualized on both T1- and T2-weighted images as it exits laterally from the pons and forms the trigeminal ganglion. Post-contrast T1-weighted images with thin (1 mm) sectioning through the skull base are ideal. High-resolution constructive interference in steady state (CISS) or 3D fast imaging employing steady-state acquisition (FIESTA) sequences can show enhanced visualization of the trigeminal nerve surrounded by CSF.
- First-line therapy for trigeminal neuralgia is pharmacologic management with carbamazepine, or second-line agents such as oxcarbazepine, lamotrigine, gabapentin, phenytoin, benzodiazepines, and baclofen—which can be used alone or in combination.
  - Patients with refractory symptoms or side effects from medication may be considered for procedural intervention, including microvascular or balloon decompression, glycerol injection or radiofrequency rhizotomy, or SRS.

Table 7.1 The diagnostic criteria for trigeminal neuralgia

Trigeminal Neuralgia Diagnostic Criteria (ICHD-3)[a]	
A	Recurrent episodes of unilateral facial pain occurring in at least one trigeminal nerve division (without radiation beyond the CN V distribution) (fulfilling criteria B and C)
B	Pain matches all of the following characteristics: 1. Lasting from a fraction of a second to 2 min (a few patients may report attacks lasting for >2 min) 2. Severe intensity (pain may become more severe over time) 3. Electric shock-like, shooting, stabbing, or sharp quality
C	Precipitated by innocuous stimuli within the affected trigeminal distribution
D	Symptoms not better accounted for by another ICHD-3 diagnosis

[a]Modified from *ICHD-3*, International classification of headache disorder, third edition, 2018, [1]

7.3 Staging, Grading, and Other Classifications

The third edition of the International Classification of Headache Disorders (ICHD-3) describes the diagnostic criteria for trigeminal neuralgia [1] (Table 7.1).

7.4 Patient Selection

- Consider SRS for patients refractory to medical therapy, or significant side effects, who are not surgical candidates, decline procedural intervention, or had microvascular decompression with failed resolution or significant improvement in facial pain.
- Factors influencing treatment recommendations include patient age, medical comorbidities, trial and/or failure of medical therapies, and the severity and/or duration of symptoms .
- In patients who are not surgical candidates, early SRS (within 3 years of pain onset) as the initial procedure may provide superior pain control as compared to later SRS treatments [2].
- Patients who already received SRS may be re-irradiated with a lower dose as a salvage treatment [3].

7.5 Treatment Planning Considerations

Treatment planning considerations, including critical components of simulation, target delineation, coverage considerations, and planning strategies are described in (Table 7.2).

Table 7.2 Treatment planning considerations

Simulation instructions	**Position**: Supine, arms at sides, head and neck neutral. **Immobilization**: A rigid (frame or frameless) stereotactic immobilization system[a] • GammaKnife: Head frame in conjunction with a metal collimator helmet • Linac-based/frameless GammaKnife/CyberKnife: Various, including rigid frame with external skull fixation, non-invasive modified GTC frame (non-invasive fixation by use of a dental plate), or a three-point thermoplastic mask with a modified stereotactic frame/moldable headrest. **CT**: Thin-cut CT images (0.625–0.8 mm slice thickness) from vertex to mid-cervical spine. **Diagnostic imaging**: Co-registration of planning CT with diagnostic MRI for target and OAR delineation. • MRI: Non-contrast, whole head, high-resolution CISS or FIESTA sequences provide enhanced visualization of the trigeminal nerve surrounded by CSF and the brainstem surface [4].
Image guidance	Imaging options include CBCT, orthogonal KV X-rays; misalignment corrections via positional systems with four or six rotational axes of the patient couch/platform.
Target delineation	The preferred target is the anterior retrogasserian part of the trigeminal nerve at the level of the pons (Fig. 7.1) [5]. A 4–6 mm segment of the nerve should be targeted [3, 6, 7]. The trigeminal nerve can be visualized on both T1- and T2-weighted images as it exits laterally from the pons and forms the trigeminal ganglion (Fig. 7.2). Note: Inferior results have been reported with SRS targeting the gasserian ganglion [5, 8]. Moreover, targeting the DREZ/proximal trigeminal nerve may cause more complications [5].
Margins	Target is the anterior retrogasserian part of the trigeminal nerve (GTV = CTV). No PTV margin is applied, therefore, on-treatment re-imaging is crucial to monitor potential motion.
Target coverage considerations	The prescription dose is centered on the nerve's cross-section. The distance from the brainstem surface, along this axis, is dictated by the modality and beam collimation hardware used, as this determines the volume of the pseudo-spherical dose distributions which abuts the brainstem. The sharper the penumbra, the closer the isocenter to the brainstem surface.
Treatment modality	GammaKnife, CyberKnife, or Linac
Planning strategies/ assessment	Steep dose gradients are generated using multiple non-coplanar beam arrangements or arcs. For linac-based SRS, the beam profile is shaped using high-definition multi-leaf collimation or static cones. The treatment isocenter is positioned along the center of the nerve cross-section and positioned as close as possible to the tangential surface of the brainstem without exceeding defined dose constraints.

[a]Based on delivery system and institutional protocol
Abbreviations: *GTC* Gill-Thomas-Cosman, *FLAIR* fluid-attenuated inversion recovery, *CISS* constructive interference in steady state, *FIESTA* 3D fast imaging employing steady-state acquisition, *Linac* linear accelerator, *DREZ* dorsal root entry zone

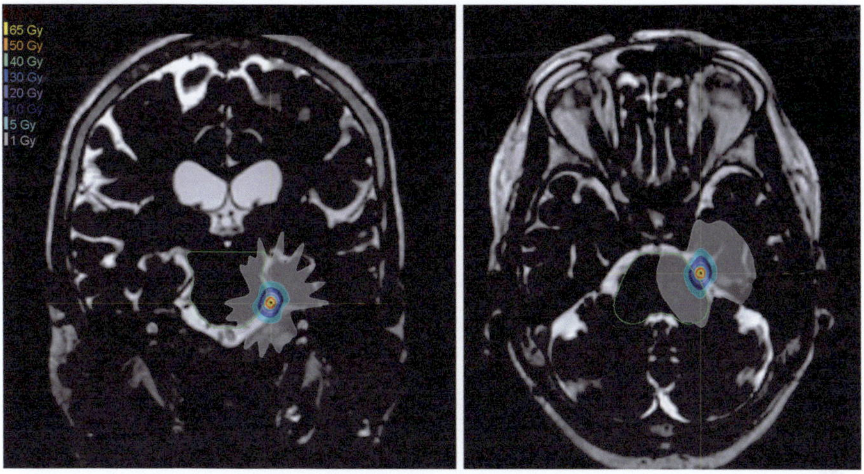

Fig. 7.1 Treatment planning MRI. Identification of the left anterior retrogasserian part of the trigeminal nerve at the level of the pons

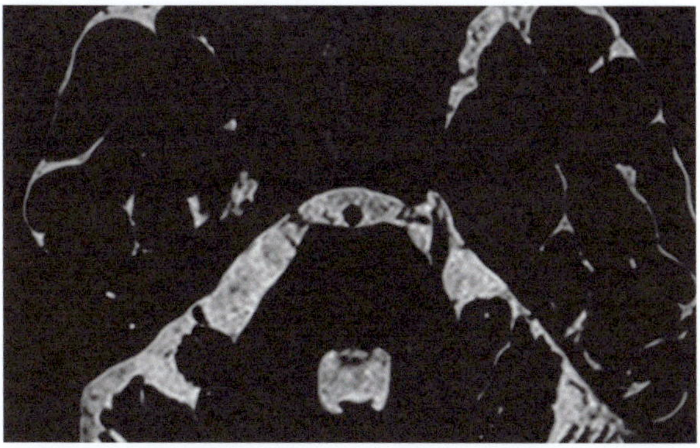

Fig. 7.2 Treatment planning for trigeminal neuralgia. A 4–6 mm anterior retrogasserian part of the trigeminal nerve at the level of the pons should be the preferred target

7.6 Commonly Used Dose/Fractionation Schemes

Commonly utilized dose/fractionation schemes are:

70–90 Gy × 1 fx, prescribed to the 100% and 80–90% prescription isodose lines for GammaKnife and linac-based SRS [5, 9–11].

60–70 Gy × 1 fx, prescribed to the 80–90% isodose line for CyberKnife [3, 5, 6, 12].

40–45 Gy × 1 fx, prescribed to the 80–90% isodose line for CyberKnife in the recurrent setting after SRS [3].

7.7 Normal Tissue Tolerances

Normal tissue tolerances for SRS are described in Table 7.3.

Table 7.3 Normal tissue tolerances for SRS

Dmax[a] (Gy) in critical structures for SRS			
Organ	Authors' recommendations	TG101 [13]	QUANTEC [14]
Brainstem			
1 fx	≤40 Gy at 0.01 cc	15 Gy	<12.5 Gy

[a]Maximum point dose
Abbreviation: *fx* fraction

7.8 Patient Management Considerations

- Premedication/prophylactic medication:
  - There is no standard premedication regimen.
- Acute toxicity:
  - Generally well tolerated; increase in trigeminal neuralgia pain within the first few hours after SRS (<5%) [15].
- Late toxicity:
  - Any paresthesia or hypesthesia: up to a maximum of 68%, mostly ranging between 19 and 29% [5].
  - Bothersome hypesthesia (Barrow Neurological Institute (BNI) numbness scale grade III and IV): up to a maximum of 17%, mostly ranging between 0 and 10% [5].
  - Anesthesia dolorosa (0–1%) [15, 16].

7.9 Follow-Up

- H&P with pain assessments (e.g., BNI Pain Intensity Scale) every 6–12 months.
- Recommend neurologist or primary care physician for long-term management of medical therapies.

7.10 Relevant Literature

- SRS is a well-established technique for treatment of trigeminal neuralgia in medically refractory patients or those who are not surgical candidates [5, 17]. Moreover, a second SRS treatment with a lower dose can be applied in selected patients with recurrent pain [3].
- Historically, GammaKnife has been the gold standard modality; however, advances in linac-based SRS and other stereotactic approaches over the past two decades have shown a comparable efficacy and safety profile [5, 6, 11] (Table 7.4).

Table 7.4 Relevant literature

Study	Patients (*n*)	Median follow-up (months)	Modality, dose	Outcomes
Riesenburger 2010 [18]	53	48	GammaKnife, median maximum dose 80 Gy × 1 fx	59% achieved initial pain relief that was adequate or better, ± medications (equivalent to BNI scores I–IIIb)
Kondziolka 2010 [9]	503	24 (107 pts >5-year follow-up)	GammaKnife, maximum dose 80 Gy × 1 fx	89% achieved initial pain relief that was adequate or better, ± medications (BNI scores I–IIIb), BNI of I–IIIb: 80% 1 year, 71% 3 years, 46% 5 years, 30% 10 years
Smith 2011 [11]	179	NA	Linac, 70 Gy × 1 fx (1995–1999), 90 Gy × 1 fx (1999–2008)	Significant pain relief in 79%, mean time to relief 1.9 month
Régis 2016 [10]	497	43	GammaKnife, median maximum dose 85 Gy × 1 fx	92% pain free in a median time of 10 days Pain free without medication at 3, 5, 7, and 10 years was 72%, 65%, 60%, and 45%, respectively
Romanelli 2017 [6]	138	52	CyberKnife, median prescription dose 60 Gy × 1 fx	Significant pain relief in 93%, median time to relief 3 weeks, BNI of I–IIIa: 85% 1 year, 79% 2 years, 76% 3 years; 20 out of 33 (61%) patients who required re-irradiation achieved pain control (BNI of I–IIIa) with SRS alone
Romanelli 2019 [3]	496	All patients minimum 6 months, 343 patients with a minimum of 36 months	CyberKnife, median dose 60 Gy × 1 fx	Pain relief rate at 6, 12, 18, 24, 30 and 36 months: 92, 87, 87, 82, 78, and 76%. Forty-four patients underwent a second SRS treatment

Abbreviations: *BNI* Barrow Neurological Institute, *fx* fraction(s), *Linac* linear accelerator

References

1. Headache Classification Committee of the International Headache Society (IHS) The International Classification of Headache Disorders, 3rd edition. Cephalalgia. 2018;38(1):211. https://doi.org/10.1177/0333102417738202.
2. Mousavi SH, Niranjan A, Huang MJ, Laghari FJ, Shin SS, Mindlin JL, Flickinger JC, Lunsford LD. Early radiosurgery provides superior pain relief for trigeminal neuralgia patients. Neurology. 2015;85(24):2159–65. https://doi.org/10.1212/WNL.0000000000002216.
3. Romanelli P, Conti A, Redaelli I, Martinotti AS, Bergantin A, Bianchi LC, Beltramo G. Cyberknife radiosurgery for trigeminal neuralgia. Cureus. 2019;11(10):e6014. https://doi.org/10.7759/cureus.6014.

4. Lee NY, Riaz N, Lu JJ. Target volume delineation and field setup: a practical guide for conformal and intensity-modulated radiation therapy. Heidelberg: Springer; 2015.
5. Tuleasca C, Régis J, Sahgal A, De Salles A, Hayashi M, Ma L, Martínez-Álvarez R, Paddick I, Ryu S, Slotman BJ, Levivier M. Stereotactic radiosurgery for trigeminal neuralgia: a systematic review. J Neurosurg. 2017;130(3):733–57. https://doi.org/10.3171/2017.9.JNS17545.
6. Romanelli P, Conti A, Bianchi L, Bergantin A, Martinotti A, Beltramo G. Image-guided robotic radiosurgery for trigeminal neuralgia. Neurosurgery. 2017;83(5):1023–30. https://doi.org/10.1093/neuros/nyx571.
7. Flickinger JC, Pollock BE, Kondziolka D, Phuong LK, Foote RL, Stafford SL, Lunsford LD. Does increased nerve length within the treatment volume improve trigeminal neuralgia radiosurgery? A prospective double-blind, randomized study. Int J Radiat Oncol Biol Phys. 2001;51(2):449–54. https://doi.org/10.1016/S0360-3016(01)01606-6.
8. Quinones-Hinojosa A. Schmidek and sweet: operative neurosurgical techniques: indications, methods and results. Elsevier Health Sciences; 2012.
9. Kondziolka D, Zorro O, Lobato-Polo J, Kano H, Flannery TJ, Flickinger JC, et al. Gamma knife stereotactic radiosurgery for idiopathic trigeminal neuralgia. J Neurosurg. 2010;112(4):758–65.
10. Regis J, Tuleasca C, Resseguier N, Carron R, Donnet A, Gaudart J, et al. Long-term safety and efficacy of gamma knife surgery in classical trigeminal neuralgia: a 497-patient historical cohort study. J Neurosurg. 2016;124(4):1079–87.
11. Smith ZA, Gorgulho AA, Bezrukiy N, McArthur D, Agazaryan N, Selch MT, et al. Dedicated linear accelerator radiosurgery for trigeminal neuralgia: a single-center experience in 179 patients with varied dose prescriptions and treatment plans. Int J Radiat Oncol Biol Phys. 2011;81(1):225–31.
12. Adler JR, Bower R, Gupta G, Lim M, Efron A, Gibbs IC, Chang SD, Soltys SG. Nonisocentric radiosurgical rhizotomy for trigeminal neuralgia. Neurosurgery. 2009;64(suppl_2):A84–90. https://doi.org/10.1227/01.NEU.0000341631.49154.62.
13. Benedict SH, Yenice KM, Followill D, Galvin JM, Hinson W, Kavanagh B, et al. Stereotactic body radiation therapy: the report of AAPM task group 101. Med Phys. 2010;37(8):4078–101.
14. Marks LB, Yorke ED, Jackson A, Haken Ten RK, Constine LS, Eisbruch A, et al. Use of normal tissue complication probability models in the clinic. Int J Radiat Oncol Biol Phys. 2010;76(3 Suppl):S10–9.
15. Kondziolka D, Perez B, Flickinger JC, Habeck M, Lunsford LD. Gamma knife radiosurgery for trigeminal neuralgia: results and expectations. Arch Neurol. 1998;55(12):1524–9.
16. Kotecha R, Kotecha R, Modugula S, Murphy ES, Jones M, Kotecha R, et al. Trigeminal neuralgia treated with stereotactic radiosurgery: the effect of dose escalation on pain control and treatment outcomes. Int J Radiat Oncol Biol Phys. 2016;96(1):142–8.
17. Leksell L. Trigeminal neuralgia. Some neurophysiologic aspects and a new method of therapy. Lakartidningen. 1971;68(45):5145–8.
18. Riesenburger RI, Hwang SW, Schirmer CM, Zerris V, Wu JK, Mahn K, et al. Outcomes following single-treatment Gamma Knife surgery for trigeminal neuralgia with a minimum 3-year follow-up. J Neurosurg. 2010;112(4):766–71.

Chapter 8
Meningioma

Felix Ehret, Katelyn M. Atkins, Marc Bussière, and Helen A. Shih

8.1 Introduction

Meningiomas are the most frequent primary intracranial neoplasm, for which the treatment strategies range from observation to surgical resection and/or radiotherapy, depending on tumor size, location, histology, and growth pattern over time. Notably, stereotactic radiosurgery (SRS) and conventionally fractionated radiotherapy are well-established techniques for the treatment of benign meningiomas with high local control rates and robust long-term follow-up data. Recent studies have applied the principles of SRS to fractionated stereotactic radiotherapy (FSRT) techniques, typically for patients with large tumors or those abutting critical organs-at-risk. Fractionation schemes are variable, though early data are promising. This chapter summarizes hypofractionated radiotherapy techniques, including SRS and FSRT, for meningiomas.

F. Ehret
Department of Radiation Oncology, Charité - Universitätsmedizin Berlin, Berlin, Germany
e-mail: felix.ehret@charite.de

K. M. Atkins
Department of Radiation Oncology, Cedars-Sinai Medical Center, Los Angeles, CA, USA
e-mail: katelyn.atkins@cshs.org

M. Bussière · H. A. Shih (✉)
Department of Radiation Oncology, Massachusetts General Hospital, Francis H. Burr Proton Therapy Center, Boston, MA, USA
e-mail: bussiere.marc@mgh.harvard.edu; hshih@mgh.harvard.edu

O. Kaidar-Person, R. Chen (eds.), *Hypofractionated and Stereotactic Radiation Therapy*, https://doi.org/10.1007/978-3-031-47701-0_8

8.2 Pearls

- Arise from arachnoid cap cells of the arachnoid villi and are the most frequent primary intracranial neoplasm, accounting for one-third of all primary brain tumors.
- The average annual age-adjusted incidence is 7.86 per 100,000 people, with a median age at diagnosis of 65 years.
- More frequently diagnosed in women; female:male ratio of 2–3:1.
- Risk factors include exposure to ionizing radiation (therapeutic or incidental) and genetic conditions such as type 2 neurofibromatosis (NF2) and schwannomatosis.
- The link between ionizing radiation exposure and risk for meningioma is well established from studies of therapeutic radiation, atomic bomb fallout, and historic use of cranial and scalp irradiation for tinea capitis.
- The role of sex hormones is less clear, although more than 70% of meningiomas express PR and nearly 40% express ER and androgen receptor.
- Meningiomas can arise from any location of the dura (see local anatomy below) and presenting symptoms depend largely on anatomic location, time course over which it developed, and presence of edema.
- While generally slow growing and clinically asymptomatic, there is a higher association with seizure in convexity and parasagittal/falcine locations and those with peritumoral edema.
- The WHO describes 3 grades (I–III, 1–3 since 2021) and 15 histologic subtypes (see Sect. 8.3) [1].
- Local anatomy:

  – Meninges: Comprised of three membranes that envelop the brain and spinal cord, including the outer dura mater (including an outer endosteal and an inner meningeal layer), the middle arachnoid mater, and the inner pia mater. The arachnoid and pia mater form the leptomeninges and CSF flows between the two.
  – The dura has four areas of infolding to form the falx cerebri (separating the cerebral hemispheres), the tentorium cerebelli (separating the occipital lobes from the cerebellum), the falx cerebelli (separating the cerebellar hemispheres), and the diaphragma sellae (covering the pituitary gland and sella turcica).
  – Meningiomas develop in various regions: parasagittal/falcine (25%), convexity (19%), sphenoid ridge (17%), suprasellar (9%), posterior fossa (8%), olfactory groove (8%), middle fossa/Meckel's cave (4%), tentorial (3%), peritorcular (3%), lateral ventricle (1–2%), foramen magnum (1–2%), and orbit/optic nerve sheath (1–2%) [2]. Of those in the parasagittal region, 49% occur in the anterior one-third of the falx cerebri.

- Medical workup:

  – History: Assessment of performance status, potential risk factors (prior therapeutic radiation exposure), genetic predisposition syndromes (NF2, schwannomatosis), conditions that can also cause a dural-based lesion (sarcoidosis,

hematologic and non-hematologic malignancy, infection/fungal/tuberculosis), and associated neurological symptoms (e.g., seizures, headaches, vision changes).
  - Physical examination: Thorough neurologic examination.

- Imaging workup:
  - CT: Meningiomas are well-circumscribed, extra-axial masses that display strong, homogenous contrast enhancement, and are iso- or hyper-dense to normal brain parenchyma—which is often displaced adjacently. Approximately 20–30% of meningiomas harbor calcifications, while approximately 50% are associated with hyperostosis or osteolysis in the adjacent bone.
  - MRI: Meningiomas are typically iso- or hypo-intense to gray matter on T1-weighted images, and hyperintense to gray matter on FLAIR sequences, and may display associated peritumoral edema. More than 90% of meningiomas display strong, homogenous contrast enhancement and approximately two-thirds demonstrate an adjacent dural thickening or "dural tail."
- Management strategies include observation, surgical resection, and/or radiotherapy, depending on tumor size, location, histology, and growth pattern over time.

8.3 Staging, Grading, and Other Classifications

Most of the available SRS and FSRT literature is based on previous WHO classifications (2007 and 2016). The most recent classification from 2021 introduces several changes and additions to the meningioma diagnosis, including molecular biomarkers and grading predominantly irrespective of the underlying histological subtype [1]. Because of the scope of this chapter, recency of the 2021 classification, and available literature, we will primarily refer to the 2016 classification. Nevertheless, we emphasize the important changes and clinical implications of the 2021 classification, especially concerning the introduction of molecular grading characteristics, for example, TERT promoter mutation.

The WHO describes 3 grades (I–III) and 15 histologic subtypes of meningioma. The WHO grade is prognostic, with strong associations between grade, progression-free survival (PFS), and OS (Table 8.1, [3]). Surgery is often an appropriate therapy for benign (WHO Grade I) meningiomas, with extent of resection based on the Simpson grade and correlating to the rate of tumor recurrence (Table 8.2, [4, 5]).

Table 8.1 The 2016 WHO meningioma grading criteria[a]

Grade	Tumor histology/features
I (benign)	1. Any major histologic subtype, ***except*** clear cell, chordoid, papillary, or rhabdoid 2. Does not otherwise meet the criteria for grade II or III
II (atypical)	1. Chordoid or clear cell subtype, ***or*** 2. Presence of brain invasion, ***or*** 3. Increased mitotic index (4–19 per 10 hpf), ***or*** 4. Three or more of the following histologic features: Sheetlike or patternless architecture, increased cellularity (focal or diffuse), prominent nucleoli, small cells with high nuclear: cytoplasmic ratio, foci of spontaneous or geographic necrosis
III (anaplastic or malignant)	1. Papillary or rhabdoid subtypes, ***or*** 2. High mitotic index (≥20 per 10 hpf), ***or*** 3. Anaplastic by the following criteria: Focal or diffuse loss of meningothelial differentiation, resembling sarcomata, carcinomata, or melanoma

[a]Modified from Louis et al. [3]
Abbreviation: *Hpf* high-power field

Table 8.2 Simpson grade of resection and recurrence risk[a]

Grade	Extent of tumor resection	Recurrence rate (%)
I	Macroscopic complete resection of tumor, dural attachments, and abnormal bone	9
II	Macroscopic complete resection of tumor, coagulation of dural attachments	19
III	Macroscopic complete resection of tumor, without resection or coagulation of dural attachments or with extradural disease	29
IV	Subtotal resection of tumor	44
V	Decompression or biopsy only	N/A

[a]Modified from Simpson et al. [4]

8.4 Patient Selection for SRS or FSRT

- Factors influencing treatment recommendations include patient age, performance status, medical comorbidities, cranial nerve deficits, tumor size, location, grading and/or growth rate, presenting symptoms, competing symptoms (i.e., contralateral hearing or vision loss), and proximity to critical organs at risk (OAR, such as brainstem, cochlea, optic apparatus, eloquent brain).
- For SRS, targets should generally be:
  - <3 cm.
  - Not directly abutting critical OAR.
  - >3 to 5 mm from the optic apparatus (optic chiasm, optic nerves) to achieve adequate dose fall-off between the prescription dose and OAR tolerance (<8 to 10 Gy for single-fraction SRS).

- For FSRT, tumors may be larger (>3 to 4 cm), in closer proximity to or involving OAR [6].
- Case-by-case consideration of SRS for parasellar meningiomas (including cavernous sinus and medial sphenoid wing) given proximity to optic apparatus.
- Optic nerve sheath and tuberculum sellae meningiomas are generally a contraindication for SRS in patients with preserved vision given that the lowest therapeutic dose (12–13 Gy) exceeds optic apparatus tolerance (8–10 Gy). However, in carefully selected cases of optic nerve sheath and orbital meningiomas after surgical resection, SRS or FSRT might be feasible. Early adjuvant SRS (within 6 months after surgery) may improve local tumor control in such cases [7].
- Given their biological aggressiveness, grade II and III meningioma require higher doses to achieve durable local control (Tables 8.4 and 8.5). However, the optimal SRS and FSRT dose for such tumors is not well established. Therefore, patient selection and treatment parameters for SRS and FSRT must be carefully considered [23, 24]. The standard of care is conventionally fractionated radiotherapy with total doses of 60 Gy [25].

8.5 Treatment Planning Considerations (Table 8.3)

Table 8.3 Treatment planning considerations

Simulation instructions	**Position**: Supine, arms at sides, head and neck neutral. **Immobilization**: A rigid (frame or frameless) stereotactic immobilization system[a]. • GammaKnife: Head frame in conjunction with a metal collimator helmet. • Linac-based: Various, including rigid frame with external skull fixation, noninvasive modified GTC frame (noninvasive fixation by use of a dental plate), or a three-point thermoplastic mask with a modified stereotactic frame. **CT**: Thin-cut CT images (1.0–1.5 mm slice thickness) ideally with IV contrast spanning from vertex to mid-cervical spine. **Diagnostic imaging**: Co-registration of planning CT with the appropriate diagnostic imaging (contrast-enhanced MRI or CT) for target and OAR delineation. MRI sequences should include pre- and post-contrast T1-weighted, pre-contrast T2-weighted and FLAIR, and multi-planar (axial, sagittal, and coronal) post-contrast T1-weighted images. Post-contrast T1-weighted images with thin (1 mm) sectioning should be obtained. High-resolution series, such as MP-RAGE, should be obtained for contrast-enhancing targets. Cranial nerves may be more readily visualized on a CISS or 3D FIESTA series as needed [26].
Image guidance	Imaging options include CBCT, orthogonal KV X-rays; misalignment corrections via positional systems with four or six rotational axes of the patient couch/platform.

(continued)

Table 8.3 (continued)

Target delineation	The tumor bed/GTV is defined as the enhancing lesion on the post-gadolinium T1-weighted MRI ([26], and see Fig. 8.1a). Target delineation may be improved with DOTATOC-/DOTATATE-PET guidance [27, 28]. The GTV does not include any surrounding edema on T2-weighted images. The linearly enhancing dura adjacent to the primary meningioma is defined as the dural tail, which can be included in the GTV electively (the proximal component only) or if there is any enhancing nodularity [26]. Dural tail: Defined as presence of ≥2 consecutive slices and > 1 imaging plane, tapering adjacently from the mass with increased contrast enhancement [29, 30]. This is most often an inflammatory effect of the tumor that does not require inclusion in grade I tumor target definition. For postoperative cases, the GTV is defined as the resection bed plus any residual nodular enhancement.
Margins	For grade I tumors, GTV = CTV. For grade II tumors, CTV = GTV plus 0–2 mm uniform expansion. CTV margins for grade III tumors must be carefully selected on a case-by-case basis. May consider an additional margin for dural tail or uncertainty in contrast enhancement on T1-weighted images. PTV = CTV plus 0–5 mm uniform expansion (depending on institutional setup error, including accuracy and reproducibility of immobilization). Generally, CTV plus 3–5 mm uniform expansion for standard thermoplastic mask or CTV plus 0–1 mm uniform expansion for a stereotactic frame.
Tumor/target coverage considerations	≥98% of the GTV/CTV should receive the prescription dose. ≥95% of the PTV should receive the prescription dose.
Treatment modality	Linac, GammaKnife, CyberKnife, proton beam
Planning strategies/ assessment	Steep PTV to OAR dose gradients are generated using multiple beam arrangements or non-coplanar arcs together with dose prescription to the steepest portion of the beam profile. For Linac-based SRS, the standard beam profile is shaped with cone collimation or MLCs. An example treatment plan is depicted in Fig. 8.1a. Notably, as target size increases, the dosimetric advantages of SRS tend to decline—As the sharp dose fall-off becomes shallower and the higher doses to adjacent normal tissue become prohibitive, thereby generally precluding safe and effective SRS delivery to targets >3 cm in diameter. The following indices should be generated [31]: **Conformality index**: Prescription isodose volume/target volume (ideally ≤1.5). **Homogeneity index**: Maximum dose to target volume/prescription dose (ideally ≤2). **Gradient index**: Volume receiving half the prescription isodose/volume receiving the full prescription isodose (ideally ≤4).

[a]Based on delivery system and institutional protocol

Abbreviations: *GTC* Gill-Thomas-Cosman, *FLAIR* fluid-attenuated inversion recovery, *MP-RAGE* magnetization-prepared rapid gradient echo, *CISS* constructive interference in steady state, *FIESTA* 3D fast imaging employing steady-state acquisition, *Linac* linear accelerator

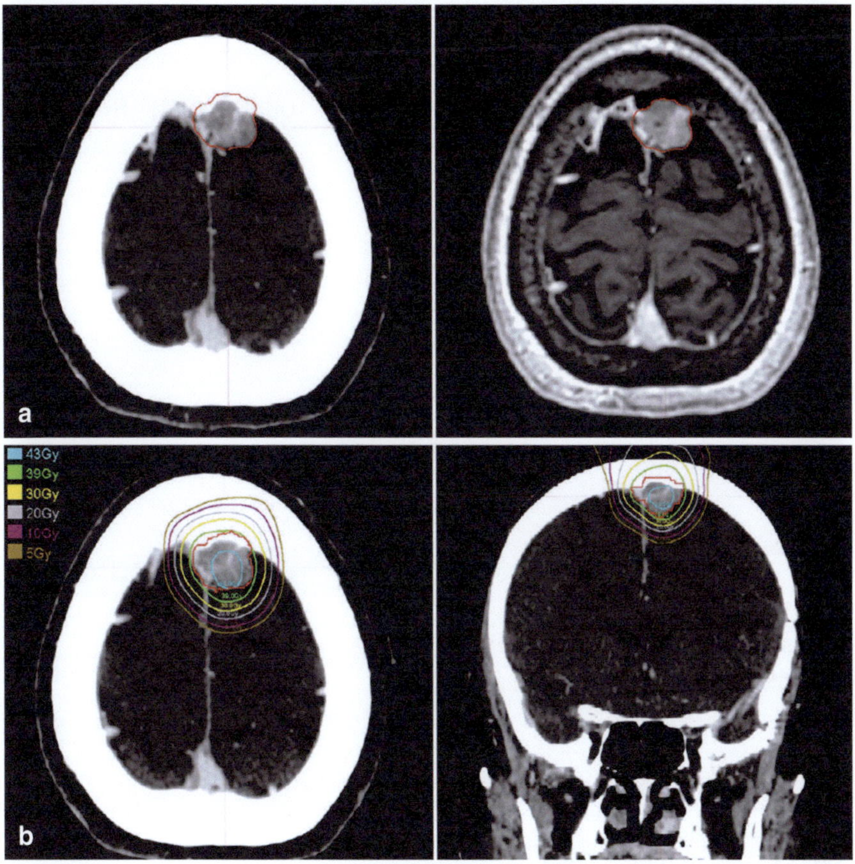

Fig. 8.1 A 2.6 cc left frontal meningioma; GTV target delineation in red. (**a**) Simulation CT (left), post-contrast T1-weighted MRI (right). (**b**) Treatment plans with prescription IDL in green, effective normalization 90%. FSRT, 3 GyRBE protons × 13 fx (39 Gy RBE total). Simulation CT axial (left) and coronal (right). IDL, isodose line

8.6 Commonly Used Dose/Fractionation Schemes (Table 8.4)

Table 8.4 Commonly used dose/fractionation schemes

Commonlyused dose/fractionation schemes		
	Patient selection considerations	Dose/fx
SRS	• More than 3–5 mm from optic apparatus • Optic nerve sheath and tuberculum sellae meningiomas are generally a contraindication to SRS (therapeutic doses exceed OAR tolerance)	WHO grade I: 12–15 Gy × 1 fx, prescribed to the 50%, 70–80%, 90% and 50–90% prescription isodose lines for GammaKnife, CyberKnife, proton beam, and Linac [8–12] WHO grade II–III: 15–21 Gy × 1 fx [13–16]
FSRT	Larger tumor and/or < 2–3 mm from optic apparatus or other critical OAR	WHO grade I: 5 Gy × 5 fx [17–19], WHO grade II–III: 7-8 Gy × 3 fx or 5 Gy × 5 fx [13, 15]

Abbreviations: *fx* fraction(s), *Linac* linear accelerator

Table 8.5 Relevant literature

Dmax[a] (Gy) in criticalstructures for SRS and FSRT				
Organ	Authors' recommendations	TG101 [20]	QUANTEC [21]	HyTEC [22]
Brainstem				
1 fx	≤12 Gy	15 Gy	<12.5 Gy	–
3 fx	≤21 Gy	23.1 Gy	–	–
5 fx	≤30 Gy	31 Gy	–	–
Cochlea				
1 fx	≤11 Gy, median <4.2 Gy [34]	9 Gy	≤14 Gy	–
3 fx	–	17.1 Gy	–	–
5 fx	–	25 Gy	–	–
Optic apparatus				
1 fx	≤8 Gy	10 Gy	–	<10 Gy
3 fx	≤16.5 Gy	17.4 Gy	–	<20 Gy
5 fx	≤25 Gy	25 Gy	–	<25 Gy
Optic chiasm				
1 fx	≤8 Gy	–	<12 Gy	–
3 fx	–	–	–	–
5 fx	–	–	–	–
Optic nerve				
1 fx	≤8 Gy	–	<12 Gy	–
3 fx	–	–	–	–
5 fx	–	–	–	–

[a]Maximum point dose

8.7 Normal Tissue Tolerances

Rates of radiation-induced optic neuropathy are very rare <8 to 10 Gy but reach >10% at single-SRS doses between 12 and 15 Gy [32, 33] (Table 8.5). In a study by Kano et al., patients with vestibular schwannomas treated with GammaKnife SRS had improved serviceable hearing preservation if they received a median central cochlea dose <4.2 Gy [34].

8.8 Patient Management Considerations

- Premedication/prophylactic medication:
  - There is no standard premedication regimen.
  - Consideration of steroids, benzodiazepines, and/or anticonvulsants is dependent on severity and progression of symptoms or neurologic deficit(s), treatment volume/location and number of fractions, if known prior seizures, as well as patient age and/or medical comorbidities.

- Acute toxicity: Side effects are tumor location dependent and include, but are not limited to, rare transient nausea, headache, alopecia, skin erythema, conjunctivitis, and fatigue.
- Late toxicity: Transient complications (3%), permanent neurologic deficits (5–9%), radionecrosis, or delayed CN deficits (<6%). Other late side effects depend on the tumor location and involved OAR [8, 35].

8.9 Follow-Up

- H&P every 6–12 months.
- Yearly imaging (ideally MRI, CT with contrast if non-tolerant or MRI contraindicated, PET imaging may be useful in selected situations) for 4–5 years, then every 2 years.
- For meningiomas close to the optic system, monitor eyesight.
- For cavernous sinus or base of skull locations, monitor for hypopituitarism with regular serum analyses annually or as needed.
  - Recommend endocrinologist for long-term management and monitoring of endocrine dysfunction.

8.10 Relevant Literatures

- SRS and conventionally fractionated radiotherapy are well-established techniques for meningiomas with high local control rates and extensive long-term follow-up data. Nevertheless, local failures may occur many years after treatment, necessitating long-term imaging follow-up [25, 36].
- For grade II and III tumors, results are less favorable and careful patient selection is crucial, especially for grade III tumors. Young patients with grade II meningiomas without previous irradiations and up to one surgical resection may be adequate candidates for SRS [37].
- While FSRT is a promising treatment modality, more mature data are needed for robust evaluation of the long-term efficacy and toxicity profile for FSRT compared to SRS or conventionally fractionated radiotherapy ([6, 17, 38], Table 8.6).

Table 8.6 Relevant literature

Study	Patients (*n*), (tumor location; histopathological grading if available)	Median follow-up (months)	Median tumor vol (cm^3)	Modality, dose, fractionation	Local Control (%)
Torres, 2003 [10]	128 with 156 tumors, SRS 79, FSRT 77 (not reported; 21 atypical meningioma, remaining considered benign)	40.6 (mean)	12.7 (mean)	Linac, 15.6 Gy × 1 fx	• 92% ~3 years
DiBiase, 2004 [39]	162 (21% cavernous sinus, 13% petroclival, 12% posterior fossa; benign tumors)	54	4.5	GammaKnife, 14 Gy × 1 fx	• DFS 86% at 5 years
Kreil, 2005 [40]	200 (34% cavernous sinus, 22% petroclival, 16% sphenoid wing; 99 grade I tumors, remaining considered benign)	95	6.5	GammaKnife, 12 Gy × 1 fx	• 98.5% at 5 years • 97% at 10 years
Kollova, 2007 [41]	368 with 400 tumors (25% cavernous sinus, 12% cerebellopontine angle, 11% tentorium; all considered benign)	60	4.4	GammaKnife, 12.5 Gy × 1 fx	• 98% at 5 years
Feigl, 2007 [42]	214 with 243 tumors (28% cavernous sinus, 13% sphenoid wing, 13% falx; 214 grade I tumors, 29 grade II tumors)	24 (mean)	6.5 (mean)	GammaKnife, mean 13.6 Gy × 1 fx	• 86% at 4 years
Kondziolka, 2008 [8]	972 (71% skull base; 54 grade II tumors, 29 grade III tumors, remaining considered benign)	48 (mean)	7.4	GammaKnife, mean 14 Gy × 1 fx	• 87% at 10 years
Gorman, 2008 [43]	38 (100% skull base; 2 grade II tumors, remaining considered benign)	47	8.3	Linac, 2.5 Gy × 15 fx	100%
Choi, 2010 [13]	25 (all grade 2 tumors)	28	5.3	CyberKnife, 21 Gy × 1 fx	• 93% at 1 year • 93% at 2 years • 54% at 3 years
Mahadevan, 2011 [9]	16 (100% skull base; not reported)	22	10.5 (mean)	CyberKnife, mean 5.62 Gy × 5 fx	100%

Table 8.6 (continued)

Study	Patients (*n*), (tumor location; histopathological grading if available)	Median follow-up (months)	Median tumor vol (cm^3)	Modality, dose, fractionation	Local Control (%)
Halasz, 2011 [11]	50 (31% cavernous sinus, 16% cerebellopontine angle, 16% falx; 6 tumors with atypical features, remaining considered benign)	32	2.1	Proton beam, 13 Gy (RBE) × 1 fx	• 94% at 3 years • 90% at last follow-up
Han, 2014 [18]	220, SRS 55, FSRT 22, conventional 143 (100% skull base; 10 grade II/III tumors, remaining considered benign)	32	2.8 4.8 11.1	Linac, 12.5 Gy × 1 fx (SRS), 5 Gy × 5 fx (FSRT), 1.8 Gy × 28 fx (conventional fx)	• SRS 91% • FSRT 94% • conventional 95%
Smith, 2014 [44]	28 (50% skull base; 2 tumors with atypical features, remaining considered benign)	32.6	14.7	CyberKnife, 4.5–6 Gy × 5 fx	100%
Navarria, 2015 [45]	26 (100% skull base; not reported)	24.5	13	Linac, 5 Gy × 5 fx	100%
Conti, 2015 [46]	39 (100% perioptic; not reported)	15	7.5	CyberKnife, 5 Gy × 5 fx	100%
Mehta, 2017 [47]	57 (100% foramen magnum; 18 grade I tumors, remaining considered benign)	36 (radiographic)	2.9	GammaKnife, 12.5 Gy × 1 fx	PFS at 5 and 10 years: 92%
Conti, 2020 [19]	156 (46% perioptic/ anterior fossa, 28% petroclival; 49 grade I tumors, remaining considered benign)	36.6	7.5	CyberKnife, 5 Gy × 5 fx	PFS: • 95% at 2 years • 90% at 5 years • 80% at 10 years
Shepherd, 2021 [14]	271 (52% convexity, 37% parasagittal; 233 grade II tumors, 38 grade III tumors)	36.2 (radiographic mean)	9.7 (mean)	GammaKnife, 14.8 Gy × 1 fx	PFS: • 83% at 1 year • 66% at 2 years • 33% at 5 years
Ehret, 2022 [12]	62 (100% foramen magnum; 22 grade I tumors, 1 grade II tumor, remaining considered benign)	29	2.6	CyberKnife, 14 Gy × 1 fx	100%
Pinzi, 2022 [17]	178 (87% skull base; all considered benign)	53	10.5	CyberKnife, 5 Gy × 5 fx	• 95% at 5 years

Abbreviations: *fx* fraction(s), *vol* volume, *Linac* linear accelerator, *PFS* progression-free survival, *DFS* disease-free survival

References

1. Louis DN, Perry A, Wesseling P, Brat DJ, Cree IA, Figarella-Branger D, Hawkins C, Ng HK, Pfister SM, Reifenberger G, Soffietti R, von Deimling A, Ellison DW. The 2021 WHO classification of tumors of the central nervous system: a summary. Neuro Oncol. 2021;23(8):1231–51.
2. Lee JH. Meningiomas: diagnosis, treatment, and outcome. London: Springer; 2008.
3. Louis DN, Perry A, Reifenberger G, von Deimling A, Figarella-Branger D, Cavenee WK, et al. The 2016 World Health Organization classification of tumors of the central nervous system: a summary. Acta Neuropathol. 2016;131(6):803–20.
4. Simpson D. The recurrence of intracranial meningiomas after surgical treatment. J Neurol Neurosurg Psychiatry. 1957;20(1):22–39.
5. Pollock BE, Stafford SL, Utter A, Giannini C, Schreiner SA. Stereotactic radiosurgery provides equivalent tumor control to Simpson grade 1 resection for patients with small- to medium-size meningiomas. Int J Radiat Oncol Biol Phys. 2003;55(4):1000–5.
6. Bin-Alamer O, Alnefaie N, Qedair J, Chaudhary A, Hallak H, Abdulbaki A, Mallela AN, Palmisciano P, Gersey ZC, Legarreta AD, Labib MA, Zada G, Sheehan JP, Couldwell WT, Lunsford LD, Abou-Al-Shaar H. Single session versus multisession stereotactic radiosurgery for the management of intracranial meningiomas: a systematic review and meta-analysis. Single session versus multisession stereotactic radiosurgery for the management of intracranial meningiomas: a systematic review and metaanalysis. J Neuro Oncol. 2021;161(2):215–24.
7. Terpolilli NA, Ueberschaer M, Niyazi M, Hintschich C, Egensperger R, Muacevic A, Thon N, Tonn JC, Schichor C. Longterm outcome in orbital meningiomas: progression-free survival after targeted resection combined with early or postponed postoperative radiotherapy. J Neurosurg. 2018;133(2):302–12.
8. Kondziolka D, Mathieu D, Lunsford LD, Martin JJ, Madhok R, Niranjan A, Flickinger JC. Radiosurgery as definitive management of intracranial meningiomas. Neurosurgery. 2008;62(1):53–8; discussion 8–60.
9. Mahadevan A, Floyd S, Wong E, Chen C, Kasper E. Clinical outcome after hypofractionated stereotactic radiotherapy (HSRT) for benign skull base tumors. Comput Aided Surg. 2011;16(3):112–20.
10. Torres RC, Frighetto L, De Salles AA, Goss B, Medin P, Solberg T, et al. Radiosurgery and stereotactic radiotherapy for intracranial meningiomas. Neurosurg Focus. 2003;14(5):e5.
11. Halasz LM, Bussière MR, Dennis ER, Niemierko A, Chapman PH, Loeffler JS, Shih HA. Proton stereotactic radiosurgery for the treatment of benign meningiomas. Int J Radiat Oncol Biol Phys. 2011;81(5):1428–35.
12. Ehret F, Kufeld M, Fürweger C, Haidenberger A, Fichte S, Lehrke R, Senger C, Kaul D, Bleif M, Becker G, Rueß D, Ruge M, Schichor C, Tonn JC, Muacevic A. The role of stereotactic radiosurgery in the management of foramen magnum meningiomas —a multicenter analysis and review of the literature. Cancers. 2022;14(2):341.
13. Choi CY, Soltys SG, Gibbs IC, Harsh GR, Jackson PS, Lieberson RE, Chang SD, Adler JR. Cyberknife stereotactic radiosurgery for treatment of atypical (WHO grade II) cranial meningiomas. Neurosurgery. 2010;67(5):1180–8.
14. Shepard MJ, Xu Z, Kearns K, Li C, Chatrath A, Sheehan K, Sheehan D, Faramand A, Niranjan A, Kano H, Gurewitz J, Bernstein K, Liscak R, Guseynova K, Grills IS, Parzen JS, Cifarelli CP, Rehman AA, Atik A, Bakhsheshian J, Zada G, Chang E, Giannotta S, Speckter H, Wu HM, Kondziolka D, Golfinos JG, Mathieu D, Lee CC, Warnick RE, Lunsford LD, Sheehan JP. Stereotactic radiosurgery for atypical (World Health Organization II) and anaplastic (World Health Organization III) meningiomas. Neurosurgery. 2021;88(5):980–8.
15. Acker G, Meinert F, Conti A, Kufeld M, Jelgersma C, Nguyen P, Kluge A, Lukas M, Loebel F, Pasemann D, Kaul D, Budach V, Vajkoczy P, Senger C. Image-guided robotic radiosurgery for treatment of recurrent grade II and III meningiomas. A singlecenter study. World Neurosurg. 2019;131:e96–e107.

16. Kano H, Takahashi JA, Katsuki T, Araki N, Oya N, Hiraoka M, Hashimoto N. Stereotactic radiosurgery for atypical and anaplastic meningiomas. J Neuro Oncol. 2007;84(1):41–7.
17. Pinzi V, Marchetti M, Viola A, Tramacere I, Cane I, Iezzoni C, Fariselli L. Hypofractionated radiosurgery for large or in critical-site intracranial meningioma: results of a phase 2 prospective study. Int J Radiat Oncol Biol Phys. 2022;115(1):153–63.
18. Han J, Girvigian MR, Chen JC, Miller MJ, Lodin K, Rahimian J, Arellano A, Cahan BL, Kaptein JS. A comparative study of stereotactic radiosurgery, hypofractionated, and fractionated stereotactic radiotherapy in the treatment of skull base meningioma. Am J Clin Oncol. 2014;37(3):255–60.
19. Conti A, Pontoriero A, Iatì G, Cardali SM, Brogna A, Friso F, Rosetti V, Zoli M, Parisi S, Cacciola A, Lillo S, Pergolizzi S, Mazzatenta D. Image-guided multisession radiosurgery of skull base meningiomas. Cancers. 2020;12(12):3569.
20. Benedict SH, Yenice KM, Followill D, Galvin JM, Hinson W, Kavanagh B, et al. Stereotactic body radiation therapy: the report of AAPM task group 101. Med Phys. 2010;37(8):4078–101.
21. Marks LB, Yorke ED, Jackson A, Haken Ten RK, Constine LS, Eisbruch A, et al. Use of normal tissue complication probability models in the clinic. Int J Radiat Oncol Biol Phys. 2010;76(3 Suppl):S10–9.
22. Milano MT, Grimm J, Soltys SG, Yorke E, Moiseenko V, Tomé WA, Sahgal A, Xue J, Ma L, Solberg TD, Kirkpatrick JP, Constine LS, Flickinger JC, Marks LB, El Naqa I. Single- and multi-fraction stereotactic radiosurgery dose tolerances of the optic pathways. Int J Radiat Oncol Biol Phys. 2018;110(1):87–99.
23. Gagliardi F, De Domenico P, Snider S, Pompeo E, Roncelli F, Barzaghi LR, Acerno S, Mortini P. Efficacy of radiotherapy and stereotactic radiosurgery as adjuvant or salvage treatment in atypical and anaplastic (WHO grade II and III) meningiomas: a systematic review and meta-analysis. Neurosurg Rev. 2023;46:1–71.
24. Bergner A, Maier AD, Mirian C, Mathiesen TI. Adjuvant radiotherapy and stereotactic radiosurgery in grade 3 meningiomas—a systematic review and meta-analysis. Neurosurg Rev. 2022;45(4):2639–58.
25. Goldbrunner R, Stavrinou P, Jenkinson MD, Sahm F, Mawrin C, Weber DC, Preusser M, Minniti G, Lund-Johansen M, Lefranc F, Houdart E, Sallabanda K, Le Rhun E, Nieuwenhuizen D, Tabatabai G, Soffietti R, Weller M. EANO guideline on the diagnosis and management of meningiomas. Neuro Oncol. 2021;23(11):1821–34.
26. Lee NY, Riaz N, Lu JJ. Target volume delineation and field setup: a practical guide for conformal and intensity-modulated radiation therapy. Heidelberg: Springer; 2015.
27. Galldiks N, Albert NL, Sommerauer M, Grosu AL, Ganswindt U, Law I, Preusser M, Le Rhun E, Vogelbaum MA, Zadeh G, Dhermain F, Weller M, Langen KJ, Tonn JC. PET imaging in patients with meningioma—report of the RANO/PET Group. Neuro Oncol. 2017;19(12):1576–87.
28. Perlow HK, Siedow M, Gokun Y, McElroy J, Matsui J, Zoller W, Beyer S, Arnett A, Blakaj D, Boulter D, Fritz J, Miller E, Raval R, Kleefisch C, Bovi J, Palmer JD. 68Ga-DOTATATE PET-based radiation contouring creates more precise radiation volumes for patients with meningioma. Int J Radiat Oncol Biol Phys. 2022;113(4):859–65.
29. Rokni-Yazdi H, Sotoudeh H. Prevalence of "dural tail sign" in patients with different intracranial pathologies. Eur J Radiol. 2006;60(1):42–5.
30. Goldsher D, Litt AW, Pinto RS, Bannon KR, Kricheff II. Dural "tail" associated with meningiomas on Gd-DTPA-enhanced MR images: characteristics, differential diagnostic value, and possible implications for treatment. Radiology. 1990;176(2):447–50.
31. Balagamwala EH, Suh JH, Barnett GH, Khan MK, Neyman G, Cai RS, et al. The importance of the conformality, heterogeneity, and gradient indices in evaluating gamma knife radiosurgery treatment plans for intracranial meningiomas. Int J Radiat Oncol Biol Phys. 2012;83(5):1406–13.
32. Mayo C, Martel MK, Marks LB, Flickinger J, Nam J, Kirkpatrick J. Radiation dose-volume effects of optic nerves and chiasm. Int J Radiat Oncol Biol Phys. 2010;76(3 Suppl):S28–35.

33. Tishler RB, Loeffler JS, Lunsford LD, Duma C, Alexander E 3rd, Kooy HM, et al. Tolerance of cranial nerves of the cavernous sinus to radiosurgery. Int J Radiat Oncol Biol Phys. 1993;27(2):215–21.
34. Kano H, Kondziolka D, Khan A, Flickinger JC, Lunsford LD. Predictors of hearing preservation after stereotactic radiosurgery for acoustic neuroma. J Neurosurg. 2009;111(4):863–73.
35. Minniti G, Amichetti M, Enrici RM. Radiotherapy and radiosurgery for benign skull base meningiomas. Radiat Oncol. 2009;4:42.
36. Lippitz BE, Bartek J Jr, Mathiesen T, Förander P. Ten-year follow-up after Gamma Knife radiosurgery of meningioma and review of the literature. Acta Neurochir. 2020;162(9):2183–96.
37. Kowalchuk RO, Shepard MJ, Sheehan K, Sheehan D, Faramand A, Niranjan A, Kano H, Gurewitz J, Bernstein K, Liscak R, Guseynova K, Grills IS, Parzen JS, Cifarelli CP, Rehman AA, Atik A, Bakhsheshian J, Zada G, Chang E, Giannotta S, Speckter H, Wu HM, Kondziolka D, Mathieu D, Lee CC, Warnick RE, Lunsford LD, Trifiletti DM, Sheehan JP. Treatment of WHO grade 2 meningiomas with stereotactic radiosurgery: identification of an optimal group for SRS using RPA. Int J Radiat Oncol Biol Phys. 2021; 110(3):804–14.
38. Fatima N, Meola A, Pollom EL, Soltys SG, Chang SD. Stereotactic radiosurgery versus stereotactic radiotherapy in the management of intracranial meningiomas: a systematic review and meta-analysis. Neurosurg Focus. 2019;46(6):E2.
39. DiBiase SJ, Kwok Y, Yovino S, Arena C, Naqvi S, Temple R, et al. Factors predicting local tumor control after gamma knife stereotactic radiosurgery for benign intracranial meningiomas. Int J Radiat Oncol Biol Phys. 2004;60(5):1515–9.
40. Kreil W, Luggin J, Fuchs I, Weigl V, Eustacchio S, Papaefthymiou G. Long term experience of gamma knife radiosurgery for benign skull base meningiomas. J Neurol Neurosurg Psychiatry. 2005;76(10):1425–30.
41. Kollova A, Liscak R, Novotny J Jr, Vladyka V, Simonova G, Janouskova L. Gamma knife surgery for benign meningioma. J Neurosurg. 2007;107(2):325–36.
42. Feigl GC, Samii M, Horstmann GA. Volumetric follow-up of meningiomas: a quantitative method to evaluate treatment outcome of gamma knife radiosurgery. Neurosurgery. 2007;61(2):281–6, discussion 6–7.
43. Gorman L, Ruben J, Myers R, Dally M. Role of hypofractionated stereotactic radiotherapy in treatment of skull base meningiomas. J Clin Neurosci. 2008;15(8):856–62.
44. Smith DE, Ghosh S, O'Leary M, Chu C, Brody D. Hypofractionated radiosurgery for meningiomas—a safer alternative for large tumors? Transl Cancer Res. 2014;3(4):367–72.
45. Navarria YY, Pessina F, Cozzi L, Clerici E, Villa E, Ascolese AM, et al. Hypofractionated stereotactic radiation therapy in skull base meningiomas. J Neuro Oncol. 2015;124(2):283–9.
46. Conti A, Pontoriero A, Midili F, Iati G, Siragusa C, Tomasello C, et al. CyberKnife multisession stereotactic radiosurgery and hypofractionated stereotactic radiotherapy for perioptic meningiomas: intermediate-term results and radiobiological considerations. Springerplus. 2015;4:37.
47. Mehta GU, Zenonos G, Patibandla MR, Lin CJ, Wolf A, Grills I, Mathieu D, McShane B, Lee JY, Blas K, Kondziolka D, Lee CC, Lunsford LD, Sheehan JP. Outcomes of stereotactic radiosurgery for foramen magnum meningiomas: an international multicenter study. J Neurosurg. 2018;129(2):383–9.

Chapter 9
Vestibular Schwannoma

Felix Ehret, Katelyn M. Atkins, Marc Bussière, and Helen A. Shih

9.1 Introduction

Vestibular schwannoma is a benign intracranial tumor, also known as acoustic neurinoma. It usually causes progressive hearing loss and tinnitus. Stereotactic radiosurgery (SRS) and conventionally fractionated radiotherapy have well-established track records with high local control rates and robust long-term follow-up data. This chapter summarizes hypofractionated radiotherapy techniques, including SRS and fractionated stereotactic radiotherapy (FSRT), for vestibular schwannomas.

9.2 Pearls

- Incidence is estimated at 0.6–0.8 per 100,000 person-years and is increasing over time.
- Increased incidence is due (at least in part) to incidental diagnosis in asymptomatic patients in the setting of widespread MRI and CT imaging—as vestibular schwannomas are identified on 0.2% of MRIs in asymptomatic patients.

F. Ehret
Department of Radiation Oncology, Charité - Universitätsmedizin Berlin, Berlin, Germany
e-mail: felix.ehret@charite.de

K. M. Atkins
Department of Radiation Oncology, Cedars-Sinai Medical Center, Los Angeles, CA, USA
e-mail: katelyn.atkins@cshs.org

M. Bussière · H. A. Shih (✉)
Department of Radiation Oncology, Massachusetts General Hospital, Francis H. Burr Proton Therapy Center, Boston, MA, USA
e-mail: bussiere.marc@mgh.harvard.edu; hshih@mgh.harvard.edu

O. Kaidar-Person, R. Chen (eds.), *Hypofractionated and Stereotactic Radiation Therapy*, https://doi.org/10.1007/978-3-031-47701-0_9

- Comprise 8% of adult intracranial tumors, 80–90% arise within the cerebellopontine angle, with more than 90% being sporadic and unilateral.
- The median age of diagnosis is 50 years; rare in children with the exception of patients with NF2.
- Both sporadic and NF2-associated vestibular schwannomas are routinely associated with biallelic inactivating mutations of the tumor-suppressor gene *NF2* (located on 22q12).
  - Bilateral vestibular schwannomas are pathognomonic for NF2 and patients with NF2 commonly manifest symptoms by 20–30 years of age.
- For sporadic lesions, the estimated average growth rate is 1–2 mm per year, while for NF2-associated lesions it is 3 mm per year.
- The cystic schwannoma subtype displays a more aggressive growth pattern, but malignant transformation is rare.
- The most common symptoms include hearing loss (95% objective, 66% subjective; usually gradual in tempo—but a subset present with sudden hearing loss), tinnitus (63%), imbalance or vertigo (61%, generally mild-to-moderate unsteadiness with ambulation, tilting, or veering, with true spinning vertigo unusual), facial paresthesias or pain (17%, typical onset more than 2 years after presence of hearing loss), facial paresis or taste disturbance (6%), and less commonly cerebellar symptoms or lower cranial nerve deficits.
- Local anatomy:
  - The cerebellopontine angle is bounded by the temporal bone laterally, the brainstem medially, the cerebellum superiorly and posteriorly, and the inferior cranial nerves inferiorly (CN IX–XI).
  - Additional structures within the cerebellopontine angle include CN VII and the anterior inferior cerebellar artery.
  - The vestibular and cochlear nerve roots arise from the vestibular and cochlear apparatus, respectively, which together form the vestibulocochlear nerve, which travels through the internal auditory canal to the cerebellopontine angle.
  - The majority of vestibular schwannomas arise within the internal auditory canal from the superior or inferior branches of the vestibular nerve, and rarely arise from the cochlear nerve.
  - The natural history is characterized by progressive growth within the internal auditory canal, extending to the cerebellopontine angle with associated compression of nearby cranial nerves—most notably the facial and trigeminal nerves—as well as the brainstem.
- Medical workup:
  - H&P, including assessment of performance status, with emphasis on preceding neurological symptoms (e.g., hearing loss, tinnitus, imbalance, facial paresthesias, or weakness) and thorough neurologic examination including detailed examination of cranial nerves, balance, and ambulation.

- Weber and Rinne testing may suggest asymmetric sensorineural hearing loss.
- Romberg and Hall-Pike maneuvers are typically normal.
- Audiometry: Initial screening test of choice, as 95% of patients will have an abnormal test, most commonly revealing asymmetric sensorineural hearing loss, preferentially at higher frequencies with impaired speech discrimination scores out of proportion to the degree of hearing loss.
- Vestibular testing: Not commonly performed as a screening modality given decreased sensitivity, but may show decreased or absent caloric response on the involved side.
- Brainstem-evoked response audiometry is less commonly performed.

- Imaging workup:
  - CT: Appear as a well-defined isodense, contrast-enhancing mass within the internal auditory canal with variable extension into the cerebellopontine angle, and rarely harbor calcifications (as opposed to meningiomas).
  - MRI: Gold standard imaging modality; typically appear iso- or hypointense to the pons on T1-weighted images, heterogeneously hyperintense on T2-weighted images, and strongly and homogenously contrast enhancing.
  - Purely intracanalicular vestibular schwannomas are usually round or oval in shape, while those extending into the cistern have a spherical extra-internal auditory canal component with a tail-like taper into the internal auditory canal.
  - Post-contrast T1-weighted images with thin (1 mm) sectioning through the internal auditory canal are ideal. High-resolution constructive interference in steady state (CISS) or 3D fast imaging employing steady-state acquisition (FIESTA) sequences can show enhanced visualization of structures surrounded by CSF, thereby assisting in delineation of the tumor and cranial nerves.
  - High-resolution CT with and without contrast can be used as an alternative in patients who cannot tolerate MRI.

- Management options include surveillance, surgical resection, SRS, FSRT, or conventionally fractionated radiotherapy.
- Goals of therapy are to maximize local tumor and preservation of function (i.e., minimizing hearing loss and other cranial nerve deficits such as facial or trigeminal nerve dysfunction).
- Surgical resection is performed via a suboccipital (retrosigmoid), middle fossa, or translabyrinthine approach. Hearing preservation rates for suboccipital and middle fossa approaches range from 20 to 71% with smaller tumor size and extent of preoperative hearing level of variable prediction for hearing preservation; the general indications and limitations for each are as follows [1–3]:

  - Suboccipital (retrosigmoid):
  - Indications: Any tumor size, can attempt hearing preservation, lower risk of facial nerve injury.
  - Limitations: Increased incidence of headache and CSF leak, incomplete visualization of the internal auditory canal fundus.
  - Middle fossa:

- Indications: Small tumors ≤1.5–2 cm and hearing preservation can be attempted (highest rates of hearing preservation among surgical approaches).
- Limitations: Increased risk of facial nerve damage, incomplete visualization of the internal auditory canal fundus.
- Translabyrinthine:
- Indications: Non-serviceable hearing in affected ear, any tumor size, and complete visualization of the internal auditory canal.
- Limitations: Hearing is inevitably sacrificed.

9.3 Staging, Grading, and Other Classifications

Vestibular schwannomas are divided into four grades based on size and location according to the Koos grading system (Table 9.1, [4]).

Table 9.1 Koos grading system for vestibular schwannomas

Koos grading system for vestibular schwannomas[a]	
Grade	Tumor localization/extension
I	Purely intracanalicular
II	Extension into the CPA (without contacting the brainstem):
IIA	≤ 10 mm from the Porus acusticus
IIB	11–18 mm from the Porus acusticus
III	Large tumor extending to the CPA cistern without brainstem displacement
IV	Very large tumor with displacement of brainstem and/or cranial nerves

[a]Modified from Koos et al. [4]
Abbreviation: *CPA* cerebellopontine angle

9.4 Patient Selection for SRS or FSRT

- Factors influencing treatment recommendations include patient age, medical comorbidities (e.g., NF2), cranial nerve deficits, tumor size and/or growth rate, presenting symptoms, competing symptoms (i.e., contralateral hearing loss), and proximity to critical organs at risk (OAR, such as brainstem, cochlea).
- Prophylactic irradiation of small tumors with stable size and good hearing should be avoided due to a high frequency of treatment-associated hearing decline [5].
- For single-fraction SRS, targets should generally be <3 cm.
- For FSRT, tumors may be larger (>3 to 4 cm), in closer proximity to or involving OAR (e.g., abutting the brainstem).
- Patients with non-serviceable hearing (typically <50% speech discrimination at >50 dB) may not benefit from therapeutic approaches to preserve hearing [6].

9.5 Treatment Planning Considerations (Table 9.2)

Table 9.2 Treatment planning considerations

Simulation instructions	**Position**: Supine, arms at sides, head and neck neutral. **Immobilization**: A rigid (frame or frameless) stereotactic immobilization system[a]. • GammaKnife: Head frame in conjunction with a metal collimator helmet. • Linac-based: Various, including rigid frame with external skull fixation, noninvasive modified GTC frame (noninvasive fixation by use of a dental plate), or a three-point thermoplastic mask with a modified stereotactic frame. **CT**: Thin-cut CT images (1.0–1.5 mm slice thickness) ideally with IV contrast spanning from vertex to mid-cervical spine. **Diagnostic imaging**: Co-registration of planning CT with the appropriate diagnostic imaging (contrast-enhanced MRI or CT) for target and OAR delineation. MRI sequences should include pre- and post-contrast T1-weighted, pre-contrast T2-weighted and FLAIR, and multi-planar (axial, sagittal, and coronal) post-contrast T1-weighted images. Post-contrast T1-weighted images with thin (1 mm) sectioning should be obtained. High-resolution series, such as MP-RAGE, should be obtained for contrast-enhancing targets. Cranial nerves may be more readily visualized on a CISS or 3D FIESTA series [7].
Image guidance	Imaging options include CBCT, orthogonal KV X-rays; misalignment corrections via positional systems with four or six rotational axes of the patient couch/platform.
Target delineation	The GTV is defined as the enhancing lesion on the post-gadolinium T1-weighted MRI ([7], and see Fig. 9.1a).
Margins	GTV = CTV. PTV = CTV plus 0–2 mm uniform expansion (depending on institutional setup error, including accuracy and reproducibility of immobilization).
Tumor/target coverage considerations	≥98% of the GTV/CTV should receive the prescription dose. ≥95% of the PTV should receive the prescription dose.

(continued)

Table 9.2 (continued)

Treatment modality	Linac, GammaKnife, CyberKnife, proton beam
Planningstrategies/ assessment	Steep PTV to OAR dose gradients are generated using multiple beam arrangements or non-coplanar arcs together with dose prescription to the steepest portion of the beam profile. For Linac-based SRS, the standard beam profile is shaped by collimation with cones or MLCs. An example treatment plan is depicted in Fig. 9.1b. Notably, as target size increases, the dosimetric advantages of SRS tend to decline—As the sharp dose fall-off becomes shallower and the higher doses to adjacent normal tissue become prohibitive, thereby generally precluding safe and effective SRS delivery to targets >3 cm in diameter. The following indices should be generated [8]: **Conformality index**: Prescription isodose volume/target volume (ideally ≤1.5). **Homogeneity index**: Maximum dose to target volume/prescription dose (ideally ≤2). **Gradient index**: Volume receiving half the prescription isodose/volume receiving the full prescription isodose (ideally ≤4).

[a]Based on delivery system and institutional protocol

Abbreviations: *GTC* Gill-Thomas-Cosman, *FLAIR* fluid-attenuated inversion recovery, *MP-RAGE* magnetization-prepared rapid gradient echo, *CISS* constructive interference in steady state, *FIESTA* 3D fast imaging employing steady-state acquisition, *Linac* linear accelerator

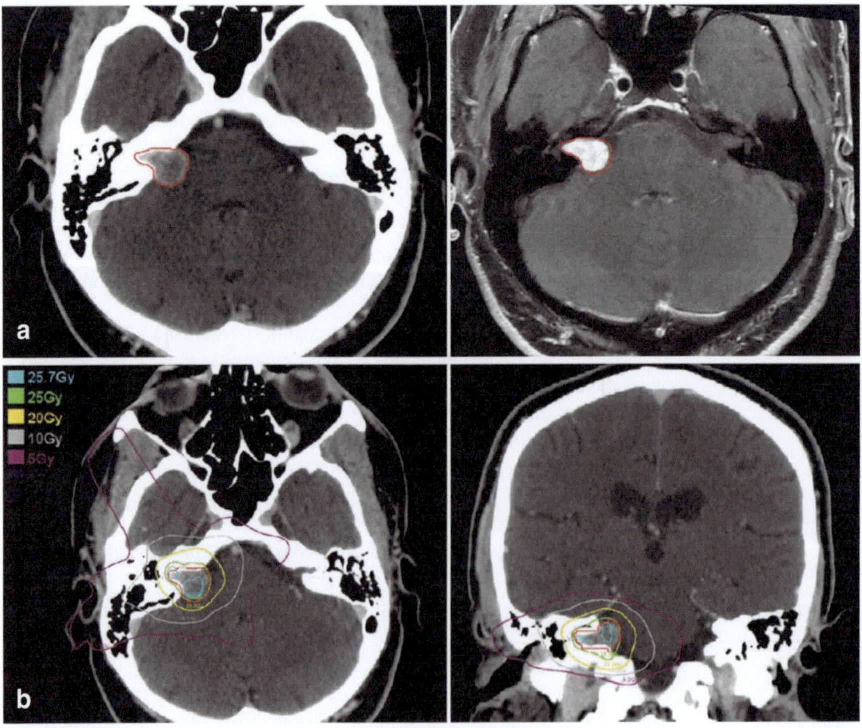

Fig. 9.1 A 1.9 cc right vestibular schwannoma; GTV target delineation in red. (**a**) Simulation CT (left), post-contrast T1-weighted MRI (right). (**b**) Treatment plans with prescription IDL in green, effective normalization 97%. FSRT, 5 Gy × 5 fx (25 Gy total) with 6 MV photon using VMAT. Simulation CT axial (left) and coronal (right). *IDL* isodose line

9.6 Commonly Used Dose/Fractionation Schemes

Commonly utilized dose/fractionation schemes for SRS and FSRT are described in Table 9.3.

Table 9.3 Commonly utilized dose/fractionation schemes for SRS and FSRT

	Patient selection considerations	Dose/fx
SRS	Small, <3 cm	12–13 Gy, prescribed to the 50%, 65%, 70%, and 70–80% prescription isodose lines for GammaKnife, CyberKnife, proton beam, and Linac [9–13]
FSRT	Larger, >3–4 cm, proximity to or involving OAR	6 Gy × 3 fx, 5 Gy × 5 fx [9, 14, 15]

Abbreviations: *fx* fraction(s), *Linac* linear accelerator

Table 9.4 Normal tissue tolerances

Dmax[a] (Gy) incritical structures for SRS and FSRT			
Organ	Authors' recommendations	TG101 [17]	QUANTEC [18]
Brainstem			
1 fx	≤12 Gy	15 Gy	<12.5 Gy
3 fx	≤21 Gy	23.1 Gy	–
5 fx	≤30 Gy	31 Gy	–
Cochlea			
1 fx	≤11 Gy, median <4.2 Gy [16]	9 Gy	≤14 Gy
3 fx	–	17.1 Gy	–
5 fx	–	25 Gy	–

[a]Maximum point dose

9.7 Normal Tissue Tolerances

Improved serviceable hearing preservation has been reported in patients with vestibular schwannomas treated with GammaKnife SRS who received a median central cochlea dose <4.2 Gy [16] (Table 9.4).

9.8 Patient Management Considerations

- Premedication/prophylactic medication:
  - There is no standard premedication regimen.
  - Consideration of steroids is dependent on severity and tempo of symptoms or neurologic deficit(s), treatment volume, number of fractions, as well as patient age and/or medical comorbidities.
- Acute toxicity: Treatment is generally well tolerated, transient dizziness reported in ~17%, hydrocephalus in less than 1% [15, 19].
- Late toxicity: Hearing loss (29–68%), CN V/VII neuropathy (<5%), dizziness (2%) [19, 20].
- Temporary tumor enlargement after irradiation may occur and usually resolves over time without a dedicated treatment [21].

9.9 Follow-Up

- H&P every 6–12 months.
- Yearly imaging (ideally MRI, CT with contrast if non-tolerant or MRI contraindicated) for 4–5 years, then every 2 years.
- Audiometry and vestibular testing as needed.

9.10 Relevant Literature

- The treatment of vestibular schwannomas with SRS and conventionally fractionated radiotherapy is well characterized with excellent local control rates and extensive long-term follow-up [9].
- In recent years FSRT has emerged as a promising treatment technique in patients with large tumors or those in close proximity to or involving critical OAR. However, more mature data are required for adequate evaluation of long-term local control rates as well as associated toxicity profiles for FSRT compared to SRS or conventionally fractionated radiotherapy (Table 9.5, [9, 26]).
- Re-irradiation with SRS for tumor recurrences seems feasible and safe, with only limited data and follow-up available [27].

Table 9.5 Relevant literature

Study	Patients (n)	Median follow-up (years)	Mean tumor vol (cm^3)	Modality, dose, fractionation	LC	Hearing preservation (%)
Prasad 2000 [22]	153	4.3 (mean)	2.8	GammaKnife, 13 Gy × 1 fx	93%	58[a]
Harsh 2002 [13]	68	2.8 (mean, radiographic)	2.4	Proton beam, 12 Gy × 1 fx	2-year: 94% 5-year: 84%	Only six patients with functional hearing before treatment, four lost hearing after irradiation
Hasegawa 2005 [23]	317	7.8	5.6	GammaKnife, 13.2 Gy × 1 fx	PFS: 5-year: 93% 10-year: 92%	13 (>13 Gy)[a] 68 (≤13 Gy)[a]
Lunsford 2005 [10]	829	≥10 for 252 patients	2.5	GammaKnife, 13 Gy × 1 fx	6-year: 98% 10-year: 97%	50–77% of patients (up to 90% in those with intracanalicular tumors)
Friedman 2006 [12]	295	3.3	2.2 (median)	Linac, 12.5 Gy × 1 fx	2-year: 98% 5-year: 90% 10-year: 90%	NA
Chopra 2007 [24]	216	5.7	1.3	GammaKnife, 13 Gy × 1 fx	10-year: 98%	44, 10 years[a]
Fukuoka 2009 [19]	152	>5	2.0	GammaKnife, 12 Gy × 1 fx	5-year: 94% 8-year: 92%	71
Murphy 2011 [20]	103	3.1	1.95	GammaKnife, 13 Gy × 1 fx	92%	NA

(continued)

Table 9.5 (continued)

Study	Patients (*n*)	Median follow-up (years)	Mean tumor vol (cm³)	Modality, dose, fractionation	LC	Hearing preservation (%)
Williams 2002 [14]	125	1.8	Vol (diameter): 1.4 (<3 cm), 8.1 (≥3 cm)	Linac, 5 Gy × 5 fx (<3 cm, *n* = 111), 3 Gy × 10 fx (≥3 cm, *n* = 14)	100%	59[a]
Meijer 2003 [25]	80	2.8 (mean)	2.5 cm (mean diameter)	Linac, 4 Gy × 5 fx (1992–1995), 5 Gy × 5 fx (1995–2000)	5-year: 94%	61
Kapoor 2011 [15]	385	4.7	0.9	Linac, 5 Gy × 5 fx (*n* = 340) or 3 Gy × 10 fx (*n* = 36)	FFS: 97%	NA
Windisch 2019 [11]	996	3.6	0.61 (median)	CyberKnife, 13 Gy × 1 fx	3-year: 97% 5-year: 92% 10-year: 90%	Median hearing loss compared to untreated ear: 17 dB; 23 dB at one year, 29 dB at 5 years
Santa Maria 2018 [5]	576 (244 tumors/ears with measurable hearing before SRS)	5.5 (mean)	2.2	CyberKnife, 6 Gy × 3 fx	NA	<70% at 1 year, 50% at 3 years, 40% at 5 years

[a]Gardner-Robertson Class I–II
Abbreviations: *vol* volume, *LC* local control, *fx* fraction(s), *PFS* progression-free survival, *NA* not available, *FFS* freedom from surgery, *Linac* linear accelerator

References

1. Brackmann DE, Owens RM, Friedman RA, Hitselberger WE, De la Cruz A, House JW, et al. Prognostic factors for hearing preservation in vestibular schwannoma surgery. Am J Otol. 2000;21(3):417–24.
2. Betchen SA, Walsh J, Post KD. Long-term hearing preservation after surgery for vestibular schwannoma. J Neurosurg. 2005;102(1):6–9.
3. Khrais T, Sanna M. Hearing preservation surgery in vestibular schwannoma. J Laryngol Otol. 2006;120(5):366–70.
4. Koos WT, Spetzler RF, Lang J. Color atlas of microneurosurgery, 2. Stuttgart: Thieme; 1993.
5. Santa Maria PL, Shi Y, Gurgel RK, Corrales CE, Soltys SG, Santa Maria C, Murray K, Chang SD, Blevins NH, Gibbs IC, Jackler RK. Long-term hearing outcomes following stereotactic radiosurgery in vestibular schwannoma patients—a retrospective cohort study. Neurosurgery. 2018;85(4):550–9.
6. Wackym PA. Stereotactic radiosurgery, microsurgery, and expectant management of acoustic neuroma: basis for informed consent. Otolaryngol Clin N Am. 2005;38(4):653–70.

7. Lee NY, Riaz N, Lu JJ. Target volume delineation and field setup: a practical guide for conformal and intensity-modulated radiation therapy. Heidelberg: Springer; 2015.
8. Balagamwala EH, Suh JH, Barnett GH, Khan MK, Neyman G, Cai RS, et al. The importance of the conformality, heterogeneity, and gradient indices in evaluating gamma knife radiosurgery treatment plans for intracranial meningiomas. Int J Radiat Oncol Biol Phys. 2012;83(5):1406–13.
9. Soltys SG, Milano MT, Xue J, Tomé WA, Yorke E, Sheehan J, Ding GX, Kirkpatrick JP, Ma L, Sahgal A, Solberg T, Adler J, Grimm J, El Naqa I. Stereotactic radiosurgery for vestibular schwannomas: tumor control probability analyses and recommended reporting standards. Int J Radiat Oncol Biol Phys. 2020;110(1):100–11.
10. Lunsford LD, Niranjan A, Flickinger JC, Maitz A, Kondziolka D. Radiosurgery of vestibular schwannomas: summary of experience in 829 cases. J Neurosurg. 2005;102(Suppl):195.
11. Windisch PY, Tonn JC, Fürweger C, Wowra B, Kufeld M, Schichor C, Muacevic A. Clinical results after single-fraction radiosurgery for 1,002 vestibular schwannomas. Cureus. 2019;11(12):e6390.
12. Friedman WA, Bradshaw P, Myers A, Bova FJ. Linear accelerator radiosurgery for vestibular schwannomas. J Neurosurg. 2006;105(5):657–61.
13. Harsh GR, Thornton AF, Chapman PH, Bussiere MR, Rabinov JD, Loeffler JS. Proton beam stereotactic radiosurgery of vestibular schwannomas. Int J Radiat Oncol Biol Phys. 2002;54(1):35–44.
14. Williams JA. Fractionated stereotactic radiotherapy for acoustic neuromas. Int J Radiat Oncol Biol Phys. 2002;54(2):500–4.
15. Kapoor S, Batra S, Carson K, Shuck J, Kharkar S, Gandhi R, et al. Long-term outcomes of vestibular schwannomas treated with fractionated stereotactic radiotherapy: an institutional experience. Int J Radiat Oncol Biol Phys. 2011;81(3):647–53.
16. Kano H, Kondziolka D, Khan A, Flickinger JC, Lunsford LD. Predictors of hearing preservation after stereotactic radiosurgery for acoustic neuroma. J Neurosurg. 2009;111(4):863–73.
17. Benedict SH, Yenice KM, Followill D, Galvin JM, Hinson W, Kavanagh B, et al. Stereotactic body radiation therapy: the report of AAPM task group 101. Med Phys. 2010;37(8):4078–101.
18. Marks LB, Yorke ED, Jackson A, Haken Ten RK, Constine LS, Eisbruch A, et al. Use of normal tissue complication probability models in the clinic. Int J Radiat Oncol Biol Phys. 2010;76(3 Suppl):S10–9.
19. Fukuoka S, Takanashi M, Hojyo A, Konishi M, Tanaka C, Nakamura H. Gamma knife radiosurgery for vestibular schwannomas. Prog Neurol Surg. 2009;22(45):62.
20. Murphy ES, Barnett GH, Vogelbaum MA, Neyman G, Stevens GH, Cohen BH, et al. Long-term outcomes of gamma knife radiosurgery in patients with vestibular schwannomas. J Neurosurg. 2011;114(2):432–40.
21. Pollock BE. Management of vestibular schwannomas that enlarge after stereotactic radiosurgery: treatment recommendations based on a 15 year experience. Neurosurgery. 2006;58(2):241–8.
22. Prasad D, Steiner M, Steiner L. Gamma surgery for vestibular schwannoma. J Neurosurg. 2000;92(5):745–59.
23. Hasegawa T, Fujitani S, Katsumata S, Kida Y, Yoshimoto M, Koike J. Stereotactic radiosurgery for vestibular schwannomas: analysis of 317 patients followed more than 5 years. Neurosurgery. 2005;57(2):257–65; discussion-65.
24. Chopra ZR, Kondziolka D, Niranjan A, Lunsford LD, Flickinger JC. Long-term follow-up of acoustic schwannoma radiosurgery with marginal tumor doses of 12 to 13 Gy. Int J Radiat Oncol Biol Phys. 2007;68(3):845–51.
25. Meijer OW, Vandertop WP, Baayen JC, Slotman BJ. Single-fraction vs. fractionated linac-based stereotactic radiosurgery for vestibular schwannoma: a single-institution study. Int J Radiat Oncol Biol Phys. 2003;56(5):1390–6.
26. Persson O, Bartek J Jr, Shalom NB, Wangerid T, Jakola AS, Förander P. Stereotactic radiosurgery vs. fractionated radiotherapy for tumor control in vestibular schwannoma patients: a systematic review. Acta Neurochir. 2017;159(6):1013–21.
27. Balossier A, Régis J, Reyns N, Roche PH, Daniel RT, George M, Faouzi M, Levivier M, Tuleasca C. Repeat stereotactic radiosurgery for progressive vestibular schwannomas after previous radiosurgery: a systematic review and meta-analysis. Neurosurg Rev. 2021;44(6):3177.

Chapter 10
Pituitary Adenoma

Carolyn Savioz, Krishna Reddy, Katelyn M. Atkins, Marc Bussière, and Helen A. Shih

10.1 Introduction

Pituitary adenomas represent a heterogeneous group of benign tumors that can present as an incidental radiographic finding or with a variety of neurologic and/or endocrine symptoms. The goals of therapy are to maximize local control, preservation of normal function, and normalization of endocrine abnormalities. Stereotactic radiosurgery (SRS) and conventionally fractionated radiotherapy are well-established treatments for pituitary adenoma with high local tumor control rates and extensive long-term follow-up data. There has also been recent clinical interest in the application of fractionated stereotactic radiotherapy (FSRT) in patients with large tumors or those abutting or involving the optic apparatus. This chapter summarizes hypofractionated radiotherapy techniques including SRS and FSRT for pituitary adenomas.

C. Savioz
Department of Radiation Oncology, University of Kansas, Kansas City, KS, USA
e-mail: csavioz@kumc.edu

K. Reddy · K. M. Atkins
Department of Radiation Oncology, Massachusetts General Hospital, Boston, MA, USA
e-mail: kreddy@kumc.edu; kmatkins@partners.org

M. Bussière · H. A. Shih (✉)
Department of Radiation Oncology, Massachusetts General Hospital, Francis H. Burr Proton Therapy Center, Boston, MA, USA
e-mail: bussiere.marc@mgh.harvard.edu; hshih@mgh.harvard.edu

O. Kaidar-Person, R. Chen (eds.), *Hypofractionated and Stereotactic Radiation Therapy*, https://doi.org/10.1007/978-3-031-47701-0_10

10.2 Pearls

- Prevalence of pituitary adenomas ranges from 1 in 865 adults to 1 in 2688 adults with approximately 50% being microadenomas (<10 mm) and the rest being macroadenomas (≥10 mm) or giant adenomas (≥40 mm) [1]. However, pooled meta-analyses of autopsy and radiological studies suggest that the estimated prevalence may be as high as one in six persons.
- Genetic predisposition has been identified in multiple endocrine neoplasia (MEN) type 1 syndrome, Carney's syndrome, and isolated familial somatotropinomas.
- Pituitary adenomas can present with a variety of neurologic and/or endocrine symptoms or as an incidental radiographic finding. Approximately, 10% of asymptomatic adults have an MRI-detectable pituitary abnormality compatible with the diagnosis of asymptomatic pituitary adenoma.
- Symptomatic pituitary adenomas usually present with hypopituitarism, hyperpituitarism, and/or symptoms related to mass effect:
  - Hypopituitarism: Short stature in children (GH), failure of postpartum lactation (PRL), hypocortisolism (ACTH), hypogonadism (LH or FSH), or hypothyroidism (thyroid-stimulating hormone, TSH).
  - Hyperpituitarism: Acromegaly or gigantism (GH), galactorrhea or amenorrhea (PRL), Cushing's disease or Nelson's syndrome (ACTH), gonadal dysfunction (LH, FSH), or hyperthyroidism (TSH).
  - Mass effect: Visual impairment is the most common presenting symptom of a nonfunctioning pituitary adenoma due to suprasellar extension with associated optic chiasm compression, classically resulting in bitemporal hemianopsia.
  - Other presenting neurologic symptoms: headaches, diplopia, or homonymous hemianopsia (due to oculomotor nerve compression).
  - Pituitary apoplexy is a rare emergency following infarction or hemorrhage of the pituitary gland and can present with headache, vomiting, altered sensorium, visual defect, and/or endocrine dysfunction [2].
  - Presenting symptoms by tumor type:
    - prolactinoma: loss of libido, infertility, and osteoporosis in both sexes, oligomenorrhea or amenorrhea, and galactorrhea in women and erectile dysfunction in men.
    - growth hormone-secreting tumor: gigantism, acromegaly, changes in facial features (tongue, lip, and nose enlargement; forehead prominence), diabetes mellitus, hypertension, arthritis, carpal tunnel syndrome, sleep apnea.
    - ACTH-secreting tumor: hypercortisolism (Cushing syndrome), which may present with weight gain, centripetal obesity, facial rounding and plethora, violaceous skin striae and ecchymoses, diabetes mellitus, hypertension, mood disorders (depression), osteoporosis.
    - thyrotropin-secreting adenomas: clinical hyperthyroidism, including a goiter.

- Pituitary subtypes in order of highest to lowest frequency are prolactinomas, nonfunctioning adenomas, growth hormone (GH)-releasing adenomas, adrenocorticotropic hormone (ACTH)-secreting adenomas, and TSH-releasing adenomas (less than 1%)
- Local anatomy:
  - The pituitary gland is an 8–10 mm structure (in the superior-inferior dimension) located in the sella turcica.
  - Boundaries of the sella turcica:
  - Anterior: tuberculum sellae and anterior clinoid process
  - Posterior: dorsum sellae and posterior clinoid process
  - Inferior: sphenoid bone (superior margin of sphenoid sinus)
  - Superior: diaphragma sellae
  - Lateral: cavernous sinuses bridging the superior orbital fissure to the petrous apex
  - Contents of the cavernous sinus: segment of internal carotid artery; and superiorly to inferiorly, CN III (oculomotor), CN IV (trochlear), CN V_1 (ophthalmic branch of trigeminal), CN V_2 (maxillary branch of the trigeminal nerve), and CN VI (abducens).
- Medical workup:
  - H&P with emphasis on thorough endocrine history and neurologic-ophthalmic examination including visual field and acuity testing.
  - Complete serum endocrine evaluation including serum prolactin, insulin-like growth factor (IGF)-1, growth hormone (after glucose load), 24-h urine cortisol, ACTH, LH, FSH, free T4, T3, and TSH.
- Imaging workup:
  - Differential diagnosis for a sellar mass is broad including pituitary adenoma, congenital lesions (craniopharyngioma or Rathke's cleft cyst), infiltrative or infectious process (e.g., granuloma, tuberculosis, lymphocytic hypophysitis), or non-adenoma neoplasm (e.g., meningioma, primary lymphoma, chordoma, germ cell tumor, or metastasis).
  - CT: Pituitary microadenomas are hypodense and less contrast enhancing than normal pituitary gland.
  - MRI: Pituitary microadenomas are typically hypointense to normal pituitary gland on T1-weighted images and can be iso-, hypo-, or hyperintense to normal pituitary on T2-weighted images. There may be hyperintensity on T1-weighted images in the setting of cystic lesions or a component of intralesional hemorrhage. In contrast to meningiomas, pituitary adenomas demonstrate partial, incomplete, or heterogenous contrast enhancement.
  - The closest distance between the tumor and optic chiasm and optic nerves should be determined, particularly when suprasellar extension is present.
- Management strategies include observation, surgical resection (standardly via transsphenoidal microsurgery), medical management, radiotherapy, or various

combinations of these depending on tumor size and location, specific endocrine abnormalities, and response to initial therapies. For prolactinomas, medical management is the first line treatment. For nonfunctioning pituitary adenomas that are symptomatic or causing mass effect, surgery is often the first-line option for pathologic confirmation and decompression.

10.3 Staging, Grading, and Other Classifications

Pituitary adenomas are broadly classified by endocrine function, anatomic size, and extent of invasiveness. There is no universally accepted staging or classification system. The first devised system was the Hardy classification, whereby pituitary tumors were described based on the extent of invasiveness (Table 10.1, [3]). Additionally, pituitary tumors can be classified based on their endocrine activity as secretory or nonsecretory, and further categorized based on the pituitary cell type, tumor type, and associated endocrine syndromes (Table 10.2, [4]).

Table 10.1 Hardy classification of pituitary adenomas[a]

Grade	Extent of invasiveness
Noninvasive	
0	Sella intact with normal contour
I	Sella intact, but with bulging of floor
II	Sella intact, with enlarged fossa
Invasive	
III	Sella with localized or focal destruction
IV	Sella with diffuse destruction

[a]Modified from Hardy [3]

Table 10.2 Pituitary classification based on cell type and endocrine syndrome

Pituitary cell type	Hormones	Endocrine syndrome	Percent of cases
Corticotroph	ACTH, POMC-derived peptides	Cushing's syndrome Nelson's syndrome	10%
Somatotroph	GH α-subunit	Gigantism (children) Acromegaly (adults)	15%
Lactotroph	Prolactin	Galactorrhea and amenorrhea (in females) Infertility, sexual dysfunction	30%
Thyrotroph	TSH α-subunit	Hypothyroidism, hyperthyroidism	<1%
Gonadotroph	FSH, LH α-subunit	Hypogonadism, hypopituitarism	10%
Nonsecretory	–	± Hypopituitarism due to mass effect	25%

[a]Modified from Stoller et al. 2009 [4]

Abbreviations: *ACTH* adrenocorticotropic hormone, *POMC* pro-opiomelanocortin, *GH* growth hormone, *TSH* thyroid-stimulating hormone, *FSH* follicle-stimulating hormone, *LH* luteinizing hormone

10.4 Patient Selection for SRS or FSRT

- Factors influencing treatment recommendations include patient age, medical comorbidities, cranial nerve deficits, tumor size and/or growth rate, presenting symptoms, competing symptoms (i.e., vision loss), and proximity to critical organs at risk (such as the optic apparatus).
- For single-fraction SRS, targets should generally be:
  - <3 cm in size.
  - Not directly abutting critical OARs.
  - >3 to 5 mm from the optic apparatus (optic chiasm, optic nerves) to achieve adequate dose fall-off between the prescription dose and OAR tolerance (<8 to 10 Gy for single-fraction SRS).
- For FSRT, tumors may be larger in size (> 3–4 cm) with closer proximity to or abutting/involving OARs.
- For secretory adenomas, SRS is associated with faster biochemical normalization [5, 6], with a mean time to normalization of 8.5 months for SRS versus 18 months for conventionally fractionated radiotherapy [7].
- For nonfunctioning pituitary adenomas that are subtotally resected, multiply recurrent, or patients who are not good surgical candidates, consider standard-fractionated radiation therapy, SRS or FSRT, depending on size and proximity to the optic apparatus.
- For prolactinomas, the first-line therapy is a dopamine agonist such as bromocriptine or cabergoline. Surgery is second line, and radiation therapy is reserved for patients who do not respond to/do not tolerate medical therapy, or patients with persistent disease without surgical options [8, 9].

10.5 Treatment Planning Considerations (Table 10.3)

Table 10.3 Guidelines for simulation, target delineation, and treatment planning

Treatment planning considerations	
Simulation instructions	**Position**: Supine, arms at sides, head and neck neutral. **Immobilization**: A rigid (frame or frameless) stereotactic immobilization system[a]. • GammaKnife: Head frame in conjunction with a metal collimator helmet. • Linac/CyberKnife based: Various, including rigid frame with external skull fixation, noninvasive modified GTC frame (noninvasive fixation by use of a dental plate), or a three-point thermoplastic mask with a modified stereotactic frame (see Fig. 10.2). **CT**: Thin-cut CT images (1.0–2.0 mm slice thickness) ideally with IV contrast from vertex to mid-cervical spine. **Diagnostic imaging**: Co-registration of planning CT with the contrast-enhanced MRI for target and OAR delineation. MRI sequences should include pre- and post-contrast T1-weighted, T2-weighted and FLAIR, with multi-planar (axial, sagittal, and coronal) post-contrast T1-weighted images. Post-contrast T1-weighted images with thin (1 mm) slices should be obtained. High-resolution series, such as MP-RAGE, should be obtained for contrast-enhancing targets. Cranial nerves may be more readily visualized on a CISS or 3D FIESTA series [10].
Image guidance	Pre-treatment CBCT and/or orthogonal KV X-rays; misalignment corrections via positional systems with four or ideally six axes (including rotational corrections) of the patient couch/platform.
Target delineation	The tumor bed/GTV is defined as the enhancing lesion on the post-gadolinium T1-weighted MRI ([10], and see Fig. 10.1a).
Margins	GTV = CTV PTV = CTV plus 0–5 mm uniform expansion (depending on institutional setup error, including accuracy and reproducibility of immobilization). Generally, CTV plus 3–5 mm uniform expansion for standard thermoplastic mask or CTV plus 0–2 mm uniform expansion for a stereotactic frame. PTV margin may be trimmed as needed (even to 0 mm) at interface with critical OARs (optic chiasm, optic nerve).
Tumor/target coverage considerations	≥98% of the GTV/CTV should receive the prescription dose. ≥95% of the PTV should receive the prescription dose.
Treatment modality	Linac, GammaKnife, CyberKnife, proton beam

Table 10.3 (continued)

Planning strategies/ assessment	Steep PTV to OAR dose gradients are generated using multiple beam arrangements or non-coplanar arcs. Dose often prescribed to the steepest portion of the beam profile (often the 50% IDL for GammaKnife). For linac-based SRS, the standard beam profile is shaped by collimation with cones or MLCs. An example treatment plan is depicted in Fig. 10.1b. Notably, as target size increases, the dosimetric advantages of SRS tend to decline (the sharp dose fall-off becomes shallower, leading to higher doses to adjacent normal tissues). FSRT in 3–5 fx is generally necessary for targets ≥ 3 cm. The following indices should be assessed: **Conformality index**: Prescription isodose volume/target volume (ideal is 1; at least 1.2–1.5 for SRS to minimize dose to surrounding tissues) **Gradient index**: Volume receiving half the prescription isodose/volume receiving the full prescription isodose (ideally 2–3 for smaller lesions; for larger lesions treated with FSRT should be ≤ 4) **Heterogeneity index**: maximum dose/prescription dose (ideally ≤ 2)

[a]Based on delivery system and institutional protocol

Abbreviations: *GTC* Gill-Thomas-Cosman, *FLAIR* fluid-attenuated inversion recovery, *MP-RAGE* magnetization-prepared rapid gradient echo, *CISS* constructive interference in steady state, *FIESTA* 3D fast imaging employing steady-state acquisition

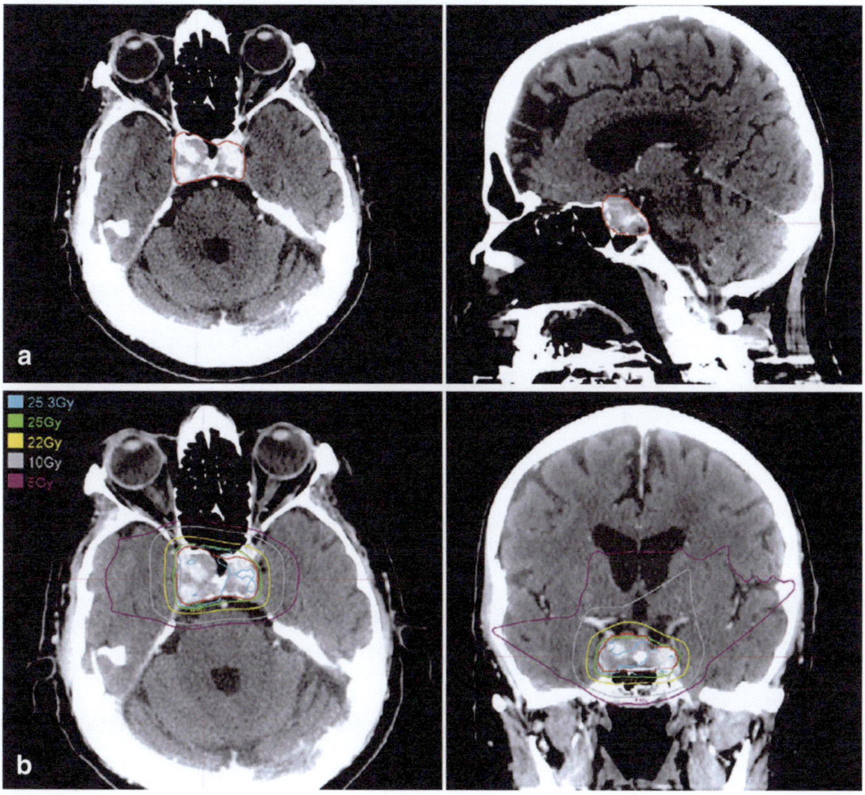

Fig. 10.1 A 9.7 cc postsurgical recurrent nonfunctioning macroadenoma; GTV target delineation in red. (**a**) Simulation CT axial (left) and sagittal (right). (**b**) Treatment plans with prescription IDL in green, effective normalization 97%. Hypofractionated stereotatctic RT, 5 GyRBE protons × 5 fx (25 GyRBE total). Simulation CT axial (left) and coronal (right). *IDL* isodose line

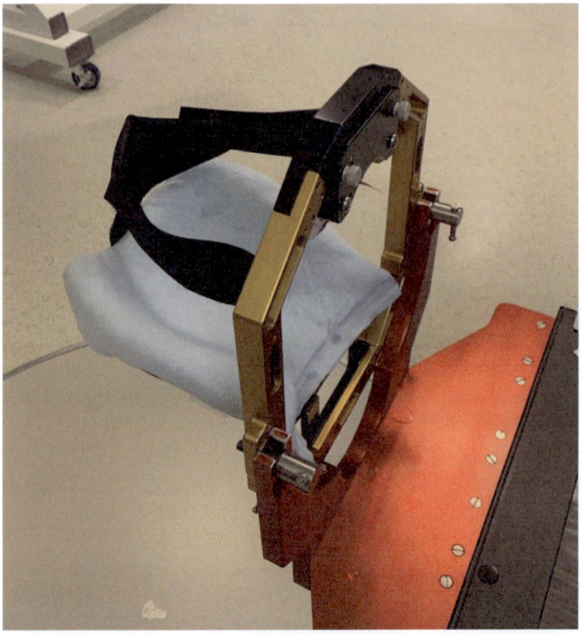

Fig. 10.2 A modified stereotactic head frame

Table 10.4 Commonly used dose/fractionation schemes (refer to Tables 10.4 and 10.5 for other fractionation regimen used at single institution studies)

	Patient selection considerations	Dose/fx
SRS	Small tumor (<3 cm), >3 to 5 mm from optic apparatus	Nonsecretory: 12–20 Gy × 1 fx (optimally 14–18 Gy × 1 fx) ACTH secreting: 15–30 Gy × 1 fx (optimally 20–25 Gy × 1 fx) GH secreting: 10–35 Gy × 1 fx (optimally 20–25 Gy × 1 fx) Other secretory: 15–25 Gy × 1 fx [9]
FSRT	Larger tumor and/or <2 to 3 mm from optic apparatus	7 Gy × 3 fx or 5 Gy × 5 fx [11]

Abbreviations: *fx* fraction(s), *ACTH* adrenocorticotropic hormone, *GH* growth hormone

10.6 Commonly Used Dose/Fractionation Schemes

Commonly utilized dose/fractionation schemes for SRS and FSRT are described in Table 10.4.

10.7 Normal Tissue Tolerances

Guidelines for contouring of optic structures:

- The anterior–posterior extent of the chiasm is variable. ESTRO-ACROP recommends that the anterior and posterior limbs extend 5 mm to include the start of the optic nerves anteriorly and optic tracts posteriorly. The optic nerves should originate from the back of the globes, entering into the skull anterior and inferior to the anterior clinoid process [12, 13].
- There should be no gap between the optic nerves and chiasm (when scrolling through CT slices in coronal plane).
- Dose constraints for optic pathway: Numerous retrospective experiences such as Mayo et al. [14] have contributed to current recommendations by multiple organizations on safe practices to minimize risk to visual function.

  Guidelines re: dose-volume constraints for optic structures:

Organization	DVH constraint guidelines for optic pathway
AAPM TG101 [15]	< 0.2 cc receives 8 Gy (single fx), 15.3 Gy (3 fx), or 23 Gy (5 fx) ≤0.035 cc) receives 10 Gy (single fx), <17.4 Gy (3 fx) or 25 Gy (5 fx)
Timmerman [16]	< 0.2 cc receives 8 Gy (single fx), 15 Gy (3 fx) or 20 Gy (5 fx) ≤0.035 cc receives <10 Gy (single fx), <19.5 Gy (3 fx) or 25 Gy (5 fx)
QUANTEC [17]	Radiation-induced optic neuropathy is rare if single fx Dmax <8 Gy, increases between 8–12 Gy, and is >10% between 12 and 15 Gy
AAPM Working Group on Stereotactic Body Radiotherapy [12]	Max dose associated with a clinically reasonable optic neuropathy risk is no more than 10 Gy in 1 fx, 20 Gy in 3 fx, and 25 Gy in 5 fx

10.8 Patient Management Considerations

- Premedication/prophylactic medication:
  - There is no standard pre-medication regimen.
  - For secretory adenomas, consider temporary discontinuation of pituitary-suppressive medications to enhance radiotherapy response. [18].
- Acute toxicity: Treatment is generally well tolerated; transient symptoms such as nausea, headache, alopecia, skin erythema, or fatigue are possible.
- Late toxicity: Hypopituitarism of single or multiple hormonal axes: 20% at 5 years; 80% by 10–15 years, 5–10% with panhypopituitarism [9].

10.9 Follow-Up

- H&P every 6–12 months.
- Yearly imaging (ideally MRI, CT with contrast if unable to tolerate MRI or MRI contraindicated) for 4–5 years, then every 2 years.
- Secretory adenomas: Monitor for biochemical normalization and hypopituitarism of other axes.
- Nonsecretory and secretory adenomas: Monitor for hypopituitarism with serum analysis every six months.
  - Recommend early referral to endocrinologist for long-term management and monitoring of endocrine dysfunction.

10.10 Relevant Literature on Outcomes

- Stereotactic radiosurgery and conventionally fractionated radiotherapy are well-established techniques for the treatment of secretory and nonsecretory pituitary adenomas with high local control rates and robust long-term follow-up data. Most data are single institutional reports. Representative large series are listed in Table 10.5. In addition, there are three meta-analyses that report outcomes of patients treated with SRS and fractionated stereotactic radiotherapy (FSRT):
  - Li et al. included 8 studies of 273 patients with secretory and nonsecretory pituitary adenomas concluded that there was no significant differences between efficacy or safety/toxicity (new-onset hypopituitarism, visual disturbance rate) between SRS and FSRT [19].
  - Singh et al. included 20 studies of 1533 patients with acromegaly treated with SRS and showed 57% 10 year endocrine remission, 70% 10 year endocrine control, 93% 10 year local control with 2.7% visual toxicity, and 27% hypopituitarism [20].
  - Albano et al. included 52 retrospective studies of 30 patients with both secretory and non-secretory adenomas treated with SRS using GammaKnife and showed 93% 5-year overall tumor control for nonsecretory adenomas and overall remission (cure without need for medication) of 45% for growth hormone-secreting adenomas, 64% for ACTH-secreting adenomas and 34% for prolactin-secreting adenomas [21].
- While initial data reporting FSRT strategies show promising results in patients with large tumors or those abutting or involving critical OARs, more mature data are required for robust characterization of the long-term efficacy and toxicity profile for FSRT compared to SRS or conventionally fractionated radiotherapy (Table 10.5).

Table 10.5 Summary of single institution retrospective studies reporting outcomes of patients treated with SRS and FSRT.

Study	Patients (*n*)	Median follow-up (years)	Mean treatment volume (cm^3)	Modality, fractionation	Local control (based on radiology)	Remission (mean time to biochemical control without medications in months unless stated otherwise)
Iwai, 2005 [22]	34 nonsecretory	5	2.5	GammaKnife, 14 Gy in 1 fx	93%	NA
Mingione, 2006 [23]	90 nonsecretory	3.7	4.8	GammaKnife, mean 18.5 Gy in 1 fx	92%	NA
Voges, 2006 [24]	175 • nonsecretory (*n* = 37) • GH (*n* = 64) • ACTH (*n* = 17) • Nelson's (*n* = 9) • PRL (*n* = 13) • TSH (*n* = 2)	6.8	4.4	Linac based, mean 15.3 Gy in 1 fx	97%	3 years 34%; 5 years 51%
Liscak, 2007 [25]	140 Nonsecretory	5	3.45	GammaKnife, 20 Gy in 1 fx	100%	NA
Pollock, 2008 [26]	62 Nonsecretory	5.3	4.0	GammaKnife, 16 Gy in 1 fx	95% (7 years)	NA
Sheehan, 2011 [27]	418 • nonsecretory (*n* = 152) • GH (*n* = 130) • ACTH (*n* = 82) • Nelson's (*n* = 22) • PRL (*n* = 32)	2.6	1.9	GammaKnife, 24 Gy in 1 fx	90%	49-month median time to remission
Iwata, 2011 [11]	100 nonsecretory	2.7	5.1	CyberKnife, 17.01–21 Gy in 4 fx or 22–25 Gy in 5 fx	97%	NA
Khattab, 2021 [28]	45 nonsecretory: SRS (*n* = 19), HSRT (*n* = 26)	5	5.34	Linac based. SRS 16 Gy in 1 fx; HSRT 20 Gy in 2–3 fx, or 25 Gy in 5 fx	SRS: 95%; HSRT: 92%	NA

(continued)

Table 10.5 (continued)

Study	Patients (*n*)	Median follow-up (years)	Mean treatment volume (cm^3)	Modality, fractionation	Local control (based on radiology)	Remission (mean time to biochemical control without medications in months unless stated otherwise)
Sherry, 2019 [29]	18 secretory (ACTH): SRS ($n = 9$), HSRT ($n = 9$)	3.4	Not reported	Linac based. SRS 20 Gy in 1 fx; HSRT 30 in 2–5 fx	SRS: 100%; HSRT: 100%	SRS: 29% (2.7 months); HSRT: 33% (44 months)
Iwata, 2016 [30]	52 secretory (GH). All treated with HSRT. Clinically silent (n = 8) Symptomatic GH (n = 44)	5	4.4	CyberKnife, 21 Gy in 3 fx or 25 Gy in 5 fx	100% at 5 years, 94% after 5 years	17% (63% in clinically silent patients, 9% in symptomatic patients)
Hata, 2021 [31]	32 nonsecretory, all treated with HSRT	8.3	5.33	Linac based. Multiple fractionations used: 33.5/6, 28.4/7, 30.8/8, 30.4/9, 32.9/10, 37.4/11, 35.7/14, 38.5/15	97%	NA
Sumodhee, 2021 [32]	18 secretory (GH, ACTH), 11 nonsecretory	3.9	4.77	CyberKnife, 35 Gy in 5 fx	96%	44%
Apaydin, 2021 [33]	38 secretory (ACTH)	6.33	17 (treated with GammaKnife), 3 (treated with CyberKnife)	GammaKnife SRS (n = 31): median dose 25.7 ± 3.71 Gy in 1 fx; CyberKnife HFRT ($n = 7$): median dose: 28 Gy (number of fractions not reported)	100% in both groups	53% had suppressed cortisol level after low dose dexamethasone (15 months); GammaKnife SRS 58% (17.5 months); CyberKnife HFRT 28.5% (4.5 months)
Puataweepong, 2016 [34, 35]	40 secretory and nonsecretory	3.35	3.2	CyberKnife. Multiple fractionations used: 24/3, 20/4, 21–25/5	97.5%	54% (28 months)

Abbreviations: *Gy* gray, *GH* growth hormone, *ACTH* adrenocorticotropic hormone, *PRL* prolactin, *TSH* thyroid-stimulating hormone, *HSRT* hypofractionated stereotactic radiotherapy, *SRS* stereotactic radiosurgery, *HFRT* hypofractionated radiation therapy

References

1. Molitch ME. Diagnosis and treatment of pituitary adenomas. JAMA. 2017;317(5):516. https://doi.org/10.1001/jama.2016.19699.
2. Baruah Manash P, Salam R. Pituitary apoplexy. Indian J Endocrinol Metab. 2011;15(7):188. https://doi.org/10.4103/2230-8210.84862.
3. Hardy J. Transphenoidal microsurgery of the normal and pathological pituitary. Clin Neurosurg. 1969;16(185):217. https://doi.org/10.1093/neurosurgery/16.CN_suppl_1.185, 1:STN:280:DyaF1M3ptFaltg%3D%3D, 5811707
4. Stoller JKM, Franklin A, Mandell BF. Pituitary disorders and multiple endocrine neoplasia syndromes. In: The cleveland clinic foundation intensive review of internal medicine. Hagerstwon, MD: Lippincott Williams & Wilkins; 2009. p. 525–35.
5. Landolt AM, Haller D, Lomax N, Scheib S, Schubiger O, Siegfried J, et al. Stereotactic radiosurgery for recurrent surgically treated acromegaly: comparison with fractionated radiotherapy. J Neurosurg. 1998;88(6):1002–8.
6. Sheehan JP, Niranjan A, Sheehan JM, Jane JA Jr, Laws ER, Kondziolka D, et al. Stereotactic radiosurgery for pituitary adenomas: an intermediate review of its safety, efficacy, and role in the neurosurgical treatment armamentarium. J Neurosurg. 2005;102(4):678–91.
7. Mitsumori M, Shrieve DC, Alexander E 3rd, Kaiser UB, Richardson GE, Black PM, et al. Initial clinical results of LINAC-based stereotactic radiosurgery and stereotactic radiotherapy for pituitary adenomas. Int J Radiat Oncol Biol Phys. 1998;42(3):573–80.
8. Gillam MP, Molitch ME, Lombardi G, Colao A. Advances in the treatment of prolactinomas. Endocr Rev. 2006;27(5):485–534. https://doi.org/10.1210/er.2005-9998, 1:CAS:528:DC%2BD28XpvVelurY%3D, 16705142
9. Loeffler JS, Shih HA. Radiation therapy in the management of pituitary adenomas. J Clin Endocrinol Metab. 2011;96(7):1992–2003. https://doi.org/10.1210/jc.2011-0251, 1:CAS:528:DC%2BC3MXptlSrs7Y%3D, 21525155
10. Lee NY, Riaz N, Lu JJ. Target volume delineation and field setup: a practical guide for conformal and intensity-modulated radiation therapy. Heidelberg: Springer; 2015. https://doi.org/10.1007/978-3-319-05726-2.
11. Iwata H, Sato K, Tatewaki K, Yokota N, Inoue M, Baba Y, et al. Hypofractionated stereotactic radiotherapy with CyberKnife for nonfunctioning pituitary adenoma: high local control with low toxicity. Neuro Oncol. 2011;13(8):916–22.
12. Milano MT, Jimm G, Soltys Scott G, Ellen Y, Vitali M, Tomé Wolfgang A, Arjun S, Jinyu X, Lijun M, Solberg Timothy D, Kirkpatrick John P, Constine Louis S, Flickinger John C, Marks Lawrence B, Issam EN. Single- and multi-fraction stereotactic radiosurgery dose tolerances of the optic pathways. Int J Radiat Oncol Biol Phys. 2021;110(1):87–99. https://doi.org/10.1016/j.ijrobp.2018.01.053.
13. Maximilian N, Michael B, Chalmers Anthony J, Combs Stephanie E, Erridge Sara C, Alba F, Grosu Anca L, Lagerwaard Frank J, Giuseppe M, René-Olivier M, Umberto R, Short Susan C, Weber Damien C, Claus B. ESTRO-ACROP guideline "target delineation of glioblastomas". Radiother Oncol. 2016;118(1):35–42. https://doi.org/10.1016/j.radonc.2015.12.003.
14. Mayo C, Martel MK, Marks LB, Flickinger J, Nam J, Kirkpatrick J. Radiation dose-volume effects of optic nerves and chiasm. Int J Radiat Oncol Biol Phys. 2010;76(3 Suppl S28):S35. https://doi.org/10.1016/j.ijrobp.2009.07.1753, 20171514
15. Benedict SH, Yenice KM, Followill D, Galvin JM, Hinson W, Kavanagh B, et al. Stereotactic body radiation therapy: the report of AAPM task group 101. Med Phys. 2010;37(8):4078–101.
16. Timmerman RD. An overview of hypofractionation and introduction to this issue of seminars in radiation oncology. Semin Radiat Oncol. 2008;18(4):215–22. https://doi.org/10.1016/j.semradonc.2008.04.001.
17. Marks LB, Yorke ED, Jackson A, Haken Ten RK, Constine LS, Eisbruch A, et al. Use of normal tissue complication probability models in the clinic. Int J Radiat Oncol Biol Phys. 2010;76(3 Suppl):S10–9.

18. Pollock BE, Jacob JT, Brown PD, Nippoldt TB. Radiosurgery of growth hormone-producing pituitary adenomas: factors associated with biochemical remission. J Neurosurg. 2007;106(5):833–8. https://doi.org/10.3171/jns.2007.106.5.833, 1:CAS:528:DC%2BD2sXlsF2msbs%3D, 17542527
19. Xuezhen L, Yanbin L, Yang C, Peiliang L, Liang B, Jidian S, Enshan F. Safety and efficacy of fractionated stereotactic radiotherapy and stereotactic radiosurgery for treatment of pituitary adenomas: a systematic review and meta-analysis. J Neurol Sci. 2017;372:110–6. https://doi.org/10.1016/j.jns.2016.11.024.
20. Raj S, Prabhanjan D, Lehrer Eric J, Darrah S, Kimball S, Trifiletti Daniel M, Sheehan Jason P. Stereotactic radiosurgery for acromegaly: an international systematic review and meta-analysis of clinical outcomes. J Neurooncol. 2020;148(3):401–18. https://doi.org/10.1007/s11060-020-03552-2.
21. Luigi A, Marco L, Raffaella BL, Ajay N, Zaid S, Flickinger JC, Dade LL, Pietro M. Gamma knife radiosurgery for pituitary tumors: a systematic review and meta-analysis. Cancers. 2021;13(19):4998. https://doi.org/10.3390/cancers13194998.
22. Iwai Y, Yamanaka K, Yoshioka K. Radiosurgery for nonfunctioning pituitary adenomas. Neurosurgery. 2005;56(4):699–705. https://doi.org/10.1227/01.NEU.0000156836.42945.28, 15792508; discussion 699-705.
23. Mingione V, Yen CP, Vance ML, Steiner M, Sheehan J, Laws ER, et al. Gamma surgery in the treatment of nonsecretory pituitary macroadenoma. J Neurosurg. 2006;104(6):876–83.
24. Voges J, Kocher M, Runge M, Poggenborg J, Lehrke R, Lenartz D, et al. Linear accelerator radiosurgery for pituitary macroadenomas: a 7-year follow-up study. Cancer. 2006;107(6):1355–64.
25. Liscak R, Vladyka V, Marek J, Simonova G, Vymazal J. Gamma knife radiosurgery for endocrine-inactive pituitary adenomas. Acta Neurochir. 2007;149(10):999–1006. https://doi.org/10.1007/s00701-007-1253-7, 1:STN:280:DC%2BD2srpslCgtg%3D%3D, 17676409; discussion
26. Pollock BE, Cochran J, Natt N, Brown PD, Erickson D, Link MJ, et al. Gamma knife radiosurgery for patients with nonfunctioning pituitary adenomas: results from a 15-year experience. Int J Radiat Oncol Biol Phys. 2008;70(5):1325–9.
27. Sheehan JP, Pouratian N, Steiner L, Laws ER, Vance ML. Gamma knife surgery for pituitary adenomas: factors related to radiological and endocrine outcomes. J Neurosurg. 2011;114(2):303–9. https://doi.org/10.3171/2010.5.JNS091635, 20540596
28. Khattab MH, Sherry AD, Xu MC, Patrick K, Anderson JL, Guozhen L, Chambless LB, Cmelak AJ, Albert A. Stereotactic radiosurgery and hypofractionated stereotactic radiotherapy for nonfunctioning pituitary adenoma. J Neurol Surg B Skull Base. 2021;82(S 03):e51–8. https://doi.org/10.1055/s-0040-1710518.
29. Sherry AD, Khattab MH, Xu MC, Patrick K, Anderson Joshua L, Guozhen L, Utz Andrea L, Chambless Lola B, Cmelak Anthony J, Albert A. Outcomes of stereotactic radiosurgery and hypofractionated stereotactic radiotherapy for refractory Cushing's disease. Pituitary. 2019;22(6):607–13. https://doi.org/10.1007/s11102-019-00992-6.
30. Hiromitsu I, Kengo S, Ryutaro N, Yusuke T, Ichiro S, Naoki Y, Mitsuhiro I, Seiji O, Shozo Y, Yuta S. Long-term results of hypofractionated stereotactic radiotherapy with CyberKnife for growth hormone-secreting pituitary adenoma: evaluation by the Cortina consensus. J Neuro Oncol. 2016;128(2):267–75. https://doi.org/10.1007/s11060-016-2105-1.
31. Aiko H, Masaya O, Takahiro O, Akira S, Noriaki H, Masataka T, Toshio S, Manabu H, Taizen N, Hiroaki S. Long-term outcomes of hypofractionated stereotactic radiotherapy for the treatment of perioptic nonfunctioning pituitary adenomas. Neurol Med Chir. 2021;61(7):404–13. https://doi.org/10.2176/nmc.oa.2020-0378.
32. Sumodhee S, Atallah V, Kinj R, Doyen J, L'Homel B, Gillon P, Paquis P, Almairac F, Hieronimus S, Schiappa R, Sadoul J-L, Sumodhee D, Pontikos N, Richier Q, Hannoun-Levi J-M, Scouarnec C, Chevalier N, Bondiau P-Y. Fractionated stereotactic radiation therapy

for pituitary adenomas: an alternative escalating protocol of hypofractionated stereotactic radiotherapy delivering 35 Gy in 5 fractions. Cancer Radiother. 2022;26(4):557. https://doi.org/10.1016/j.canrad.2021.08.021.
33. Tugce A, Mefkure OH, Memis DS, Rasim M, Pinar K. Efficacy and safety of stereotactic radiotherapy in cushing's disease: a single center experience. Exp Clin Endocrinol Diabetes. 2021;129(07):482–91. https://doi.org/10.1055/a-1217-7365.
34. Putipun P, Mantana D, Ake H, Somjai D, Thiti S, Chomporn S, Chuleeporn J, Patamintita V, Pornpan Y. The clinical outcome of hypofractionated stereotactic radiotherapy with cyberknife robotic radiosurgery for perioptic pituitary adenoma. Technol Cancer Res Treat. 2016;15(6):NP10–5. https://doi.org/10.1177/1533034615607113.
35. Puataweepong P, Dhanachai M, Hansasuta A, Dangprasert S, Swangsilpa T, Sitathanee C, et al. The clinical outcome of hypofractionated stereotactic radiotherapy with cyberknife robotic radiosurgery for perioptic pituitary adenoma. Technol Cancer Res Treat. 2016;15(6):NP10.

Part II
Malignant Central Nervous System Tumors

Chapter 11
Glioblastoma

Dominic H. Moon, Dat Vo, and Timothy M. Zagar

11.1 Introduction

Glioblastoma (WHO 4), previously known as glioblastoma multiforme (GBM), is the most common and most aggressive primary malignant brain tumor in adults. Because glioblastoma is commonly a diagnosis of older patients, many with compromised performance status, balancing the therapeutic benefit with toxicity and quality of life is an especially important consideration. Hypofractionated RT has an important role in the treatment of many patients with glioblastoma with best data supporting its use in the older population above age 65–70 years.

11.2 Pearls

- Glioblastoma is the most common adult primary malignant brain tumor accounting for about 55% of all gliomas.
- Incidence is approximately 3 per 100,000 adults per year in the USA with a male:female ratio of 3:2.
- Median age at diagnosis is 64 years. The incidence rises with age and peaks at age 75–84.
- The vast majority of glioblastomas are sporadic. Genetic predisposition has been shown with *TP53* gene mutation (Li- Fraumeni syndrome), neurofibromatosis I, and Turcot's syndrome.

D. H. Moon (✉) · D. Vo
Department of Radiation Oncology, UT Southwestern Medical Center, Dallas, TX, USA
e-mail: dominic.moon@utsouthwestern.edu

T. M. Zagar
Northeastern Radiation Oncology, PLLC, Saratoga Springs, NY, USA

O. Kaidar-Person, R. Chen (eds.), *Hypofractionated and Stereotactic Radiation Therapy*, https://doi.org/10.1007/978-3-031-47701-0_11

- There is insufficient evidence that exposure to electromagnetic fields or cell phones increase the risk of brain tumors.
- Median survival of all patients with glioblastoma is approximately 16 months with a 2-year survival of 25–30%, but the prognosis varies based on age, performance status, extent of resection, and location of the tumor (refer to Sect. 11.3).
- For patients 65 years of age and older with glioblastoma, the median survival is approximately 6 months.
- Methylation of the O-6-methylguanine-DNA methyltransferase (MGMT) promoter is both predictive for response to DNA alkylating agents (e.g., temozolomide) and prognostic for survival.
- Presenting symptoms can include headaches, nausea/vomiting, neurologic deficits, and/or seizures.
- Brain tumors are classified based on the World Health Organization (WHO) classification system, revised in 2021. By definition, glioblastoma lacks mutations in isocitrate dehydrogenase (i.e., IDH-wild type) and is WHO grade IV.
- MRI brain with contrast is part of a standard work-up. Glioblastoma is typically ring-enhancing or heterogeneously enhancing. Post-operative MRI brain completed within 48 hours helps to evaluate the extent of resection and the tumor bed for treatment planning.
- Tissue diagnosis is required and can be obtained via stereotactic biopsy, open biopsy, or gross resection.

11.3 Prognosis

Recursive partitioning analysis (RPA) based on RTOG glioma database of patients receiving RT alone [1]

RPA class	Defining variables	Median survival (mo)
III	Age <50, KPS ≥90	17.1
IV	Age <50, KPS <90 Age ≥50, KPS ≥70, resection, working	11.2
V or VI	Age ≥50, KPS ≥70, resection, not working Age ≥50, KPS ≥70, biopsy only Age ≥50, KPS <70	7.5

Abbreviations: *mo* months, *KPS* Karnofsky performance status

RPA of patients ≥70 years of age and receiving RT alone [2]

		Median survival (mo)	
RPA class	Defining variables	US data	French data
I	GTR/PR, age <75.5	9.3	8.5
II	GTR/PR, age >75.5	6.4	7.7
III	Biopsy, KPS ≥70	4.6	4.3
IV	Biopsy, KPS <70	2.3	3.1

Abbreviations: *mo* months, *GTR* gross total resection, *PR* partial resection, *KPS* Karnofsky performance status

RPA of patients receiving RT with concurrent and adjuvant temozolomide [3, 4]

RPA class	Defining variables	Median survival (mo)	
		Original	Validation
I	• MGMT methylation +, IDH1 mutation + • MGMT methylation +, IDH1 mutation –, GTR, KPS ≥90	67.2	49.7
II	• MGMT methylation +, IDH1 mutation –, GTR, KPS <90 • MGMT methylation +, IDH1 mutation –, PR/biopsy • MGMT methylation –, age <50 • MGMT methylation –, age ≥50, GTR	24.0	19.2
III	• MGMT methylation –, age ≥50, PR/biopsy	15.2	13.6

Abbreviations: *mo* months, *MGMT* methylguanine-DNA-methyltransferase, *IDH* isocitrate dehydrogenase, + positive, – negative, *GTR* gross total resection, *PR* partial resection

Validated nomogram in the temozolomide era based on RTOG trial data [5]

11.4 Tumor/Patient Selection

- The first step in management is maximal safe surgical resection, as gross total resection is associated with better survival outcomes [6].
- In general, patients aged 65 and younger with KPS ≥60 should receive standard fractionation RT (e.g., 60 Gy in 30 fractions) + concurrent and adjuvant temozolomide.
- Patients older than 65–70 with KPS ≥60 can be considered for hypofractionated RT ± concurrent and adjuvant temozolomide.
- -Patients of any age with KPS <60 can be considered for hypofractionated RT alone, temozolomide alone, or palliative/best supportive care based on MGMT methylation status, and comorbidities.

11.5 Treatment Planning Considerations

Simulation instructions	• Timing: Simulate patient 10–14 days after surgery/biopsy • Position: Supine • Immobilization: Customized head cast/mask (Fig. 11.1) • Pituitary board can be considered to allow for vertex beams • 3D-CRT or IMRT should be used • Fuse postoperative MRI brain (T1 post-gadolinium contrast and T2/FLAIR) to help delineate target volume
Image guidance	Cone beam CT or kV on-board imaging as appropriate (1–5 times a week)

Margins	GTV: T1 post-contrast volume (resection bed and any residual tumor) CTV1*: T2 or FLAIR volume (edema) + 1–2 cm margin CTV2*: GTV + 1–2 cm margin PTV: CTV + 0.3–0.5 cm margin *CTV expanded as above excluding brainstem, chiasm, nerve, and bone (Figs. 11.2 and 11.3). Anatomic barriers to spread such as the interhemispheric falx and tentorium cerebelli may also be taken into account if clearly not involved
Dosimetric considerations	95% of the PTV receives 100% of the prescription dose ≤1% of non-PTV tissue receives > 110% of the prescription dose

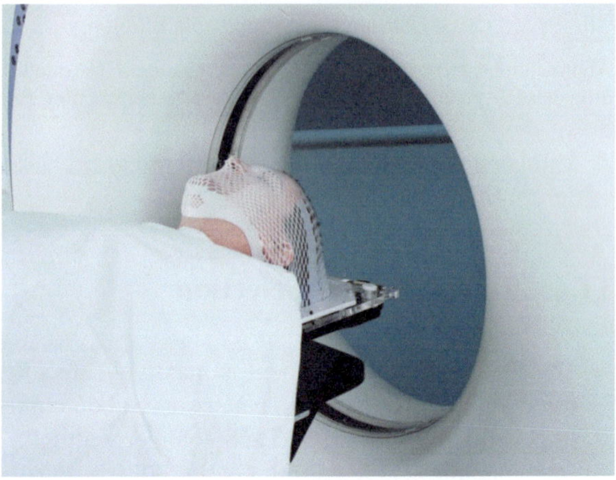

Fig. 11.1 CT simulation with a customized head cast/mask

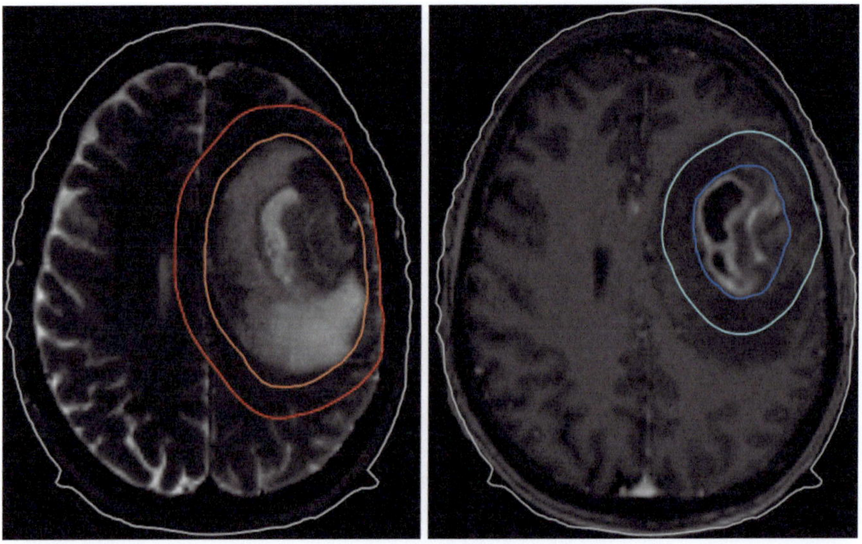

Fig. 11.2 Target delineation. CTV1 based on the volume of edema (orange) with a 1 cm margin excluding the skull (red) on MRI T2 sequence (left image). GTV volume (blue) with a 1 cm margin for CTV2 (turquoise) based on post-contrast MRI T1 sequence (right image). For hypofractionated RT, either CTV1 or CTV2 volume can be used for the entire treatment course per the discretion of the treating physician. The authors most commonly use CTV2 in clinical practice

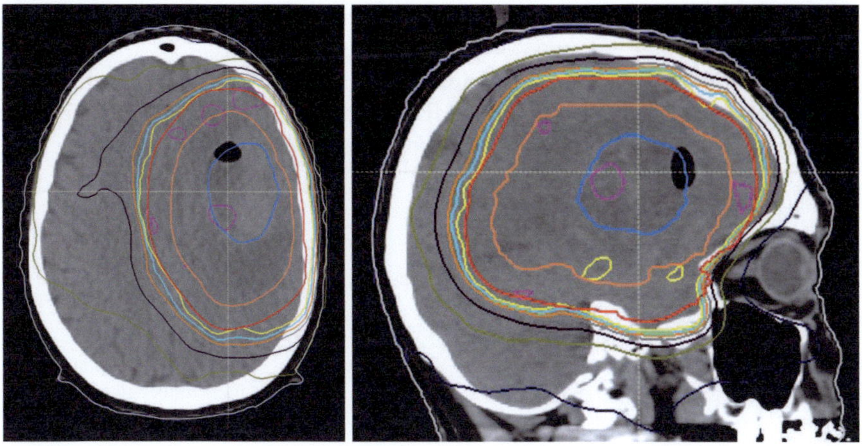

Fig. 11.3 Treatment plan using intensity-modulated RT (IMRT) to spare optic structures, brainstem, and normal brain in the setting of a large treatment volume

11.6 Commonly Used Dose/Fractionation Schemes

Target	Dose/fx (Gy)	# of fx	Total dose (Gy)	Notes
Standard fractionation				
PTV1 PTV2 Total	2 2 2	23 7 30	46 14 60	Age ≤65, KPS ≥60 Generally with concurrent temozolomide Either volume/fractionation is acceptable without any perceptible differences in outcomes
PTV2	2	30	60	
Hypofractionation				
PTV1 [7] or PTV2 [8]	2.67	15	40.05	Age >65 to 70, KPS ≥60, ± temozolomide Any age, KPS <60
PTV2 [9]	3.4	10	34	
PTV2 [10]	5	5	25	In elderly and/or frail patients, if longer course is not feasible
Whole brain [11]	3	10	30	Alternative to involved-field radiation for elderly patients with poor performance status

Abbreviation: *KPS* Karnofsky performance

- At our institutions, patients aged 65–70 with good performance status (KPS ≥60) receive standard RT (2 Gy × 30 = 60 Gy) or hypofractionated RT with concurrent and adjuvant temozolomide.
- Patients older than 70 with good performance status receive hypofractionated RT (2.67 Gy × 15 = 40.05 Gy) with concurrent and adjuvant temozolomide, unless

concurrent temozolomide is considered inappropriate by the multidisciplinary team.

- Patients with poor performance status (KPS <60) regardless of age receive hypofractionated RT alone (especially if MGMT unmethylated), temozolomide alone (only if MGMT methylated), or best supportive care.

11.7 Normal Tissue Tolerances

Organ	QUANTEC for standard fractionation (constraints and endpoints)	NCIC for 40 Gy in 15 fx regimen [8]	Our institutional practice[a] (constraints and endpoints)	
			10 fx	15 fx
Brain parenchyma	Dmax < 60 Gy <3% symptomatic necrosis	N/A	N/A	N/A
	Dmax = 72 Gy 5% symptomatic necrosis			
Brainstem	Dmax < 54 Gy Point dose Dmax < 64 Gy <5% permanent cranial neuropathy or necrosis	Dmax < 40 Gy	Dmax < 38 Gy V32 Gy < 5 cc Cranial neuropathy	Dmax < 44 Gy V40 Gy < 5 cc Cranial neuropathy
Optic nerve/chiasm	Dmax < 55 Gy <3% optic neuropathy	Dmax < 40 Gy	Dmax < 33.1 Gy V30.6 Gy < 0.5 cc Neuritis	Dmax < 42 Gy V39 Gy < 0.5 cc Neuritis
	Dmax = 55–60 Gy 3–7% optic neuropathy			
	Dmax > 60 Gy >7% optic neuropathy			
Spinal cord	Dmax = 50 Gy 0.2% myelopathy	Dmax < 40 Gy	Dmax < 36 Gy V31 Gy< 5 cc Myelitis	Dmax < 42 Gy V39 Gy < 5 cc Myelitis
	Dmax = 60 Gy 6% myelopathy			
	Dmax = 69 Gy 50% myelopathy			
Cochlea	Mean dose ≤ 45 Gy <30% sensorineural hearing loss	N/A	Dmax < 27 Gy V25 Gy < 0.5 cc Hearing loss	Dmax < 33 Gy V30 Gy < 0.5 cc Hearing loss
Eyes	N/A	Dmax < 40 Gy	Dmax < 30 Gy Dmean < 26 Gy	Dmax < 37.5 Gy Dmean < 33 Gy
Lens	N/A	Dmax < 4 Gy	Dmax < 7 Gy	Dmax < 9 Gy

Abbreviations: *NCIC* National Cancer Institute of Canada, *Dmax* maximum point dose, *N/A* not available, *VX Gy* volume in cc receiving ≥ X Gy, *Dmean* mean dose

[a]No standard constraints have been established in the setting of hypofractionated RT to doses ≤40 Gy. The constraints listed are Timmerman dose parameters [12]

11.8 Patient Management Considerations

- Premedication: Patients should be evaluated for steroids as appropriate based on the patient's symptoms. Routine premedication is not indicated.
- Acute toxicity: Acute symptoms are generally self-limited and mild. Pain and nausea medications are used as needed.
  - Fatigue: Up to 90% of patients. Many patients recover over several weeks, but some may experience chronic fatigue.
  - Nausea: ~ 30% of patients. Generally well-controlled on antiemetics (e.g., ondansetron 4–8 mg q8h prn).
  - Headaches: Symptoms may occur due to inflammation and potential transient increase in cerebral edema. Headaches can be managed with OTC pain medications as needed. Patients with significant pretreatment cerebral edema should be placed on dexamethasone (4 mg BID-QID) prior to RT.
  - Scalp erythema: Generally mild and treated with topical emollients or moisturizing cream (e.g., calendula cream or Aquaphor) as needed.
  - Alopecia: Hair loss occurs at the site of radiation treatment. Severity and permanence are dose dependent.
  - Thrombocytopenia: In patients receiving concurrent temozolomide, blood counts should be monitored regularly. For patients with severe thrombocytopenia (<10,000–20,000/μL), RT may need to be held until counts recover.
- Late toxicity: Difficult to attribute to treatment due to multiple confounding factors including disease progression, medications (e.g., anticonvulsants), systemic therapy, and comorbidities.
  - Neurocognitive decline: Patients receiving RT may experience decline in memory and executive functioning. Retrospective and small prospective studies suggest bevacizumab may improve or preserve neurocognitive function in poor-prognosis glioblastoma patients [13].
  - Radiation necrosis: Radiation necrosis typically occurs 1–3 years after RT at or adjacent to the original tumor, which can cause neurologic symptoms based on the location. It is often difficult to distinguish recurrence from radiation necrosis. Radiation necrosis is managed conservatively if asymptomatic or with moderate dose steroids (e.g., dexamethasone 4 mg BID) if symptomatic. Accumulating data suggest bevacizumab may also provide symptomatic relief [14]. Surgical resection for palliation may be needed in severe cases, with increasing data demonstrating the utility of laser interstitial thermal therapy (LITT) for the management of radiation necrosis [15].

11.9 Follow-Up

- According to NCCN guidelines [16]
  - First brain MRI 2–8 weeks after RT
  - Follow-up q2–4 months with brain MRI for the first 3 years
  - Follow-up q3–6 months with brain MRI after 3 years

11.10 Relevant Literature

Study	Patients	Treatment	Median follow-up	Outcomes
Randomized trials				
Roa 2004 [7]	*N* = 100 Age ≥60 KPS ≥50	(1) 2 Gy × 30 = 60 Gy (2) 2.67 Gy × 15 = 40 Gy	Not reported	**(1) Standard fx:** • 5.1 mo median OS • 49% required post-RT steroid dose increase **(2) Hypofx:** • 5.6 mo median OS (p = NS) • 23% required post-RT steroid dose increase (p = 0.02)
Souhami 2004 (RTOG 93-05) [17]	*N* = 206 Size ≤4 cm KPS ≥60	(1) Post-op SRS (15–24 Gy x 1) + EBRT (60 Gy) + carmustine (2) EBRT (60 Gy) + carmustine	61 mo	**(1) Post-op SRS:** • 13.5 mo median OS **(2) No post-op SRS:** • 13.6 mo median OS (p = NS)
Malmstrom 2012 [9]	*N* = 342 Age ≥60 WHO PS 0–2	(1) Temozolomide (2) 3.4 Gy × 10 = 34 Gy alone (3) 2 Gy × 30 = 60 Gy alone	Not reported	**(1) Temozolomide:** • 8.3 mo median OS • 9.0 mo median OS (age >70) **(2) Hypofx:** • 7.5 mo median OS • 7.0 mo median OS (age >70) **(3) Standard fx:** • 6 mo median OS (p = NS vs. hypofx, p = 0.01 vs. temozolomide) • 5.2 mo median OS (age >70) (p = 0.02 vs. hypofx, p < 0.0001 vs temozolomide)

Study	Patients	Treatment	Median follow-up	Outcomes
Roa 2015 [10]	$N = 98$ Frail: age ≥50 and KPS 50–70% Elderly and frail: age ≥65 and KPS 50–70% Elderly: age ≥65 and KPS 80–100%	(1) 5 Gy × 5 = 25 Gy (2) 2.67 Gy × 15 = 40 Gy	6.3 mo	**(1) 5 Gy × 5** • 7.9 mo median OS • 4.2 mo median PFS **(2) 2.67 Gy × 15** • 6.4 mo median OS (p = NS) • 4.2 mo median PFS (p = NS)
Perry 2017 [8]	$N = 562$ Age ≥65 ECOG 0-2	(1) 2.67 Gy × 15 = 40 Gy (2) 2.67 Gy × 15 = 40 Gy + temozolomide	17 mo	**(1) Hypofx** • 7.6 mo median OS • 7.7 mo median OS (MGMT methylated) • 7.9 mo median OS (MGMT unmethylated) • 3.9 mo median PFS **(2) Hypofx + temozolomide** • 9.3 mo median OS ($p < 0.001$) • 13.5 mo median OS (MGMT methylated) ($p < 0.001$) • 10 mo median OS (MGMT unmethylated) ($p = 0.055$) • 5.3 mo median PFS ($p < 0.001$)
Prospective non-randomized studies				
Bauman 1994 [11] (Phase II)	$N = 29$ Age ≥65 KPS ≤50	3 Gy × 10 = 30 Gy (whole brain RT)	Not reported	• 6.0 mo median OS
Azoulay 2020 [18] (Phase I/II)	$N = 30$ Age ≥18 PTV ≤150 cc	Dose levels: 5 Gy × 5 = 25 Gy ($N = 6$) 6 Gy × 5 = 30 Gy ($N = 6$) 7 Gy × 5 = 35 Gy ($N = 6$) 8 Gy × 5 = 40 Gy ($N = 12$) + temozolomide	13.8 mo	• 14.8 mo median OS • 19.9 mo median OS (MGMT methylated) • 11.3 mo median OS (MGMT unmethylated) ($p = 0.03$) • 8.2 mo median PFS • MTD: 8 Gy × 5 = 40 Gy

Abbreviations: *KPS* Karnofsky performance status, *fx* fractionation, *mo* months, *OS* overall survival, *SRS* stereotactic radiosurgery, *EBRT* external beam RT, *PFS* progression-free survival, *NS* not significant, *MTD* maximum tolerated dose

References

1. Li J, Wang M, Won M, et al. Validation and simplification of the Radiation Therapy Oncology Group recursive partitioning analysis classification for glioblastoma. Int J Radiat Oncol Biol Phys. 2011;81:623–30. https://doi.org/10.1016/j.ijrobp.2010.06.012.
2. Scott JG, Bauchet L, Fraum TJ, et al. Recursive partitioning analysis of prognostic factors for glioblastoma patients aged 70 years or older. Cancer. 2012;118:5595–600. https://doi.org/10.1002/cncr.27570.
3. Wee CW, Kim E, Kim N, et al. Novel recursive partitioning analysis classification for newly diagnosed glioblastoma: A multi-institutional study highlighting the MGMT promoter methylation and IDH1 gene mutation status. Radiother Oncol J Eur Soc Ther Radiol Oncol. 2017;123:106–11. https://doi.org/10.1016/j.radonc.2017.02.014.
4. Wee CW, Kim IH, Park C-K, et al. Validation of a novel molecular RPA classification in glioblastoma (GBM-molRPA) treated with chemoradiation: A multi-institutional collaborative study. Radiother Oncol J Eur Soc Ther Radiol Oncol. 2018;129:347–51. https://doi.org/10.1016/j.radonc.2018.09.001.
5. Gittleman H, Lim D, Kattan MW, et al. An independently validated nomogram for individualized estimation of survival among patients with newly diagnosed glioblastoma: NRG Oncology RTOG 0525 and 0825. Neuro Oncol. 2017;19:669–77. https://doi.org/10.1093/neuonc/now208.
6. Brown TJ, Brennan MC, Li M, et al. Association of the extent of resection with survival in glioblastoma: a systematic review and meta-analysis. JAMA Oncol. 2016;2:1460–9. https://doi.org/10.1001/jamaoncol.2016.1373.
7. Roa W, Brasher PMA, Bauman G, et al. Abbreviated course of radiation therapy in older patients with glioblastoma multiforme: a prospective randomized clinical trial. J Clin Oncol. 2004;22:1583–8. https://doi.org/10.1200/JCO.2004.06.082.
8. Perry JR, Laperriere N, O'Callaghan CJ, et al. Short-course radiation plus temozolomide in elderly patients with glioblastoma. N Engl J Med. 2017;376:1027–37. https://doi.org/10.1056/NEJMoa1611977.
9. Malmström A, Grønberg BH, Marosi C, et al. Temozolomide versus standard 6-week radiotherapy versus hypofractionated radiotherapy in patients older than 60 years with glioblastoma: the Nordic randomised, phase 3 trial. Lancet Oncol. 2012;13:916–26. https://doi.org/10.1016/S1470-2045(12)70265-6.
10. Roa W, Kepka L, Kumar N, et al. International atomic energy agency randomized phase III study of radiation therapy in elderly and/or frail patients with newly diagnosed glioblastoma multiforme. J Clin Oncol. 2015;33:4145–50. https://doi.org/10.1200/JCO.2015.62.6606.
11. Bauman GS, Gaspar LE, Fisher BJ, et al. A prospective study of short-course radiotherapy in poor prognosis glioblastoma multiforme. Int J Radiat Oncol Biol Phys. 1994;29:835–9. https://doi.org/10.1016/0360-3016(94)90573-8.
12. Timmerman R. A story of hypofractionation and the table on the wall. Int J Radiat Oncol Biol Phys. 2022;112(1):4–21. https://doi.org/10.1016/j.ijrobp.2021.09.027.
13. Henriksson R, Asklund T, Poulsen HS. Impact of therapy on quality of life, neurocognitive function and their correlates in glioblastoma multiforme: a review. J Neurooncol. 2011;104:639–46. https://doi.org/10.1007/s11060-011-0565-x.
14. Xu Y, Rong X, Hu W, et al. Bevacizumab monotherapy reduces radiation-induced brain necrosis in nasopharyngeal carcinoma patients: a randomized controlled trial. Int J Radiat Oncol Biol Phys. 2018;101:1087–95. https://doi.org/10.1016/j.ijrobp.2018.04.068.
15. Ahluwalia M, Barnett GH, Deng D, et al. Laser ablation after stereotactic radiosurgery: a multicenter prospective study in patients with metastatic brain tumors and radiation necrosis. J Neurosurg. 2018;130:804–11. https://doi.org/10.3171/2017.11.JNS171273.
16. Nabors LB, Portnow J, Ahluwalia M, et al. Central nervous system cancers, version 3.2020, NCCN clinical practice guidelines in oncology. J Natl Compr Cancer Netw. 2020;18:1537–70. https://doi.org/10.6004/jnccn.2020.0052.

17. Souhami L, Seiferheld W, Brachman D, et al. Randomized comparison of stereotactic radiosurgery followed by conventional radiotherapy with carmustine to conventional radiotherapy with carmustine for patients with glioblastoma multiforme: report of Radiation Therapy Oncology Group 93-05 protocol. Int J Radiat Oncol Biol Phys. 2004;60:853–60. https://doi.org/10.1016/j.ijrobp.2004.04.011.
18. Azoulay M, Chang SD, Gibbs IC, et al. Phase I/II trial of 5-fraction stereotactic radiosurgery with 5-mm margins with concurrent temozolomide in newly diagnosed glioblastoma: primary outcomes. Neuro Oncol. 2020;22(8):1182–9. https://doi.org/10.1093/neuonc/noaa019.

Chapter 12
Secondary Malignant (Metastases)

Dominic H. Moon, Dat Vo, and Timothy M. Zagar

12.1 Introduction

Brain metastasis is the most common indication for stereotactic radiosurgery (SRS). SRS is a safe and effective treatment modality for patients with good performance status and limited number and volume of brain metastases. In addition, SRS serves as adjuvant therapy for resected brain lesions. Accumulating studies also support the use of hypofractionated stereotactic radiotherapy (HSRT) delivering treatments in 3–5 fractions for relatively large brain lesions and resection beds.

12.2 Pearls

- Brain metastases are the most common intracranial tumors in adults.
- Incidence of brain metastases has been increasing due to improvement in detection with MRI and improvement in extracranial disease control with systemic therapy.
- Up to 30% of patients with cancer develop brain metastases.
- Common primary malignancies metastasizing to the brain include lung cancer, breast cancer, melanoma, and renal cell cancer.
- Metastases are most commonly located at the gray-white matter junction.

D. H. Moon (✉) · D. Vo
Department of Radiation Oncology, UT Southwestern Medical Center, Dallas, TX, USA
e-mail: dominic.moon@utsouthwestern.edu

T. M. Zagar
Northeastern Radiation Oncology, PLLC, Saratoga Springs, NY, USA

O. Kaidar-Person, R. Chen (eds.), *Hypofractionated and Stereotactic Radiation Therapy*, https://doi.org/10.1007/978-3-031-47701-0_12

- Distribution of metastases is approximately proportional to the blood flow to the different parts of the brain: cerebral hemispheres (80%), cerebellum (15%), and brainstem (5%).
- Patients commonly present with headaches, focal neurologic dysfunction, cognitive dysfunction, seizures, and/or stroke.
- The imaging study of choice is a contrast-enhanced brain MRI. Brain metastases are suspected by the presence of multiple lesions, localization at the gray-white matter junction, circumscribed margins, and the presence of vasogenic edema.

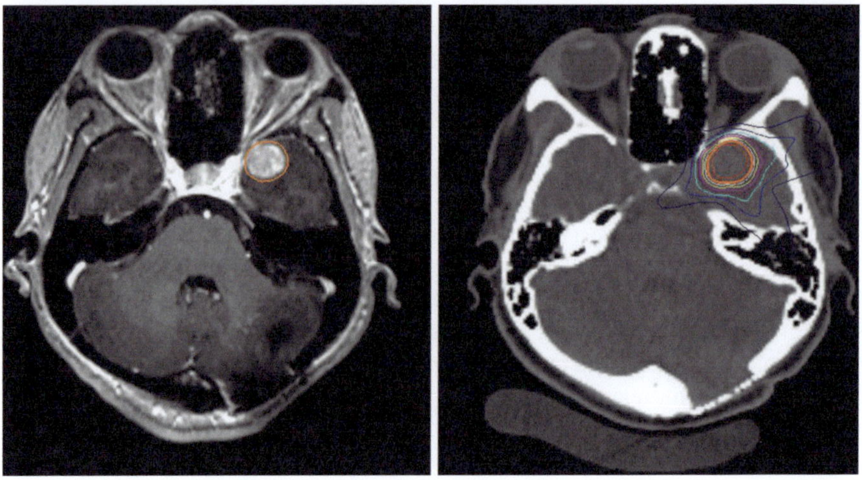

Fig. 12.1 Contouring of a left temporal lobe metastasis based on contrast-enhanced MRI brain (left) and the treatment plan sparing optic structures (right)

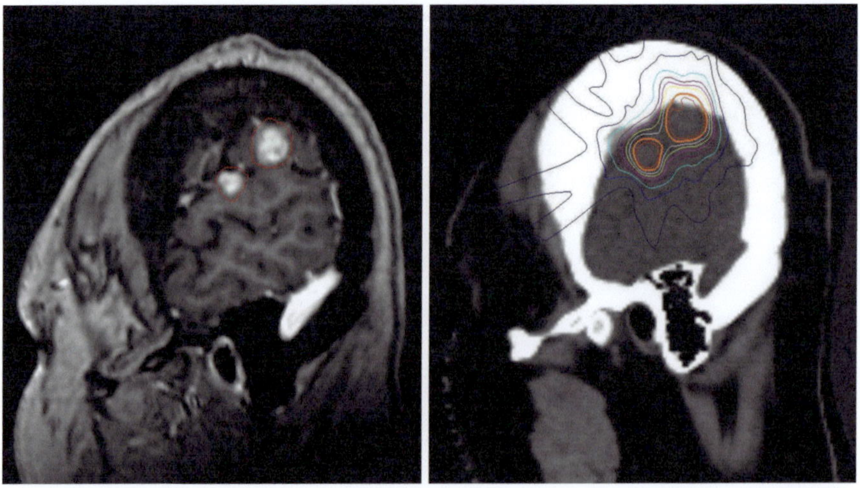

Fig. 12.2 Sagittal view of two adjacent left temporal brain metastases (left) and the treatment plan targeting both lesions (right)

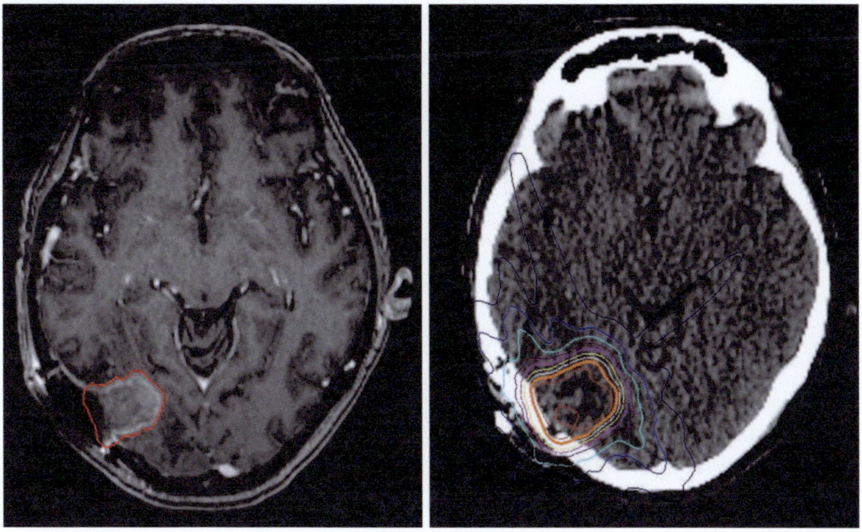

Fig. 12.3 Contouring of a right occipital surgical bed following a resection of a renal cell metastasis based on the post-operative contrast-enhanced MRI brain (left) and the treatment plan (right)

12.3 Prognosis

Diagnosis-specific graded prognostic assessment (GPA) has been developed and updated for common malignancies metastasizing to the brain [1]:

Breast cancer

Prognostic factor	GPA scoring criteria 0	0.5	1.0	1.5
KPS	≤60	70–80	90–100	–
Age (years)	≥60	<60	–	–
# of brain mets	≥2	1	–	–
Extracranial mets	Present	Absent	–	–
Subtypea	Basal	Luminal A	–	HER2 or Luminal B
Median survival (mo) by GPA score	0–1.0 = 6; 1.5–2.0 = 13; 2.5–3.0 = 24; 3.5–4.0 = 36			

[a]Basal = triple negative; Luminal A = ER/PR+, Her2-; Luminal B = triple positive; HER2 = ER/PR-, Her2+

Non-small cell lung cancer: adenocarcinoma

Prognostic factor	GPA scoring criteria 0	0.5	1.0
KPS	≤70	80	90–100
Age (years)	≥70	<70	–

Prognostic factor	GPA scoring criteria		
	0	0.5	1.0
# of brain mets	≥5	1–4	–
Extracranial mets	Present	–	Absent
EGFR and ALK	Both negative or unknown	–	EGFR or ALK positive
Median survival (mo) by GPA score	0–1.0 = 7; 1.5–2.0 = 13; 2.5–3.0 = 25; 3.5–4.0 = 46		

Non-small cell lung cancer: non-adenocarcinoma

Prognostic factor	GPA scoring criteria		
	0	0.5	1.0
KPS	≤70	80	90–100
Age (years)	≥70	<70	–
# of brain mets	≥5	1–4	–
Extracranial mets	Present	–	Absent
Median survival (mo) by GPA score	0–1.0 = 5; 1.5–2.0 = 10; 2.5–3.0 = 13		

Renal cell carcinoma

Prognostic factor	GPA scoring criteria				
	0	0.5	1.0	1.5	2.0
KPS	<70	–	80	–	90–100
# of brain mets	≥ 5	1–4	–	–	–
Extracranial mets	Present	Absent	–	–	–
Hemoglobin level	<11.1	11.1–12.5 or unknown	>12.5	–	–
Median survival (mo) by GPA score	0–1.0 = 4; 1.5–2 = 12; 2.5–3.0 = 17; 3.5–4.0 = 35				

Melanoma

Prognostic factor	GPA scoring criteria		
	0	0.5	1.0
KPS	≤70	80	90–100
Age (years)	≥70	<70	–
# of brain mets	≥5	2–4	1
Extracranial mets	Present	–	Absent
BRAF	Negative or unknown	Positive	–
Median survival (mo) by GPA score	0–1.0 = 5; 1.5–2.0 = 8; 2.5–3.0 = 16; 3.5–4 = 34		

GI cancers

Prognostic factor	GPA scoring criteria				
	0	0.5	1.0	1.5	2.0
KPS	≤70	–	80	–	90–100
Age (years)	≥60	<60	–	–	–

Prognostic factor	GPA scoring criteria 0	0.5	1.0	1.5	2.0
# of brain mets	≥4	2–3	1	–	–
Extracranial mets	Present	Absent	–	–	–
Median survival (mo) by GPA score	0–1.0 = 3; 1.5–2.0 = 7; 2.5–3.0 = 11; 3.5–4.0 = 17				

Abbreviation: *KPS* Karnofsky performance score

12.4 Tumor/Patient Selection

- SRS is generally recommended for patients with good performance status (KPS ≥70).
- Patients with brain metastases and a KPS <70 have poor overall prognosis, and could be considered for whole brain radiotherapy (WBRT) vs. best supportive care [2]. Whenever possible, hippocampal-sparing WBRT with memantine should be used to reduce cognitive side effects [3].
- Indications for SRS:
  - 1–4 brain metastases and surgery is not feasible/indicated secondary to location, comorbidities, or patient preference
  - Post-operative treatment status post resection of a dominant or a limited number of brain metastases
  - 5–10 brain metastases with low tumor burden in the brain (i.e., total volume of disease in the brain is limited) [4]
- The use of SRS in patients with relatively poor performance status is increasing at many institutions, especially for those with limited tumor burden in the brain, controlled systemic disease, and the poor performance status is thought to be contributed by the brain metastases.
- The use of SRS in patients with >10 brain metastases is also increasing as data accumulate suggesting the overall tumor volume rather than number of metastases may be more predictive of outcomes after SRS [5], and SRS for 10+ brain metastases is safe and effective [6]. A distributed approach can be considered in patients with 10+ brain metastases where the metastases are treated over 2–5 treatment sessions, as opposed to a single treatment session, to reduce the potential risk of long-term toxicities.
- For patients with a limited number of brain metastases, adding WBRT to SRS is generally not recommended. Although SRS with WBRT improves local and distant brain control, it leads to significant cognitive decline without an improvement in overall survival [7, 8].
- Dose and fractionation are selected based on size and setting (refer to Sects. 12.6 and 12.10 for details)
  - For lesions up to 40 mm or relatively small post-operative bed, a single fraction SRS is given with doses of 15–24 Gy based on size/volume.

  - For larger lesions, lesions near critical structures such as the brainstem and optic apparatus, or resected lesions with a sizeable post-operative bed, hypofractionated stereotactic radiotherapy (HSRT) is generally recommended (commonly 27 Gy in 3 fractions or 30 Gy in 5 fractions).
- Re-irradiation with SRS is used in some institutions as salvage therapy for local failure after initial SRS. Several retrospective series report good local control rates but relatively high risk of radiation necrosis [9]. For select patients (e.g., surgically inaccessible local recurrence, small and limited number of lesions, etc.), repeat SRS may be an option, but the authors urge caution.

12.5 Treatment Planning Considerations

Simulation instructions	• Position: Supine • Immobilization: customized head cast/mask • 1 mm thick CT slices • Fuse MRI brain (1 mm slices preferred, T1 post-gadolinium contrast) to help delineate target volume • Fuse pre- and post-operative MRI for surgical bed treatment
Image guidance	Linac: daily cone beam CT CyberKnife: continuous skull tracking GammaKnife: cone beam CT (if treated on the GammaKnife Icon)
Margins	• The authors use no CTV or PTV expansions for intact brain metastases (Figs. 12.1 and 12.2) • Consider 1–2 mm expansion of post-operative bed CTV for resected brain metastasis (Fig. 12.3) • Consensus contouring guidelines are available for delineating the postoperative bed [10]
Tumor coverage considerations	• 100% of GTV (or CTV for post-operative cases) receives 100% of prescription dose (if GTV/CTV ≤ 20 mm) • ≥95% of GTV (or CTV for post-operative cases) receives 100% of prescription dose (if GTV/CTV >20 mm)

12.6 Commonly Used Dose/Fractionation Schemes

Dose/fx (Gy)	# of fx	Total dose (Gy)	Notes
SRS for intact lesions			
RTOG 90-05 [11]			
20–24	1	20–24	≤ 20 mm
18	1	18	21–30 mm
15	1	15	31–40 mm
Hypofractionated stereotactic radiotherapy			
Manning 2000 [12]			
9	3	27	≤ 3 brain mets

Dose/fx (Gy)	# of fx	Total dose (Gy)	Notes
Aoyama 2003 [13]			
8.75	4	35	≤ 4 brain mets
Ernst-Stecken 2006 [14]			
6	5	30	If combined with WBRT (2 Gy × 20 fx = 40 Gy on trial, but 3 Gy × 10 fx = 30 Gy commonly used)
7	5	35	HSRT alone
Murai 2014 [15]			
9–10	3	27–30	25–39 mm
6.2–7	5	31–35	≥40 mm
Post-operative SRS			
Minniti 2013 [16]			
9	3	27	>30 mm
N107C/CEC.3 [17]			
20	1	20	<4.2 cc
18	1	18	≥4.2 and <8.0 cc
17	1	17	≥8.0 and <14.4 cc
15	1	15	≥14.4 and <20 cc
14	1	14	≥20 and <30 cc
12	1	12	≥30 cc and <5 cm
Mahajan 2016 [18]			
16	1	16	≤10 cc
14	1	14	10.1–15 cc
12	1	12	>15 cc

- At our institutions, intact lesions are generally treated with 20 Gy in a single fraction if ≤ 20 mm, 18 Gy in a single fraction if 21–30 mm, and 30 Gy in 5 fractions or 27 Gy in 3 fractions if >30 mm.
- Post-operative CTV is generally >30 mm and 30 Gy in 5 fractions or 27 Gy in 3 fractions is frequently used. To improve local control in the postoperative setting, we advise using the Consensus Contouring Guidelines for Postoperative Completely Resected Cavity Stereotactic Radiosurgery for Brain Metastases by Soliman et al. (2018) [10], based on the N107C/CEC.3 trial outcomes [17]

12.7 Normal Tissue Tolerances

	TG101	QUANTEC	Our institutional practice[a]
Brain parenchyma			
1 fx	N/A	V12 < 5–10 cc	N/A
Toxicity	N/A	<20% symptomatic necrosis	N/A

	TG101	QUANTEC	Our institutional practice[a]
Brainstem			
1 fx 3 fx 5 fx	Dmax ≤ 15 Gy, V10 < 0.5 cc Dmax ≤ 23.1 Gy, V18 < 0.5 cc Dmax ≤ 31 Gy, V23 < 0.5 cc	Dmax < 12.5 Gy	Dmax < 15 Gy, V10 < 0.5 cc Dmax < 23.1 Gy, V15.9 < 0.5 cc Dmax < 31 Gy, V23 < 0.5 cc
Toxicity	≥grade 3 cranial neuropathy	<5% permanent cranial neuropathy or necrosis	Cranial neuropathy
Optic pathway			
1 fx 3 fx 5 fx	Dmax ≤ 10 Gy, V8 < 0.2 cc Dmax ≤ 17.4, V15.3 < 0.2 cc Dmax ≤ 25, V23 < 0.2 cc	Dmax < 12 Gy	Dmax < 10 Gy, V8 < 0.2 cc Dmax < 17.4, V15.3 < 0.2 cc Dmax < 25, V23 < 0.2 cc
Toxicity	≥grade 3 neuritis	<10% optic neuropathy	Neuritis
Spinal cord			
1 fx 3 fx 5 fx	Dmax ≤ 14 Gy, V10 < 0.35 cc, V7 < 1.2 cc Dmax ≤ 21.9 Gy, V18 < 0.35 cc, V 12.3 < 1.2 cc Dmax ≤ 30 Gy, V23 < 0.35 cc, V 14.5 < 1.2 cc	Dmax = 13 Gy	Dmax < 14 Gy, V10 < 0.35 cc Dmax < 22.5 Gy, V15.9 < 0.35 cc Dmax <28 Gy, V22< 0.35 cc
Toxicity	≥grade 3 myelitis	1% myelopathy	Myelitis
Cochlea			
1 fx 3 fx 5 fx	Dmax ≤ 9 Gy Dmax ≤ 17.1 Gy Dmax ≤ 25 Gy	Dose ≤ 14 Gy (prescription dose)	Dmax < 9 Gy Dmax < 14.4 Gy Dmax < 22 Gy
Toxicity	≥grade 3 hearing loss	<25% sensory neural hearing loss	Hearing loss

[a]Timmerman dose parameters [19]

12.8 Patient Management Considerations

- Premedication: if the patient is not already on steroids, premedicate with dexamethasone 4 mg PO prior to each fraction. Lorazepam 0.5–1 mg PO can be used prior to each fraction.
- Acute toxicities can include mild nausea, headaches, and new-onset seizures in rare cases.
- The main dose-limiting late toxicity of SRS is radiation necrosis, which occurs in 5–10% of cases, 6 months to years after treatment.

- Factors associated with increased risk of radiation necrosis include larger size of the brain metastasis and a history of prior radiation to the same region. Other tumor biology characteristics including renal cell or lung adenocarcinoma histology, HER2 amplification, and ALK/BRAF mutation may increase the risk of radiation necrosis [20].
- Radiation necrosis is managed conservatively if asymptomatic or with moderate dose steroids (e.g., dexamethasone 4 mg BID) if symptomatic. Accumulating data suggest bevacizumab may also provide symptomatic relief [21]. Surgical resection for palliation may be needed in severe cases, with increasing data demonstrating the utility of laser interstitial thermal therapy (LITT) for the management of radiation necrosis [22].

12.9 Follow-Up

- According to NCCN guidelines [23]:
  - Follow-up with brain MRI q2–3 months for the first 2 years
  - Follow-up with brain MRI q4–6 months after 2 years

12.10 Relevant Literature

Study	Patients	Treatment	Median follow-up	Outcomes
Dose escalation				
RTOG 90-05 [11] (Phase I trial)	$N = 156$ patients previously treated with WBRT	SRS dose escalation: ≤ 20 mm: 18 → 21 → 24 Gy 21–30 mm: 15 → 18 → 21 → 24 Gy 31–40 mm: 12 → 15 → 18 Gy	3 years	• Maximum tolerated dose: ≤ 20 mm: 24 Gy 21–30 mm: 18 Gy 31–40 mm: 15 Gy • Total grade 3–5 toxicity: ≤ 20 mm: 18 Gy (8%), 21 Gy (11%), 24 Gy (10%) 21–30 mm: 15 Gy (13%), 18 Gy (20%), 21 Gy (38%), 24 Gy (58%) 31–40 mm: 12 Gy (10%), 15 Gy (14%), 18 Gy (50%)

Study	Patients	Treatment	Median follow-up	Outcomes
WBRT ± SRS boost				
RTOG 95-08 [24] (Randomized trial)	*N* = 333 KPS ≥ 70, 1–3 mets ≤40 mm	(1) WBRT (37.5 Gy) (2) WBRT + SRS boost (15–24 Gy per RTOG 90-05)	Not reported	**(1) WBRT** • 5.7 mo median OS • 4.9 mo median OS (single met) • 71% 1-year LC • 27% stable/improved KPS at 6 mo **(2) WBRT + SRS** • 6.5 mo median OS (p = NS) • 6.5 mo (single met) ($p = 0.039$) • 82% 1-year LC ($p = 0.013$) • 43% stable/improved KPS at 6 mo ($p = 0.03$)
SRS ± WBRT				
JROSG 99-1 [25] (Randomized trial)	*N* = 132 KPS ≥ 70, 1–4 mets ≤30 mm	(1) SRS (18–25 Gy) (2) SRS (30% reduction) + WBRT (30 Gy)	7.8 mo (entire study) 49.2 mo (survivors)	**(1) SRS** • 8 mo median OS • 73% 1-year LC • 76% 1-year brain tumor recurrence **(2) SRS + WBRT** • 7.5 mo median OS (p = NS) • 89% 1-year LC ($p = 0.002$) • 47% 1-year brain tumor recurrence ($p < 0.001$)
Chang 2009 [7] (Randomized trial)	*N* = 58 KPS ≥ 70, 1–3 mets	(1) SRS (15–20 Gy) (2) SRS + WBRT (30 Gy)	9.5 mo	**(1) SRS** • 15.2 mo median OS • 67% 1-year LC • 24% mean probability of neurocognitive decline at 4 mo **(2) SRS + WBRT** • 5.7 mo median OS ($p = 0.003$) • 100% 1-year LC ($p = 0.01$) • 52% mean probability of neurocognitive decline at 4 mo
EORTC22952-26001 [26] (Randomized trial)	*N* = 359 ECOG 0-2, 1–3 mets ≤35 mm	(1) SRS (14–25 Gy) (2) SRS + WBRT (30 Gy)	(1) SRS: 40 mo (2) SRS + WBRT: 49 mo	**(1) SRS:** • 10.7 mo median OS • 69% 2-year LC **(2) SRS + WBRT** • 10.9 mo median OS (p = NS) • 81% 2-year LC ($p = 0.04$)

Study	Patients	Treatment	Median follow-up	Outcomes
Brown 2016 [8] (Randomized trial)	$N = 213$ ECOG 0-2, 1–3 mets <30 mm	(1) SRS (20–24 Gy) (2) SRS (18–22 Gy) + WBRT (30 Gy)	7.2 mo	**(1) SRS** • 10.4 mo median OS • 73% 1-year LC • 64% cognitive deterioration at 3 mo • 0.1 mean decline from baseline in overall quality of life score **(2) SRS + WBRT** • 7.4 mo median OS (p = NS) • 90% 1-year LC ($p = 0.003$) • 92% cognitive deterioration at 3 mo ($p < 0.001$) • 12 mean decline from baseline in overall quality of life score ($p = 0.001$)
Number of metastases				
Likhacheva 2013 [27] (Retrospective study)	$N = 251$ brain mets (median 2, range 1–9)	• SRS alone (62% of patients, median dose: 20 Gy) • SRS + salvage SRS (22%), WBRT (13%) or surgery (3%)	9.4 mo	• 11.1 mo median OS • 94.6% 1-year LC • Factors associated with OS on multivariable analysis: total tumor volume > 2 cc, age ≥60, diagnosis-specific graded prognostic assessment, and extracranial disease • Number of brain mets not associated with OS
JLGK0901 [4] (Prospective observational cohort study)	$N = 1194$ KPS ≥ 70, 1–10 brain mets <3 cm each, <10 cc each, ≤15 cc total volume	SRS: <4 cc: 22 Gy 4–10 cc: 20 Gy	20.9 mo (survivors)	**1 metastasis** • 13.9 mo median OS • 7% any grade toxicity **2–4 metastases** • 10.8 mo median OS • 9% any grade toxicity **5–10 metastases** • 10.8 mo median OS (p = NS vs. 2–4 metastases) • 9% any grade toxicity (p = NS vs. 2–4 metastases)
Yamamoto 2014 [6] (Retrospective study: case-matched)	$N = 720$ 2–9 brain mets ($N = 360$) vs ≥10 brain mets ($N = 360$)	SRS with Gamma Knife	Not reported	**2–9 metastases** • 6.8 mo median OS • 10.0% neurological death **≥10 metastases** • 6.0 mo median OS (p = NS) • 9.4% neurological death (p = NS) • No difference in neurologic deterioration (HR 0.994, p = NS) and SRS-related complications (HR 0.541, p = NS)

Study	Patients	Treatment	Median follow-up	Outcomes
Hypofractionated stereotactic radiotherapy				
Manning 2000 [12] (Phase II)	*N* = 32 ≤3 brain mets	HSRT with a linac Median 9 Gy × 3 = 27 Gy to the 80–90% isodose line	37 weeks (survivors)	• 11.8 mo median OS • Acute toxicity: none • Late toxicity: seizures (13%), radionecrosis (6%)
Ernst-Stecken 2006 [14] (Phase II)	*N* = 51 KPS ≥ 60, ≤3 brain mets	HSRT with a linac 7 Gy × 5 = 35 Gy to the 90% isodose line 6 Gy × 5 = 30 Gy if additional WBRT	7 mo	• 11 mo median OS • 76% 1-year LC • Acute toxicity: none • Increasing rates of edema and necrosis if V4 ≥ 23 cc
Ammirati 2014 [28] (Phase II)	*N* = 40 KPS ≥ 60, ≤3 brain mets	HSRT with a linac 6 Gy × 5 = 30 Gy Definitive or adjuvant following a surgical resection	16 mo	• 16 mo median OS • 11 mo median PFS • 13% neurological death rate • Acute toxicity: none • Late toxicity: 8% radiation necrosis
Aoyama 2003 [13] (Retrospective)	*N* = 87 ≤4 brain mets	HSRT with a linac Median 35 Gy/4 fx to the 80–90% isodose line	6.3 mo (entire study) 7.6 mo (survivors)	• 8.7 mo median OS • 81% 1-year LC • Acute toxicity: 2% nausea, 1% hypomnesia, 1% seizure • Late toxicity: 1% nausea, 1% hemiparesis
Murai 2014 [15] (Retrospective)	*N* = 54 brain mets ≥2.5 cm	HSRT with a linac Dose escalation: 3 fx (2.5–3.9 cm): 18–22 Gy to 27–30 Gy 5 fx (≥4 cm): 21–25 Gy to 31–35 Gy	Not reported	• 6 mo median OS • 78% 1-year LC • No ≥ grade 3 toxicity at every level of dose
Post-operative SRS				
Mahajan 2016 [18] (Randomized trial)	*N* = 131 1–3 mets, ≥1 met with complete resection, ≤4 cm resection cavity	(1) SRS (12–16 Gy) (2) Observation of the resection cavity	11.1 mo	**(1) SRS** • 17 mo median OS • 72% 1-year LC **(2) Observation** • 18 mo median OS (p = NS) • 43% 1-year LC ($p = 0.015$)

Study	Patients	Treatment	Median follow-up	Outcomes
N107C/CEC.3 [17] (Randomized trial)	$N = 194$ 1–4 mets, s/p surgical resection of 1 met, <5 cm resection cavity	(1) SRS (12–20 Gy) (2) WBRT (30 or 37.5 Gy) Unresected mets treated with SRS in both arms	11.1 mo	**(1) SRS** • 12.2 mo median OS • 3.7 mo cognitive deterioration free survival • 60.5% 1-year surgical bed control • 36.6% 1-year overall brain control **(2) WBRT** • 11.6 mo median OS (p = NS) • 3.0 mo cognitive deterioration free survival ($p < 0.0001$) • 80.6% 1-year surgical bed control ($p = 0.00068$) • 72.1% 1-year overall brain control ($p < 0.0001$)
Brennan 2014 [29] (Phase II)	$N = 49$ 1–2 brain mets s/p resection	SRS with a linac ≤2 cm: 22 Gy 2.1–3 cm: 18 Gy 3.1–4 cm: 15 Gy	12 mo	• 78% 1-year LC • 56% 1-year distant brain control • Toxicity: 17.5% with radionecrosis
Jensen 2011 [30] (Retrospective)	$N = 106$ s/p surgical resection, no prior WBRT	SRS with Gamma Knife Median dose of 17 Gy to the 50% isodose line	Not reported	• 10.9 mo median OS • 80.3% 1-year LC • 35.4% 1-year distant brain control • 37% received salvage WBRT at a median of 12.6 mo
Choi 2012 [31] (Retrospective)	$N = 112$ s/p surgical resection	SRS with Cyber Knife Median dose of 20 Gy in 1–5 fx to a median 79% isodose line, 2 mm margin	11 mo	• 17 mo median OS • 90.5% 1-year LC • 46% 1-year distant brain control • 28% received salvage WBRT at a median on 7 months
Minniti 2013 [16] (Retrospective)	$N = 101$ s/p surgical resection (resection cavity > 3 cm)	SRS with a linac 9 Gy × 3 = 27 Gy to a median 83% isodose line, 2 mm margin	16 mo	• 17 mo median OS • 93% 1-year LC • 50% 1-year distant brain control • 24% received salvage WBRT

Abbreviations: *WBRT* whole brain RT, *SRS* stereotactic radiosurgery, *KPS* Karnofsky performance status, *OS* overall survival, *LC* local control, *NS* not significant, *HSRT* hypofractionated stereotactic RT, *fx* fraction, *mo* months

References

1. Sperduto PW, Mesko S, Li J, et al. Survival in patients with brain metastases: summary report on the updated diagnosis-specific graded prognostic assessment and definition of the eligibility quotient. J Clin Oncol. 2020;38:3773–84. https://doi.org/10.1200/JCO.20.01255.
2. Mulvenna P, Nankivell M, Barton R, et al. Dexamethasone and supportive care with or without whole brain radiotherapy in treating patients with non-small cell lung cancer with brain metastases unsuitable for resection or stereotactic radiotherapy (QUARTZ): results from a phase 3, non-inferiority, randomised trial. Lancet. 2016;388:2004–14. https://doi.org/10.1016/S0140-6736(16)30825-X.
3. Brown PD, Gondi V, Pugh S, et al. Hippocampal avoidance during whole-brain radiotherapy plus memantine for patients with brain metastases: phase III Trial NRG oncology CC001. J Clin Oncol. 2020;38:1019–29. https://doi.org/10.1200/JCO.19.02767.
4. Yamamoto M, Serizawa T, Shuto T, et al. Stereotactic radiosurgery for patients with multiple brain metastases (JLGK0901): a multi-institutional prospective observational study. Lancet Oncol. 2014;15:387–95. https://doi.org/10.1016/S1470-2045(14)70061-0.
5. Baschnagel AM, Meyer KD, Chen PY, et al. Tumor volume as a predictor of survival and local control in patients with brain metastases treated with Gamma Knife surgery. J Neurosurg. 2013;119:1139–44. https://doi.org/10.3171/2013.7.JNS13431.
6. Yamamoto M, Kawabe T, Sato Y, et al. Stereotactic radiosurgery for patients with multiple brain metastases: a case-matched study comparing treatment results for patients with 2-9 versus 10 or more tumors. J Neurosurg. 2014;121(Suppl):16–25. https://doi.org/10.3171/2014.8.GKS141421.
7. Chang EL, Wefel JS, Hess KR, et al. Neurocognition in patients with brain metastases treated with radiosurgery or radiosurgery plus whole-brain irradiation: a randomised controlled trial. Lancet Oncol. 2009;10:1037–44. https://doi.org/10.1016/S1470-2045(09)70263-3.
8. Brown PD, Jaeckle K, Ballman KV, et al. Effect of radiosurgery alone vs radiosurgery with whole brain radiation therapy on cognitive function in patients with 1 to 3 brain metastases: a randomized clinical trial. JAMA. 2016;316:401–9. https://doi.org/10.1001/jama.2016.9839.
9. McKay WH, McTyre ER, Okoukoni C, et al. Repeat stereotactic radiosurgery as salvage therapy for locally recurrent brain metastases previously treated with radiosurgery. J Neurosurg. 2016;127(1):148. https://doi.org/10.3171/2016.5.JNS153051.
10. Soliman H, Ruschin M, Angelov L, et al. Consensus contouring guidelines for postoperative completely resected cavity stereotactic radiosurgery for brain metastases. Int J Radiat Oncol Biol Phys. 2018;100:436–42. https://doi.org/10.1016/j.ijrobp.2017.09.047.
11. Shaw E, Scott C, Souhami L, et al. Single dose radiosurgical treatment of recurrent previously irradiated primary brain tumors and brain metastases: final report of RTOG protocol 90-05. Int J Radiat Oncol Biol Phys. 2000;47:291–8.
12. Manning MA, Cardinale RM, Benedict SH, et al. Hypofractionated stereotactic radiotherapy as an alternative to radiosurgery for the treatment of patients with brain metastases. Int J Radiat Oncol Biol Phys. 2000;47:603–8.
13. Aoyama H, Shirato H, Onimaru R, et al. Hypofractionated stereotactic radiotherapy alone without whole-brain irradiation for patients with solitary and oligo brain metastasis using noninvasive fixation of the skull. Int J Radiat Oncol. 2003;56:793–800. https://doi.org/10.1016/S0360-3016(03)00014-2.
14. Ernst-Stecken A, Ganslandt O, Lambrecht U, et al. Phase II trial of hypofractionated stereotactic radiotherapy for brain metastases: results and toxicity. Radiother Oncol J Eur Soc Ther Radiol Oncol. 2006;81:18–24. https://doi.org/10.1016/j.radonc.2006.08.024.
15. Murai T, Ogino H, Manabe Y, et al. Fractionated stereotactic radiotherapy using Cyber Knife for the treatment of large brain metastases: a dose escalation study. Clin Oncol (R Coll Radiol). 2014;26:151–8. https://doi.org/10.1016/j.clon.2013.11.027.

16. Minniti G, Esposito V, Clarke E, et al. Multidose stereotactic radiosurgery (9 Gy × 3) of the postoperative resection cavity for treatment of large brain metastases. Int J Radiat Oncol Biol Phys. 2013;86:623–9. https://doi.org/10.1016/j.ijrobp.2013.03.037.
17. Brown PD, Ballman KV, Cerhan JH, et al. Postoperative stereotactic radiosurgery compared with whole brain radiotherapy for resected metastatic brain disease (NCCTG N107C/CEC·3): a multicentre, randomised, controlled, phase 3 trial. Lancet Oncol. 2017;18:1049–60. https://doi.org/10.1016/S1470-2045(17)30441-2.
18. Mahajan A, Ahmed S, McAleer MF, et al. Post-operative stereotactic radiosurgery versus observation for completely resected brain metastases: a single-centre, randomised, controlled, phase 3 trial. Lancet Oncol. 2017;18:1040–8. https://doi.org/10.1016/S1470-2045(17)30414-X.
19. Timmerman R. A story of hypofractionation and the table on the wall. Int J Radiat Oncol Biol Phys. 2022;112(1):4–21. https://doi.org/10.1016/j.ijrobp.2021.09.027.
20. Miller JA, Bennett EE, Xiao R, et al. Association between radiation necrosis and tumor biology after stereotactic radiosurgery for brain metastasis. Int J Radiat Oncol Biol Phys. 2016;96(5):1060. https://doi.org/10.1016/j.ijrobp.2016.08.039.
21. Xu Y, Rong X, Hu W, et al. Bevacizumab monotherapy reduces radiation-induced brain necrosis in nasopharyngeal carcinoma patients: a randomized controlled trial. Int J Radiat Oncol Biol Phys. 2018;101:1087–95. https://doi.org/10.1016/j.ijrobp.2018.04.068.
22. Ahluwalia M, Barnett GH, Deng D, et al. Laser ablation after stereotactic radiosurgery: a multicenter prospective study in patients with metastatic brain tumors and radiation necrosis. J Neurosurg. 2018;130:804–11. https://doi.org/10.3171/2017.11.JNS171273.
23. Nabors LB, Portnow J, Ahluwalia M, et al. Central nervous system cancers, version 3.2020, NCCN clinical practice guidelines in oncology. J Natl Compr Cancer Netw. 2020;18:1537–70. https://doi.org/10.6004/jnccn.2020.0052.
24. Andrews DW, Scott CB, Sperduto PW, et al. Whole brain radiation therapy with or without stereotactic radiosurgery boost for patients with one to three brain metastases: phase III results of the RTOG 9508 randomised trial. Lancet. 2004;363:1665–72. https://doi.org/10.1016/S0140-6736(04)16250-8.
25. Aoyama H, Shirato H, Tago M, et al. Stereotactic radiosurgery plus whole-brain radiation therapy vs stereotactic radiosurgery alone for treatment of brain metastases: a randomized controlled trial. JAMA. 2006;295:2483–91. https://doi.org/10.1001/jama.295.21.2483.
26. Kocher M, Soffietti R, Abacioglu U, et al. Adjuvant whole-brain radiotherapy versus observation after radiosurgery or surgical resection of one to three cerebral metastases: results of the EORTC 22952-26001 study. J Clin Oncol. 2011;29:134–41. https://doi.org/10.1200/JCO.2010.30.1655.
27. Likhacheva A, Pinnix CC, Parikh NR, et al. Predictors of survival in contemporary practice after initial radiosurgery for brain metastases. Int J Radiat Oncol Biol Phys. 2013;85:656–61. https://doi.org/10.1016/j.ijrobp.2012.05.047.
28. Ammirati M, Kshettry VR, Lamki T, et al. A prospective phase II trial of fractionated stereotactic intensity modulated radiotherapy with or without surgery in the treatment of patients with 1 to 3 newly diagnosed symptomatic brain metastases. Neurosurgery. 2014;74:586–94; discussion 594. https://doi.org/10.1227/NEU.0000000000000325.
29. Brennan C, Yang TJ, Hilden P, et al. A phase 2 trial of stereotactic radiosurgery boost after surgical resection for brain metastases. Int J Radiat Oncol Biol Phys. 2014;88:130–6. https://doi.org/10.1016/j.ijrobp.2013.09.051.
30. Jensen CA, Chan MD, McCoy TP, et al. Cavity-directed radiosurgery as adjuvant therapy after resection of a brain metastasis. J Neurosurg. 2011;114:1585–91. https://doi.org/10.3171/2010.11.JNS10939.
31. Choi CYH, Chang SD, Gibbs IC, et al. Stereotactic radiosurgery of the postoperative resection cavity for brain metastases: prospective evaluation of target margin on tumor control. Int J Radiat Oncol Biol Phys. 2012;84:336–42. https://doi.org/10.1016/j.ijrobp.2011.12.009.

Part III
Head and Neck Tumors

Chapter 13
Nasopharynx

Jacob T. Hall, Gregory D. Judy, and Bhishamjit S. Chera

13.1 Introduction

Radiation therapy is the primary treatment for nasopharyngeal carcinoma given its difficult anatomical location for surgical resection and the knowledge of it being a radiosensitive tumor that demonstrates a dose-response to radiation. Traditionally, more advanced tumors have a significant local failure rate, in part because the dose of radiation that can be delivered is limited by critical adjacent normal structures. Various methods including brachytherapy and SBRT allow for dose escalation while also minimizing dose to the surrounding normal tissue, with SBRT also providing the benefit of being noninvasive. This chapter summarizes the use of hypofractionated RT, focusing on SBRT, for nasopharyngeal carcinoma in the definitive setting where it is used as a boost to traditional EBRT, as well as in the re-irradiation setting. Brachytherapy for H&N cancers is covered in a separate chapter.

J. T. Hall
Department of Radiation Oncology, University of North Carolina School of Medicine, Chapel Hill, NC, USA
e-mail: jacob.hall@unchealth.unc.edu

G. D. Judy (✉)
Department of Radiation Oncology, University of North Carolina School of Medicine, Chapel Hill, NC, USA

Lineberger Comprehensive Cancer Center, University of North Carolina School of Medicine, Chapel Hill, NC, USA
e-mail: gregory.judy@unchealth.unc.edu

B. S. Chera
Department of Radiation Oncology, MUSC, Medical University of South Carolina, Charleston, USA
e-mail: Bchera@med.unc.edu

O. Kaidar-Person, R. Chen (eds.), *Hypofractionated and Stereotactic Radiation Therapy*, https://doi.org/10.1007/978-3-031-47701-0_13

13.2 Pearls

- ~86,000 annual cases worldwide. Distinct geographic distribution with high incidence in southern China and Hong Kong (25–50 cases/100,000 people), while less common in the USA and Western Europe (0.2–0.5 cases/100,000 people).
- More common in men (2–3:1). Two age peaks: 15–25 years and 50–60 years.
- Strong association with EBV (70–80% of patients); other risk factors include tobacco, alcohol, and preserved or fermented food consumption.
  - p16 positive, EBV negative in approximately 20% of the cases.
- Higher incidence with known first-degree relative.
- Most common presenting symptoms include headache, diplopia, facial numbness (cranial nerve involvement), and neck mass (nodal involvement). Other symptoms can include nasal pain/obstruction, epistaxis, serous otitis media, tinnitus, hearing loss, or other cranial nerve involvement (III, IV, V, VI most common).
- Local anatomy:
  - Arises from epithelial lining of the nasopharynx.
  - Three histological subtypes: WHO I (keratinizing SCC, ~25% of US cases), WHO II (nonkeratinizing, differentiated SCC, ~12% of US cases), and WHO III (nonkeratinizing, undifferentiated, ~63% US of cases vs. 95% of Chinese cases). There is also a basaloid SCC, noted to be more aggressive with poor survival.
  - Anatomical borders of nasopharynx:

    Anterior—posterior nasal septum and nasal choanae
    Posterior—pharyngeal mucosa
    Superior—sphenoid bone
    Inferior—roof of the soft palate

  - The lateral wall contains pharyngeal opening of the Eustachian tubes; a protuberance (torus tubarius) is created at the posterior aspect of the orifice. Posterior to the torus tubarius is the fossa of Rosenmüller (most common primary site).
- Common pathways of local spread include along the walls of the nasopharynx, superiorly through sphenoid bone (can involve CN III, IV, V, VI), and laterally to involve parapharyngeal space (including CN IX–XII).
- High incidence of lymph node metastases at diagnosis—70–80% clinical, 90% subclinical, and up to 50% bilateral. Cervical levels II and V most commonly involved.
- Distant metastases present in 5–10%; most common sites are bone, lung, and liver.
- Medical workup:
  - H&P, focusing on assessment of cranial nerves and cervical lymph node assessment

  - Fiberoptic nasopharyngolaryngoscopy
  - Lab work: CBC, metabolic panel, liver function tests, TSH, and EBV DNA viral load
  - Dental and baseline speech/swallowing evaluations

- Imaging workup: Crucial to determine the extent of tumor invasion and detecting nodal metastases

  - MRI head/neck w/wo contrast, CT neck w/ contrast, chest CT wo contrast. Additionally, strongly consider PET/CT to assess distant metastases.

    MRI: Appear as heterogeneous-enhancing mass on T1 post-contrast image; T1 pre- and T2 images reveal isointense tumor compared to muscle; also good to delineate PNI and medullary bone invasion.
    CT: Appear as soft-tissue mass; will show heterogeneous enhancement post-contrast; optimal for assessing cortical bone involvement.
    PET/CT: Both primary and nodal metastases will show FDG avidity.

- Pathology workup:

  - EBV FISH or PCR.
  - HPV and p16 can also test positive, but no prognostic/predictive value in nasopharynx cancer.

- Treatment strategies: Radiation therapy with EBRT alone for early stage tumors (stage I). Radiation with EBRT + concurrent chemotherapy for locally advanced tumors (stage 2–4). SBRT can be used as a boost following EBRT for primary treatment, or as sole therapy in the re-irradiation setting. Surgery not typically recommended due to anatomic location.

13.3 Patient Selection for SBRT

- Definitive setting: EBRT (5–7 weeks) followed by SBRT boost (1–6 weeks later) to radiographically residual tumor.
- Re-irradiation setting:

  - Small (≤3.5 cm diameter or ≤5 cc tumor volume), single lesion preferred; node negative.
  - Biopsy or radiographic-proven local persistence or recurrence.
  - Not directly encasing cavernous sinus and/or internal carotid artery or within 9 mm of optic chiasm/optic nerve (or use multiple fractions to reduce late complications).

13.4 Treatment Planning

Simulation instructions	SBRT boost • 1–6 weeks post conventionally fractionated chemoradiation • Repeat diagnostic MRI w/wo contrast – Use T1 post-contrast MRI to aid in tumor delineation and planning – T2 sequences are helpful to distinguish between inflammation/fluid and gross tumor • Use adaptive planning: – Re-simulate patient: Supine, immobilized with head and neck thermoplastic mask or stereotactic frame • Planning CT performed with IV contrast, 1–3 mm slices • Fuse pretreatment and post EBRT MRI to CT sim to delineate residual tumor after initial EBRT • Post-EBRT GTV is the target (residual tumor). Re-irradiation: • Simulate supine immobilized with head and neck thermoplastic mask or stereotactic frame • Planning CT performed with IV contrast, 1–3 mm slices • Fuse updated diagnostic MRI (should be within 2 weeks of CT simulation) to planning CT to delineate recurrent tumor
Image guidance	• CyberKnife: skull and spine tracking • Linac: CBCT
Margins	PTV = GTV + 3–5 mm
Dosimetric considerations	Dose prescribed to periphery of lesion. Goal = 95% of PTV covered by 80% IDL Depending upon technique, target shape, and proximity to critical structures, prescribing to lower IDL may be necessary Conformity index for the PTV should be ≤2 (preferably ≤1.5)

13.5 Common Dose/Fractionation Schemes

13.5.1 Definitive EBRT + SBRT Boost

There is a range of doses used in the literature. EBRT doses typically range from 2 Gy × 25 to 35 fx with SBRT boost doses ranging from 7–15 Gy × 1 fx to 12–15 Gy total in 3–5 fx.

Dose/fx	# of fx	Total dose	Notes
EBRT—2 Gy SBRT boost—11–12 Gy	EBRT—33 SBRT boost—1	EBRT—66 Gy SBRT boost—11–12 Gy	Use SBRT boost for small amount of residual tumor, away from critical OAR(s) [1]
EBRT—2 Gy SBRT boost—4–5 Gy	EBRT—33 SBRT boost—3	EBRT—66 Gy SBRT boost—12–15 Gy	For use when nearby critical OAR(s); treat boost QOD [2, 3]
EBRT—2 Gy SBRT boost—5 Gy	EBRT—25 SBRT boost—3	EBRT—50 Gy SBRT boost—15 Gy	Alternative for use when nearby critical OAR(s); treat boost QOD [2, 3]

13.5.2 *Definitive Hypofractionated EBRT*

Hypofractionated RT either alone or with concurrent chemotherapy have been described. There may be a higher rate of temporal lobe necrosis with these regimens.

Dose/fx	# of fx	Total dose	Notes
2.34 Gy	30	70.2 Gy	Treat QD [4]
2.25–2.27	30	67.5–68 Gy	Tread QD ± concurrent chemotherapy [5, 6]

13.5.3 *Re-irradiation SBRT*

Wide range of fractionation schedules in the literature. Re-irradiation dose depends on tumor size, dose to nearby OARs, cumulative RT already received, and time interval from previous RT.

Dose/fx	# of fx	Total dose	Notes
9 Gy	2	18 Gy	Treat QOD [7]
11 Gy	3	33 Gy	Treat QOD [8]
12 Gy	4	48 Gy	Treat QOD [7]
6 Gy	5	30 Gy	Treat QOD [9]
6 Gy	8	48 Gy	Treat QOD [7]
8 Gy	6	48 Gy	Treat QOD [10]

13.6 Normal Tissue Tolerances

	TG101[a] [11]	
Organ	Dmax	Volumetric
Brainstem		
1 fx	15 Gy	<0.5 cc
3 fx	23 Gy	<0.5 cc
5 fx	31 Gy	<0.5 cc
DLT	Cranial neuropathy	
Optic nerves/chiasm		
1 fx	10 Gy	<0.2 cc
3 fx	17 Gy	<0.2 cc
5 fx	25 Gy	<0.2 cc
DLT	Neuritis	
Spinal cord		
1 fx	14 Gy	<0.35 cc
3 fx	22 Gy	<0.35 cc
5 fx	30 Gy	<0.35 cc
DLT	Myelitis	

	TG101[a] [11]	
Organ	Dmax	Volumetric
Cochlea		
1 fx	9 Gy	NA
3 fx	17 Gy	NA
5 fx	25 Gy	NA
DLT	Hearing loss	

[a]At UNC we follow TG101 constraints. However, TG101 dose constraints were *not* created from nasopharynx patients who received SBRT following EBRT or SBRT alone. Thus while the constraints may not directly apply to nasopharynx patients, they are a good reference

13.7 Patient Management

1. Premedicate for SBRT with single-dose 4 mg PO dexamethasone. May consider premedicating with antiemetic (e.g., Zofran 4 mg PO × 1 or Phenergan 12.5 mg PO × 1, 30 min before treatment) for nausea or anxiolytic (e.g., Ativan 0.5–1 mg PO × 1, 30 min before treatment) for claustrophobia and/or anxiety.
2. Toxicity

   (a) Definitive (EBRT + SBRT boost)

   - Acute:

     – Skin/soft tissue (dermatitis, alopecia, xerostomia, mucositis, dysgeusia, dysphagia, odynophagia)

       Emollients (Aquaphor, calendula): remove prior to RT treatment
       Baking soda/salt rinses up to 12x/day
       Oral solutions (first BLM, magic mouthwash): use prior to meals
       Pain medication: long-acting example—fentanyl patch 25–100 mcg q72 h; short-acting example—oxycodone 5–20 mg q4–6 h

     – Nausea/vomiting

       – Zofran 4 mg q8 h; can increase to 8 mg q8 h
       – Phenergan 12.5 mg q4–6 h; can increase to 25 mg q4–6 h
       – Compazine 5 mg q6 h; can increase to 10 mg q6 h

   - Subacute/late:

     – Skin/soft tissue (ulceration, fistula, necrosis, <10%)
     – Tinnitus/hearing loss (variable, worse when receiving cisplatin chemotherapy): Discontinue offending drug; Refer to neurology
     – Trismus (<10%)
     – Cranial nerve neuropathy (<10%)
     – Nasopharyngeal hemorrhage (<5%)

- Pharyngeal stricture/stenosis (<10%)
- Temporal lobe necrosis/osteoradionecrosis of skull base (<15%)
- Carotid aneurysm/blowout (~1%): Emergent surgery
- For above late complications, recommend referral to appropriate specialty for management (ENT, surgery, neurology, etc.).

(b) Re-irradiation (SBRT alone)

- Acute:
  - Patients unlikely to experience symptoms during treatment
  - In the 2–4 weeks posttreatment, patients can experience dysphagia, odynophagia, dysgeusia, fatigue, or nausea/vomiting

    Management similar to definitive treatment setting (above)

- Subacute /late:
  - Mucosal necrosis (<10%)
  - Trismus (<10%)
  - Nasopharyngeal hemorrhage (10%)
  - Pharyngeal stricture/stenosis (<15%)
  - Temporal lobe necrosis/ORN skull base (<15%)
  - Carotid aneurysm/blowout (5–10%)
  - Cranial nerve neuropathies [] (<15%)
  - *For above late complications, recommend referral to appropriate specialty for management (ENT, surgery, neurology, etc.).*

3. Systemic therapy:

(a) There are minimal to no data addressing the use of concurrent chemotherapy/systemic therapy with SBRT boost, in either the definitive setting or the re-irradiation setting. When used in the definitive setting, neoadjuvant, concurrent, or adjuvant chemotherapy was frequently given with EBRT; however, its use was held during the SBRT boost. When used in the re-irradiation setting, chemotherapy is typically not given concurrently with radiation; if given at all, typically following completion of radiation.

(b) We recommend against the use of concurrent systemic therapy off-study due to the concern of increasing toxicity and lack of data on benefit of this combination.

13.8 Follow-Up

- The authors generally see patient at 1 month posttreatment to assess acute toxicity.
- H&P, fiber-optic nasopharyngoscopy every 2–3 months for first 2 years, q6 months years 3–5, then annually.

- PET/CT and MRI w/wo contrast at 3 months posttreatment, then q6 months for first 2 years, then as clinically indicated. Chest CT w/o contrast annually.
- If pretreatment EBV viral load is elevated, follow posttreatment EBV DNA plasma levels at 3 and 6 months, then as clinically indicated.

13.9 Relevant Literature

- There are no published guidelines on the recommended dose/fractionation of SBRT for both definitive boost following chemoradiation or in the re-irradiation setting; however, there are several studies demonstrating its efficacy.
- There is wide variation in published studies with regard to dose, fraction size, prescribed IDL, use of concurrent chemotherapy, and timing of when boost is delivered. Overall promising results with small but concerning late toxicity.

13.9.1 Definitive EBRT + SBRT Boost

Study	Patients	Treatment	Median follow-up	Outcomes
Prospective studies				
Hara (2008) [1]	*n* = 82, stage IIA-IVb 85% with concurrent cisplatin chemotherapy during EBRT	EBRT to 66 Gy + single fx SBRT boost Boost 2–6 weeks post-EBRT (reimaged prior to boost) Boost: Median 11 Gy (range 7–15 Gy) × 1 fx Dose Rx to 80% IDL	40 months	98% 5-year LC 69% 5-year OS Late toxicity: Carotid aneurysm (1%), temporal lobe necrosis (12%)
Chen (2006) [2]	*n* = 64, majority stage III–IVb 60% with concurrent cisplatin chemotherapy during EBRT	EBRT 64–68 Gy + fractionated SBRT boost Boost 1 week post-EBRT Boost: 4–5 Gy × 3 fx GTV + 2–3 mm Dose Rx to 85% IDL	31 months	93% 3-year LC 84% 3-year OS Late toxicity: No grade 4 toxicity. 3 pts died from nasal bleeding, unclear if related to SBRT
Retrospective studies				
Yamazaki (2014) [3]	*n* = 25, stage IIA–IVb Majority with concurrent cisplatin or 5FU chemotherapy during EBRT	EBRT to 50 Gy (median) in 1.8–2 Gy/fx + SBRT boost Boost: 5 Gy × 3 fx (median) Dose Rx to 80% IDL	28 months	71% 5-year LC 70% 5-year OS Late toxicity: grade 2 ulcerations (12%), grade 3+ fistula (8%)

Study	Patients	Treatment	Median follow-up	Outcomes
Yau (2004) [12]	*n* = 52, majority stage II–IV 23% with concurrent cisplatin chemotherapy during EBRT	EBRT to 66 Gy + either brachytherapy or SBRT boost Boost: 7.5 Gy × 2 fx or 2.5 Gy × 8 fx Brachytherapy: ^{192}Ir HDR, median 4–10 Gy × 2–5 fx, twice weekly GTV + 3–5 mm Dose Rx to 100% IDL	36 months	**Overall**: 71% 3-year LC 82% 3-year OS **Brachytherapy**: 71% 3-year LC **SBRT**: 82% 3-year LC Late toxicity: Transient soft-tissue necrosis (3%)

Abbreviations: *EBRT* external beam radiotherapy, *fx* fraction, *Rx* prescription, *IDL* isodose line, *LC* local control, *OS* overall survival

13.9.2 Definitive Hypofractionated EBRT

Study	Patients	Treatment	Median follow-up	Outcomes
Prospective studies				
Bakst (2011) [4]	*n* = 25	Dose painting EBRT with concurrent chemotherapy 2.34 Gy × 30 fx PTV = GTV + 1 cm	33 months	91% 3-year LC 89% 3-year OS Late toxicity: 12% temporal lobe necrosis
Miao (2019) [5]	*n = 254*	Dose painting EBRT with or without concurrent chemotherapy 2.27 Gy × 30 fx	62 months	**With chemotherapy** 74% 5-year OS 94% 5-year LRRFS **Without chemotherapy** 72% 5-year OS 94% 5-year LRRFS
Du (2017) [6]	*n = 296*	Dose painting EBRT with concurrent chemotherapy 2.12 Gy × 33 fx or 2.25 Gy × 30 fx	33 months	**2.12 Gy/fx** 94.0% 3-year LRRFS 93.9% 3-year OS **2.25 Gy/fx** 92.7% 3-year LRRFS 90.4% 3-year OS No statistically significant differences in oncologic outcomes or acute and late toxicity

Abbreviations: *EBRT* external beam radiotherapy, *LC* local control, *OS* overall survival, *LRRFS* local-regional recurrence-free survival

13.9.3 Re-irradiation

Study	Patients	Treatment	Median follow-up	Outcomes
Retrospective studies				
Chua (2009) [7]	*n* = 125 Previous EBRT 66–70 Gy. ~25% concurrent chemotherapy Median time to recurrence 10 months	Single fx SBRT: 12.5 Gy median Multiple fx SBRT: 18 Gy total in 2–4 fx qod (persistent disease), or 48 Gy total in 4–6 fx (recurrent disease) PTV = GTV + 2–3 mm Dose Rx to 80% IDL (single fx) or 90% IDL (multiple fx) Median tumor volume 5.2 cc	40 months	**Single fraction**: 51% 3-year LC 66% 3-year OS 33% late toxicity (16% brain necrosis, 2% hemorrhage) **Multiple fraction**: 83% 3-year LC 61% 3-year OS 21% late toxicity (12% brain necrosis, 4% hemorrhage)
Seo (2009) [8]	*n* = 35 Previous EBRT + cisplatin. Median RT dose 70 Gy Median time to recurrence 26 months	Median 33 Gy total in 3 fx or 5 fx, qd PTV = GTV + 2 mm Dose Rx to 80% IDL Median tumor volume 8 cc	25 months	84% 5-year LC 60% 5-year OS 5 patients with late grade 4-5 toxicity: mucosal necrosis (5%), hemorrhage (9%)
Ozyigit (2011) [9]	*n* = 51 Previous EBRT 67–70 Gy. ~60% concurrent chemotherapy Median time to recurrence 36 months	SBRT: 30 Gy in 5 fx qd 3DCRT: 60 Gy in 30 fx PTV = GTV (SBRT) Dose Rx to 95–99% IDL Median tumor volume 63 cc	24 months	**SBRT**: 82% 2-year LC 64% 2-year CSS 21% late toxicity (17% carotid blowout, 12% cranial neuropathy, 4% brain necrosis) **3DCRT**: 80% 2-year LC 47% 2-year CSS 48% late toxicity (4% carotid blowout, 26% cranial neuropathy, 19% brain necrosis, 18% trismus)

Study	Patients	Treatment	Median follow-up	Outcomes
Wu (2007) [10]	$n = 90$ (majority had single lesion, ≤4 cm) Previous EBRT 60–74 Gy Median time to recurrence 23 months	Persistent disease: median 6 Gy × 3 fx qd Recurrent: median 8 Gy × 6 fx qd PTV = GTV + 2–3 mm Dose Rx to 90% IDL Tumor volume 5–6 cc	20 months	**Persistent disease**: 89% 3-year LFFS 81% 3-year DMFS 72% 3-year PFS 8.8% late toxicity: temporal lobe necrosis (3%) **Recurrent disease**: 75% 3-year LFFS 67% 3-year DMFS 43% 3-year PFS 25% late toxicity: mucosal necrosis (7%), Grade 5 hemorrhage (2%), brainstem necrosis (3%), temporal lobe necrosis (3%)
Pai (2002) [13]	$n = 36$ Previous EBRT 64–81 Gy Median time to recurrence 16 months	3DCRT (median 2 Gy × 25 fx) + SBRT (median 12 Gy × 1 fx) PTV = GTV Dose Rx to 80% IDL Median tumor volume 16.8 cc	22 months	57% 3-year LC 54% 3-year OS Late toxicity: mucosal necrosis (11%) and nasal bleeding (8%)

Abbreviations: *EBRT* external beam radiotherapy, *fx* fraction, *IDL* isodose line, *LC* local control, *OS* overall survival, *CSS* cancer-specific survival, *LFFS* local failure-free survival, *DMFS* distant metastasis-free survival, *PFS* progression-free survival

13.10 Summary

There is wide variation in published studies with regard to dose, fraction size, prescribed IDL, use of concurrent chemotherapy, and volume irradiated. Results are promising; however, there remains a relatively high rate of grade 3+ toxicity, including some grade 5.

13.11 UNC Experience

At our institution, we do not routinely perform SBRT boost in the definitive setting, as the LC and OS rates are similar to those of definitive EBRT alone with chemotherapy, and SBRT boost has a higher risk of severe late effects (e.g. carotid blowout, temporal lobe necrosis).

For patients with persistent/recurrent local disease, we re-irradiate with SBRT at 6 Gy/fx for five fractions for a total dose of 30 Gy. Radiation is given every other day using the CyberKnife radiosurgery system. The GTV is expanded 3–5 mm to make a PTV (no CTV is created). We typically track on the skull base and prescribe to the 80% IDL. We counsel the patient regarding risk for carotid artery blowout: this is an emergency and, if it occurs, patients should seek emergency care.

References

1. Hara W, Loo BW Jr, Goffinet DR, et al. Excellent local control with stereotactic radiotherapy boost after external beam radiotherapy in patients with nasopharyngeal carcinoma. Int J Radiat Oncol Biol Phys. 2008;71:393–400.
2. Chen HH, Tsai ST, Wang MS, et al. Experience in fractionated stereotactic body radiation therapy boost for newly diagnosed nasopharyngeal carcinoma. Int J Radiat Oncol Biol Phys. 2006;66:1408–14.
3. Yamazaki H, Ogita M, Himei K, et al. Hypofractionated stereotactic radiotherapy using CyberKnife as a boost treatment for head and neck cancer, a multi-institutional survey: impact of planning target volume. Anticancer Res. 2014;34:5755–9.
4. Bakst RL, Lee N, Pfister DG, et al. Hypofractionated dose-painting intensity modulated radiation therapy with chemotherapy for nasopharyngeal carcinoma: a prospective trial. Int J Radiat Oncol Biol Phys. 2011;80:148–53.
5. Miao J, Wang L, Zhu M, Xiao W, Wu H, Di M, Huang Y, Huang S, Han F, Deng X, Guo X. Long-term survival and late toxicities of elderly nasopharyngeal carcinoma (NPC) patients treated by high-total- and fractionated-dose simultaneous modulated accelerated radiotherapy with or without chemotherapy. Oral Oncol. 2019;89:40–7. https://doi.org/10.1016/j.oraloncology.2018.12.008.
6. Du L, Zhang XX, Feng LC, Qu BL, Chen J, Yang J, Liu HX, Xu SP, Xie CB, Ma L. Propensity score matching analysis of a phase II study on simultaneous modulated accelerated radiation therapy using helical tomotherapy for nasopharyngeal carcinomas. BMC Cancer. 2017;17(1):1–11. https://doi.org/10.1186/s12885-017-3581-1.
7. Chua DT, Wu SX, Lee V, Tsang J. Comparison of single versus fractionated dose of stereotactic radiotherapy for salvaging local failures of nasopharyngeal carcinoma: a matched-cohort analysis. Head Neck Oncol. 2009;1:13.
8. Seo Y, Yoo H, Yoo S, et al. Robotic system-based fractionated stereotactic radiotherapy in locally recurrent nasopharyngeal carcinoma. Radiother Oncol. 2009;93:570–4.
9. Ozyigit G, Cengiz M, Yazici G, et al. A retrospective comparison of robotic stereotactic body radiotherapy and three-dimensional conformal radiotherapy for the reirradiation of locally recurrent nasopharyngeal carcinoma. Int J Radiat Oncol Biol Phys. 2011;81:e263–8.
10. Wu SX, Chua DT, Deng ML, et al. Outcome of fractionated stereotactic radiotherapy for 90 patients with locally persistent and recurrent nasopharyngeal carcinoma. Int J Radiat Oncol Biol Phys. 2007;69:761–9.
11. Benedict SH, Yenice KM, Followill D, et al. Stereotactic body radiation therapy: the report of AAPM task group 101. Med Phys. 2010;37:4078–101.
12. Yau TK, Sze WM, Lee WM, et al. Effectiveness of brachytherapy and fractionated stereotactic radiotherapy boost for persistent nasopharyngeal carcinoma. Head Neck. 2004;26:1024–30.
13. Pai PC, Chuang CC, Wei KC, Tsang NM, Tseng CK, Chang CN. Stereotactic radiosurgery for locally recurrent nasopharyngeal carcinoma. Head Neck. 2002;24:748–53.

Chapter 14
Larynx

Jacob T. Hall, Gregory D. Judy, and Bhishamjit S. Chera

14.1 Introduction

Early stage glottic SCC carries a favorable prognosis with low rates of long-term complications when treated with RT. One particular advantage to using RT is improved preservation of voice quality compared to laryngectomy. Historically, small, daily fractions were used to treat this disease; however, treatment has evolved to a more hypofractionated, shorter overall treatment course which improves local control without increasing complications. This chapter summarizes the use of hypofractionated RT for the treatment of early stage SCC of the glottic larynx.

J. T. Hall
Department of Radiation Oncology, University of North Carolina School of Medicine, Chapel Hill, NC, USA
e-mail: jacob.hall@unchealth.unc.edu

G. D. Judy (✉)
Department of Radiation Oncology, University of North Carolina School of Medicine, Chapel Hill, NC, USA

Lineberger Comprehensive Cancer Center, University of North Carolina School of Medicine, Chapel Hill, NC, USA
e-mail: gregory.judy@unchealth.unc.edu

B. S. Chera
Department of Radiation Oncology, MUSC, Medical University of South Carolina, Charleston, USA
e-mail: Bchera@med.unc.edu

O. Kaidar-Person, R. Chen (eds.), *Hypofractionated and Stereotactic Radiation Therapy*, https://doi.org/10.1007/978-3-031-47701-0_14

14.2 Pearls

- 13,000 annual estimated cases in the USA (~3.4 cases/100,000 people).
- Predominately affects men; median age at diagnosis is 65.
- Etiologies include tobacco, alcohol, betel nut consumption, and deficiencies in iron, vitamin B12, and vitamin C.
- Common presenting symptoms include hoarseness, dysphagia, odynophagia, chronic cough, and referred otalgia; can be location-dependent.
- 90–95% are SCC; can also see verrucous carcinoma, adenocarcinoma, adenoid cystic carcinoma, and mucoepidermoid carcinomas.
- Local anatomy:
  - Divided into three subsites:

    Supraglottis: includes supra- and infrahyoid epiglottis, aryepiglottic folds, arytenoids, ventricles, and false vocal cords.
    Glottis: true vocal cords, infraglottis (free edge of true vocal cord to within 5 mm inferior), and mucosa of the anterior and posterior commissures.
    Subglottis: lower border of glottis to inferior border of cricoid cartilage.

  - Intrinsic muscles of the larynx are innervated by recurrent laryngeal nerve, except for cricothyroid muscle, which is innervated by the superior laryngeal nerve and is solely responsible for producing tension of the vocal cords.
- Lymph node drainage:
  - Glottis has sparse lymphatic supply, and thus rarely spreads to lymph nodes (T1–2: <5%; T3–4: ~20%). If involved, typically bilateral levels II, III, IV, and VI.
  - Supraglottis has richer lymphatic supply and is thus more common to have nodal metastases at presentation (~50%); drains to bilateral levels II, III, IV, and VI.
  - Subglottis typically drains to levels II, III, IV, VI, and VII.
- Incidence of distant metastases is low (≤10%); common sites include lungs>liver>bone.
- Medical workup:
  - H&P; physical exam requires thorough cervical lymph node assessment.
  - Fiberoptic nasopharyngolaryngoscopy.
  - Biopsy and basic lab work (CBC, metabolic panel, liver function tests, TSH).
  - Dental and baseline speech/swallowing evaluations.
- Imaging workup:
  - CT neck w/wo contrast: look for enhancing mass at level of laryngeal sides (supraglottis), true vocal fold (glottis), or cricoid cartilage (subglottis).
  - CT chest w/wo contrast.

  - Additionally may consider PET/CT: look for primary disease and nodal metastases with FDG avidity.

- Treatment strategies: radiation therapy alone or surgery for early stage, T1–2 tumors. Radiation therapy with concurrent chemotherapy or surgical resection for locally advanced stage III–IVB tumors. Surgical resection recommended for T4 tumors.

14.3 Patient Selection for Hypofractionation Treatment

- T1–2 tumors of the glottic larynx

14.4 Treatment Planning

Simulation instructions	• Supine, immobilized with head and neck thermoplastic mask • Head/neck hyperextended (position submandibular glands outside of lateral fields) • Autotraction straps to immobilize and pull shoulders down • Opposed lateral fields typically utilized • 3DCRT plan to minimize normal tissue injury – IMRT is an option: reduces dose to carotid arteries, but there is lack of data to demonstrate benefit in patient outcomes • Daily bolus: over anterior larynx for patients with thin necks and anterior commissure involvement to ensure adequate coverage. 2 cm wide × 5 cm long
Image guidance	• At least weekly portal imaging • Daily clinical verification of light field in the treatment room. See Figs. 14.1 and 14.2: palpate thyroid notch = superior field border, cricoid = inferior field border, thyroid alae = posterior field border
Margins	3DCRT • T1 tumors: 4 × 4 cm or 5 × 5 cm (preferred) field • T2 tumors: 5 × 5 cm (preferred) or 6 × 6 cm field • Borders: *Superior*: bottom/mid-thyroid notch (top of notch if there is supraglottic extension) *Inferior*: bottom of cricoid cartilage (1 cm inferior to cricoid cartilage if subglottic extension) *Posterior*: anterior edge of vertebral body (split vertebral body if there is posterior commissure involvement) *Anterior*: 2 cm skin flash IMRT • CTV = entire larynx (includes anterior/posterior commissures, arytenoids from top of thyroid cartilage to inferior cricoid cartilage) • PTV = CTV + 0–10 mm (wide range in literature)

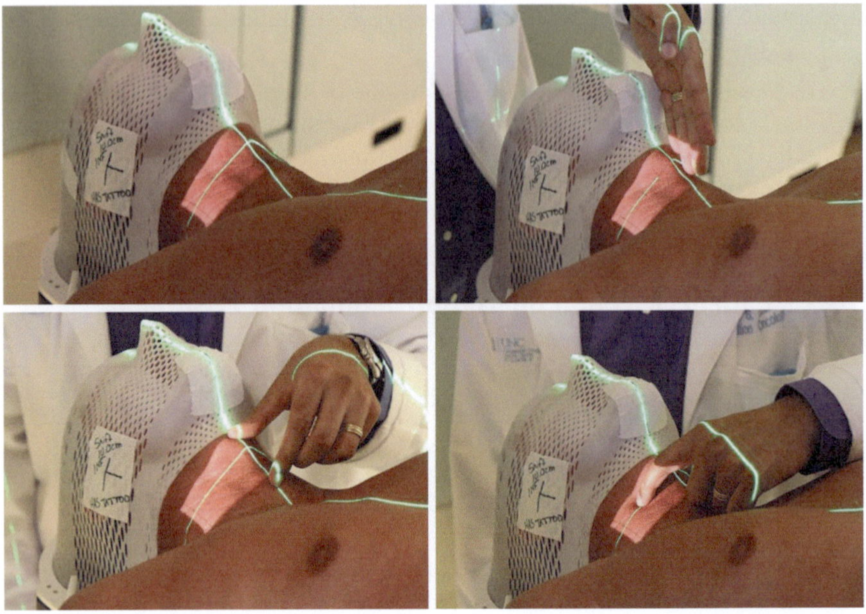

Fig. 14.1 Light field images showing daily verification of light field in the treatment room

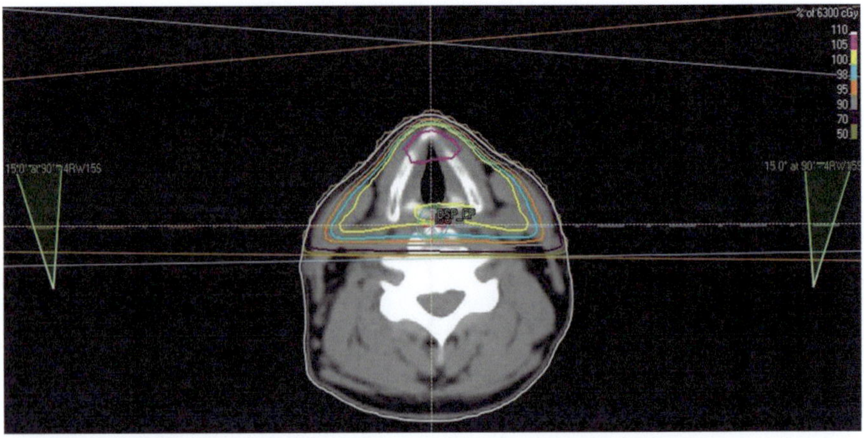

Fig. 14.2 Plan design showing isodose lines

14.5 Common Dose/Fractionation Schemes

Dose/fx	# of fx	Total dose	Notes
2.25 Gy	28	63 Gy	T1 tumors; treat daily [1–6]
2.25 Gy	29	65.25 Gy	T2 tumors; treat daily [1, 3, 4]
2.4 Gy	25	60 Gy	T1–T2 tumors: treat daily [7]

14.6 SBRT

- SBRT for early stage laryngeal cancer has been recently explored following data showing an improvement in local control with hypofractionation.
- Results of two Phase I dose-escalation studies of SBRT for laryngeal cancer have been published.
- SBRT is feasible but likely leads to increased toxicity and possible increased risk of marginal misses, especially when including large laryngeal volumes.
- To our knowledge, there are no phase II or III data comparing SBRT to conventionally or moderately hypofractionated techniques for early stage laryngeal cancer.
- Further investigation is needed to determine if there is a local control benefit that outweighs the increased toxicity with SBRT for early stage laryngeal cancer. The authors do not recommend using SBRT.

14.7 Normal Tissue Tolerances

- The main relevant dose constraint is to ensure that overall plan is not too hot to minimize the risk for laryngeal edema and necrosis: goal of ≤105% of the prescription with a max point dose (0.1–0.3 cc) of ≤110%.
- Several studies have reported increased risk of carotid artery-related adverse events after radiation therapy.
  - We interpret the studies on cerebrovascular disease to show that the risk of moderate and severe carotid complications from neck radiotherapy with 3DCRT is so low that very few patients will end up with a better clinical outcome as a result of changing the radiotherapy modality (e.g., using carotid-sparing IMRT).
  - There is no specific study associating dose volume data with clinical outcomes of carotid artery stenosis/stroke.

14.8 Patient Management

1. No premedications required.
   (a) Tobacco cessation is important—smoking during treatment increases acute toxicities and decreases local control.

2. Toxicity.

   (b) Acute:

   - Skin/soft tissue (dermatitis, mucositis, dysphagia, laryngeal edema).
     - Emollients (Aquaphor, calendula): Remove 4 h prior to RT treatment.
     - Oral solutions (first BLM, magic mouthwash): Use TID prior to meals.
     - Pain medication: typically not needed, or use NSAIDS and acetaminophen.
   - Late:
     - Skin/soft tissue (fibrosis, laryngeal edema, fistula) (<10%).
     - Hypothyroidism (<5%, majority of thyroid is excluded).
     - Laryngeal necrosis (<5%).
     - *For above late complications, recommend referral to appropriate specialty for management (ENT, surgery, PCP, etc.).*

14.9 Follow-Up

- H&P with fiberoptic nasopharyngoscopy every 3 months for first 2 years, q6 months years 3–5, then annually.
- TSH q6–12 months.
- Lung cancer screening as appropriate for patients with smoking history.

14.10 Relevant Literature

Study	Patients	Treatment	Median follow-up	Outcomes
Randomized controlled trials				
Moon (2014) [1]	$n = 156$ T1–2 N0 glottic SCC	(1) 2 Gy × 33–35 fx (2) 2.25 Gy × 28–30 fx Opposed laterals	67 months	**2.25 Gy/fx**: 88.5% 5-year LPFS **2 Gy/fx**: 77.8% 5-year LPFS ($p = 0.213$) Toxicity: No difference between arms
Yamazaki (2006) [2]	$n = 180$ T1 glottic SCC	(1) 2 Gy × 30–33 fx (2) 2.25 Gy × 25–28 fx	64 months	**2.25 Gy/fx**: 92% 5-year LC 100% 5-year CSS **2 Gy/fx**: 77% 5-year LC ($p = 0.004$) 97% 5-year CSS (p = NS) Toxicity: No difference between arms

Study	Patients	Treatment	Median follow-up	Outcomes
Kodaira (2018) [7]	$n = 370$	(1) 2 Gy × 33–35 fx (2) 2.4 Gy × 25–27 fx	36 months	**2 Gy/fx** 79.9% 3-year PFS 98.4% 3-year OS **2.4 Gy/fx** 81.7% 3-year PFS ($p = 0.047$) 93.5% 3-year OS (p = NS) No difference in toxicity
Prospective non-randomized studies				
Sher (2019) [8] Phase I trial	$n = 29$ Tis–T2 glottic SCC	Level 0: 50 Gy in 15 fx ($n = 4$) Level 1: 45 Gy in 10 fx ($n = 13$) Level 2: 42.5 Gy in 5 fx ($n = 12$)	39 months	Level 0: 2 patients with local recurrence Level 1: 1 patient grade 4 laryngeal edema and grade 3 dysphagia. 3 patients with local recurrence Level 2: 1 patient grade 3 laryngeal necrosis and dysphagia. No local recurrence
Kang (2019) [9] Phase I trial	$n = 13$ cT1–2 N0 glottic SCC	Arm 1: 59.5 Gy to GTV with 47.6 Gy to the entire larynx in 17 fx ($n = 7$) Arm 2: 55 Gy to the GTV with 40.7 Gy to the entire larynx in 11 fx ($n = 6$)	37 months for arm 1 and 15 months for arm 2	Arm 1: Grade 1 laryngeal edema in 1 patient. No local recurrence. Arm 2: Grade 3 chronic laryngeal inflammation (laryngeal ulcer, arytenoid necrosis requiring supraglottic laryngectomy) in 2 patients. 1 patient with recurrence
Szutkowski (2016) [5]	$n = 223$	2.25 Gy × 28 fx	60 months	87.5% 5-year OS 73.6% 5-year PFS
Salas-Salas (2019) [6]	$n = 138$	2 Gy × 35 fx vs. 2.2–2.25 Gy × 28–29 fx	120 months	2 Gy/fx vs. 2.2–2.25 Gy/fx No significant difference in LRFS, OS, or late toxicity Increased rate of acute laryngeal toxicity with hypofractionation
Retrospective studies				
Chera (2010) [3]	$n = 585$ T1–2 N0 glottic SCC	2.25 Gy × 28–29 fx (T2 lesions offered 1.2 Gy/fx BID) Opposed laterals	144 months	**Local control**: 93% 10 years (T1a) 91% 10 years (T1b) 80% 10 years (T2a) 67% 10 years (T2b) **Overall survival**: 62% 10 years (T1a) 57% 10 years (T1b) 51% 10 years (T2a) 49% 10 years (T2b) Toxicity: 10 patients with grade 4–5; one fatal RT-induced carotid artery angiosarcoma

Study	Patients	Treatment	Median follow-up	Outcomes
Gowda (2003) [10]	$n = 200$ T1 N0 glottic SCC	3.12 or 3.28 Gy × 16 fx Opposed laterals	72 months	93% 5-year LC 80% 5-year OS Toxicity: No severe acute toxicity; 1 patient with severe late toxicity (continued to smoke following treatment)
Le (1997) [4]	$n = 398$ T1–2 glottic SCC	Total dose: T1 63 Gy, T2 65 Gy Fx sizes: <1.8 Gy, 1.8–1.99 Gy, 2–2.24 Gy, ≥2.25 Gy Opposed laterals	116 months	**T1 tumors** ≥ 2.25 Gy/fx: 94% 5-year LC <1.8 Gy/fx: 79% 5-year LC (p = NS on multivariable analysis) **T2 tumors** ≥ 2.25 Gy/fx: 100% 5-year LC <1.8 Gy/fx: 44% 5-year LC ($p = 0.003$ on multivariable analysis)

Abbreviations: *SCC* squamous cell carcinoma, *fx* fraction, *LPFS* local progression-free survival, *CSS* cancer-specific survival, *PFS* progression-free survival, *OS* overall survival, *LC* local control, *NS* not significant, *LRFS* local recurrence-free survival

14.11 Summary

Hypofractionation improves local control versus standard fractionation with similar rates of severe complications. SBRT may have lower local control and increased toxicity in phase I studies, especially when including the entire larynx; more data on SBRT are needed.

14.12 UNC Experience

Our standard is to treat with 5 × 5 cm opposed lateral fields with daily clinical verification of the light field by the physician. Our interpretation of the published literature on the potential increase in carotid artery-related adverse events is that the risk, if any, is small. We do not treat with carotid-sparing IMRT because the added complexity and cost are not clearly justified until there are data demonstrating a patient outcome benefit. We do not recommend SBRT.

References

1. Moon SH, Cho KH, Chung EJ, et al. A prospective randomized trial comparing hypofractionation with conventional fractionation radiotherapy for T1-2 glottic squamous cell carcinomas: results of a Korean radiation oncology group (KROG-0201) study. Radiother Oncol. 2014;110:98–103.
2. Yamazaki H, Nishiyama K, Tanaka E, Koizumi M, Chatani M. Radiotherapy for early glottic carcinoma (T1N0M0): results of prospective randomized study of radiation fraction size and overall treatment time. Int J Radiat Oncol Biol Phys. 2006;64:77–82.
3. Chera BS, Amdur RJ, Morris CG, Kirwan JM, Mendenhall WM. T1N0 to T2N0 squamous cell carcinoma of the glottic larynx treated with definitive radiotherapy. Int J Radiat Oncol Biol Phys. 2010;78:461.
4. Le QT, Fu KK, Kroll S, et al. Influence of fraction size, total dose, and overall time on local control of T1-T2 glottic carcinoma. Int J Radiat Oncol Biol Phys. 1997;39:115–26.
5. Szutkowski Z, Kawecki A, Jarząbski A, Laskus Z, Krajewski R, Michalski W, Kukołowicz P. Hypofractionated accelerated radiotherapy in T1–3 N0 cancer of the larynx: a prospective cohort study with historical controls. Rep Pract Oncol Radiother. 2016;21(6):537–43. https://doi.org/10.1016/j.rpor.2016.08.001.
6. Salas-Salas BG, Domínguez-Nuez DJ, Cabrera R, Ferrera-Alayón L, Lloret M, Lara PC. Hypofractionation vs. conventional radiotherapy fractionation in the conservative treatment of T1 glottic cancer: a prospective cohort study. Clin Transl Oncol. 2020;22(1):151–7. https://doi.org/10.1007/s12094-019-02118-7.
7. Kodaira T, Kagami Y, Shibata T, Shikama N, Nishimura Y, Ishikura S, Nakamura K, Saito Y, Matsumoto Y, Teshima T, Ito Y. Results of a multi-institutional, randomized, non-inferiority, phase III trial of accelerated fractionation versus standard fractionation in radiation therapy for T1-2N0M0 glottic cancer: Japan Clinical Oncology Group Study (JCOG0701). Ann Oncol. 2018;29(4):992–7. https://doi.org/10.1093/annonc/mdy036.
8. Sher DJ, Timmerman RD, Nedzi L, Ding C, Pham NL, Zhao B, Sumer BD. Phase 1 Fractional dose-escalation study of equipotent stereotactic radiation therapy regimens for early-stage glottic larynx cancer. Int J Radiat Oncol Biol Phys. 2019;105(1):110–8. https://doi.org/10.1016/j.ijrobp.2019.03.010.
9. Kang BH, Yu T, Kim JH, Park JM, Kim JI, Chung EJ, Kwon SK, Kim JH, Wu HG. Early closure of a phase 1 clinical trial for SABR in early-stage glottic cancer. Int J Radiat Oncol Biol Phys. 2019;105(1):104–9. https://doi.org/10.1016/j.ijrobp.2019.03.011.
10. Gowda RV, Henk JM, Mais KL, Sykes AJ, Swindell R, Slevin NJ. Three weeks radiotherapy for T1 glottic cancer: the Christie and Royal Marsden Hospital experience. Radiother Oncol. 2003;68:105–11.

Chapter 15
Other Head and Neck Sites

Jacob T. Hall, Gregory D. Judy, and Bhishamjit S. Chera

15.1 Introduction

Data regarding the use of hypofractionated chemoradiation in the definitive management of head and neck squamous cell carcinoma are increasing. Several prospective and retrospective series have shown local control/response rates comparable to conventional fractionation but increased rates of acute toxicity. There are minimal to no data regarding the use of SBRT as definitive primary treatment in other head and neck disease sites. Limited data support the use of brachytherapy or SBRT as a boost to EBRT in the definitive setting for nasopharyngeal (Chap. 13), paranasal sinus, and oropharyngeal SCC.

J. T. Hall
Department of Radiation Oncology, University of North Carolina School of Medicine, Chapel Hill, NC, USA
e-mail: jacob.hall@unchealth.unc.edu

G. D. Judy (✉)
Department of Radiation Oncology, University of North Carolina School of Medicine, Chapel Hill, NC, USA

Lineberger Comprehensive Cancer Center, University of North Carolina School of Medicine, Chapel Hill, NC, USA
e-mail: gregory.judy@unchealth.unc.edu

B. S. Chera
Department of Radiation Oncology, MUSC, Medical University of South Carolina, Charleston, USA
e-mail: Bchera@med.unc.edu

O. Kaidar-Person, R. Chen (eds.), *Hypofractionated and Stereotactic Radiation Therapy*, https://doi.org/10.1007/978-3-031-47701-0_15

15.2 Patient Selection

- Locally advanced squamous cell carcinoma of the head and neck.
- Many of the studies referenced below included a large proportion of patients with primary oropharyngeal SCC.

15.3 Dose and Fractionation Schemes for Hypofractionated RT with Concurrent Chemotherapy

# of fx	Dose/fx	Total dose
20	2.75 Gy	55 Gy [1–3]
25	2.56 Gy	64 Gy [4]
30	2.33 Gy	70 Gy [5]
30	2.2 Gy	66 Gy [6]

15.4 Relevant Studies

Conventionally fractionated RT plus brachytherapy or SBRT boost

Study	Patients	Treatment	Median follow-up	Outcomes
Retrospective studies				
Al-Mamgani (2013) [7]	$n = 250$ Oropharynx SCC, T1–2 N0-3 Chemotherapy given for N2c/N3	EBRT + brachytherapy or SBRT boost EBRT: 2 Gy × 23 fx Brachytherapy: ^{192}Ir source; PDR: total dose 22 Gy given in 8 fx/day SBRT boost: 5.5 Gy × 3 fx	66 months	**Brachytherapy**: 94% 3-year LC 86% 3-year DFS 83% 3-year OS 31% acute grade 3 toxicity 4% late grade 3 toxicity **SBRT**: 97% 3-year LC 92% 3-year DFS 81% 3-year OS 23% acute grade 3 toxicity 5% late grade 3 toxicity
Lee (2012) [8]	$n = 26$ Locally advanced H&N SCC (nasopharynx, oropharynx, paranasal sinus, tongue)	EBRT + SBRT boost EBRT: Median 50 Gy in 2 Gy/fx SBRT: 5 Gy × 2–5 fx (median 21 Gy/ median 5 fx)	56 months	100% response rate (21 CR, 5 PR) 86% 2-year LRRFR ~35% late grade ≥ 3 toxicities; boost volume significant predictor
Baker (2019) [9]	*n = 195* Oropharynx SCC T1–T3 N0-N2c	EBRT + SBRT boost EBRT: 2 Gy × 23 SBRT: 5.5 Gy × 3	51 months	67% 5-year OS 62% 5-year DFS 84% 5-year LRC 33% required feeding tube 28% late grade ≥ 3 toxicity

Chemoradiation with hypofractionated EBRT

Study	Patients	Treatment	Median follow-up	Outcomes
Prospective studies				
Grover (2021) [6]	$n = 100$ Locally advanced (oropharynx, hypopharynx, and larynx)	Randomized: SIB-IMRT: 2.2 Gy × 30 fx SEQ-IMRT: 2 Gy × 35 fx	3 months	**SIB-IMRT** 72% acute grade 3 dysphagia 72% CR **SEQ-IMRT** 41% acute grade 3 dysphagia 73% CR No difference in other acute toxicity
Jacinto (2018) [1]	$n = 20$ Locally advanced H&N SCC	2.75 Gy × 20 fx	24 months	85% CR 5% grade 4 hematologic toxicity 40% grade 3 mucositis
Meade (2018) [4]	$n = 15$ Oropharyngeal SCC	2.56 Gy × 25 fx	24 months	93% 2-year OS 100% CR Acute toxicity: 90% grade 3 mucositis, 80% grade 3 pharyngeal dysphagia
Retrospective studies				
Iqbal (2015) [2]	$n = 63$ Buccal mucosa SCC Induction chemotherapy then EBRT with chemotherapy	2.75 Gy × 20 fx	~24 months	30% 5-year OS 49% 5-year DFS 30% 5-year PFS 2–13% grade 3 toxicity No grade 4 toxicity
Benghiat (2014) [3]	$n = 85$ Oropharyngeal SCC	2.75 Gy × 20 fx	26 months	68% 2-year LRRFS 100% grade 3 mucositis 45% unplanned hospital admissions

Abbreviations: *EBRT* external beam radiotherapy, *H&N* head and neck, *SCC* squamous cell carcinoma, *SIB* simultaneous integrated boost, *SEQ* sequential boost, *fx* fractions, *CR* complete response, *OS* overall survival, *DFS* disease-free survival, *PFS* progression-free survival, *LRRFS* local-regional recurrence-free survival, *SBRT* stereotactic body radiotherapy, *PDR* pulse dose rate, *LC* local control, *PR* partial response, *LRRFR* local-regional recurrence-free rate, *LRC* local-regional control

15.5 Summary

There are variable dose fractionation schemes and responses to treatment, with limited numbers of patients in published studies. Overall, complication rates (especially acute toxicity) from hypofractionated RT are higher compared to conventionally fractionated RT. However, oncologic outcomes appear to be similar.

References

1. Jacinto AA, Batalha Filho ES, Viana LD, De Marchi P, Capuzzo RD, Gama RR, Boldrini Junior D, Santos CR, Pinto GD, Dias JM, Canton HP. Feasibility of concomitant cisplatin with hypofractionated radiotherapy for locally advanced head and neck squamous cell carcinoma. BMC Cancer. 2018;18(1):1–9. https://doi.org/10.1186/s12885-018-4893-5.
2. Iqbal H, Jamshed A, Bhatti AB, Hussain R, Jamshed S, Irfan M, Hameed N, Illyas A. Five-year follow-up of concomitant accelerated hypofractionated radiation in advanced squamous cell carcinoma of the Buccal Mucosa: a retrospective cohort study. BioMed Res Int. 2015:1–8. https://doi.org/10.1155/2015/963574.
3. Benghiat H, Sanghera P, Cashmore J, Hodson J, Mehanna H, Simmons R, Massey P, Sangha G, Bode C, Cooper P, Glaholm J, Hartley A. Four week hypofractionated accelerated intensity modulated radiotherapy and synchronous carboplatin or cetuximab in biologically staged oropharyngeal carcinoma. Cancer Clin Oncol. 2014;3(2):1. https://doi.org/10.5539/cco.v3n2p1.
4. Meade S, Gaunt P, Hartley A, Robinson M, Harrop V, Cashmore J, Wagstaff L, Babrah J, Bowden SJ, Mehanna H, Sanghera P. Feasibility of dose-escalated hypofractionated chemoradiation in human papilloma virus-negative or smoking-associated oropharyngeal cancer. Clin Oncol. 2018;30(6):366–74. https://doi.org/10.1016/j.clon.2018.01.015.
5. Bourhis J, Sire C, Graff P, Grégoire V, Maingon P, Calais G, Gery B, Martin L, Alfonsi M, Desprez P, Pignon T. Concomitant chemoradiotherapy versus acceleration of radiotherapy with or without concomitant chemotherapy in locally advanced head and neck carcinoma (GORTEC 99-02): an open-label phase 3 randomised trial. Lancet Oncol. 2012;13(2):145–53. https://doi.org/10.1016/S1470-2045(11)70346-1.
6. Grover A, Soni TP, Patni N, Singh DK, Jakhotia N, Gupta AK, Sharma LM, Sharma S, Gothwal RS. A randomized prospective study comparing acute toxicity compliance and objective response rate between simultaneous integrated boost and sequential intensity-modulated radiotherapy for locally advanced head and neck cancer. Radiation Oncology Journal. 2021;39(1):15–23. https://doi.org/10.3857/roj.2020.01018.
7. Al-Mamgani A, Van Rooij P, Sewnaik A, et al. Brachytherapy or stereotactic body radiotherapy boost for early-stage oropharyngeal cancer: comparable outcomes of two different approaches. Oral Oncol. 2013;49:1018–24.
8. Lee DS, Kim YS, Cheon JS, et al. Long-term outcome and toxicity of hypofractionated stereotactic body radiotherapy as a boost treatment for head and neck cancer: the importance of boost volume assessment. Radiat Oncol. 2012;7:85.
9. Baker S, Verduijn GM, Petit S, Sewnaik A, Mast H, Koljenović S, Nuyttens JJ, Heemsbergen WD. Long-term outcomes following stereotactic body radiotherapy boost for oropharyngeal squamous cell carcinoma. Acta Oncol. 2019;58(6):926–33. https://doi.org/10.1080/0284186X.2019.1581375.

Chapter 16
Intraoral Cone (IOC)

Jacob T. Hall, Gregory D. Judy, and Bhishamjit S. Chera

16.1 Introduction

This chapter is included for a historical perspective as intraoral cone is rarely used today for head and neck tumors such as floor of mouth, oral tongue, buccal mucosa, gingiva, and retromolar trigone.

16.2 General Utilization

1. Mainly for floor of mouth, oral tongue, buccal mucosa, gingiva, and retromolar trigone.
   (a) Indications:
      - Small, superficial, early stage disease.

J. T. Hall
Department of Radiation Oncology, University of North Carolina School of Medicine, Chapel Hill, NC, USA
e-mail: jacob.hall@unchealth.unc.edu

G. D. Judy (✉)
Department of Radiation Oncology, University of North Carolina School of Medicine, Chapel Hill, NC, USA

Lineberger Comprehensive Cancer Center, University of North Carolina School of Medicine, Chapel Hill, NC, USA
e-mail: gregory.judy@unchealth.unc.edu

B. S. Chera
Department of Radiation Oncology, MUSC, Medical University of South Carolina, Charleston, USA
e-mail: Bchera@med.unc.edu

O. Kaidar-Person, R. Chen (eds.), *Hypofractionated and Stereotactic Radiation Therapy*, https://doi.org/10.1007/978-3-031-47701-0_16

(b) Technique:

- Administered with orthovoltage X-rays or electrons.
- Orthovoltage preferred due to less beam constriction and higher surface dose (obviating the need for bolus).
- If electrons are utilized, bolus is needed for adequate surface dose and a larger margin is necessary due to beam constriction (intermediate and high isodoses "bowing in").
- Daily setup verification is necessary to ensure position of tumor relative to the cone.

16.3 Specific Disease Sites

1. Floor of mouth

(a) Indications:

- Superficial (≤4 mm thick), well-differentiated tumors.
- Alone or as a boost with EBRT:
  - If used as a boost, IOC will precede EBRT (can optimally define the extent of tumor and procedure is difficult when following EBRT due to patient discomfort and tumor regression).

(b) Dose:

- Monotherapy = 45 Gy over 3 weeks (55 Gy over 4 weeks if palpable induration or positive margins).
- Boost with EBRT = 15–24 Gy in 10 fx followed by 45–50 Gy EBRT.

2. Oral tongue

(a) Indications:

- Early T1 and superficial T2 N0 tumors if patient declines surgery or is at high surgical risk.
- Typically used as a boost with EBRT.
- Daily setup/reproducibility can be an issue due to difficulty with immobilization of the lesion.

(b) Dose:

- 21–27 Gy in 7–9 fx followed by 30–50 Gy EBRT.

16.4 Relevant Literature

Study	Patients	Treatment	Outcomes
Wang (1989) [1]	*n* = 142 Oral tongue SCC (93 treated with IOC)	EBRT + brachytherapy or IOC boost IOC: 24–27 Gy in 8–9 fx EBRT: 51.4 Gy in 32 fx BID	**Brachytherapy boost**: 54% 5-year LC **IOC boost (orthovoltage)** 50% 5-year LC **IOC (electrons)**: 86% 5-year LC Toxicity: osteoradionecrosis, ulceration

Abbreviations: *IOC* intraoral cone, *SCC* squamous cell carcinoma, *fx* fractions

16.5 Summary

IOC is no longer commonly used. It has variable LC rates, and the literature is limited. The types of severe complications are similar to brachytherapy (osteoradionecrosis, ulceration) and generally acceptable, but, like brachytherapy, are also likely related to clinician experience and expertise in performing the procedure.

Reference

1. Wang CC. Radiotherapeutic management and results of T1N0, T2N0 carcinoma of the oral tongue: evaluation of boost techniques. Int J Radiat Oncol Biol Phys. 1989;17(2):287–91.

Chapter 17
Brachytherapy

Jacob T. Hall, Gregory D. Judy, and Bhishamjit S. Chera

17.1 Introduction

This chapter is included for a historical perspective as brachytherapy is not commonly performed anymore with the advent of more sophisticated linear accelerators and lower toxicities obtained with IMRT. However, brachytherapy literature is the foundation on which SBRT is justified and brachytherapy can be utilized in a number of H&N sites to treat early stage tumors, primarily in the oral cavity. Brachytherapy can be used as sole treatment or in combination with EBRT for definitive, small, early stage tumors or in re-irradiation setting.

J. T. Hall
Department of Radiation Oncology, University of North Carolina School of Medicine, Chapel Hill, NC, USA
e-mail: jacob.hall@unchealth.unc.edu

G. D. Judy (✉)
Department of Radiation Oncology, University of North Carolina School of Medicine, Chapel Hill, NC, USA

Lineberger Comprehensive Cancer Center, University of North Carolina School of Medicine, Chapel Hill, NC, USA
e-mail: gregory.judy@unchealth.unc.edu

B. S. Chera
Department of Radiation Oncology, MUSC, Medical University of South Carolina, Charleston, USA
e-mail: Bchera@med.unc.edu

O. Kaidar-Person, R. Chen (eds.), *Hypofractionated and Stereotactic Radiation Therapy*, https://doi.org/10.1007/978-3-031-47701-0_17

17.2 Lip

- Indications:
  - Monotherapy for T1–T2 tumors (but often performed as a boost after initial 50 Gy EBRT).
  - Boost treatment following EBRT in low-volume T3–T4 tumors.
  - Use of EBRT is necessary to treat lymphatics for upper lip lesions, poorly differentiated lesions, presence of PNI, or recurrent disease.
- Technique:
  - Typically performed under local anesthesia.
  - Uses single-plane interstitial catheter technique: sources arranged horizontally (10–12 mm apart) with crossing sources over lateral aspect; the number of sources used depends on tumor size.
  - Place gauze between lip and gum to increase distance between alveolar ridge and sources (to minimize osteoradionecrosis).
- Dose:
  - Definitive:

    LDR implant alone: 60–70 Gy at dose rate of 0.4–0.5 Gy/h (~5-day implant).
    HDR: 45 Gy in 9 fractions, BID [1].
  - Boost: 35–40 Gy at dose rate 0.4–0.5 Gy/h (EBRT dose 45–50 Gy, 1.8–2 Gy/fx).

    Duration: approximately 2–3-day implant.
- Complications: dermatitis, mucosal necrosis (10%), osteoradionecrosis (<10%), or acute hemorrhage.

Study	Patients	Treatment	Median follow-up	Outcomes
Retrospective studies				
Guinot (2003) [2]	$n = 39$ T1–4 SCC lip	^{192}Ir HDR brachytherapy BID Total dose 40.5–45 Gy in 8–10 fx	18 months	88% 3-year LC 91% 3-year CSS Very good cosmetic result
Tombolini (1998) [3]	$n = 57$ T1–3 N+, SCC lower lip	^{192}Ir LDR brachytherapy alone (cN+ patients also received EBRT) Median dose 62 Gy (range 44–96 Gy)	Not specified	90% 5-year LC 81% 5-year DFS 76% 5-year OS

Study	Patients	Treatment	Median follow-up	Outcomes
Orecchi (1991) [4]	$n = 47$ T1–2 N0 SCC lower lip	^{192}Ir LDR brachytherapy alone 60–80 Gy	Not specified	94% 5-year LC 92% 5-year DFS 85% 10-year DFS Toxicity: 10% mucosal necrosis Excellent/good cosmetic result 92%
Mut (2016) [1]	$n = 68$ T1–2 SCC lip	HDR brachytherapy alone Median dose 45 Gy	56 months	97% 5-year LC 93.8% 5-year RC T1 80.8% 5-year RC T2 All achieved good or excellent cosmetic result No soft tissue or bone necrosis

Abbreviations: *SCC* squamous cell carcinoma, *fx* fractions, *EBRT* external beam radiotherapy, *LC* local control, *CSS* cancer-specific survival, *DFS* disease-free survival, *OS* overall survival, *RC* regional control

17.3 Floor of the Mouth

(a) Indications:

- Monotherapy for well-differentiated, superficial (≤ 4 mm) T1–T2 tumors.
- Boost treatment following EBRT in T1–2 tumors with thickness > 4 mm and/or poorly differentiated (higher risk for nodal spread).
- Not recommended when tumor extends to mandibular alveolar ridge due to increased risk of osteoradionecrosis.
- Post-operative therapy for those with high-risk features, such as a positive or close margin.

(b) Technique:

- Interstitial catheter technique (discussed above).

(c) Dose:

- LDR implant alone: 60–70 Gy at dose rate of 0.4–0.5 Gy/h over 5–7 days.
- LDR implant boost: 10–25 Gy at dose rate 0.4–0.5 Gy/h (EBRT dose 46–50 in 2 Gy/fx).
- HDR: 10–48 Gy total in 1–15 fractions.

(d) Complications: mucosal necrosis (<5%), osteoradionecrosis (2.5%), or acute hemorrhage.

Study	Patients	Treatment	Median follow-up	Outcomes
Retrospective studies				
Marsiglia (2002) [5]	$n = 160$ T1–2 N0–1 SCC of FOM	^{192}Ir LDR brachytherapy alone (cT2 or N1 also received surgery) Median 70 Gy (58–80 Gy)	108 months	93% LC (T1) 88% LC (T2) Toxicity: mucosal necrosis and osteoradionecrosis (2.5% grade 3 osteoradionecrosis)
Lapeyre (2000) [6]	$n = 36$ T1–2 N0 SCC tongue or FOM	Surgery ± ^{192}Ir brachytherapy (if close or + margins) Mean 60 Gy (50–67.4 Gy)	80 months	88.5% 2-year LC Toxicity: grade 2–3 in 16% FOM cases
Pernot (1995) [7]	$n = 207$ T1–4 N0–3 SCC of FOM	EBRT (50 Gy) + ^{192}Ir brachytherapy or brachytherapy alone	60 months	**T1 tumors**: 97% 5-year LC 88% 5-year CSS **T2 tumors**: 72% 5-year LC 47% 5-year CSS **T3 tumors**: 51% 5-year LC 36% 5-year CSS Toxicity: 1% grade ≥ 3 soft-tissue necrosis; 6% grade ≥ 3 bone necrosis
Ferenczi (2021) [8]	$n = 44$ T1–3 N0–1 SCC of FOM	Surgery + HDR brachytherapy Mean dose 22.7 Gy (10–45 Gy)	122 months	32% 10-year OS 89% 10-year LC 16 patients received salvage surgery, EBRT, or both 11% grade 3 mucositis 9% soft tissue necrosis

Abbreviations: *SCC* squamous cell carcinoma, *FOM* floor of mouth, *EBRT* external beam radiotherapy, *LC* local control, *CSS* cancer-specific survival, *OS* overall survival

17.4 Oral Tongue

(a) Indications:

- Monotherapy for well-differentiated, superficial (≤3 mm) T1–2 tumors.
- Boost treatment following EBRT for T1–2 tumors with thickness > 3 mm and/or poorly differentiated.
- Post-operative therapy for those with high-risk features, such as a positive or close margin.

(b) Technique:

- Interstitial catheter technique (discussed above).

(c) Dose:

- LDR implant alone: 65–70 Gy at dose rate of 0.4–0.5 Gy/h over 5–7 days.

- LDR implant boost: 25–30 Gy at dose rate 0.4–0.5 Gy/h (EBRT dose 40–45 Gy in 1.8–2 Gy/fx).
- HDR implant alone: All administered BID, 5 days per week.
  - 39 Gy in 13 fractions
  - 40–52 Gy in 10–12 fractions
  - 50 Gy in 10 fractions
  - 40.8 Gy in 12 fractions.
- HDR implant boost:
  - 15–16 Gy in 3–4 fractions, BID after EBRT
  - 18–24 Gy in 6–8 fractions, BID after EBRT.

(d) Complications: mucosal necrosis (<5%), osteoradionecrosis (<5%), or acute hemorrhage.

Study	Patients	Treatment	Median follow-up	Outcomes
Prospective studies				
Inoue (1996) [9] Randomized trial	$n = 29$ T1–2 N0 SCC tongue	^{192}Ir LDR vs. HDR brachytherapy alone LDR: 70 Gy, 4–9 days HDR: 60 Gy, 6 days	24 months	**LDR**: 86% 2-year LC **HDR**: 100% 2-year LC Toxicity: ulcer (3%), necrosis (3%)
Ianovski (2020) [10]	$n = 41$ T1–3 N0–2 SCC tongue	Surgery and postoperative brachytherapy 40.8 Gy/12 fx for positive margins 34 Gy/10 fx for narrow margins ± neck EBRT	25 months	59% 5-year OS 86% 3-year LC 7% late grade 2 toxicity
Retrospective studies				
Matsuura (1998) [11]	$n = 173$ T1–3 N0–3 SCC tongue	EBRT +^{192}Ir LDR brachytherapy or brachytherapy alone Brachytherapy alone: 60–84 Gy Total EBRT + brachytherapy dose: 38–136 Gy	24 months	**T1 tumor**: 93% 5-year LC **T2 tumor**: 78% 5-year LC Tumor thickness < 8 mm: 92% 5-year LC Tumor thickness > 8 mm: 28% 5-year LC
Wendt (1990) [12]	$n = 103$ T1–2 N0 SCC tongue	EBRT + ^{192}Ir LDR brachytherapy or brachytherapy alone EBRT + brachytherapy: 40–50 Gy + 20–40 Gy	159 months	**Brachytherapy alone**: 67% 2-year LC **EBRT + brachytherapy**: 92% 2-year LC (EBRT dose >40 Gy) 65% 2-year LC (EBRT dose <40 Gy) Toxicity: moderate-severe complications ~15%
Kazemian (2017) [13]	$n = 78$ SCC oral cavity	HDR brachytherapy alone (39–45 Gy) or EBRT + brachytherapy (46 Gy + 9–40 Gy)	37 months	83% 4-year OS 90% 4-year LC 3.8% total complication rate other than xerostomia

Study	Patients	Treatment	Median follow-up	Outcomes
Bansal (2016) [14]	$n = 92$ T1–2 SCC tongue	HDR brachytherapy alone (40–52 Gy) or EBRT + brachytherapy (40 Gy + 18–24 Gy)	53 months	73% 5-year OS 64% 5-year LC 87% grade ≥ 2 mucositis brachytherapy alone 66% grade ≥ 2 mucositis EBRT + brachytherapy 28% grade ≥ 3 acute or late toxicity
Potharaju (2018) [15]	$n = 73$ T1–2 SCC tongue	Brachytherapy alone vs. surgery + brachytherapy	74 months	**Brachytherapy alone** 74% 6-year OS 55% 6-year DFS **Surgery and brachytherapy** 92% 6-year OS 92% 6-year DFS

Abbreviations: *SCC* squamous cell carcinoma, *LC* local control, *OS* overall survival, *DFS* disease-free survival

17.5 Buccal Mucosa

(a) Indications:

- Combination therapy with EBRT in T1–2 tumors.

(b) Technique:

- Interstitial catheter technique: single plane of 3–5 horizontal tubes (10–12 mm apart); crossing tubes at either end of the horizontal tubes.

(c) Dose:

- LDR boost: 25–30 Gy at dose rate 0.4–0.5 Gy/h following EBRT (45–50 Gy in 1.8–2 Gy/fx).
- HDR boost: 48 Gy in 8 fractions.

(d) Complications: mucosal necrosis, trismus, and acute hemorrhage.

Study	Patients	Treatment	Median follow-up	Outcomes
Retrospective studies				
Nair (1988) [16]	$n = 52$ T1–4 N0–3 (33% T1–2 N0) Majority buccal mucosa	^{192}Ir LDR brachytherapy alone: 65 Gy over 6 days	36 months	85% 3-year OS Toxicity: mucositis, mild-moderate xerostomia in most patients. No osteoradionecrosis

Study	Patients	Treatment	Median follow-up	Outcomes
Kotsuma (2017) [17]	*n* = 36 T1–4 buccal mucosa SCC	Interstitial brachytherapy: HDR (24 – 60 Gy) vs. LDR (42–110 Gy) ± EBRT to regional lymphatics and/or boost to primary (24.5–70 Gy)	99 months	**HDR** 82% 5-year LC 0% grade 3 toxicity **LDR** 72% 5-year LC 13% grade 3 toxicity

Abbreviations: *SCC* squamous cell carcinoma, *EBRT* external beam radiotherapy, *OS* overall survival, *LC* local control

17.6 Oropharynx

(a) Indications:

- Combination therapy with EBRT for small (<5 cm), node-negative tonsillar fossa, base of tongue, or soft palate tumors.
- Contraindicated if tumor invades underlying structures or bone.

(b) Technique:

- Interstitial catheter technique (described above).

(c) Dose:

- LDR boost: 25–35 Gy at dose rate 0.4–0.5 Gy/h following EBRT (45–50 Gy in 1.8–2 Gy/fx).
- HDR boost: 21–30 Gy in 3 Gy/fx or 21–24 Gy in 4 Gy/fx following EBRT (45–50 Gy in 1.8–2 Gy/fx).

(d) Complications: ulceration (10–20%), mucosal necrosis (<5%), pain (20%), trismus (<2%), and acute hemorrhage (3%).

Study	Patients	Treatment	Median follow-up	Outcomes
Prospective studies				
Levendag (2004) [18]	*n* = 248 T1–3, N0–N+ SCC tonsillar fossa or soft palate	EBRT + brachytherapy boost (if brachytherapy not possible, patient underwent surgery) EBRT 46 Gy in 2 Gy/fx ^{192}Ir LDR/HDR brachytherapy: 20–36 Gy (LDR) or 15–30 Gy (HDR)	24 months	88% 5-year LC Brachytherapy toxicity: mucosal ulcer (39%), pain (20%), trismus (1%)

Study	Patients	Treatment	Median follow-up	Outcomes
Harrison (1998) [19]	$n = 68$ T1–3, N0–N+ SCC base of tongue	EBRT + brachytherapy boost (+neck dissection if N+) EBRT 54 Gy in 2 Gy/fx ^{192}Ir LDR brachytherapy 20–30 Gy	36 months	89% 5-year LC 80% 5-year DFS Toxicity: soft tissue ulceration (13%), osteoradionecrosis (3%), hemorrhage (3%)

Abbreviations: *SCC* squamous cell carcinoma, *EBRT* external beam radiotherapy, *LC* local control, *DFS* disease-free survival

17.7 Nasopharynx

(a) Indications:

- Brachytherapy monotherapy or in combination with EBRT for small, superficial, well-circumscribed T1–2 tumors and/or in the re-irradiation setting.
- Contraindicated if tumor extends into nasal cavities or the oropharynx.
- As a boost for T1 disease.

(b) Technique:

- Intracavitary or interstitial techniques.
- Applicator should be used. The Rotterdam nasopharyngeal applicator is commonly used with a HDR afterloading device.
- Shaped to conform to nasopharynx, guided through oral cavity to correct position; once immobilized, X-rays are performed to confirm location and define anatomy for treatment planning.

(c) Dose

- HDR boost: 5–6 Gy in 2 fx (5–6 h apart) following EBRT (40–50 Gy).
- LDR interstitial for recurrent disease: 120 Gy.

(d) Complications: hemorrhage (<5%), cranial nerve neuropathies (<10%), trismus (10–20%), osteoradionecrosis (<5%), and soft-tissue necrosis (10–15%).

Study	Patients	Treatment	Median follow-up	Outcomes
Retrospective studies				
Koutcher (2010) [20]	$n = 29$ Recurrent T1–4 Median 3.9 years between primary treatment and re-treatment	EBRT alone = median 59.4 Gy Chemotherapy given to all patients EBRT + ^{125}I or ^{192}Ir brachytherapy: 40 Gy total median (20 Gy EBRT, 20 Gy brachytherapy)	45 months	52% 5-year LC 69% 5-year OS Toxicity: hemorrhage (4%), cranial nerve neuropathy (9%), trismus (17%), soft tissue necrosis (13%)

Study	Patients	Treatment	Median follow-up	Outcomes
Lee (1997) [21]	$n = 654$ Recurrent T1–3 Median 2 years between primary treatment and re-treatment	EBRT alone = median 46.5 Gy EBRT + brachytherapy: 40 Gy EBRT, 20 Gy brachytherapy Intracavitary ^{137}Cs alone = median 40 Gy	1.4 years	23% 5-year LC 16% 5-year OS Toxicity: trismus/soft tissue necrosis (16%), osteoradionecrosis (3%), neuropathies (7%), fatal hemorrhage (<1%)
Yan (2017) [22]	$n = 81$ Locally recurrent following EBRT ± chemo	LDR brachytherapy (120–140 Gy) vs. EBRT (60–70 Gy)	30 months	**Brachytherapy** 31% 3-year OS 25% grade ≥ 3 toxicity 0% grade 5 toxicity **EBRT** 33% 3-year OS 67% grade ≥ 3 toxicity 14% grade 5 toxicity
Chao (2017) [23]	$n = 232$	IMRT (70 Gy) ± HDR brachytherapy boost (6 Gy in 2 fx) ± chemotherapy	63 months	Brachytherapy boost: Improved 5-year LC for T1 patients (98% vs. 86% EBRT alone) No LC benefit for T2–4 patients No increase in toxicity

Abbreviations: *EBRT* external beam radiotherapy, *fx* fractions, *LC* local control, *OS* overall survival

17.8 Paranasal Sinuses

(a) Indications:

- Nasal vestibule and nasal cavity tumors.
  - Nasal vestibule: monotherapy for small lesions (<2 cm) or in combination with EBRT for larger (≥2 cm) lesions.
  - Nasal cavity: monotherapy for small (≤1.5 cm) anteroinferior septal lesions (better cosmetic outcome vs. surgery).

(b) Technique:

- Interstitial technique with ^{192}Ir wire implant is typically used.
- Afterloading needles inserted under general anesthesia (to visualize tumor and protect airway in case of hemorrhage).

- For HDR, custom mold of nasal vestibule is made.
  - Tumor is marked and 2–4 plastic tubes with 1 cm spacing inserted.
  - Lateral vestibule tumors: two tubes placed on inner aspect of vestibule.
  - Medial tumors: 2–4 tubes placed on both sides of tumor.

(c) Dose

- LDR
  - Monotherapy: 60–65 Gy at dose rate of 0.4 – 0.6 Gy/h over 5–7 days.
  - Boost: 20–25 Gy at 0.4–0.6 Gy/h following EBRT (50 Gy in 2 Gy/fx).
- HDR:
  - Monotherapy: 42–54 Gy in 10–18 fractions, BID, 5–7 days per week.
  - Boost: 18 Gy in 3 Gy/fx BID following EBRT (50 Gy in 2 Gy/fx).

(d) Complications: hemorrhage (<5%), rhinorrhea (40%), nasal dryness (40–50%), and osteoradionecrosis (<5%).

Study	Patients	Treatment	Median follow-up	Outcomes
Retrospective studies				
Langendijk (2004) [24]	*n* = 56 T1–2 SCC nasal vestibule	EBRT or EBRT + brachytherapy EBRT alone: median 52.5 Gy EBRT + brachytherapy: ^{137}Cs LDR: 16 Gy at 2.7 Gy/h ^{192}Ir HDR: 18 Gy in 3 fx, BID	24 months	80% 2-year LC, 95% 5-year LC (some patients were salvaged with surgery) **Tumor diameter < 1.5 cm**: 83% 2-year LC **Tumor diameter ≥ 1.5 cm**: 74% 2-year LC Toxicity: rhinorrhea (45%), nasal dryness (39%), epistaxis (15%), adhesions (4%)
Chobe (1988) [25]	*n* = 32 SCC nasal vestibule	EBRT or brachytherapy alone EBRT: 55–70 Gy LDR brachytherapy: 60–75 Gy	Not specified	**Brachytherapy**: 100% LC **EBRT**: 95% LC Toxicity: osteoradionecrosis (3%), hemorrhage (3%)
Czerwinksi (2019)[26]	*n* = 102 T1–2 nasal vestibule	^{192}Ir HDR interstitial or intracavitary mold 49 Gy total in 3.5 Gy/fx	42 months	74% 5-year OS 92% 5-year LC Patient-reported QOL rated as high

Abbreviations: *SCC* squamous cell carcinoma, *EBRT* external beam radiotherapy, *LC* local control, *OS* overall survival, *QOL* quality of life

17.9 Summary: Brachytherapy

Overall, while brachytherapy is no longer commonly utilized, it does offer good local control in a variety of disease sites of the head and neck (with exception of the nasopharynx, where control rates are variable). Complication rates are generally acceptable but are likely also related to clinician experience and expertise in performing the procedure.

References

1. Mut A, Guinot JL, Arribas L, Díez-Presa L, Tortajada MI, Santos MÁ, Samper J, Santamaría P, Vendrell JB. Braquiterapia de alta tasa en el carcinoma escamoso de labio en estadios iniciales. Acta Otorrinolaringol Española. 2016;67(5):282–7. https://doi.org/10.1016/j.otorri.2015.12.003.
2. Guinot JL, Arribas L, Chust ML, et al. Lip cancer treatment with high dose rate brachytherapy. Radiother Oncol. 2003;69:113–5.
3. Tombolini V, Bonanni A, Valeriani M, Zurlo A, Vitturini A. Brachytherapy for squamous cell carcinoma of the lip. The experience of the Institute of Radiology of the University of Rome "La Sapienza". Tumori. 1998;84:478–82.
4. Orecchia R, Rampino M, Gribaudo S, Negri GL. Interstitial brachytherapy for carcinomas of the lower lip. Results of treatment. Tumori J. 1991;77:336–8.
5. Marsiglia H, Haie-Meder C, Sasso G, Mamelle G, Gerbaulet A. Brachytherapy for T1-T2 floor-of-the-mouth cancers: the Gustave-Roussy Institute experience. Int J Radiat Oncol Biol Phys. 2002;52:1257–63.
6. Lapeyre M, Hoffstetter S, Peiffert D, et al. Postoperative brachytherapy alone for T1–2N0 squamous cell carcinomas of the oral tongue and floor of mouth with close or positive margins. Int J Radiat Oncol Biol Phys. 2000;48:37–42.
7. Pernot M, Hoffstetter S, Peiffert D, et al. Epidermoid carcinomas of the floor of mouth treated by exclusive irradiation: statistical study of a series of 207 cases. Radiother Oncol. 1995;35:177–85.
8. Ferenczi Ö, Major T, Akiyama H, Fröhlich G, Oberna F, Révész M, Poósz M, Polgár C, Takácsi-Nagy Z. Results of postoperative interstitial brachytherapy of resectable floor of mouth tumors. Brachytherapy. 2021;20(2):376–82. https://doi.org/10.1016/j.brachy.2020.10.008.
9. Inoue T, Inoue T, Teshima T, et al. Phase III trial of high and low dose rate interstitial radiotherapy for early oral tongue cancer. Int J Radiat Oncol Biol Phys. 1996;36:1201–4.
10. Ianovski I, Mlynarek AM, Black MJ, Bahoric B, Sultanem K, Hier MP. The role of brachytherapy for margin control in oral tongue squamous cell carcinoma. J Otolaryngol Head Neck Surg. 2020;49(1):1–11. https://doi.org/10.1186/s40463-020-00467-w.
11. Matsuura K, Hirokawa Y, Fujita M, Akagi Y, Ito K. Treatment results of stage I and II oral tongue cancer with interstitial brachytherapy: maximum tumor thickness is prognostic of nodal metastasis. Int J Radiat Oncol Biol Phys. 1998;40:535–9.
12. Wendt CD, Peters LJ, Delclos L, et al. Primary radiotherapy in the treatment of stage I and II oral tongue cancers: importance of the proportion of therapy delivered with interstitial therapy. Int J Radiat Oncol Biol Phys. 1990;18:1287–92.
13. Kazemian A, Babaei M, Lashkari M, Ghalehtaki R, Garajei A, Motiee-Langroudi M, Sebzari A, Jaberi R, Gholami S, Babaloui S, Aghili M. Adjuvant high-dose-rate brachytherapy in the management of oral cavity cancers: 5 years of experience in Iran. J Contemp Brachyther. 2017;9(4):323–9. https://doi.org/10.5114/jcb.2017.69806.

14. Bansal A, Ghoshal S, Oinam AS, Sharma SC, Dhanireddy B, Kapoor R. High-dose-rate interstitial brachytherapy in early stage oral tongue cancer—15-year experience from a tertiary care institute. J Contemp Brachyther. 2016;8(1):156–65. https://doi.org/10.5114/jcb.2016.58082.
15. Potharaju M, Raj H, Muthukumaran M, Venkataraman M, Ilangovan B, Kuppusamy S. Long-term outcome of high-dose-rate brachytherapy and perioperative brachytherapy in early mobile tongue cancer. J Contemp Brachyther. 2018;10(1):64–72. https://doi.org/10.5114/jcb.2018.74139.
16. Nair MK, Sankaranarayanan R, Padmanabhan TK, Madhu CS. Oral verrucous carcinoma. Treatment with radiotherapy. Cancer. 1988;61:458–61.
17. Kotsuma T, Yamazaki H, Masui K, Yoshida KE, Shimizutani K, Akiyama H, Murakami S, Isohashi F, Yoshioka Y, Ogawa K, Tanaka E. Brachytherapy for buccal cancer: from conventional low dose rate (LDR) or mold technique to high dose rate interstitial brachytherapy (HDR-ISBT). Anticancer Res. 2017;37(12):6887–92. https://doi.org/10.21873/anticanres.12151.
18. Levendag P, Nijdam W, Noever I, et al. Brachytherapy versus surgery in carcinoma of tonsillar fossa and/or soft palate: late adverse sequelae and performance status: can we be more selective and obtain better tissue sparing? Int J Radiat Oncol Biol Phys. 2004;59:713–24.
19. Harrison LB, Lee HJ, Pfister DG, et al. Long term results of primary radiotherapy with/without neck dissection for squamous cell cancer of the base of tongue. Head Neck. 1998;20:668–73.
20. Koutcher L, Lee N, Zelefsky M, et al. Reirradiation of locally recurrent nasopharynx cancer with external beam radiotherapy with or without brachytherapy. Int J Radiat Oncol Biol Phys. 2010;76:130–7.
21. Lee AW, Foo W, Law SC, et al. Reirradiation for recurrent nasopharyngeal carcinoma: factors affecting the therapeutic ratio and ways for improvement. Int J Radiat Oncol Biol Phys. 1997;38:43–52.
22. Yan H, Mo Z, Xiang Z, Rong D, Zhang Y, Chen G, Zhong Z, Zhang F, Gao F. CT-guided 125I brachytherapy for locally recurrent nasopharyngeal carcinoma. J Cancer. 2017;8(11):2104–13. https://doi.org/10.7150/jca.19078.
23. Chao HL, Liu SC, Tsao CC, Lin KT, Lee SP, Lo CH, Huang WY, Liu MY, Jen YM, Lin CS. Dose escalation via brachytherapy boost for nasopharyngeal carcinoma in the era of intensity-modulated radiation therapy and combined chemotherapy. J Radiat Res. 2017;58(5):654–60. https://doi.org/10.1093/jrr/rrx034.
24. Langendijk JA, Poorter R, Leemans CR, de Bree R, Doornaert P, Slotman BJ. Radiotherapy of squamous cell carcinoma of the nasal vestibule. Int J Radiat Oncol Biol Phys. 2004;59:1319–25.
25. Chobe R, McNeese M, Weber R, Fletcher GH. Radiation therapy for carcinoma of the nasal vestibule. Otolaryngol Head Neck Surg. 1988;98:67–71.
26. Czerwinski MD, van Leeuwen RG, Kaanders JH, Zwijnenburg EM, Lipman D, Takes RP, Verhoef CG. Image guided brachytherapy for cancer of the nasal vestibule: local control and cosmesis. Int J Radiat Oncol Biol Phys. 2019;103(4):913–21. https://doi.org/10.1016/j.ijrobp.2018.11.018.

Chapter 18
Intraoperative Radiotherapy (IORT)

Jacob T. Hall, Gregory D. Judy, and Bhishamjit S. Chera

18.1 Introduction

IORT can be used in conjunction with surgery to provide additional local disease control. In certain situations where a maximum surgical resection is the primary treatment, IORT can be used, location permitting, to deliver RT to an area of high concern for recurrence (e.g., possible positive margins).

J. T. Hall
Department of Radiation Oncology, University of North Carolina School of Medicine, Chapel Hill, NC, USA
e-mail: jacob.hall@unchealth.unc.edu

G. D. Judy (✉)
Department of Radiation Oncology, University of North Carolina School of Medicine, Chapel Hill, NC, USA

Lineberger Comprehensive Cancer Center, University of North Carolina School of Medicine, Chapel Hill, NC, USA
e-mail: gregory.judy@unchealth.unc.edu

B. S. Chera
Department of Radiation Oncology, MUSC, Medical University of South Carolina, Charleston, USA
e-mail: Bchera@med.unc.edu

O. Kaidar-Person, R. Chen (eds.), *Hypofractionated and Stereotactic Radiation Therapy*, https://doi.org/10.1007/978-3-031-47701-0_18

18.2 IORT Using Electrons

- Technique:
  - Sterile applicator and cone required.
  - Attaches to the head of linac.
  - Collimate the electron beam to define treatment field and retract, shield normal tissue.
  - Typical margin 1–2 cm. A 5 mm water equivalent bolus is used.
  - The target area should be defined with the surgeon, as it is typically the high-risk, postoperative bed where the tumor was in close proximity to normal tissue structures (and likely where there is a positive margin).
  - Must be performed in shielded OR or special IORT suite.
- Dose:
  - Ranges between 10 and 25 Gy × 1 fx prescribed to 80–100% IDL.
- Advantages: area at risk directly visible, better sparing of normal tissue/overlying tissue.
- Complications: major organ at risk is the spinal cord and cranial nerves.

18.3 Intraoperative Brachytherapy

- Use of radioactive source (^{192}Ir, ^{125}I, ^{137}Cs) to deliver RT in or < 5 cm from the tumor.
- Technique:
  - ^{192}Ir: requires afterloading catheters to be placed in applicator
  - ^{125}I, ^{131}Cs: permanently inserted at time of surgery.
- Dose:
  - HDR 10–20 Gy × 1 fx.
  - LDR 40–50 Gy over 4–10 days.
- Advantages: meticulous placement of catheters or implants within tumor bed (ability to conform to irregular surfaces), sparing of normal tissue.
- Disadvantage: if LDR, catheters remain in place for several days = increase risk of infection (HDR can be done the same day in the OR); additional hospital personnel exposed to radiation.
- Complications: osteoradionecrosis (up to ~15%), fistula (1–2%), hemorrhage, and infection (<5%).

18.4 Relevant Literature

Study	Patients	Treatment	Median follow-up	Outcomes
Prospective studies				
Nag (1996) [1]	$n = 29$, recurrent SCC	Surgery + intraoperative brachytherapy (additional adjuvant EBRT given in RT naïve areas) ^{192}Ir HDR: 15 Gy (if previous RT given) 7.5–12.5 Gy to RT naïve areas + EBRT 45–50 Gy	21 months	67% 2-year LC 72% 2-year OS No intraoperative complications. Delayed toxicity: CSF leak (3%), septicemia (3%), otitis media (3%), xerostomia (3%)
Retrospective studies				
Perry (2010) [2]	$n = 34$, recurrent SCC (majority in the neck) All pts received definitive EBRT previously (median 63 Gy) Median time to recurrence 16 months	Surgery + IORT ^{192}Ir HDR: 10–20 Gy (median 15) × 1	23 months	66% 2-year LC 55% 2-year OS Toxicity: fibrosis (30–40%), fistula (<10%), wound infection (<10%), osteoradionecrosis (<5%)
Chen (2007) [3]	$n = 137$, recurrent SCC	Surgery + IORT Electrons: 10–18 Gy (median 15 Gy) × 1 Median cone size 5 cm Rx 90% IDL	41 months	61% 3-year LC 36% 3-year OS No perioperative complications Delayed complications: wound infection (<5%), fistula (1–2%), necrosis (<1%), neuropathy (<1%), trismus (<1%)
Rate (1991) [4]	$n = 126$, recurrent SCC (majority in the neck); 47 recurred in area with previous RT Median time to recurrence 18 months	Surgery + IORT (for R1, R2 resections) Electrons: 15, 20, 25 Gy × 1 Rx to Dmax	14 months	62% 2-year LC 55% 2-year OS Toxicity: osteoradionecrosis (1%), fistula (2%)
Vikram (1985) [5]	$n = 21$, recurrent SCC Median time to recurrence 36 months	Surgery + IORT ^{192}Ir LDR: 40–56 Gy over 4–10 days	35 months	81% 2-year LC 55% 2-year DFS Toxicity: osteoradionecrosis (14%)

Study	Patients	Treatment	Median follow-up	Outcomes
Khan (2019) [6]	$n = 51$, regional lymphatic recurrences from H&N SCC primary	Salvage surgery with intraoperative interstitial brachytherapy ^{192}Ir (mean dose 60 Gy, 0.6 Gy/h)	41 months	38% 10-year LRC 46% 10-year OS 15% acute grade 3–4 toxicity 11% late grade 3–4 toxicity
Wald (2019) [7]	$n = 61$, recurrent H&N SCC	Salvage surgery with electron IORT 10–17.5 Gy × 1 Rx to 90% IDL, 6 MeV	16 months	35% 2-year LRC 42% 2-year OS 1 patient with carotid rupture (grade 5 toxicity)

Abbreviations: *SCC* squamous cell carcinoma, *EBRT* external beam radiotherapy, *H&N* head and neck, *Rx* prescription, *IDL* isodose line, *LC* local control, *OS* overall survival, *DFS* disease-free survival, *LRC* local-regional control

18.5 Summary: IORT

Most studies have small sample sizes and LC rates vary from 60% to 80%. Complication rates are generally low, with intraoperative brachytherapy showing a higher complication rate with regard to fistula, osteoradionecrosis, and wound infection.

References

1. Nag S, Schuller D, Pak V, et al. Pilot study of intraoperative high dose rate brachytherapy for head and neck cancer. Radiother Oncol. 1996;41(2):125–30.
2. Perry DJ, Chan K, Wolden S, et al. High-dose-rate intraoperative radiation therapy for recurrent head-and-neck cancer. Int J Radiat Oncol Biol Phys. 2010;76(4):1140–6.
3. Chen AM, Bucci MK, Singer MI, Chen AM, Bucci MK, Singer MI, Garcia J, Kaplan MJ, Chan AS, Phillips TL. Intraoperative radiation therapy for recurrent head-and-neck cancer: the UCSF experience. Int J Radiat Oncol Biol Phys. 2007;67(1):122–9.
4. Rate WR, Garrett P, Pugh N, Ross D, Haerr R, Hamaker R, Singer M, Charles G. Intraoperative radiation therapy for recurrent head and neck cancer. Cancer. 1991;67(11):2738–40.
5. Vikram B, Strong EW, Shah JP, Spiro R. Intraoperative radiotherapy in patients with recurrent head and neck cancer. Am J Surg. 1985;150:485–7.
6. Khan N, Clemens M, Liu J, Garden AS, Lawyer A, Weber R, Gunn GB, Morrison WH, Kupferman ME. The role of salvage surgery with interstitial brachytherapy for the Management of Regionally Recurrent Head and Neck Cancers. Cancers Head Neck. 2019;4(1):1–9. https://doi.org/10.1186/s41199-019-0043-2.
7. Wald P, Grecula J, Walston S, Wei L, Bhatt A, Martin D, Bonomi M, Rocco J, Old M, Teknos T, Blakaj D. Intraoperative electron beam radiotherapy for locoregionally persistent or recurrent head and neck cancer. Head Neck. 2019;41(7):2148–53. https://doi.org/10.1002/hed.25673.

Chapter 19
Re-irradiation of Head and Neck Malignancies

Gregory N. Gan and Christopher Lominska

19.1 Introduction

Loco-regional recurrence and development of second primary head and neck cancers remain significant issues for patients with locally advanced head and neck cancer following definitive treatment and contribute to substantial morbidity and early mortality (Pignon et al. Radiother Oncol 92(1):4-14, 2009; Chao et al. Int J Radiat Oncol Biol Phys 55(2):312–21, 2003). Up to 50% of patients develop a local recurrence within 5 years. Both scenarios may warrant consideration of re-irradiation with or without systemic therapy but should be discussed in a multidisciplinary head and neck cancer tumor board. Patients with recurrent disease or second primary head and neck cancers who are appropriate and amenable for salvage surgery should receive this as first line therapy. There is an accumulating literature reporting the safety and efficacy of re-irradiation for head and neck cancer patients. Multiple therapeutic techniques for salvage re-irradiation or for management of second primary are available and include conventionally fractionated photon or proton radiotherapy with or without systemic therapy or SBRT with or without biotherapy or checkpoint inhibitor.

G. N. Gan (✉) · C. Lominska
Department of Radiation Oncology, University of Kansas Medical Center, Kansas City, KS, USA
e-mail: ggan@kumc.edu

O. Kaidar-Person, R. Chen (eds.), *Hypofractionated and Stereotactic Radiation Therapy*, https://doi.org/10.1007/978-3-031-47701-0_19

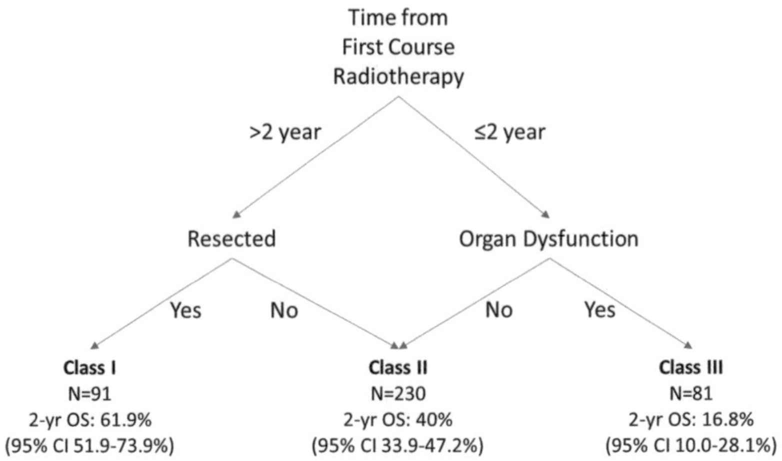

Fig. 19.1 Recursive partitioning analysis for overall survival

19.2 Prognosis

- The Multi-Institutional Re-Irradiation (MIRI) consortium has developed a recursive partitioning analysis algorithm for prognosticating outcomes for patients with recurrent disease based on time from original radiotherapy course to surgery or re-irradiation (if not a surgical candidate) and whether they have organ dysfunction (Fig. 19.1, adapted from [3]).
- Organ dysfunction as defined by the MIRI consortium included patients with tracheostomy tube and/or PEG tube dependence at time of recurrence or new primary.

19.3 Patient Selection (Fig. 19.2)

- Patients should be evaluated in a multidisciplinary tumor board setting and those amenable to surgical resection should consider surgery (gross total or maximally safe resection) as this has been reported as providing the best outcomes. Adjuvant radiotherapy can be considered primarily in those with high-risk features including gross residual disease, positive margins, extracapsular extension, and perineural invasion.
- Table 19.1 summarizes the authors' recommendations for patients who are eligible for re-irradiation.

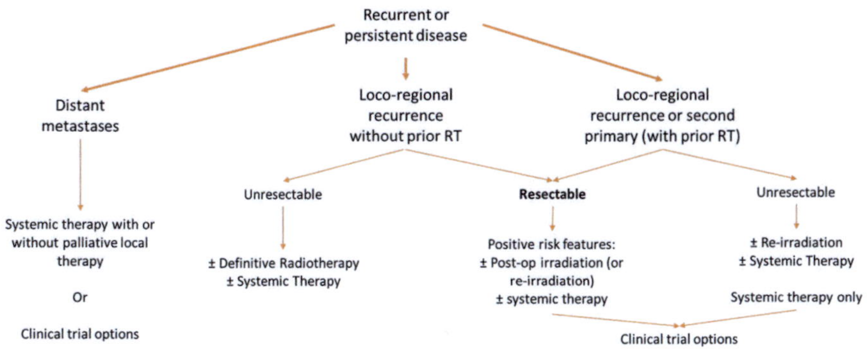

Fig. 19.2 Suggested re-irradiation algorithm

Table 19.1 Patient characteristics amenable for re-irradiation

No distant metastases
Good performance status (KPS ≥ 80%)
No severe post-radiation treatment issues (i.e., tracheotomy tube, osteoradionecrosis, feeding tube dependence)
At least 6-month interval from initial radiotherapy to surgery (longer preferred)
Recovered from salvage surgery (i.e., wound healing, dehiscence)
Presence high risk feature(s) (i.e., gross residual, positive margin, ECE, PNI)

19.4 Treatment Planning considerations

Simulation instructions	• Position: Supine • Immobilization: customized head and shoulder mask or SRT rated mask • Additional immobilization of tongue or displacement of the tongue for recurrences within the oral cavity-oropharynx • ≤ 1 mm thick CT slices • Fusion of high-resolution diagnostic imaging to assist with target delineation (i.e., MRI, CT neck, PET-CT)
Image guidance	Daily cone beam CT
Margins	3 mm with daily cone beam CT; adjust off critical structures as necessary (i.e., spinal cord; optic apparatus)
Tumor coverage considerations	Tumor coverage while balancing neighboring normal organs at risk (i.e., cranial nerve, carotid artery, mandible); elective nodal coverage should be avoided

- Treatment restricted to gross disease/high risk microscopic volumes with small margins is generally preferable with low total treatment volume in the re-irradiation setting.

- For short interval recurrence (<1 year), planning will typically emphasize minimizing cord and brainstem dose (cumulative cord dose under 50 Gy preferred) and conformality which may result in a hotter than normal plan, especially for conventional fractionation standards.
- For patients with longer interval recurrence (>2 years), animal models (i.e., monkey, mini pig) indicate spinal cord and brainstem normal tissue recovery. However, doses should still be kept as low as possible to minimize risk of complications.
- Acute grade $\geq$ 3 toxicity and complications were the same irrespective of re-radiation treatment modality (SBRT, hypofractionated, and conventionally fractionated) and cumulative dose. In a meta-analysis review [1], the risk of on treatment (and up to 30 days post-treatment) associated death was very low (0.9%). Notable acute treatment-related toxicities associated with death included neutropenia, fatal hemorrhage (due to rapid tumor regression in an area of compromised vasculature like previously irradiated carotid artery), and aspiration pneumonia.
- Late grade $\geq$ 3 treatment associated toxicities were observed in almost 1/3 of all patients undergoing re-irradiation. Common toxicities included radionecrosis, dysphagia requiring feeding tube placement, and trismus. Carotid blowout remains an uncommon but relevant late toxicity reported in this meta-analysis review [1] and this risk is impacted based on the re-irradiation volume and proximity to the carotid.

19.5 Commonly Used Dose/Fractionation Schemes

- Re-irradiation for head and neck cancers is still an evolving area with little literature to guide optimal radiation dose.
- For conventionally-fractionated re-irradiation, a total dose of 60–66 Gy has been used.
- For SBRT, 35–40 Gy in 5 fractions has been used.

19.6 Normal Tissue Tolerances

- Literature resources to help provide modern dose guidelines for organs at risk in the re-irradiation setting are limited. The need to consider time from original course of (chemo)radiotherapy to time of planned re-irradiation (conventional, hypofractionated, or SBRT) must consider the potential for normal tissue recovery (i.e., spinal cord, brachial plexus) as this can directly impact choice of re-irradiation dose.

	TG101	QUANTEC	Our institutional practice
Brain parenchyma			
1 fx	N/A	V12 < 5–10 cc	N/A
Toxicity	N/A	<20% symptomatic necrosis	N/A
3–5 fx	N/A	N/A	Conversion of multi-fraction dose to single fraction equivalent dose, total brain V14 Gy associated with grade 3 necrosis: 5 cc = 0.4%, 10 cc = 0.8%, 20 cc = 3.4% [2]
Toxicity	N/A	N/A	Symptomatic radiation necrosis requiring surgery
Brainstem			
1 fx	Dmax ≤15 Gy, V10 < 0.5 cc	Dmax <12.5 Gy	Dmax <15 Gy, V10 < 0.5 cc
3 fx	Dmax ≤23.1 Gy, V18 < 0.5 cc		Dmax <23.1 Gy, V15.9 < 0.5 cc
5 fx	Dmax ≤31 Gy, V23 < 0.5 cc		Dmax <31 Gy, V23 < 0.5 cc
Toxicity	Grade ≥ 3 cranial neuropathy	<5% permanent cranial neuropathy or necrosis	Cranial neuropathy
Optic pathway			
1 fx	Dmax ≤10 Gy, V8 < 0.2 cc	Dmax <12 Gy	Dmax <10 Gy, V8 < 0.2 cc
3 fx	Dmax ≤17.4, V15.3 < 0.2 cc		Dmax <17.4 Gy, V15.3 < 0.2 cc
5 fx	Dmax ≤25, V23 < 0.2 cc		Dmax <25 Gy, V23 < 0.2 cc
Toxicity	Grade ≥ 3 neuritis	<10% optic neuropathy	Neuritis
Spinal cord			
1 fx	Dmax ≤14 Gy, V10 < 0.35 cc, V7 < 1.2 cc	Dmax <13 Gy	Dmax <14 Gy, V10 < 0.35 cc
3 fx	Dmax ≤21.9 Gy, V18 < 0.35 cc, V 12.3 < 1.2 cc		Dmax <22.5 Gy, V15.9 < 0.35 cc
5 fx	Dmax ≤30 Gy, V23 < 0.35 cc, V 14.5 < 1.2 cc		Dmax <28 Gy, V22 < 0.35 cc
Toxicity	Grade ≥ 3 myelitis	1% myelopathy	Myelitis
Cochlea			
1 fx	Dmax ≤9 Gy	Dose ≤14 Gy (prescription dose)	Dmax <9 Gy
3 fx	Dmax ≤17.1 Gy		Dmax <14.4 Gy

	TG101	QUANTEC	Our institutional practice
5 fx	Dmax ≤25 Gy		Dmax <22 Gy
Toxicity	Grade ≥ 3 hearing loss	<25% sensory neural hearing loss	Hearing loss
Carotid vessel			
Toxicity	N/A	N/A	Attempts at correlating dosimetric characteristics (i.e., D0.1cc, D1cc, D2cc) [3], tumor characteristics (i.e., >180°, >270° carotid involvement) or total carotid lifetime dose provide metrics to guide re-irradiation planning but have not been validated in larger studies. For large volume disease surrounding the carotid, we recommend conventional or hypofractionated re-irradiation regimens over SBRT
Brachial plexus			
1 fx	Dmax <17.5 Gy, V14 < 3 cc	N/A	V17.5 < 0.03 cc, V14 < 3 cc (NRG BR001/002 constraints)
3 fx	Dmax <24 Gy, V20.4 < 3 cc	N/A	V26 < 0.03 cc, V22 < 3 cc (NRG BR001/002 constraints)
5 fx	Dmax 30.5 Gy, V27 < 3 cc	N/A	V32 < 0.03 cc, V30 < 3 cc
Toxicity	Neuropathy		Brachial plexopathy
Skin			
1 fx	Dmax <26 Gy, V23 < 10 cc		V27.5 < 0.03 cc, V25.5 < 10 cc (NRG BR001/002 constraints)
3 fx	Dmax <33 Gy, V30 < 10 cc		V33 < 0.03 cc, V31 < 10 cc (NRG BR001/002 constraints)
5 fx	Dmax <39.5 Gy, V36.5 < 10 cc		V38.5 < 0.03 cc, V36.5 < 10 cc (NRG BR001/002 constraints)
Toxicity			Ulceration

19.7 Patient Management Considerations

- Premedication: likely to be site and patient dependent but consideration of aggressive pain control with narcotics, gabapentin (or pregabalin) may help with patient tolerance during re-irradiation.
- Common acute toxicities.
  - Pain: narcotics, steroids, NSAIDs as needed.
  - Radiation dermatitis: OTC water-based lotions for grade 1 desquamation; Rx silvadene 1% for grade 2 desquamation.
  - Soft tissue mucositis: salt water gargles, lidocaine-magic mouth wash rinses prn, short course steroid taper (Medrol dosepak).

- Late toxicities.
  - Soft tissue fibrosis: Trental 400 mg tid and Vitamin E 400 IU qd or pravastatin 40 mg qd or best supportive care (massage, acupuncture).
  - Trismus (re-irradiation dependent location): Trental 400 mg tid and Vitamin E 400 IU qd or pravastatin 40 mg qd or best supportive care (massage, acupuncture).
  - Wound skin complications: evaluation by wound care specialist.
  - Chronic pain: evaluation by pain clinic and/or need for long term pain control with narcotics or nerve block.
  - Osteoradionecrosis, dental complications: hyperbaric oxygen in the absence of disease progression, anti-fibrotic therapy (as above), dental reconstructive surgery in the absence of disease progression.
  - Malnutrition, weight loss secondary to esophageal stricture, loss of appetite, fibrotic impairment limiting oral intake: consideration of Marinol 5–10 mg tid, permanent feeding tube, anti-fibrotic therapy as noted above.
  - Lymphedema: evaluation by physical therapist specializing in lymphedema management, specialized compression sleeve, massage.

19.8 Relevant Literature

- For further information about definition, reporting, and clinical decision making in re-irradiation, please refer to EORTC-ESTRO consensus recommendation on re-irradiation (Andratschke et al., Lancet Onc, 2022).

Study	Patient	Treatment	Median follow-up	Outcomes
Conventionally fractionated re-irradiation				
Ward 2017 [4] (MIRI Consortium, retrospective)	$N = 412$ from 7 institutions Prior RT ≥ 40 Gy Recurrence or second primary without distant mets New re-irradiation fields had to overlap the prior 40 Gy portion by ≥40 Gy	Re-irradiation 1–3 Gy/fx Median dose 60 Gy Chemotherapy used in 76% of patients	10.4 months (range, 0–129.7) for all patients 22.9 months (0–129.7) for survivors	2-year OS: post-op 45.2%, definitive re-RT 35.5% 2-year LRF: post-op 39.9%, definitive re-RT 46.3% grade ≥ 3 late toxicity 14.2%

Study	Patient	Treatment	Median follow-up	Outcomes
Vargo 2017 [5] (MIRI Consortium, retrospective)	$N = 414$ (re-IMRT $N = 217$, SBRT $N = 197$) Unresectable recurrence Prior RT ≥40 Gy	IMRT: ≥40 Gy or SBRT: 1–5 fx with ≥5 Gy/fx	For all patients: 8.4 months IMRT, 7.1 months SBRT For survivors: 28 months IMRT, 24 months SBRT	2-year OS: Overall: 35.4% IMRT and 16.3% SBRT. Small tumors (≤25 cc): 50.3% IMRT, 38.5% SBRT (NS) Large tumors (>25 cc): 50.3% IMRT, 14.4% SBRT ($p < 0.001$) Acute grade ≥ 4 toxicity: 5.1% IMRT, 0.5% SBRT No significant difference in late toxicity
Takier 2016 [6] (Retrospective)	$N = 227$ Median initial RT dose: 65 Gy (range 30–79)	Median dose: definitive re-IMRT 66 Gy, after salvage resection 60 Gy $N = 104$ had salvage resection $N = 135$ received chemotherapy	24.7 months	5-year LRC, PFS, and OS were 53%, 22% and 32% for HNSCC vs 74%, 59%, 79% for non-HNSCC pts grade ≥ 3 toxicity: 2-year 32%, 5-year 48% (dysphagia or odynophagia) Increased grade ≥ 3 toxicity associated with RT volume > 50 cc and concurrent chemotherapy
SBRT				
Lartigau 2013 [7] (Phase II trial)	$N = 56$ Mean time from between initial RT to recurrence: 38 months	36 Gy in 6 fx, every other day Prescription to 85% IDL covering 95% PTV Concurrent cetuximab	11.4 months	Median OS 11.8 months 1-year OS 47.5%. 3-month ORR 58.4% Median PFS 7.1 months grade ≥ 3 toxicity 32% (mucositis, dysphagia, induration, fibrosis) grade 5 toxicity 2% (1 patient died from hemorrhage and malnutrition) Cutaneous toxicity noted in 41 patients (grade 1, 25%; grade 2, 48%; grade 3, 9%)

Study	Patient	Treatment	Median follow-up	Outcomes
Vargo 2015 [8] (Phase II trial)	$N = 50$ Unresectable recurrent HNSCC Median time between initial RT to recurrence: 26 months Median tumor volume 36 cc	40–44 Gy in 5 fx, every other day 95% PTV coverage with no more than 20% of PTV receiving >110% of prescription dose Concurrent cetuximab	18 months (range 10–70) for surviving patients	1-year LC 60%, LR PFS 37%, distant PFS 71% Median OS 10 months 1-year OS 40% grade 3 toxicity 6%
Heron 2009 [9] (Phase I)	$N = 25$ Unresectable recurrence Median initial RT dose: 65 Gy Median time between initial RT and recurrence: 13 months Median tumor volume 45 cc	5 Gy x 5–9 fx, every other day. Prescription to 80% IDL	10 months	1-year LC 59% 1-year OS 59% No grade 3–4 toxicity
Rwigema 2011 [10] (Retrospective)	$N = 96$ Median initial RT dose: 68.4 Gy (range, 32–170 Gy) Median tumor volume 24.3 cc	Mean dose 35 Gy (20–50 Gy) in 5 fx, every other day	14 months overall; 17.6 months for survivors	Doses ≥40 Gy: LRC 69.4% 1-year, 58% 2-year, 41% 3-year Doses <40 Gy: LRC 52% 1-year, 32% 2-year, 16% 3-year ($p = 0.02$) Overall survival: 59% 1-year, 28% 2-year Acute grade 3 toxicity 5.2% (dysgeusia, dysphagia, xerostomia) Late Grace 3 toxicity 3.1% (dysphagia, fibrosis) No grade 4–5 toxicity
Kawaguchi 2010 [11] (Retrospective)	$N = 22$	20–42 Gy in 2–5 fx	24 months	Complete response 64%, partial response 7% OS 55% No grade ≥ 3 toxicity

Study	Patient	Treatment	Median follow-up	Outcomes
Heron 2011 [12] (Retrospective)	*N* = 35	40 Gy (20–44 Gy) in 5 fx, every other day SBRT only (*N* = 13) SBRT plus cetuximab (*N* = 22)	For survivors: SBRT only 21.3 months, SBRT plus cetuximab 24.8 months	1-year OS: SBRT 53%, SBRT/cetuximab 66% 2-year OS: SBRT 21%, SBRT/cetuximab 53% (log rank $p = 0.031$) grade 3 toxicity 9% (xerostomia, dysphagia)
Cengiz 2011 [13] (Retrospective)	*N* = 46 (65% with SCC histology)	30 Gy (range 25–35 Gy) in 5 fx, daily treatment Prior to SBRT re-irradiation, 19 pts received chemo, 22 pts received surgery, 6 pts underwent re-irradiation	11.9 months	Complete response 27%, partial response 30% 1-year OS 47% grade 5 toxicity 15% Carotid artery rupture 18% (more likely in patients with tumor ≥180° carotid involvement)
Vargo 2012 [14] (Retrospective)	*N* = 34 Unresectable recurrent HNSCC Median initial RT dose: 61 Gy Median time between initial RT to recurrence: 53 months Median tumor volume 19 cc	Median 40 Gy in 5 fx, every other day. Prescription to 80% IDL covering 95% PTV	10 months	LC: 77% 6 months, 59% 12 months OS: 75% 6 months, 69% 12 months Acute grade 3 toxicity: 15% Late grade 3 toxicity: 6% (associated with GTV ≥ 25 cc)

Study	Patient	Treatment	Median follow-up	Outcomes
Yamazaki 2016 [15] (Retrospective)	$N = 107$ All recurrences occurred in prior irradiated volume with ≥40 Gy	Median dose 30 Gy (range, 15–39 Gy) in 5 fx (range, 3–8) Minimum dose 90% of prescription; 95% prescription dose coverage to PTV	15 months	2-year OS 35% Presence of mucosal ulceration was prognostic of 2-year OS (8% v 43%, $p < 0.0001$ UVA) MVA of OS after re-irradiation: nasopharynx vs other [HR 2.42, 95% CI 1.37–4.28, $p = 0.002$]; PTV ≤40 cc v > 40 cc [HR 1.96, 95% CI 1.19–3.21, $p = 0.007$]; ulceration yes v no [HR 2.7, 95% CI 1.53–4.76, $p = 0.0006$] Late grade ≥ 3 toxicity was 21%; carotid blowout syndrome occurred in 11 patients, 9 fatal

Abbreviations: *OS* overall survival, *RT* radiotherapy, *LRF* local regional failure, *LRC* local regional control, *PFS* progression-free survival, *ORR* overall response rate, *LC* local control, *LRPFS* local regional progression-free survival

References

1. Dionisi F, et al. Organs at risk's tolerance and dose limits for head and neck cancer re-irradiation: a literature review. Oral Oncol. 2019;98:35–47.
2. Peng L, et al. Updated risk models demonstrate low risk of symptomatic radionecrosis following stereotactic radiosurgery for brain metastases. Surg Neurol Int. 2019;10:32.
3. Gebhardt BJ, et al. Carotid dosimetry and the risk of carotid Blowout syndrome after reirradiation with head and neck stereotactic body radiation therapy. Int J Radiat Oncol Biol Phys. 2018;101(1):195–200.
4. Ward MC, et al. Refining patient selection for reirradiation of head and neck squamous carcinoma in the IMRT Era: a multi-institution cohort study by the MIRI collaborative. Int J Radiat Oncol Biol Phys. 2018;100(3):586–94.
5. Vargo JA, et al. A Multi-institutional comparison of SBRT and IMRT for definitive reirradiation of recurrent or second primary head and neck cancer. Int J Radiat Oncol Biol Phys. 2018;100(3):595–605.
6. Takiar V, et al. Reirradiation of head and neck cancers with intensity modulated radiation therapy: outcomes and analyses. Int J Radiat Oncol Biol Phys. 2016;95(4):1117–31.
7. Lartigau EF, et al. Multi institutional phase II study of concomitant stereotactic reirradiation and cetuximab for recurrent head and neck cancer. Radiother Oncol. 2013;109(2):281–5.
8. Vargo JA, et al. A prospective phase 2 trial of reirradiation with stereotactic body radiation therapy plus cetuximab in patients with previously irradiated recurrent squamous cell carcinoma of the head and neck. Int J Radiat Oncol Biol Phys. 2015;91(3):480–8.

9. Heron DE, et al. Stereotactic body radiotherapy for recurrent squamous cell carcinoma of the head and neck: results of a phase I dose-escalation trial. Int J Radiat Oncol Biol Phys. 2009;75(5):1493–500.
10. Rwigema JC, et al. The impact of tumor volume and radiotherapy dose on outcome in previously irradiated recurrent squamous cell carcinoma of the head and neck treated with stereotactic body radiation therapy. Am J Clin Oncol. 2011;34(4):372–9.
11. Kawaguchi K, et al. Stereotactic radiosurgery may contribute to overall survival for patients with recurrent head and neck carcinoma. Radiat Oncol. 2010;5:51.
12. Heron DE, et al. Concurrent cetuximab with stereotactic body radiotherapy for recurrent squamous cell carcinoma of the head and neck: a single institution matched case-control study. Am J Clin Oncol. 2011;34(2):165–72.
13. Cengiz M, et al. Salvage reirradiation with stereotactic body radiotherapy for locally recurrent head-and-neck tumors. Int J Radiat Oncol Biol Phys. 2011;81(1):104–9.
14. Vargo JA, et al. Stereotactic body radiation therapy for locally recurrent, previously irradiated nonsquamous cell cancers of the head and neck. Head Neck. 2012;34(8):1153–61.
15. Yamazaki H, et al. Reirradiation using robotic image-guided stereotactic radiotherapy of recurrent head and neck cancer. J Radiat Res. 2016;57(3):288–93.

Part IV
Skin

Chapter 20
Skin (Melanoma and Nonmelanoma Skin Cancers)

Jacob T. Hall, Gregory D. Judy, and Bhishamjit S. Chera

20.1 Introduction

Radiation therapy is commonly used to treat nonmelanoma skin cancer (NMSC) and melanoma. In general, definitive and postoperative radiation is mainly used in skin cancers located in high-risk locations (i.e., mask region of head and neck) and in immunocompromised patients (e.g., patients with organ transplants). Historically, there have been a wide range of doses utilized for NMSC, depending on tumor location, age/performance status of patients, desired cosmetic outcome, and presence of high-risk features such as PNI. Melanoma has been thought of as a more radioresistant tumor; however, this thinking is changing based on newer data. This chapter summarizes the use of hypofractionated RT for both NMSC and melanoma in the definitive setting.

J. T. Hall
Department of Radiation Oncology, University of North Carolina School of Medicine, Chapel Hill, NC, USA
e-mail: jacob.hall@unchealth.unc.edu

G. D. Judy (✉)
Department of Radiation Oncology, University of North Carolina School of Medicine, Chapel Hill, NC, USA

Lineberger Comprehensive Cancer Center, University of North Carolina School of Medicine, Chapel Hill, NC, USA
e-mail: gregory.judy@unchealth.unc.edu

B. S. Chera
Department of Radiation Oncology, MUSC, Medical University of South Carolina, Charleston, USA
e-mail: Bchera@med.unc.edu

O. Kaidar-Person, R. Chen (eds.), *Hypofractionated and Stereotactic Radiation Therapy*, https://doi.org/10.1007/978-3-031-47701-0_20

20.2 Pearls

- Nonmelanoma skin cancer (NMSC) is the most common malignancy with an estimated 5.4 million cases annually in the United States.
- The incidence of melanoma doubled from 1982 to 2011 and continues to rise; estimated incidence in 2019 is 96,480 cases.
- NMSC is more common in males (4:1); melanoma is site-dependent (men = trunk; women = extremities).
- Caucasians are at highest risk for both melanoma and NMSC.
- Risk factors:
  - NMSC: Most common risk factor is UV exposure. Other risk factors include chronic irritation, chronic arsenic exposure, immunosuppression, radiation exposure, occupational exposure, and genetic disorders (e.g., basal cell nevus syndrome, xeroderma pigmentosum).
  - Melanoma: UV exposure, atypical nevi/high nevus count, familial, immunosuppression, and phenotypic traits (light skin, blond hair, light-colored eyes, and high freckle density).
- Histology:
  - NMSC: basal cell carcinoma (BCC, ~65%), squamous cell carcinoma (SCC, ~30%), Merkel cell carcinoma (MCC) and adnexal (<5%).

    BCC subtypes include nodulo-ulcerative, superficial, morpheaform, infiltrative, pigmented, fibroepithelial tumor of Pinkus, and basosquamous.

    SCC subtypes include invasive, Bowen's disease (carcinoma in situ), erythroplasia of Queyrat (Bowen's of penis), Marjolin's ulcer (arises within chronic wound/scar), verrucous (typically anogenital or plantar of foot), and spindle cell (sun-exposed areas, Caucasian, >40 age).
  - Melanoma: superficial spreading (65%), nodular (25%), lentigo maligna (~7%), and acral lentiginous (<5%; most common type among dark-skinned individuals). Also desmoplastic (typically occurs in H&N, low likelihood for nodal metastases).
- Presenting symptoms:
  - NMSC:

    BCC: pearly papule, pruritic plaque, or bleeding ulcer (waxes/wanes). Typically slow growing.

    In situ SCC: typically soft, erythematous, scaly, well-circumscribed patch.

    Invasive SCC: firm, ulcerative mass with elevated border; signs of PNI include pain, tingling, and hypesthesia.
  - Melanoma: ABCDEs = A, asymmetry; B, irregular borders; C, color; D, diameter > 6 mm; E, evolving lesion (color, shape, size). Acral lentiginous typically presents on palms, soles, or subungual.
- Local anatomy:
  - BCC and SCC typically arise in sun-exposed areas on H&N.
  - H zone of the face (periauricular, glabella, medial canthus, nose, nasolabial region, and columella) is a high-risk area (disease extent often underestimated).

- Areas of spread:
  - NMSC:
    Spreads laterally and deep.
    BCC: low propensity for PNI (~1–2% usually in setting of recurrent or locally advanced disease), nodal spread, and distant metastases (<0.01%: regional nodes > lung > liver > bone).
    SCC: more aggressive, with ~7% PNI, nodal spread up to 10–20% in poorly differentiated, recurrent, >3 cm or > 4 mm depth; distant metastases remain low, <5%, to the lungs, liver, and bones.
  - Melanoma:
    Regional nodal metastases at presentation: <10% for T1 lesions, ~25–30% > T1.
    Sentinel lymph node status is the best prognostic factor for recurrence and survival; ulceration and tumor thickness are best prognostic factors when node negative.
    ~5% with distant metastases at presentation.
- Medical workup:
  - H&P: thorough CN exam for head/face tumors and regional nodal evaluation.
  - Biopsy.
  - Basic lab work (CBC, metabolic panel, liver function tests).
- Imaging workup:
  - CT or MRI w/wo contrast for suspected/known nodal involvement.
  - MRI w/wo contrast for suspected PNI or medial/lateral canthi lesions (rule out orbital involvement).
    CT: best to assess nodal or bone involvement.
    MRI: best to assess PNI; seen as enhancement of nerve on post contrast scan; can also see thickening along nerve or loss of fat surrounding nerve.
- Treatment strategies: surgical resection and/or RT, depending on location, disease extent, performance status [1–4].

20.3 Patient Selection for Hypofractionated RT

1. NMSC: T1–2 tumors, node negative; exact fractionation scheme utilized depends on lesion location, patient age/functional status, and cosmetic outcome considerations.

   (a) Cosmesis improved with more protracted course.
   (b) Close proximity to the eye, eyelid, nose, or ear = lower dose/fraction.
   (c) Dorsum of hands/feet = generally avoid RT (elevated risk of necrosis).
   (d) Hypofractionation not suited for larger lesions or locally advanced disease (T3/4, N+, PNI) due to large treatment fields.
   (e) Postoperative treatment = indications include gross residual disease, close or positive margins, PNI, pT3/4, node positive, or recurrent disease.

(f) Treatment of lymphatics = indications include positive nodes, PNI, T3/4, recurrent disease, or primary in close proximity to the lip, immunocompromised patients.
(g) Frail patients with a poor performance status or those treated with palliative intent are suitable for hypofractionated RT.
(h) HDR brachytherapy: suited for small tumors, abutting fields, or sloping surfaces.
  - Allows for high-dose concentration in target volumes with rapid dose fall-off at the periphery.
  - Techniques: Freiburg flap, Valencia or Leipzig applicators, or other custom surface mold.
  - Delivered with Ir^{192} afterloader.

2. Melanoma:
   (a) Primary site: Postoperative indications include desmoplastic/neurotropic features, >4 mm thick (especially if ulcerated), and close/positive margins.
   (b) Nodal basin: post-op indications include positive nodes (≥2 cervical, ≥3–4 axillary/inguinal), ECE, size ≥3 cm, recurrent disease, or SLNB+ without plan for completion dissection.
   (c) Small case series have shown radiation to be effective for melanoma in-situ.

20.4 Treatment Planning

Simulation instructions	• Location-dependent: – H&N: Clinical setup in treatment room for superficial lesions; may need CT scan w/immobilization mask when treating deep lesions/nodes – Axilla: Supine, arm akimbo, or above head (use wingboard) – Groin: Unilateral frog leg • Lead shields (lens, nasal septum, oral cavity, ear, etc.) as needed if near OAR. Use beeswax coating to minimize backscatter
Image guidance	• Weekly port films • CBCT for pelvic nodes • Weekly clinical verification for electrons • Clinical verification for HDR brachytherapy
Margins	• NMSC: GTV + 1–2 cm • Melanoma: Primary site + 2–3 cm
Tumor coverage	NMSC: Treat with orthovoltage or electrons • Orthovoltage Rx = Dmax • Electrons Rx = 90–95% IDL • Daily bolus (0.5–1 cm) to achieve adequate skin dose • If clinical PNI present (i.e., symptomatic or named nerve involvement on imaging or pathology), include nerve retrograde to skull base. Treat with EBRT and conventional or BID fractionation • HDR brachytherapy = 5–10 mm depth (depending on tumor thickness) • Melanoma: Nodal volume, location-dependent • H&N: Cover ipsilateral levels 1–5 + supraclavicular fossa. For scalp/high-facial lesions, cover pre–/postauricular nodes • Axilla: Levels 1–3 + supraclavisular (for high-axillary disease) • Groin: Include all confirmed locations; if positive inguinal nodes can treat back to external iliac

20.5 Common Dose/Fractionation Schemes

NMSC

Dose/fx	# of fx	Total dose	Notes[a]
15–20 Gy	1	15–20 Gy	Palliative (symptom relief); older patients, poor health [5]
8 Gy	4	32 Gy	QD; older patients, poor health [5]
7 Gy	3	21 Gy	QD; older patients, poor health [5]
6 Gy	5	30 Gy	QD; older patients, poor health [5, 6]
5.25 Gy	7	36.75 Gy	Weekly; older patients, poor health [7]
4 Gy	10	40 Gy	QD; older patients, poor health [5, 8]
3 Gy	15	45 Gy	QD; older patients, poor health [5, 7, 8]
2.5 Gy	20	50 Gy	QD; [5, 8, 9]

[a]Lesions with PNI need to treat the affected nerve back to skull base. In these situations, recommend using EBRT and more conventional or BID fractionation schemes (e.g., 2 Gy × 30–35 fx QD or 1.2 Gy × 38–64 fx BID) to minimize late normal tissue side effects

Melanoma is conventionally thought of as a more radioresistant tumor, potentially benefiting from higher dose/fraction.

Dose/fx	# of fx	Total dose	Notes[a]
6 Gy	4	24 Gy	Twice weekly [10]
6 Gy	5	30 Gy	Twice weekly [10–12]
2.4 Gy	20	48 Gy	QD [13–15]

[a]Daily conventional fractionation can be used (2 Gy × 25–35 fx). However, hypofractionation is believed to be more efficacious

20.6 Normal Tissue Tolerances

	TG101 [16]		
Organ	Dmax	Volumetric	OTHER[a] [17]
Cartilage			<3 Gy/day
• DLT			Chondritis
Spinal cord			Max <45–50 Gy
• 1 fx	14 Gy	<0.35 cc	
• 3 fx	22 Gy	<0.35 cc	
• 5 fx	30 Gy	<0.35 cc	
• DLT	Myelitis		Myelitis
Skin			Max 30 cc 60 Gy Max 10 cc 70 Gy
• 1 fx	26 Gy	<10 cc	
• 3 fx	33 Gy	<10 cc	
• 5 fx	39.5 Gy	<10 cc	
• DLT	Ulceration		Ulceration

[a]At UNC, we follow the above dose constraints

20.7 Patient Management

1. No premedication required.
2. Toxicity.
   (a) Acute:
   - Dermatitis ± desquamation (~100%; desquamation 5–10% but depends on location and dose).
     - Manage with emollients (e.g., Aquaphor, calendula, aloe).
     - If moist desquamation occurs, use 1% Silvadene cream on affected area.

   (b) Late:
   - Skin (hypo–/hyperpigmentation, telangiectasia, skin atrophy, fibrosis up to 50% grade 1/2, <10% grade 3/4).
     - Vast majority do not cause problems.
     - Continue use of emollients.
     - Refer to dermatology and/or surgery if causing symptoms.
   - Lymphedema (especially groin, axilla, and extremity) (~10%).
     - Refer to lymphedema physical therapy.
     - Compression sleeve.
     - Avoid vaccinations, BP readings in affected arm/leg.
   - Osteoradionecrosis (site-dependent, <5%)[*].
   - Cartilage (site-dependent, chondritis <5%, cartilage necrosis <5%)[*].
   - Neuropathy (site-dependent, 2–3%)[*].

   [*]*For above late complications, recommend referral to appropriate specialist for management (dermatology, ENT, surgery, neurology, etc.).*

   (c) Systemic therapy: limited data regarding combined radiation and systemic treatments.
   - *BRAF inhibitors*—can act as radiosensitizers and, therefore, increase acute radiation toxicity. Recommend holding systemic therapy at least 3 days before and after fractionated radiation and at least 1 day before and after SBRT/SRS.
   - *Immunotherapy* (PD-1/PDL-1 or CTLA-4 inhibitors): abscopal effects have been seen when given concurrently with radiation in retrospective studies and a small prospective phase II single-arm trial, but there are no prospective randomized data to guide decisions. Recommend sequential (giving before or after radiation therapy) rather than concurrent treatment. However, concurrent administration appears not to increase toxicity.

20.8 Follow-Up

- H&P with skin exam every 3 months for first year, q6 months years 3–5, and then annually.
- Melanoma: PET/CT at 3 months posttreatment and then restaging CT scans as clinically indicated.
- NMSC with PNI: can repeat MRI at 3 months posttreatment with subsequent scans as clinically indicated.

20.9 Relevant Literature

- NMSC—The use of 2.5 Gy/fx or lower generally gives better cosmetic result compared to larger fractionation schemes. The risk of skin ulceration and lymphedema increases proportionately with the surface area treated and is also more likely to occur in areas with poor circulation and thin skin (i.e., lower extremities and sun-damaged skin of the scalp in older patients).

Study	Patients	Treatment	Median follow-up	Outcomes
Prospective studies				
Ferro (2015) [6] Phase II trial	$n = 31$	30 Gy in 5 fx	30 months	96.8% CR 88% 3-year LC No grade ≥ 2 toxicity 96% good or excellent cosmetic result
Retrospective studies				
Gunaratne (2018) [18] Systematic review, 33 publications	75% SCC, 24% BCC	EBRT or brachytherapy Mean 38.15 Gy total dose Mean 7.95 Gy/fx	2–64 months	>90% LC in 29 publications
Zaorsky (2017) [19] Meta-analysis	$n = 9729$ T1–2 SCC/BCC Definitive radiation	45 Gy/11 fx 50 Gy/15 fx 36.75 Gy/7 fx 35 Gy/7 fx	36 months	14% 5-year LR "Good" cosmesis in 80%
Pampena (2016) [7]	$n = 385$	Orthovoltage 36.75 Gy/7 fx weekly vs. 45 Gy/15 fx daily	31 months	88.8% vs. 77.1% excellent cosmetic outcome in 45 Gy vs. 36.75 Gy No difference in LC or acute toxicity

Study	Patients	Treatment	Median follow-up	Outcomes
Grossi (2016) [9]	$n = 597$	Orthovoltage 2.5 Gy × 22 2.5 Gy × 20 2.0 Gy × 30	44 months	96% 10-year LC for BCC 87% 10-year LC for SCC Trend towards increased LC with >2.0 Gy/fx Similar rates of grade ≥ 3 toxicity across dose/fx schemes
Van Hezewijk (2010) [20]	$n = 333$ Majority head/face	Electrons to primary site 3 Gy × 18 fx, 4×/week 4.4 Gy × 10 fx, 4×/week GTV + 1 cm margin	43 months	**54 Gy**: 98% 3-year LRC (BCC) 97% 3-year LRC (SCC) 62% good cosmetic result **44 Gy**: 97% 3-year LRC (BCC) 94% 3-year LRC (SCC) 62% good cosmetic result
Abbatucci (1989) [21]	$n = 675$ Facial skin cancers (excluding lips, ears, eyelids, melanoma, and stage IV disease) Mostly elderly population	Superficial RT to primary lesion 10.2 Gy × 3 fx, once/week	24 months	96% 2-year LC 90% good cosmetic result 3% complication rate: ulcerations (2–3%), epiphora (<1%)
Kohler-Brock (1999) [22]	$n = 520$, BCC, SCC, Kaposi Sarcoma	HDR-BT w/Leipzig applicator 30–40 Gy / 5–10 fx, 1–2×/week	120 months	92% LC Low grade 1–2 late complication rates
Guix (2000) [23]	$n = 136$, BCC/SCC	HDR-BT w/custom surface molds. Treat daily	60 months	98% LC Grade 1–2 late complications (0.84%) 98% excellent cosmetic result
Gauden (2013) [24]	$n = 200$, BCC/SCC	HDR-BT w/Leipzig applicator. 36 Gy/12 fx. Treat daily	66 months	98% LC grade 1–2 late toxicity (20%) 62% excellent cosmetic result 26% good cosmetic result

Abbreviations: *CR* complete response, *LC* local control, *LR* local recurrence, *LRC* local-regional control, *SCC* squamous cell carcinoma, *BCC* basal cell carcinoma, *fx* fractions, *EBRT* external beam radiotherapy, *BT* brachytherapy

Melanoma

Study	Patients	Treatment	Median follow-up	Outcomes
Randomized controlled trials				
Burmeister (2012) [13]	$n = 217$; one nodal basin, completely resected High risk of relapse: ≥1 parotid node, ≥2 cervical/axillary nodes, ≥3 inguinal nodes, ECE, nodal size (≥3 cm cervical, ≥4 cm axilla/inguinal)	Lymphadenectomy then randomized to: (1) 2.4 Gy × 20 fx (2) observation	40 months	LN field failure improved with adjuvant RT (20 vs. 34 relapses, HR 0.56) No difference in RFS/OS Toxicity: 22% grade 3/4 toxicity; mainly skin/subcutaneous
Sause (1991) [25]	$n = 126$, definitive treatment Measurable lesions	(1) 8 Gy × 4 fx, 1×/week (2) 2.5 Gy × 20 fx, daily	24 months	**32 Gy**: 24% complete remission rate 4% grade ≥ 3 toxicity **50 Gy**: 23% complete remission rate 3% grade ≥ 3 toxicity
Prospective non-randomized studies				
Burmeister (2006) [14]	$n = 234$ N+ melanoma Nodal ECE, ≥1 LN+, or recurrent disease	Resection + adjuvant RT (1 patient received systemic therapy) 2.4 Gy × 20 fx	58 months	91% 5-year LRC 27% 5-year PFS 36% 5-year OS Grade 3 lymphedema 9% in axillary patients, 19% in ilioinguinal patients
Ang (1990) [10]	$n = 83$ Melanoma (>1.5 mm or cLN+) of H&N region Three groups: 1 = WLE + adjuvant RT; 2 = pre- vs. post-op RT w/ WLE; 3 = recurrent disease after node dissection + adjuvant RT or preoperative RT	6 Gy × 4 fx, 2×/week (RT given prior to surgery) 6 Gy × 5 fx, 2×/week (RT given after surgery)	16 months	**Group 1**: 95% 2-year LC 80% 2-year OS **Group 2**: 90% 2-year LC 71% 2-year OS **Group 3**: 83% 2-year LC 69% 2-year OS
Retrospectivestudies				
Lansu (2018) [15]	$n = 63$ Sinonasal melanoma	Resection and adjuvant radiation 2 Gy × 30 or 2.4 Gy × 20 vs. 4 Gy × 12 or 6 Gy × 6	23 months	**Conventional** 47% 5-year LC **Hypofractionation** 53% 5-year LC 1 grade ≥ 3 toxicity in each group

Study	Patients	Treatment	Median follow-up	Outcomes
Chang (2006) [11]	$n = 56$ High-risk melanoma (gross disease, close or positive margins, recurrent disease, satellitosis, nodal metastases, ECE) 87% in H&N area	WLE, node dissection, adjuvant RT (hypofractionation vs. conventional) Hypofractionation: 6 Gy × 5 fx, 2×/week Conventional: 2 Gy × 30 fx, daily	52 months	**Hypofractionation**: 87% 5-year LC 3% late toxicity (osteoradionecrosis of temporal bone and RT plexopathy) **Conventional**: 87% 5-year LC
Ballo (2006) [12]	$n = 466$ N+ melanoma Nodal ECE, ≥4 LN+, size ≥3 cm, or recurrent disease	Lymphadenectomy + adjuvant RT (33% had systemic therapy) RT: 6 Gy × 5 fx, 2×/week	48 months	89% 5-year LC 49% 5-year DSS 10-year symptomatic lymphedema 11%

Abbreviations: *WLE* wide local excision, *ECE* extracapsular extension, *LN* lymph node, *H&N* head and neck, *RT* radiotherapy, *fx* fractions; *RFS* recurrence-free survival, *OS* overall survival, *LC* local control, *DSS* disease-specific survival

20.10 Summary

Hypofractionated regimens offer good rates of tumor control with relatively low rates of toxicity. The likelihood of common toxicities such as lymphedema is related to which lymph node chains are irradiated.

20.11 UNC Experience

At our institution, we typically treat melanoma with either the 6 Gy × 5 fx or 2.4 Gy × 20 fx regimen. For NMSC, it will depend on location, patient's age, performance status, and presence of PNI. If it is an older patient who has transportation issues and a poor performance status, we will often treat with 4 Gy × 10 fx or 15–20 Gy × 1 fx. If PNI is present, we will treat with conventional dosing (2 Gy × 30–35 fx) and treat involved nerve back to the base of skull. We are very careful to consider dose and amount of skin surface area treated when treating primaries of lower extremity and scalp, as the risk of non-healing dermatitis/ulceration and lymphedema is higher in these clinical situations. Also, we try to avoid radiating the dissected groin because of a substantial risk of lymphedema.

References

1. Ballo MT. Malignant melanoma. Clinical radiation oncology. 5th ed. Philadelphia: Saunders/Elsevier; 2021. p. 806–16.
2. Screening and early detection of melanoma. Accessed Sept 2021.
3. Radiation therapy in the management of melanoma. Accessed Sept 2021.
4. Veness MJ, Howle J. Cutaneous carcinoma. Clinical radiation oncology. 5th ed. Philadelphia: Saunders/Elsevier; 2021. p. 792–805.
5. Million RR, Cassisi NJ. Management of head and neck cancer: a multidisciplinary approach. 2nd ed. Philadelphia: Lippincott; 1994.
6. Ferro M, Deodato F, Macchia G, Gentileschi S, Cilla S, Torre G, Padula GD, Nuzzo M, Massaccesi M, Valentini V, Morganti AG. Short-course radiotherapy in elderly patients with early stage non-melanoma skin cancer: a phase II study. Cancer Investig. 2014;33(2):34–8. https://doi.org/10.3109/07357907.2014.998835.
7. Pampena R, Palmieri T, Kyrgidis A, Ramundo D, Iotti C, Lallas A, Moscarella E, Borsari S, Argenziano G, Longo C. Orthovoltage radiotherapy for nonmelanoma skin cancer (NMSC): comparison between 2 different schedules. J Am Acad Dermatol. 2016;74(2):341–7. https://doi.org/10.1016/j.jaad.2015.09.031.
8. Likhacheva A, Awan M, Bhatnagar A, Bradfield L, Brady MS, Buzurovic I, et al. Definitive and postoperative radiation therapy for basal and squamous cell cancers of the skin: an ASTRO Clinical Practice Guideline. Pract Radiat Oncol. 2020;10(1):8–20.
9. Grossi Marconi D, da Costa Resende B, Rauber E, de Cassia Soares P, Fernandes JM, Mehta N, Lopes Carvalho A, Kupelian PA, Chen A. Head and neck non-melanoma skin cancer treated by superficial X-ray therapy: an analysis of 1021 cases. PLoS One. 2016;11(7):e0156544. https://doi.org/10.1371/journal.pone.0156544.
10. Ang KK, Byers RM, Peters LJ, et al. Regional radiotherapy as adjuvant treatment for head and neck malignant melanoma. Preliminary results. Arch Otolaryngol Head Neck Surg. 1990;116:169–72.
11. Chang DT, Amdur RJ, Morris CG, Mendenhall WM. Adjuvant radiotherapy for cutaneous melanoma: comparing hypofractionation to conventional fractionation. Int J Radiat Oncol Biol Phys. 2006;66:1051–5.
12. Ballo MT, Ross MI, Cormier JN, et al. Combined-modality therapy for patients with regional nodal metastases from melanoma. Int J Radiat Oncol Biol Phys. 2006;64:106–13.
13. Burmeister BH, Henderson MA, Ainslie J, et al. Adjuvant radiotherapy versus observation alone for patients at risk of lymph-node field relapse after therapeutic lymphadenectomy for melanoma: a randomised trial. Lancet Oncol. 2012;13:589–97.
14. Burmeister BH, Mark Smithers B, Burmeister E, et al. A prospective phase II study of adjuvant postoperative radiation therapy following nodal surgery in malignant melanoma-Trans Tasman Radiation Oncology Group (TROG) Study 96.06. Radiother Oncol. 2006;81:136–42.
15. Lansu J, Klop WM, Heemsbergen W, Navran A, Al-Mamgani A, Langendijk JA, Kaanders JH, Terhaard C, Karakullukcu B, Hamming-Vrieze O. Local control in sinonasal malignant melanoma: comparing conventional to hypofractionated radiotherapy. Head Neck. 2018;40(1):86–93. https://doi.org/10.1002/hed.24979.
16. Benedict SH, Yenice KM, Followill D, et al. Stereotactic body radiation therapy: the report of AAPM Task Group 101. Med Phys. 2010;37:4078–101.
17. Marks LB, Yorke ED, Jackson A, et al. Use of normal tissue complication probability models in the clinic. Int J Radiat Oncol Biol Phys. 2010;76:S10–9.
18. Gunaratne Dakshika A, Veness Michael J. Efficacy of hypofractionated radiotherapy in patients with non-melanoma skin cancer: results of a systematic review. J Med Imaging Radiat Oncol. 2018;62(3):401–11. https://doi.org/10.1111/1754-9485.12718.
19. Zaorsky NG, Lee CT, Zhang E, Keith SW, Galloway TJ. Hypofractionated radiation therapy for basal and squamous cell skin cancer: a meta-analysis. Radiother Oncol. 2017;125(1):13–20. https://doi.org/10.1016/j.radonc.2017.08.011.

20. van Hezewijk M, Creutzberg CL, Putter H, et al. Efficacy of a hypofractionated schedule in electron beam radiotherapy for epithelial skin cancer: analysis of 434 cases. Radiother Oncol. 2010;95:245–9.
21. Abbatucci JS, Boulier N, Laforge T, Lozier JC. Radiation therapy of skin carcinomas: results of a hypofractionated irradiation schedule in 675 cases followed more than 2 years. Radiother Oncol. 1989;14:113–9.
22. Köhler-Brock A, Prager W, Pohlmann S, Kunze S. The indications for and results of HDR afterloading therapy in diseases of the skin and mucosa with standardized surface applicators (the Leipzig applicator). Strahlenther Onkol. 1999;175(4):170–4.
23. Guix B, Finestres F, Tello JI, Palma C, Martinez A, Guix JR, Guix R. Treatment of skin carcinomas of the face by high-dose-rate brachytherapy and custom-made surface molds. Int J Radiat Oncol Biol Phys. 2000;47(1):95–102. https://doi.org/10.1016/S0360-3016(99)00547-7.
24. Gauden R, Pracy M, Avery AM, Hodgetts I, Gauden S. HDR brachytherapy for superficial non-melanoma skin cancers. J Med Imaging Radiat Oncol. 2013;57(2):212–7. https://doi.org/10.1111/j.1754-9485.2012.02466.x.
25. Sause WT, Cooper JS, Rush S, et al. Fraction size in external beam radiation therapy in the treatment of melanoma. Int J Radiat Oncol Biol Phys. 1991;20:429–32.

Part V
Lung Tumors

Chapter 21
Hypofractionation for Lung Tumors (Primary Malignant, Secondary Malignant)

Shalina Gupta-Burt, Rajeev Badkul, Shahid Awan, Shary Shelton, and Fen Wang

21.1 Introduction

Worldwide, lung cancer is the second highest in incidence and highest cause of cancer death [1]. Surgery has historically been the standard of care for early-stage (T1–T2 N0) NSCLC. SBRT has been established to be superior to conventional external beam radiation therapy (EBRT), achieving local control rates of >80–95% for both early-stage NSCLC and lung metastases. Less extreme hypofractionation (10–25 fractions of 2.5–6.0 Gy/fx) regimens are being evaluated to escalate the BED of radiation for more advanced (stages III–IV) NSCLC. This chapter will cover hypofractionation RT and SBRT for lung lesions.

21.2 Pearls: NSCLC

NSCLC:

- Incidence [1]:
  - 2.2 million new cases each year globally, and 1.8 million deaths US: 237,000 new cases in 2021 and 130,180 deaths

    New US cases of lung cancer (combined small cell and non-small cell lung cancer): 237,000 cases
    Male-to-female ratio ~ 1:1
    Approximately 15–20% present with Stage I (T1–T2N0) disease, 30–40% with Stage II–III disease, 40–50% with stage IV disease, with a 5-year

S. Gupta-Burt (✉) · R. Badkul · S. Awan · S. Shelton · F. Wang
Department of Radiation Oncology, University of Kansas Hospital, Kansas City, KS, USA
e-mail: sguptaburt@kumc.edu; RBADKUL@kumc.edu; sawan@kumc.edu; sshelton@kumc.edu; FWANG1@kumc.edu

O. Kaidar-Person, R. Chen (eds.), *Hypofractionated and Stereotactic Radiation Therapy*, https://doi.org/10.1007/978-3-031-47701-0_21

survival of approximately 60% for Stage I disease, 33% for Stage II–III, and 6% for IV disease

- Potential causes or risk factors
  - Smoking associated with a 10–20-fold increased risk
  - Radon, secondhand smoke, prior radiation, asbestos, inhaled chemicals (polycyclic aromatic hydrocarbons), heavy metals, and pulmonary fibrosis.
- Genetic risk factors
  - Twofold increase in incidence of lung cancer in first degree relatives.
  - Identified hereditary conditions (<1% of all NSCLCs)
    - α1-Antitrypsin deficiency
    - Li-Fraumeni syndrome
    - Hereditary lung cancer syndrome (EGFR T790 M, HER2 G660D) [2, 3].
  - Acquired mutations are more common: need to define targetable mutations as they may impact systemic treatment options
    - Frequently mutated/rearranged genes: ALK, PIK3C, EGFR, FGF, MEK1, MET, KRAS, NRAS, RET, PTEN, BRAF, DDR2, and ROS1 [4].
- Symptoms at Presentation:
  - Primary tumor: cough, dyspnea, shortness of breath, chest pain, weight loss, hoarseness, pneumonia, hemoptysis, hypercalcemia
  - NSCLC with regional and/or distant metastasis: vocal cord paralysis, headaches, seizure, pathologic fracture, SVC syndrome, dysphagia/odynophagia, paraneoplastic syndrome
- Pathology subtypes
  - Adenocarcinoma
    - Approximately 50–60% of new NSCLC diagnosis
    - Most likely histology in never/minimal smokers
    - Associated with actionable mutation (EGFR, ALK)
  - Squamous cell carcinoma
    - 60–80% centrally located
    - Strongly associated with smoking
    - Tend to be more aggressive locally
  - Large cell neuroendocrine tumors
    - Clinically less aggressive than SCLC
- Thoracic anatomy
  - Right lung divided into three lobes: RUL, RML, and RLL
    - RUL and RML separated by horizontal fissure
    - RLL separated from RML and RUL by oblique fissure
  - Left lung divided into two lobes: LUL and LLL
    - Separated by oblique fissure
    - Lingula is a projection of LUL
    - Mediastinal structures include the heart, great vessels, esophagus, trachea, and thymus
  - Nerves at risk: clinical presentation
    - Recurrent laryngeal nerve: hoarseness and vocal cord paralysis
    - Diaphragmatic nerve: elevated hemidiaphragm
    - Sympathetic ganglion (apical tumors): Horner's syndrome
    - Vagus nerve: hoarseness and pain are most common

- Regional nodal areas of likely spread: (Fig. 21.1)
  Intralobar/peribronchial/perihilar nodes (N1)
  Mediastinal nodes (N2 ipsilateral, N3 contralateral)
  Supraclavicular nodes (N3)
- Distant regions of potential spread:
  Common sites: brain, liver, bone, adrenal, ipsilateral lung lobes, and contralateral lung
  Rare sites: skin, muscle, kidney, bladder, and GI organs

• Diagnostic and staging work-up:
  - Pulmonary function tests: spirometry and DLCO.
  - Bronchoscopy
  - Mediastinal lymph node evaluation
  - FDG PET/CT scan
  - Brain MRI with contrast for stage II–IV.
  - Laboratory tests: baseline CBC, CMP, serum calcium, LFTs, coagulation studies
• Primary lesion tissue biopsy:
  - With central masses or concern for endobronchial involvement, bronchoscopy preferred
  - With peripheral masses/nodules defined as outer 1/3 of lung, preference is for navigational bronchoscopy, radial EBUS, or transthoracic needle aspiration/biopsy (Interventional Radiology)

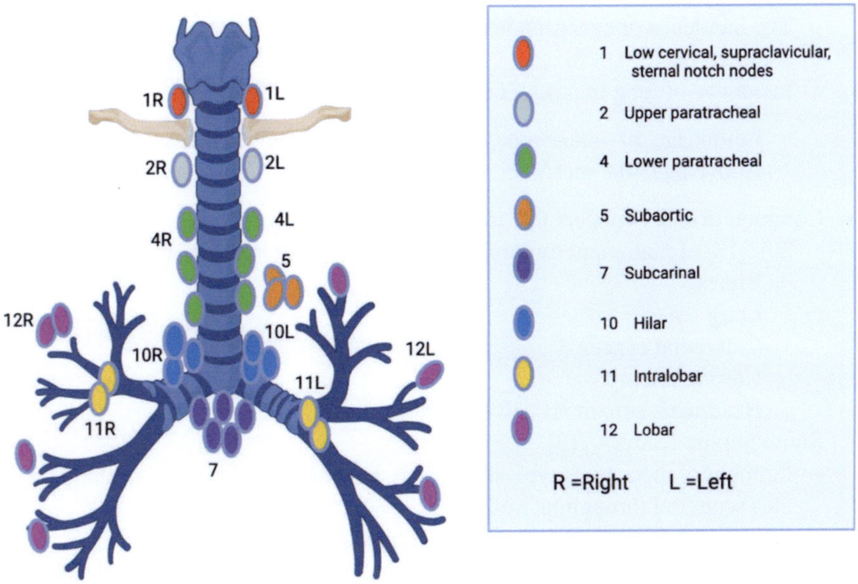

Fig. 21.1 Nodal Stations [7, 8]

- If amendable, obtain adequate amount of tissue for next generation sequencing to assess for acquired mutations
- Consider placement of fiducials at time of biopsy

  Suspected Nodal Disease: (Fig. 21.1)

  - EBUS gives access for station 2R/2L, 4R/4L, 7, 10R/10L and remainder hilar regions as indicated
  - Endobronchial ultrasound-guided transbronchial needle aspiration (EBUS-TBNA) with positive PET/CT mediastinal disease: mediastinoscopy prior to surgery needed.
  - EUS guided biopsy if stations 5, 7, 8, and 9 nodal regions clinically positive
  - Transthoracic needle aspiration-biopsy (TTNA-BX) or Chamberlain procedure is needed if anterior mediastinal station 5 and 6 are suspected
- Pleural Effusion: Thoracentesis with cytology to rule out malignant pleural involvement

  Metastatic sites: Ideally, at least one site should undergo histologic confirmation. However, empiric treatment without histologic confirmation may be considered if biopsy is difficult or carries significant risk [9].

21.3 Pearls: Lung Metastases

Lung Metastases:

- Incidence [10].
  - The incidence of synchronous lung metastasis at initial cancer presentation is about 18 per 100,000.
  - Incidence of lung metastasis increases with age

    Below age 40—incidence is 1 in 100,000
    Above age 40—incidence is 40 in 100,000
- Common primary cancers that metastasize to the lung [11, 12].
  - 20–54% of malignant tumors will have pulmonary metastasis

    Breast
    Lung
    Colorectal cancer
    Uterine leiomyosarcoma
    Head/neck squamous cell carcinomas.
- Radiographic features [13].
  - Pulmonary metastases typically appear as: multiple, peripheral, rounded nodules scattered throughout both lungs
  - Larger nodules and masses may be termed cannonball metastases.
  - Atypical features include consolidation, cavitation, cystic change, calcification, ossification, hemorrhage, and secondary pneumothorax

- Treatment.
  - Two large surgical studies (6000 patients) demonstrated feasibility and potential survival benefit of metastasectomies for patients with lung metastasis. They demonstrated a 5-year actuarial survival rate of approximately 50%. They demonstrated not only underlying histology and DFI (disease free interval) [14] but also number of metastases as predictors of outcome [15].
  - There is a growing body of level I evidence demonstrating the benefits of not only progression free survival but also overall survival by using surgery or an ablative dose of radiotherapy to treat all sites of metastasis for patients with small number of metastases who had reasonable prognosis and were responding to systemic therapy [16, 17].
  - Given such success in ablating local tumor with minimal toxicity of SBRT or hypofractionated SBRT, it is very reasonable to consider treating lung metastasis with SBRT or hypofractionated SBRT.

21.4 Patient Selection

- Clinical practice guidelines references.
  - Executive Summary of ASTRO Evidence-Based Guideline 2017 [18, 19].
  - National Comprehensive Cancer Network (NCCN) Clinical Practice Guidelines for Lung Cancer 2022 [20].
  - Patterns of Care and Outcome Analysis: Safety and Efficacy of SBRT for Stage 1 NSCLC 2013 [21].
  - ESTRO-ACORP Guidelines [22].
  - ESMO Guidelines [23].
- Consensus guidelines do not routinely endorse SBRT/SABR as primary treatment for patients who are surgical candidates despite clinical experience indicating high surgical related morbidity and mortality with standard curative lobectomy. Several cohorts of selected operable patients who underwent SBRT rather than surgery have shown 3-year overall survival rates of 75–85% [24, 25].
- A meta-analysis by Chang et al. [26] showed no significant differences in disease free survival (DFS) or overall survival (OS) comparing surgery to SBRT when adjusted for age and comorbidities.
- For patients deemed medically inoperable or those unwilling to undergo surgery, SBRT is the treatment of choice if feasible. Less aggressive hypofractionated radiation therapy could be used if SBRT is not feasible.
- Reduction of dose per fraction with 7–12 fraction regimens delivering BED >100 Gy have been used with acceptable toxicity as initial local treatment for tumors not amenable to 3–5 fractions SBRT schedules [24, 27, 28].
- Peripheral NSCLC (Table 21.1) or lung metastases:
  - At least 2 cm from the hilum, major bronchus, heart, great vessel, and esophagus

Table 21.1 Prospective trials for SBRT for early-stage NSCLC

Study	Patients (*N*)	Treatments (Gy/fx)	Median follow-up (months)	Outcomes
Ricardi (2010) [29]	*N* = *62* < 5 cm Peripheral tumors only	15 Gy/3	28	3-year LC: 88% 3-year OS: 57% Grade 3 toxicity: 10% Rib fracture: 1.6%
Bauman (2009) [30]	*N* = 57 *T1–T2 N0*	15 Gy/3	35	3-year LC: 92% 3-year OS: 60% Grade 3+ toxicity: 38% No grade 5 toxicity
Fakiris (2009) [31]	*N* = 70 < *7 cm*	20–22 Gy/3	50	3-year LC: 88% 3-year OS: 42% Grade 3+ toxicity: 10% for peripheral tumors and 27% for central tumors
Timmerman (2006) [31]	*N* = 70 < *7 cm*	20–22 Gy/3	18	2-year LC: 95% 2-year OS: 55% Grade 3+ toxicity: 17% for peripheral tumors and 40% for central tumors
Nagata (2015) [32]	*N* = *169 T1 N0* Medically operable and inoperable	12 Gy/4	47–67	3-year LC: 90% 3-year OS: 76% operable and 60% inoperable Grade 3+ toxicity: 10.6% Inoperable and 6.2% Operable (no grade 4–5)
Shibamoto (2012) [33]	*N* = *180* < 5 cm Medically operable and inoperable	11–13 Gy/4	40	3-year LC: 86% if <3 cm; 74% if >3 cm 3-year OS: 74% operable; 59% inoperable Grade 2+ pneumonitis: 13% (44–48 Gy); 21% (52 Gy)
Baba (2010) [34]	*N* = *124* < 5 cm	11–13 Gy/4	26	3-year LC: 91% (IA); 74% (IB) 3-year OS: 79% (IA); 56% (IB) Grade 3 toxicity: 2.5%-8 rib fractures Note, only 1 symptomatic

Table 21.1 (continued)

Study	Patients (*N*)	Treatments (Gy/fx)	Median follow-up (months)	Outcomes
Nagata (2005) [35]	*N = 45 T1–T2 N0*	12 Gy/4	30	5-year LC: 98% 5-year OS: 72–83% No grade 3 toxicity Grade 2 pneumonitis (requiring steroids): 4%
Sun (2017) [36]	*N = 60*	50 Gy/5	58	5-year LC: 94.8% 5-year RR: 10.3% Grade 2 pneumonitis 24% Grade 3 AE 8%
Chang (2015) [37]	*N = 58*	54 Gy/3, 50 Gy/4, 60 Gy/5	40	3-year OS 95% 3-year RFS 86% Grade 3 AE: 10% No Grade 4 AE
Grills (2010) [38]	*N = 58*	48 Gy/4, 60 Gy/5	31	2.5-year OS: 72% 2.5-year RR 4% Grade 2/3 pneumonitis: 11% Rib fracture 11% No Grade 4 AE
Lin (2019) [25]	*N = 70*	50 Gy/5,50 Gy/4, 55 Gy/5,60 Gy/8, 60 Gy/6,70 Gy/10	31	3-year OS 79.7% 3-year CSS 82.5% 3-year LRFS 91.7%

Abbreviations: *LC* Local control, *OS* overall survival, *RR* recurrence rate, *RFS* recurrence-free survival, *LRFS* local-recurrence free survival, *AE* adverse event

For NSCLC: either T1–T2 and N0 or N1–N2 and small primary distant (>5–7 cm) from nodal disease

Can consider for localized recurrence/residual disease of SCLC after definitive therapy [3].

- Central and Ultracentral NSCLC (Table 21.2 and 21.3):
  - Within 2 cm of the hilum, major bronchus, heart, great vessels, and esophagus, “no fly zone” (Fig. 21.2) [2, 4, 26].
  - Tumors ≤5 cm
  - Primary treatment for locally advance NSCLC with or without systemic therapy (Table 21.3)

    A significant subset of patients with stage II/III non–small cell lung cancer (NSCLC) cannot receive standard concurrent chemoradiotherapy owing to the risk of toxic effects outweighing potential benefits. The efficacy of conventional radiotherapy is reduced without concurrent chemotherapy.

    Hypofractionated radiotherapy (shorter course) provided at least similar treatment outcome as conventional radiotherapy (longer course) without increased treatment related toxicity.

Table 21.2 Central and ultracentral tumors treated with hypofractionated SBRT

Study	Patients (*N*)	Tumor location	Dose fractionation (Gy/fx)	BED_{10} (Gy)	Efficacy	Toxicity
Tekatli (2016) [27] Retrospective	*N = 47* Primary/Recurrent NSCLC	Ultra-central (PTV overlapped the trachea or main bronchi)	5 Gy/12	90	• Follow-up 29.3 months • LC 100% • OS 15.3 months • 3-year OS 20%	• ≥ G3 38% • 21% possible/likely treatment related death • Fatal pulmonary Hemorrhage 15%
Lischalk (2016) [39] Retrospective	*N = 20* Metastatic	Ultra-central (Abutment and/or invasion of the mainstem bronchus)	7–8 Gy/5	59.5–72	• Follow-up 19 months • 1-year LC 70% • 1-year OS 75%	• ≥ G3 10% • No reported treatment related death
Chaudhuri (2015) [40] Retrospective	*N = 68* Primary NSCLC/ Metastatic	Central (*N* = 34) Ultra-central (*N* = 7) (GTV directly abutting the central airway)	12.5 Gy/4 10 Gy/5	112.5 100	• Follow-up 18.4 months • 2-year LC 100% (UC), 90% (central) • 2-year OS 80% (UC), 63.2% (central)	• No G2 or higher toxicity for UC tumors
Taremi (2012) [41] Retrospective	*N = 20* Primary NSCLC	Central (*N* = 20)	5 Gy/10 7.5 Gy/8	75 105	• Follow-up 19.1 months • 16/20 central tumors controlled	• No grade 4/5 toxicity

Abbreviations: *NSCLC* non-small cell lung cancer, *Gy* gray, *PTV* planning target volume, *GTV* gross tumor volume, *LC* local control, *OS* overall survival, *UC* ultracentral

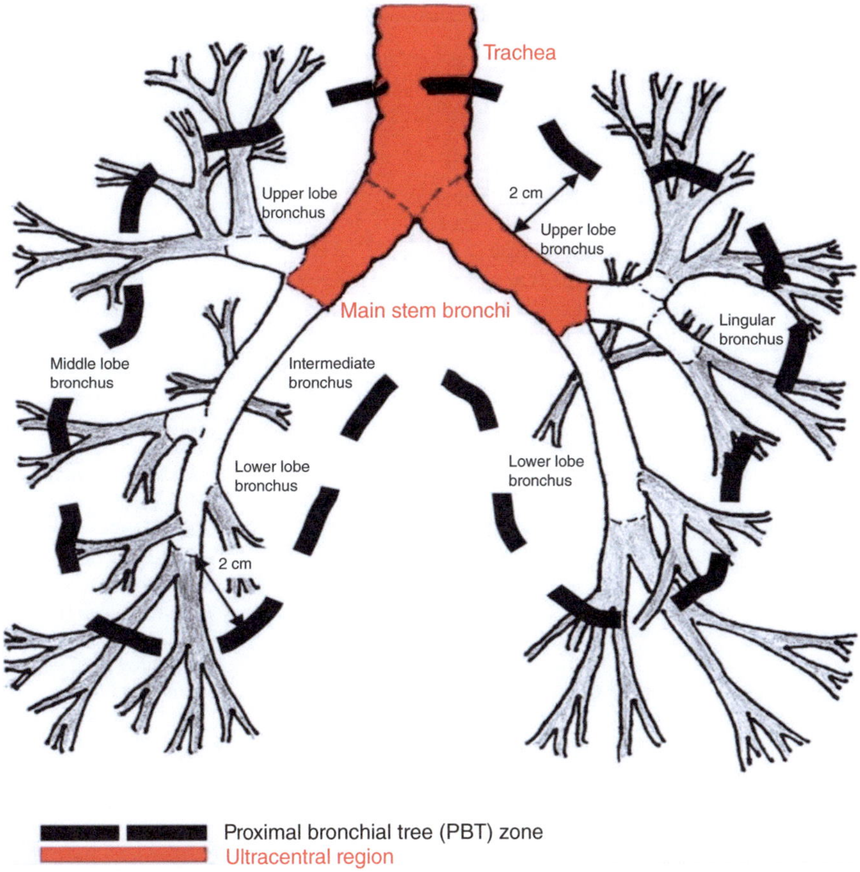

Fig. 21.2 "No Fly Zone"

Table 21.3 Studies using hypofractionated radiation for lung cancer

Study	Patients	Treatments	Median follow-up (months)	Outcomes
Prospective				
Walraven (2016) [42]	*N* = 102. *Stage II–III NSCLC*	2.75 Gy × 24 fx + concurrent cisplatin ± weekly cetuximab	60	5-year OS: 37%
Maguire (2014) [43]	*N* = 130. *Inoperable stage III NSCLC*	2.75 Gy × 20 fx with concurrent or sequential cisplatin + vinorelbine	35	2-year OS: 50% Grade 3+ esophagitis: 8% Grade 5 toxicity: 5%
Cheung (2014) [44]	*N* = 80 *T1–T3 N0*	3 Gy × 20 fx	49	2-year LC: 88% 2-year OS: 68% Grade 3 dyspnea: 14% Grade 3 pneumonitis: 10%
Cannon (2013) [45]	*N* = 79 *Stage III NSCLC*	Dose escalation 2.2–3.4 Gy × 25 fx	17	No grade 3+ esophagitis or pneumonitis 6 patients died from damage to central structures, all treated with >2.5 Gy/fx
Liu (2013) [46]	*N* = 26 *IIIa or IIIb NSCLC*	3 Gy × 20–25 fx with concurrent vinorelbine and carboplatin	11.5	Absolute response rate: 80% mPFS 11.5 months Any esophagitis: 88% Grade 3 esophagitis: 15% Grade 3 pneumonitis: 7%
Osti (2013) [46]	*N* = 30 *IIIa–VI NSCLC*	3 Gy × 20 fx	13	2-year PFS: 36% 2-year OS: 38% Grade 3 esophagitis: 7% Grade 3 pneumonitis: 3.5%
Cho (2009) [47]	*N* = 49 *Unresectable stage III NSCLC*	2.4 Gy × 25 fx	37	3-year LC: 54% 3-year OS: 44% Grade 2+ esophagitis: 60% 2 grade 5 toxicities (hemoptysis)
Belderbos (2007) [48]	*N* = 158 *Stage III NSCLC*	Induction gem + Cis followed by 2.75 Gy × 24 fx vs. 2.75 Gy × 24 fx with concurrent cis	39	mOS 16 months (both arms) Grade 3 esophagitis: 14% (C) 5% (S) Grade 3 pneumonitis: 18% (C) 14% (S)

Table 21.3 (continued)

Study	Patients	Treatments	Median follow-up (months)	Outcomes
Katsuta (2021) [49]	*N = 36. Stage IIIA and/or Stage IIIB NSCLC*	2.5 Gy × 27 fx. Concurrent chemotherapy with platinum-based therapy	60	5-year OS: 54% 5-year PFS: 36% No grade 4 or 5 toxicites Grade 3 toxicities: 14% Grade 3 pneumonitis: 8.3%
Zhang (2022) [50]	*N = 25 Unresectable stage III NSCLC*	Dose escalation—PTV-G (Levels 1–4): (1) 5 pts—60 Gy/30 fx (2 Gy/fx) (2) 5 pts—60 Gy/24 fx (2.5 Gy/fx) (3) 5 pts—60.5 Gy/22 fx (2.75 Gy/fx) (4) 10 pts—60 Gy/20 fx (3 Gy/fx)	77.1	Response rate: 92% Complete response rate: 4% Partial response rate: 88% Grade I/II Radiation pneumonities: 14 patients Grade IV/V Radiation pneumonitis: 1 patient
Parisi (2019) [51]	*N = 17. Locally advanced NSCLC*	Induction cisplatin and docetaxel. Followed with 60 Gy	87	Response rate: 42% 2-year OS: 39% Grade 5 pulmonary hemorrhage: 1 patient No grade 4 toxicities grade 3 toxicities: 4 patients Grade 1 and 2 toxicities: 12 patients
Retrospective				
Jiang (2016) [52]	*N* = 65 *Stage I NSCLC*	4–6 Gy × 12–15 fx	24	3-year LC: 90% 3-year OS: 88% Symptomatic pneumonitis: 17%
Agolli (2015) [53]	*N* = 60 IIIa–IV NSCLC	3 Gy × 20 fx	30	mPFS: 12 months mOS: 13 Grade 3 esophagitis: 6% Grade 3 pneumonitis: 5% No grade 4–5 toxicities
Chang (2012) [54]	*N* = 33 *Lung metastases or NSCLC*	4.5–7.0 Gy × 8–16 fx (50 Gy median total dose)	26	mOS: 32 months (NSCLC) mOS: >40 months (metastases) Grade 3+ pneumonitis: 6%

(continued)

Table 21.3 (continued)

Study	Patients	Treatments	Median follow-up (months)	Outcomes
Massaro (2022) [55]	*N = 210. Stage IIA-IVA NSCLC*	50–60 Gy/20 fx 2.5–3 Gy fx	24	2-year LC: 55.3%. 2-year OS: 36% Grade 4+ Pneumonitis: 3 patients
Kong (2020) [56]	*N* = 42 Unresectable stage III NSCLC	Induction platinum based doublet chemotherapy followed by radiation. 60 Gy/15 fx. (4 Gy/fx)	46	3-year OS: 64% 3-year PFS: 25% Grade 3+ toxicities: 14% Grade 3 toxicites: 9.5% Grade 5 Toxicities: 4.8%

Abbreviations: *NSCLC* non-small cell lung cancer, *Gy* gray, *OS* overall survival, *fx* fraction(s), *LC* local control, *mPFS* median progression-free survival, *PFS* progression-free survival, *mOS* median overall survival

For selected patients, hypofactionated radiotherapy with concurrent chemotherapy or immunotherapy has been studied, which demonstrated feasibility and safety of this combination regiment.

- Re-irradiation (Table 21.4 and 21.5)

  Solitary lesion <3–5 cm.

  Strongest predictors of treatment failure are tumor size >2 cm and time to recurrence <18 months (Table 21.4) [65, 66].

  Re-irradiation with SBRT for centrally located failures appears feasible with fraction sizes <10–12 Gy [61] (Table 21.5).

- Oligo-metastases/progression (Table 21.6).

  Advanced systemic therapies such as mutation driven targeted therapy and immunotherapy have resulted in significant improvement of overall survival [76] and have increased the clinical relevance of oligo-metastasis or oligo-progression [22, 77, 78].

  Defined as a limited number of metastases or sites of progression (usually 1–5) noted in only a few organs (usually 1–3) with a clinically indolent behavior [5]. Does not include serosal metastasis.

  Use of local therapy, such as SBRT, allows continuation of current systemic treatment or bridge it to new therapeutic agents.

- Baseline patient characteristics:

  Comorbidities and concomitant lung disease very common.

  Baseline PFTs

  - Continuous supplemental O_2 is not an absolute contraindication to treatment
  - Minimal PFT parameters not defined for SBRT.

Must be able to tolerate some deterioration in lung function, evaluate baseline performance status

If ECOG performance status 2 or greater *due to* baseline lung dysfunction, treatment related lung toxicity may be unacceptable

Consider deferring biopsy and/or fiducial placement if complications of pneumothorax are unlikely to be tolerated and clinical suspicion of malignancy is sufficiently high to proceed without tissue.

Patient-specific factors (e.g., medical comorbidities, systemic connective tissue disorder, pulmonary fibrosis, immunosuppression, prior radiation, etc.) can increase risk of unacceptable toxicity

Table 21.4 Clinical outcomes of lung re-irradiation using SBRT

Study	Patients (*N*)	Tumor location	Prior RT	Dose fractionation (Gy/fx)	BED_{10} (Gy)	Efficacy	Toxicity
Peulen (2011) [57] Retrospective	*N = 29*	Peripheral (*N* = 21) Central (*N* = 11)	BED_{10} = 109 Gy (median)	8–15 Gy/3–5	69.3–112.5	• Follow-up 12 months • 5 mo LC, 52% • 1-year OS 59%	• 3 of 11 patients with central tumors died of hemoptysis
Kelly (2010) [58] Retrospective	*N = 36*	Peripheral and central	36 61.6 Gy (median)	12.5 Gy/4 (median)	112.5 (median)	• Follow-up 15 months • LC 92% • 2-year OS 59%	• 28% G3 pneumonitis • 8% G3 esophagitis • No grade 4/5 toxicity
Oshiro (2010) [59] Retrospective	*N = 21*	Central	*N* = 14 Dose = NA	3–26 Gy/1–13 (10 Gy/5 & 6 Gy/10 most common)	100 (median) (50.7–157.5)	• Follow-up 20 months • 1-year LC 74% • 1-year OS 90%	• 3 patients with ≥ G3 late toxicity (2 had previous RT) • 1 patient died of hemoptysis (intrabronchial brachy therapy and two SBRT
Trovo (2014) [60] Retrospective	*N = 17*	Central	50–60 Gy/ 20–30	6 Gy/5	48	• Follow-up 18 months • 1-year LC 86% • 1-year OS 59%	• 23% G3 pneumonitis • 12% G5 (one fatal pneumonitis and one fatal hemoptysis)
Killburn (2014) [61] Retrospective	*N = 33*	Peripheral (*N* = 16) Central (*N* = 17)	SBRT 50 Gy/5 EBRT 66 Gy/33	10 Gy/5 (median) (Range, 22.5 Gy/1–18 Gy/3)	100 (median)	• Follow-up 17 months • 2-year LC 67% • 2-year OS 45%	• 3% G3–4 (pneumonitis) • 3% G5 (aortaesophageal fistula)

Parks (2016) [62] Retrospective	*N* = 27	Peripheral Ultra-central (*N* = 18) (media-stinum)	64.8 Gy	10 Gy/5 (median) (Range, 6 Gy/ to 18 Gy/3)	100 (median)	• Follow-up 22 months • 2-year LC 72% • 2-year OS 79%	• 30% G3–4 (6 pneumonitis and 2 chest wall) • 0% G5
Repka (2017) [63] Retrospective	*N* = 20	Ultra-central (Abutting the trachea, mainstem bronchus, or esophagus and included both parenchy-mal and nodal recurrences)	63 Gy	5–8 Gy/ 5	37.5–72	• Follow-up 23.3 months • 1-year LC 67% (dose ≥40 Gy) • 1-year OS 78 (dose ≥40 Gy)	• 5% G3–4 (recurrent laryngeal paralysis) • 5% G5 (hemo-ptysis)
Sood (2020) [64] Retrospective	*N* = 20 Re-current NSCLC/ Meta-static	Ultra-central (PTV in the mediastinum and hilum with directly abutting main airways, great vessels, or esophagus)	EBRT 66 Gy SBRT 50 Gy	6.5 Gy/10 (median) (range 4–7 Gy/10)	56–119 (107.5 median)	• Follow-up 17.8 months • 1-year LC 83% • 1-year OS 68%	• ≥ G3 lung 5%; 1 x grade 3 GI (tumor abutment) • 2 patients with fatal hemo-ptysis (1 tumor pro-gression on bronch & 1 with pro-gression on imaging), "unlikely" related to treatment • No G4–5

Abbreviations: *RT* radiotherapy, BED_{10} biological effective dose with the alpha/beta ratio of, *Gy* gray, *fx* fraction(s), *LC* local control, *OS* overall survival, *SBRT* stereotactic body radiotherapy, *EBRT* external beam radiation therapy, *PTV* planning target volume, *NSCLC* non-small cell lung cancer

Table 21.5 Dose constraints of OARs for retreatment of recurrence

Re-irradiation						
OAR	Reference	*N*	Time interval (months)	Doses constraint (cumulative EQD2, except lung)	G3–4 toxicity	G5 toxicity
Lung	Liu [46]	72	>12	Total lung volume = 30–35% if 20 Gy to lung	14	1
Heart	Sumita [67]	21	>24	70 Gy (Dmax)	0	0
Great vessels	Evans [67]	35	>12	Aorta pulmonary artery <110 Gy (Dmax)	0	2
Esophagus	Binkley [68]	38	>12	100 Gy (Dmax)	0	0
PBT	Feddock [68]	17	>12	<105 Gy (Dmax)	0	0
Brachial plexus	Chen [69]	43	>24	95 Gy (Dmax) >24 m 80 Gy (Dmax) <24 m	NR	NR
Spinal cord	Nieder [69]	38	>6	67.5 Gy (Dmax)-non-SBRT	1	0
	Sahgal [70]	14	>5	75 Gy (Dmax)-SBRT	5	0

Table 21.6 SBRT and oligo-metastatic NSCLC

Study	Patients (*N*)	Control treatment	Intervention treatment	RT dose (Gy/fx)	Report outcomes
Gomez (2019) [16] RCT phase II	*N = 74* NSCLC with 3 or few sites of metastasis	Maintenance chemotherapy or observation	RT or Surgery + maintenance chemotherapy	SBRT dose or 45 Gy/15 To all sites	PFS 14.2 m vs. 4.4 m OS 41.2 m vs. 17 m
Iyengar (2018) [71] RTC phase II	*N = 29* NSCLC with up to 5 sites of metastasis	Maintenance chemotherapy	SBRT + maintenance chemotherapy	21–27 Gy/1 26.5–33 Gy/3 30–37.5/5 45 Gy/15 To all sites	PFS[a] 9.7 m vs. 3.5 m
Wang (2022) [72] RCT Phase III	*N = 133*	First-line TKI	SBRT + TKI	5–8 Gy × 5 to all sites	PFS 20.2 m vs. 12.5 m OS 25.5 m vs. 17.4 m
Xu (2018) [73] Retrospective	*N = 145*	First-line TKI	RT or surgery + TKI	21–27 Gy/1 26.5–33 Gy/3 30–37/5 Gy/5 45 Gy/15 60 Gy/30 to all sites	PFS 20.6 m vs. 13.9 m OS 40.5 m vs. 31.5 m
Theelen (2021) [74] RTC phase II	*N = 92*	Pembrolizumab	SBRT + Pembrolizumab	8 Gy × 3 to all sites	PFS 6.6 m vs. 1.9 m OS[b] 15.9 m vs 7.6 m

Table 21.6 (continued)

Study	Patients (*N*)	Control treatment	Intervention treatment	RT dose (Gy/fx)	Report outcomes
Welsh (2020) [75] RCT Phase I/II	*N = 100*	Pembrolizumab	SBRT or TFRT + Pembrolizumab	12 Gy × 4 Or 3 Gy × 15 To all sites	Out-of-field ORR SBRT 38% vs. TFRT 10% PFS RT 9.1 m vs. no RT 5.1 m PFS RT 20.8 m vs. no RT 4.6 m (low PD-L1 patients, $p = 0.004$)

Abbreviations: *TFRT* traditional fractionated radiotherapy Gy × 15 fx, *RT* radiotherapy, *SBRT* stereotactic body radiotherapy, *RCT* randomized control trial, *PFS* progression free survival, *OS* overall survival, *ORR* overall response rate

[a]The trial was stopped to accrual early after an interim analysis found a significant improvement in PFS in the SBRT + maintenance chemotherapy arm

[b]Largest benefit from the addition of radiotherapy in patients with PD-L1-negative tumors

21.5 Treatment Planning Considerations

Simulation instructions	**SBRT/hypofractionation** • Patient supine, arms over head, and scanned headfirst • Respiratory motion management recommended • Abdominal compression recommended (unless other respiratory gaiting or motion management systems utilized) • 4D scan 0–90% phases with retrospective binning using appropriate respiratory monitoring, system (e.g., RGSC, RPM) • Scan with 2 mm CT slice thickness with a minimum of 3 cm superior and inferior to the thoracic cavity with helical mode. Entire lung volume must be scanned to determine if OAR dose constraints are satisfied. 4D CT used to incorporate tumor motion, create average intensity projection (AIP), and maximum intensity projection (MIP) CT series. MIP is generated from 4D CT data series, whose voxel values have the highest voxel intensity throughout the 4D CT dataset. Whereas AIP data series is a 3D CT data series whose voxel values are the arithmetic mean of the 4D CT scans. • Gated treatment if available for large motions and bigger tumors, preferably gated during the exhale part of the breathing cycle (e.g., 30–60%). Gated treatment allows smaller PTV margins. • If deep inspiration breath-hold (DIBH) technique is utilized, CT in breath-hold mode should be acquired; no 4D CT acquisition is required. DIBH RPM signal should be recorded for reference purpose during treatment. • IV contrast may be used especially for central or ultra-central tumors for better delineation between tumor, atelectasis, and vascular structures as well as better definition of normal tissue contours. Oral contrast can be used at the discretion of the treating physician.

Image guidance	**SBRT conventional linac:** • Daily CBCT for patient setup and register with AIP/free breathing CT by physician • Use image fusion for whole body to match the bony anatomy first then confine the fusion range around the tumor and refuse for final shifts. Can be manually fine-tunned for ITV to encompass all visible tumor on CBCT under lung window. • If shifts are more than 1 cm, repeat second CBCT to fine tune the small shifts • 4D CBCT if available **SBRT gated/ DIBH treatment:** • Use the reference respiratory signal from CT sim to match the patient's breathing signals. • Select the planned gated window to get the CBCT in the gated phases; only match with the gated AIP scan (same as above). • Turn on the beam with auto gating mode so it turns on only during the phases selected for gating. • For DIBH treatments, use breath-hold RPM signal from CT sim as reference, match with patient DIBH signal on the machine and use auto gated mode to treat the patient. • Perform CBCT during breath-hold and match with planning DIBH CT as above to perform the shifts. **SBRT CyberKnife:** • **Fiducial-based tracking** [5] – Wait at least 7 days between fiducial placement and sim – More than 3 markers are recommended to implant to improve translation and rotation tracking accuracy (e.g., 0.2 mm with three gold fiducial markers vs. 0.1 mm with five gold markers). – Use Accuracy software to build a synchrony model correlating target motion with external respiratory markers. – Realtime kV planar imaging confirms tracking alignment and updates synchrony model • **Spine tracking** – This method is offered to patients with distant tumors >50 mm from the middle of the posterior wall of the vertebra. – Used for patients who are not candidates for fiducial placement • **Tumor tracking** – Used for solid nodules that are "floating" in the lung and easily distinguished from the lung – The Xsight Lung technique is an option to avoid fiducial implantation when the tumor is in peripheral lung location, exceeds 15 mm, and the imaging control during treatment does not overlap with the vertebrae. – In this technique, algorithm searches the shadow of the tumor projected on each image. Tracking is like Synchrony but replaces the tracking of the tumor shadow instead of fiducial markers

Margins	CTV, PTV, ITV—Recommendations dependent on type of image guidance or motion management systems utilized **SBRT conventional linac:** • ITV: Delineated based upon tumor motion assessed during 4DCT – Combination of GTV on 0% and 90% scans or on Maximum Intensity projection (MIP) • CTV: Not typically recommended • PTV: At least a uniform 5 mm expansion of the ITV – Larger expansion (frequently 8 mm) in direction of greatest motion – Example: For a tumor with 1 cm superior-inferior displacement, consider 5 mm radial expansion with 8 mm superiorly and inferiorly **SBRT CyberKnife fiducial:** • No ITV or CTV • PTV: 5 mm expansion of GTV with 8 mm in direction of maximal displacement (see above example) **SBRT CyberKnife spine tracking:** • ITV: Union of the inspiration, expiration, and simulation GTV • PTV: 5 mm uniform expansion of the ITV with 8 mm expansion in direction of maximal displacement **Hypofractionated conventional linac:** • ITV: Delineated based upon tumor motion assessed during 4DCT – Combination of GTV on 0 and 50% scans (or MIP and FB) • CTV: 5–8 mm uniform expansion around ITV – CTV is not expanded into the bone or esophagus – Elective nodal regions are generally not included in CTV • PTV: Generally, a 3–5 mm uniform expansion around CTV • PTV is expanded into OAR including the esophagus and bone
Dosimetric consideration (RTOG 0813) [6]	• Prescription Isodose Surface Coverage: (Table 21.7) – The prescription isodose surface covers 95% of PTV. – Minimum dose to PTV is greater than 90% of the prescribed dose. • Target dose heterogeneity: – The prescription isodose surface selected should be 60-80% of the dose at the center of PTV so hot spots inside the GTV/ITV are preferably greater than 120% (dose peaking). • High Dose Spillage: – Any dose >105% of the prescription dose should be within the PTV. – The total volume of normal tissue outside the PTV receiving a dose of >105% should be less than 15% of the PTV volume. • Low dose spillage: – The falloff gradient beyond the PTV must be rapid in all directions. D2cm and R50% should be clearly defined. – The plan quality should be assessed using Table 21.8 from RTOG 0813.

Table 21.7 PTV Dose coverage metrics: (RTOG 0813)

Metric	Guideline value
PTV—D95% (i.e., Dose covering 95% of PTV)	≥100% of Rx dose
PTV—D99% (i.e., Dose covering 99% of PTV)	≥90% Rx dose
Dose heterogeneity within PTV	Typical normalization 60–80% with hotspot within GTV. For inverse planning techniques, effort should be made to design the cost function to try to mimic a 3DCRT dose distribution with a hotspot within the core of the ITV
Conformality Index (CI) defined as prescription isodose volume/PTV volume	<1.2 Desired. Exceptions can be made for small PTVs requiring a block margin to satisfy field size criteria. Effort should be made to minimize dose > 105% of the prescription dose outside of the PTV
Gradient Index (GI)/R50% (50% prescription isodose volume/PTV volume)	Effort should be made to have the 50% isodose surface be as small as possible

Table 21.8 Conformality of prescribed dose for calculations based on deposition of photon beam energy in heterogeneous tissue (RTOG 0813)

PTV volume (cc)	Ratio of prescription isodose volume to the PTV volume		Ratio of 50% prescription isodose volume to the PTV volume, $R_{50\%}$		Maximum dose (in % of dose prescribed) @ 2 cm from PYTV in any direction, $D_{2\,cm}$ (Gy)		Percent of lung receiving 20 Gy total or more, V_{20} (%)	
	Deviation		Deviation		Deviation		Deviation	
	None	Minor	None	Minor	None	Minor	None	Minor
1.8	<1.2	<1.5	<5.9	<7.5	<50.0	<57.0	<10	<15
3.8	<1.2	<1.5	<5.5	<6.5	<50.0	<57.0	<10	<15
7.4	<1.2	<1.5	<5.1	<6.0	<50.0	<58.0	<10	<15
13.2	<1.2	<1.5	<4.7	<5.8	<50.0	<58.0	<10	<15
22.0	<1.2	<1.5	<4.5	<5.5	<54.0	<63.0	<10	<15
34	<1.2	<1.5	<4.3	<5.3	<58.0	<68.0	<10	<15
50	<1.2	<1.5	<4.0	<5.0	<62.0	<77.0	<10	<15
70	<1.2	<1.5	<3.5	<4.8	<66.0	<86.0	<10	<15
95	<1.2	<1.5	<3.3	<4.4	<70.0	<89.0	<10	<15
126	<1.2	<1.5	<3.1	<4.0	<73.0	>91.0	<10	<15
163	<1.2	<1.5	<2.9	<3.7	<77.0	>94.0	<10	<15

Note 1: For values of PTV dimension or volume not specified, linear interpolation between table entries is required

Note 2: Protocol deviations greater than listed here as "minor" will be classified as "major" for protocol compliance

Contouring/Planning Considerations

1. 4D conventional linac SBRT (Fig. 21.3)
   GTV/ITV/PTV Contouring:

   (a) Utilize windowing tools **(A–C)**

   - Extent of parenchymal lesion best visualized on lung windowing **(A).**
   - Soft-tissue windowing allows for improved visualization of adjacent structures such as chest wall **(B)** but can underestimate the extent of parenchymal disease **(C).**

   (b) Delineate on different phases of breathing **(A, D, E)**

   - Contour GTV on free breathing and MIP (or 0 and 50%, etc.) **(A, D).**
   - Combine GTVs to form ITV **(E–F).**
   - Evaluate tumor motion and generate PTV **(E–F).**
     - PTVs do expand into critical structures including chest wall **(E)**
     - Non-isotropic expansion of 5 mm anterior/posterior, medial/lateral, and 8 mm superior/inferior commonly utilized as lung tumors generally show more superior/inferior displacement with breathing **(F).**

   (c) Always review 4D tumor movement. Consider changing PTV expansions based on principle direction and extent of tumor displacement with breathing.
   Contouring Normal Structures:
   (a) All normal structures should be contoured on Average Intensity Projection (AIP) CT/Free breathing CT set (free breathing CT is done with slow gantry rotation/less number of slices per revolution to capture all the breathing cycle in the scan).
   (b) For Gated treatment normal structures should be contoured on AIP which was created using gated phases.
   (c) Dose calculations should be done on AIP/Free breathing, AIP/gated, and breath-hold CT for ITV, gated and DIBH treatments respectively.
   (d) Evaluate plan in multiple planes **(G–H).**

   - Make sure lower (10–20%) isodose lines are visible.
   - Evaluate for hot spots or dose streaking.
   - Review DVHs for critical structures.
   - Consider changing isodose prescription line based on proximity to organs/structures at risk.

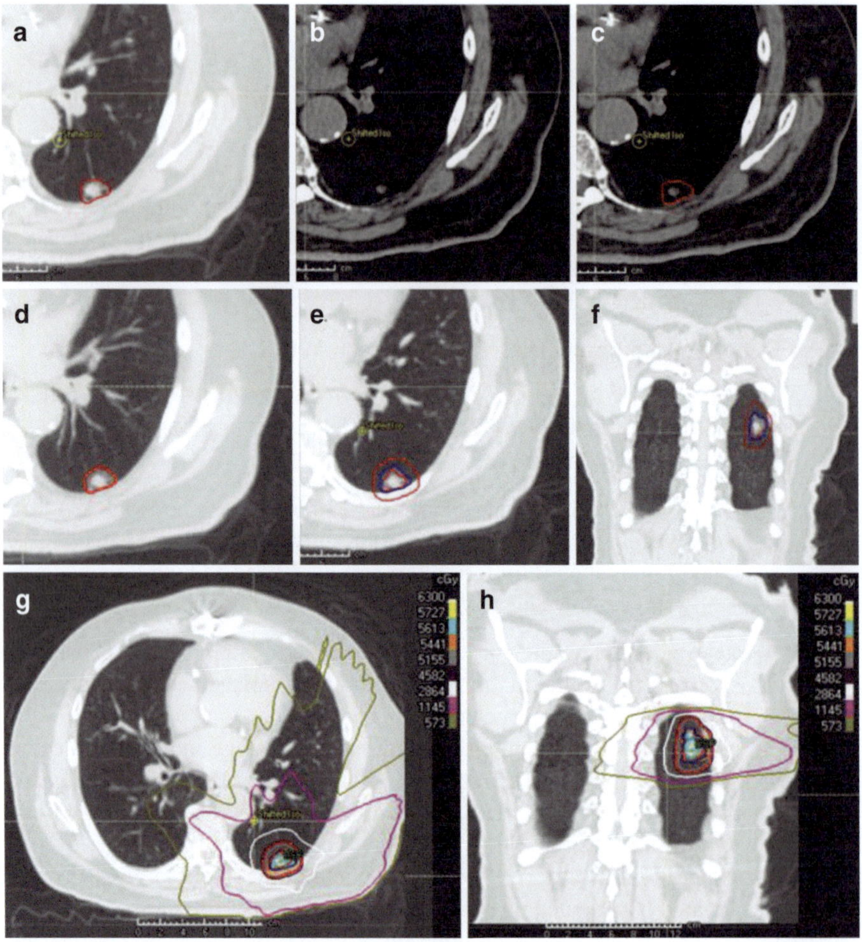

Fig. 21.3 Contouring and planning considerations for conventional linac-based lung SBRT

2. Non-fiducial based CyberKnife SBRT (Fig. 21.4).

   (a) Obtain 4D CT and delineate GTV on multiple phases (0%, 50%, free breathing, breath-hold) **(A–C):**

   - Use lung windows to delineate parenchymal disease.
   - Evaluated for bony or soft-tissue involvement on appropriate window levels.
   - PTV expansion of ITV should be based on extent and direction of tumor motion—8 mm superior/inferior with 5 mm in all other directions is common but may not be appropriate for tumor with substantial axial displacement.

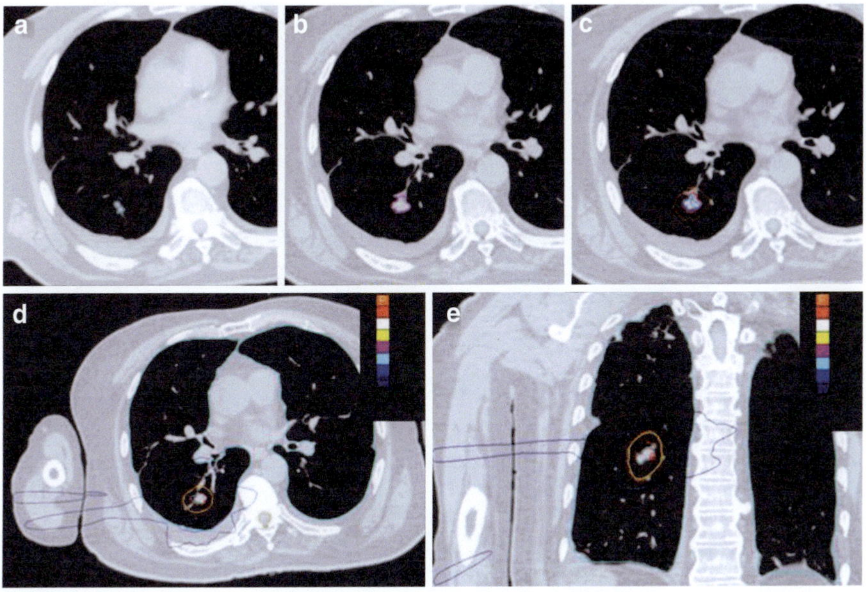

Fig. 21.4 Contouring and planning considerations for non-fiducial-based lung SBRT with CyberKnife radiosurgery

   (b) Evaluate plan in multiple planes **(D–E):**
      - Check for hot spots, dose distribution, and dose streaking.

3. Fiducial-based CyberKnife SBRT (Fig. 21.5).
4. Requires 4D scan to evaluate tracking but only requires delineating in one phase:
   (a) Yellow arrow highlights fiducial marker in the tumor **(A)**.
   (b) PTV expansion of GTV is based on tumor motion as above **(B)**.
   (c) Plan evaluation in multiple planes **(C–D)**.

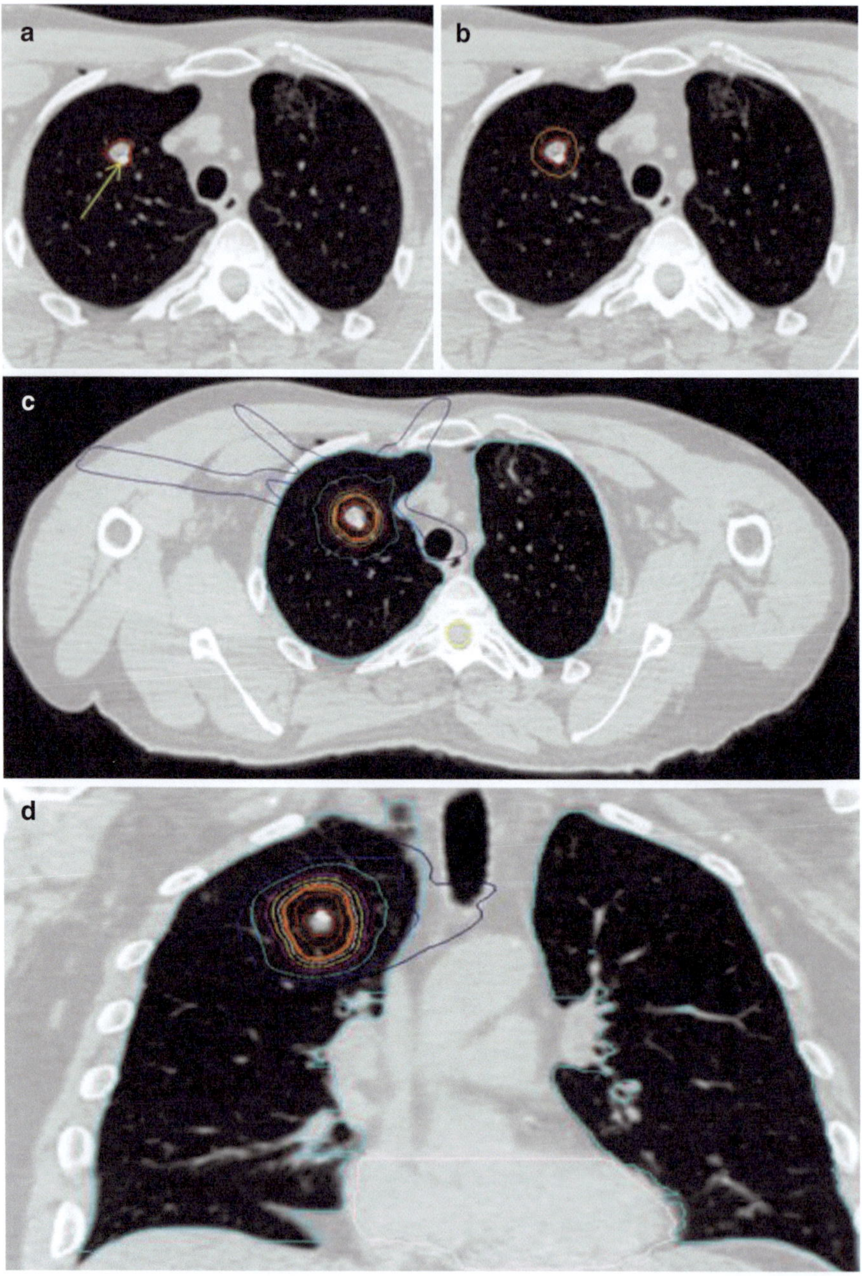

Fig. 21.5 Contouring and planning considerations for fiducial-based lung SBRT with CyberKnife

21.6 Commonly Used Dose/Fractionation Schemes

Dose/fx	# of fx	BED_{10} (Gy)	Total dose	Notes
SBRT/hypofractionated SBRT				
5–7.5 Gy	8–10 QD	5 Gy × 10 = 75 7.5 Gy × 8 = 105 6.5 Gy × 10 = 107.3	50–65 Gy	Re-irradiation, central location, patient-specific factor concerning for excess toxicity [18, 79]
10 Gy	5 QD or QOD	100	50 Gy	Centrally located (within 2 cm of major bronchus), re-irradiation [19, 21]
12–12.5 Gy	4 QD or QOD	105.6–112.5	48–50 Gy	Peripherally located (within 2 cm of chest wall or plexus) [22, 23, 26]
15–20 Gy	3 QOD	15 Gy × 3 = 112.5 20 Gy × 3 = 180	45–60 Gy	>2 cm from central structures, chest wall, and plexus [22, 23, 26]
34 Gy	1	149.6	34 Gy	Small (<2–3 cm), >2 cm from central structures, chest wall, and plexus and minimal tumor motion
Hypofractionation				
2.5–3.0 Gy	15–20 QD without concurrent chemotherapy	2.5 Gy × 20 = 62.5 3 Gy × 15 = 45	50–60 Gy	Peripheral (>2 cm from central structures) T1–T3 N0 NSCLC or metastases where SBRT is not available [6]
2.4–3.0 Gy	15–25 QD ± concurrent chemotherapy	2.4 Gy × 25 = 60 3 Gy × 15 = 45	45–60 Gy	Inoperable, stage IIIa–IV NSCLC, limited to tumors where total PTV (no ENI, involved nodes and primary tumor only) is <200–250 cc to achieve V20 < 20–30% [80–82]

21.7 Normal Tissue Tolerances

SBRT: based on NRG trials								
		# of fx						
Serial tissue	Volume CC	1	2	3	5	8	10	Endpoint (grade ≥ 3)
		Gy	Gy	Gy	Gy	Gy	Gy	
Spinal cord and medulla	<0.35 cc/<0.5 cc*	10	13	15.9	22	26.4	31*	Myelitis
	Max Point	14	18.3	22.5	28	33.6	26*	
Esophagus[a]	<5 cc	20	24.3	27.9	32.5	36.8	40	Esophagitis
	Max Point	24	28.3	32.4	38	43.2	48	

SBRT: based on NRG trials								
		# of fx						
Serial tissue	Volume CC	1	2	3	5	8	10	Endpoint (grade ≥ 3)
		Gy	Gy	Gy	Gy	Gy	Gy	
Brachial plexus	<3ccc	13.6	17.8	22	27	32.8	37	Neuropathy
	Max Point	16.4	21.2	26	32.5	39.2	43	
Heart/ pericardium	<15 cc	16	20	24	32	34.4	36.6	Pericarditis
	Max Point	22	26	30	38	40	42.5	
Great vessels	<10 cc	31	35	39	47	55.2	55.7	Aneurysm
	Max Point	37	41	45	53	62	62.9	
Trachea and large bronchus[a]	<4 cc*/<5 cc**	27.5*	34.5*	39**	45**	50**	52**	Impairment of pulmonary toilet
	Max Point	30	38	43	50	56	39	
Bronchus-smaller airways	<0.5 ccc	17.4	21.6	25.8	32	38.4	–	Stenosis with atelectasis
	Max Point	20.2	25.1	30	40	48.8	–	
Rib	<5 cc	28	34	40	45	50	–	Pain or fracture
	Max Point	33	41.5	50	57	63	–	
Skin	<10 cc	25.5	28.3	31	36.5	43.2	46.3	Ulceration
	Max Point	27.5	30.3	33	38.5	45.6	48.9	
Stomach	<5 cc/<50 cc**	17.4	20	22.5	26.5	31.2	33.9**	Ulceration/ fistula
	Max Point	22	26	30	35	42	45	
Bile duct	Max Point	30	33	36	41	48	–	Stenosis
Duodenum[a]	<5 cc	17.4	20	22.5	26.5	31.2	33.9	Ulceration
	Max Point	22	26	30	35	42	45	
Lung (right and left)	1500 cc for males and 950 cc for females	**7.2**	**9.4**	**10.8**	**12.5**	**14.4**	**15**	Basic lung function
	VxGy<37%	**8**	**10**	**11.4**	**13.5**	**15.2**	**16**	
Liver	700 cc	11.6	15.1	17.7	21.5	24.8	27	Basic Liver Function
Renal cortex (right and left)	200 cc	9.5	12.5	14.7	17.5	20	21	Basic renal function

[a]Avoid circumferential irradiation for 1–5 fx

21.8 Patient Management Considerations

1. Premedication/prophylactic medication
   (a) Patient-specific, and many patients require no premedication.
   (b) Medications to consider as needed:
      - Benzodiazepines
        – Lorazepam (Ativan) 0.5–1 mg before treatment
        – Diazepam (Valium) 10–20 mg before treatment

- Oral analgesics
  - Oxycodone 5–10 mg before treatment
  - Hydrocodone/acetaminophen (Percocet 5–10/325mg or Vicoden 5–10/300 mg) before treatment
- Oral steroids
  - Dexamethasone 4–8 mg before treatment.
- Antiemetics
  - Ondansetron (Zofran) 8 mg before treatment
  - Promethazine 25 mg before treatment [70].
  - Should consider prescribing q8–12 h for 24–72 h after treatment if nausea during treatment is problematic
- Cough suppressants.
  - Morphine 5–15 mg oral or 1–4 mg IV before treatment
  - Benzonatate (Tessalon Perles) 100 mg tid or 100–200 mg before treatment

2. Common acute and late toxicities

   (a) General acute toxicities:

   - Fatigue: 50%+ [31, 42, 83].
   - Dyspnea: 10–30% [31, 42, 83].
   - Cough: 10–30% [61, 84, 85].
   - Nausea: 10–20%
   - Chest pain: 5–10% [34, 38, 86].
   - Odynophagia: 5–10% [58, 87].

   (b) Mild-moderate late toxicities

   - Chest wall pain:
     - 5–10% incidence for non-peripheral (>2–3 cm from chest wall) lesions [84, 88]
     - Up to 30–50% incidence if abutting chest wall [84, 88].
     - 50–75% of cases are transient

       Management
       Observation
       Non-narcotic pain medications (e.g., NSAIDs)

       - Ensure patients do not overuse OTC analgesics
       - Have low threshold for narcotics if there is a history of comorbidities (upper GI ulcers, hepatic dysfunction, renal disease, etc.) which increase the risk of non-narcotic pain medications

Narcotic pain medications:

- Oxycodone 5–10 mg q4–6 h prn
- Percocet 5–10/325 mg q4–5 prn
- Vicodin 5–10/300 mg q4–6 prn
- OxyContin 10–20 mg q12 h
- Duragesic (fentanyl) patches 25–75 mcg q72 h

Neuropathic medications:

- Gabapentin 100 mg TID (can be titrated up to 1800 mg TID)
- Lyrica 75 mg BID (can be titrated up to 300 mg BID)

Orthopedic/interventional referral if fracture present

- Rib fracture:
  - Up to 20% incidence if proximal to chest wall [89].
  - Roughly half will be symptomatic [38].
  - Management: same as chest wall pain
- Pneumonitis:
  - Radiographic only: 50–80% incidence
  - Symptomatic: 10–20% incidence [38].

    Management

    - Rule out other causes (e.g., COPD exacerbation)

    Observation
    Oral prednisone, 60 mg daily for 2 weeks followed by slow taper over 2–4 weeks

  - Worsening dyspnea: 10–20% incidence [38].

    Management

    - Rule out pneumonitis and pneumonia
    - Optimize management of concomitant lung diseases
    - Symptomatic therapies
      - Short acting beta-agonists
      - Opioids
      - Steroids
    - Supplemental oxygen
    - Pulmonary rehab

(c) Severe late toxicities: overall incidence <5%, dependent on tumor location [31, 58, 83, 90, 91].

- Bronchial/tracheal stenosis
  - Stenting
  - Surgical management
- Bronchial/tracheal necrosis
  - Surgical management
- Esophageal perforation
  - Emergency surgical management
- Massive hemoptysis
  - Emergency surgery or embolization
- Impaired cardiac function
  - Medical optimization

    ACE inhibitors, angiotensin receptor blockers.
    Beta-blockers
    Loop diuretics
  - Pacemaker or AICD implantation
  - Cardiac rehabilitation
- Pulmonary necrosis.
  - Surgical options:

    Lobectomy
    Pneumonectomy
    Debridement
  - Bronchoscopy for culture
  - Long-term (4–12 weeks) antibiotic therapy, preferably driven by culture detected sensitivity analysis
- Bacterial superinfections
  - Antibiotics, initially broad spectrum followed by culture-directed sensitivity for 10–14 days. Examples include:

    Vancomycin + Zosyn
    Meropenem
    Ceftriaxone + metronidazole
- Esophageal-aortic and tracheal-esophageal fistulas
  - Surgical management

- Cord injury/myelitis
  - Generally irreversible
  - Symptomatic therapies include:

    Neuropathic medications

    - Gabapentin 100 mg TID (can be titrated up to 1800 mg TID)
    - Lyrica 75 mg BID (can be titrated up to 300 mg BID as needed)
  - Physical medicine/rehabilitation.

21.9 Follow-Up

- Clinic evaluation with physical exam every 3–4 months
- CT chest ± contrast
  - Every 3–6 months for 2 years
  - Every 6 months years 3–5
  - Consider annual after year 5
- PET-CT
  - Not indicated for NSCLC unless clinical suspicion for recurrence (e.g., growing mass on CT or symptomatic worsening) or metastatic spread.
  - For lung metastases, regular PET-CT every 3–6 months may be reasonable to assess for new metastatic lesions
- MRI or CT of brain not indicated unless symptomatic
- Blood tests
  - No routine blood work for NSCLC unless clinically indicated.
  - For lung metastases, following tumor-specific biomarkers for the primary cancer (e.g., CEA, CA19-9, CA-125) as indicated.

21.10 Relevant Literature

See Tables 21.1, 21.2, 21.3, 21.4, and 21.6.

References

1. Sung H, et al. Global cancer statistics 2020: GLOBOCAN estimates of incidence and mortality worldwide for 36 cancers in 185 countries. CA Cancer J Clin. 2021;71(3):209–49.
2. de Alencar VTL, Formiga MN, de Lima VCC. Inherited lung cancer: a review. Ecancermedicalscience. 2020;14:1008.

3. Yamamoto H, Yatabe Y, Toyooka S. Inherited lung cancer syndromes targeting never smokers. Transl Lung Cancer Res. 2018;7(4):498–504.
4. Seegobin K, et al. Immunotherapy in non-small cell lung cancer with actionable mutations other than EGFR. Front Oncol. 2021;11:750657.
5. Weickhardt AJ, et al. Local ablative therapy of oligoprogressive disease prolongs disease control by tyrosine kinase inhibitors in oncogene-addicted non-small-cell lung cancer. J Thorac Oncol. 2012;7(12):1807–14.
6. Bradley JD, et al. Standard-dose versus high-dose conformal radiotherapy with concurrent and consolidation carboplatin plus paclitaxel with or without cetuximab for patients with stage IIIA or IIIB non-small-cell lung cancer (RTOG 0617): a randomised, two-by-two factorial phase 3 study. Lancet Oncol. 2015;16(2):187–99.
7. Colella S, et al. Endoscopic ultrasound in the diagnosis and staging of lung cancer. Endosc Ultrasound. 2014;3(4):205–12.
8. Nair A, et al. Multidetector CT and postprocessing in planning and assisting in minimally invasive bronchoscopic airway interventions. Radiographics. 2012;32(5):E201–32.
9. Ma SJ, et al. Comparison of single- and three-fraction schedules of stereotactic body radiation therapy for peripheral early-stage non-small-cell lung cancer. Clin Lung Cancer. 2018;19(2):e235–40.
10. Chen H, et al. The epidemiology of lung metastases. Front Med (Lausanne). 2021;8:723396.
11. Jamil A, Kasi A. Lung metastasis. In: StatPearls. Treasure Island (FL): StatPearls Publishing LLC; 2022.
12. Riihimaki M, et al. Metastatic sites and survival in lung cancer. Lung Cancer. 2014;86(1):78–84.
13. Seo JB, et al. Atypical pulmonary metastases: spectrum of radiologic findings. Radiographics. 2001;21(2):403–17.
14. Casiraghi M, et al. A 10-year single-center experience on 708 lung metastasectomies: the evidence of the "international registry of lung metastases". J Thorac Oncol. 2011;6(8):1373–8.
15. Pastorino U, et al. Long-term results of lung metastasectomy: prognostic analyses based on 5206 cases. J Thorac Cardiovasc Surg. 1997;113(1):37–49.
16. Gomez DR, et al. Local consolidative therapy vs. maintenance therapy or observation for patients with oligometastatic non-small-cell lung cancer: long-term results of a multi-institutional, phase II, randomized study. J Clin Oncol. 2019;37(18):1558–65.
17. Palma DA, et al. Stereotactic ablative radiotherapy for the comprehensive treatment of oligometastatic cancers: long-term results of the SABR-COMET phase II randomized trial. J Clin Oncol. 2020;38(25):2830–8.
18. Cornwell LD, Korb ML, Burt BM. Guidelines for stereotactic body radiation therapy treatment of lung cancer highlight important research questions: what is the next step? J Thorac Dis. 2018;10(3):1339–42.
19. Schneider BJ, et al. Stereotactic body radiotherapy for early-stage non-small-cell lung cancer: American Society of Clinical Oncology endorsement of the American Society for Radiation Oncology evidence-based guideline. J Clin Oncol. 2018;36(7):710–9.
20. Ganti AKP, et al. Small cell lung cancer, version 2.2022, NCCN clinical practice guidelines in oncology. J Natl Compr Cancer Netw. 2021;19(12):1441–64.
21. Guckenberger M, et al. Safety and efficacy of stereotactic body radiotherapy for stage 1 non-small-cell lung cancer in routine clinical practice: a patterns-of-care and outcome analysis. J Thorac Oncol. 2013;8(8):1050–8.
22. Basler L, Kroeze SG, Guckenberger M. SBRT for oligoprogressive oncogene addicted NSCLC. Lung Cancer. 2017;106:50–7.
23. Vansteenkiste J, et al. Early and locally advanced non-small-cell lung cancer (NSCLC): ESMO Clinical Practice Guidelines for diagnosis, treatment and follow-up. Ann Oncol. 2013;24(Suppl. 6):vi89–98.
24. Li Q, et al. Stereotactic ablative radiotherapy (SABR) using 70 Gy in 10 fractions for non-small cell lung cancer: exploration of clinical indications. Radiother Oncol. 2014;112(2):256–61.
25. Lin Q, et al. Outcomes of stereotactic body radiotherapy versus lobectomy for stage I non-small cell lung cancer: a propensity score matching analysis. BMC Pulm Med. 2019;19(1):98.

26. Chang JY, et al. Stereotactic ablative radiotherapy for operable stage I non-small-cell lung cancer (revised STARS): long-term results of a single-arm, prospective trial with prespecified comparison to surgery. Lancet Oncol. 2021;22(10):1448–57.
27. Tekatli H, et al. Outcomes of hypofractionated high-dose radiotherapy in poor-risk patients with "ultracentral" non-small cell lung cancer. J Thorac Oncol. 2016;11(7):1081–9.
28. Yoo YJ, et al. Safety and efficacy of 10-fraction hypofractionated radiation therapy for non-small cell lung cancer. Radiat Oncol J. 2021;39(3):202–9.
29. Ricardi U, et al. Stereotactic body radiation therapy for early stage non-small cell lung cancer: results of a prospective trial. Lung Cancer. 2010;68(1):72–7.
30. Baumann P, et al. Outcome in a prospective phase II trial of medically inoperable stage I non-small-cell lung cancer patients treated with stereotactic body radiotherapy. J Clin Oncol. 2009;27(20):3290–6.
31. Fakiris AJ, et al. Stereotactic body radiation therapy for early-stage non-small-cell lung carcinoma: four-year results of a prospective phase II study. Int J Radiat Oncol Biol Phys. 2009;75(3):677–82.
32. Nagata Y, et al. Prospective trial of stereotactic body radiation therapy for both operable and inoperable T1N0M0 non-small cell lung cancer: Japan Clinical Oncology Group Study JCOG0403. Int J Radiat Oncol Biol Phys. 2015;93(5):989–96.
33. Shibamoto Y, et al. Stereotactic body radiotherapy using a radiobiology-based regimen for stage I nonsmall cell lung cancer: a multicenter study. Cancer. 2012;118(8):2078–84.
34. Baba F, et al. Clinical outcomes of stereotactic body radiotherapy for stage I non-small cell lung cancer using different doses depending on tumor size. Radiat Oncol. 2010;5:81.
35. Nagata Y, et al. Clinical outcomes of a phase I/II study of 48 Gy of stereotactic body radiotherapy in 4 fractions for primary lung cancer using a stereotactic body frame. Int J Radiat Oncol Biol Phys. 2005;63(5):1427–31.
36. Sun B, et al. Long-term outcomes of salvage stereotactic ablative radiotherapy for isolated lung recurrence of non-small cell lung cancer: a phase II clinical trial. J Thorac Oncol. 2017;12(6):983–92.
37. Chang JY, et al. Stereotactic ablative radiotherapy versus lobectomy for operable stage I non-small-cell lung cancer: a pooled analysis of two randomised trials. Lancet Oncol. 2015;16(6):630–7.
38. Grills IS, et al. Outcomes after stereotactic lung radiotherapy or wedge resection for stage I non-small-cell lung cancer. J Clin Oncol. 2010;28(6):928–35.
39. Lischalk JW, et al. Stereotactic body radiotherapy (SBRT) for high-risk central pulmonary metastases. Radiat Oncol. 2016;11:28.
40. Chaudhuri AA, et al. Stereotactic ablative radiotherapy (SABR) for treatment of central and ultra-central lung tumors. Lung Cancer. 2015;89(1):50–6.
41. Taremi M, et al. Stereotactic body radiotherapy for medically inoperable lung cancer: prospective, single-center study of 108 consecutive patients. Int J Radiat Oncol Biol Phys. 2012;82(2):967–73.
42. Walraven I, et al. Long-term follow-up of patients with locally advanced non-small cell lung cancer receiving concurrent hypofractionated chemoradiotherapy with or without cetuximab. Radiother Oncol. 2016;118(3):442–6.
43. Maguire J, et al. SOCCAR: a randomised phase II trial comparing sequential versus concurrent chemotherapy and radical hypofractionated radiotherapy in patients with inoperable stage III Non-Small Cell Lung Cancer and good performance status. Eur J Cancer. 2014;50(17):2939–49.
44. Cheung P, et al. Phase II study of accelerated hypofractionated three-dimensional conformal radiotherapy for stage T1-3 N0 M0 non-small cell lung cancer: NCIC CTG BR.25. J Natl Cancer Inst. 2014;106(8):dju164. https://doi.org/10.1093/jnci/dju164.
45. Cannon DM, et al. Dose-limiting toxicity after hypofractionated dose-escalated radiotherapy in non-small-cell lung cancer. J Clin Oncol. 2013;31(34):4343–8.

46. Liu YE, et al. High-dose accelerated hypofractionated three-dimensional conformal radiotherapy (at 3 Gy/fraction) with concurrent vinorelbine and carboplatin chemotherapy in locally advanced non-small-cell lung cancer: a feasibility study. Radiat Oncol. 2013;8(1):198.
47. Cho WC. Cancer research on non-small cell lung cancer in smokers and non-smokers: snapshots from the AACR annual meeting 2009. Cancer Biol Ther. 2009;8(14):1309–12.
48. Belderbos J, et al. Randomised trial of sequential versus concurrent chemo-radiotherapy in patients with inoperable non-small cell lung cancer (EORTC 08972-22973). Eur J Cancer. 2007;43(1):114–21.
49. Katsuta T, et al. Phase II Study: the outcome of hypofractionated involved-field radiation therapy with concurrent chemotherapy for the treatment of locally advanced non-small cell lung cancer. Pract Radiat Oncol. 2021;11(1):35–43.
50. Zhang Q, et al. Dose-escalation by hypofractionated simultaneous integrated boost IMRT in unresectable stage III non-small-cell lung cancer. BMC Cancer. 2022;22(1):96.
51. Parisi E, et al. Accelerated hypofractionated radiotherapy plus chemotherapy for inoperable locally advanced non-small-cell lung cancer: final results of a prospective phase-II trial with a long-term follow-up. Radiat Oncol. 2019;14(1):112.
52. Jiang W, et al. Hypofractionated radiotherapy for medically inoperable stage I non-small cell lung cancer. Thorac Cancer. 2016;7(3):296–303.
53. Agolli L, et al. Hypofractionated image-guided radiation therapy (3 Gy/fraction) in patients affected by inoperable advanced-stage non-small cell lung cancer after long-term follow-up. Anticancer Res. 2015;35(10):5693–700.
54. Chang HJ, et al. Hypofractionated radiotherapy for primary or secondary oligometastatic lung cancer using Tomotherapy. Radiat Oncol. 2012;7:222.
55. Massaro M, et al. Locally advanced non-small cell lung cancer: clinical outcome, toxicity and predictive factors in patients treated with hypofractionated sequential or exclusive radiotherapy. Curr Oncol. 2022;29(7):4893–901.
56. Kong C, et al. Survival and toxicity of hypofractionated intensity modulated radiation therapy in 4 Gy fractions for unresectable stage III non-small cell lung cancer. Int J Radiat Oncol Biol Phys. 2020;107(4):710–9.
57. Peulen H, et al. Toxicity after reirradiation of pulmonary tumours with stereotactic body radiotherapy. Radiother Oncol. 2011;101(2):260–6.
58. Kelly P, et al. Stereotactic body radiation therapy for patients with lung cancer previously treated with thoracic radiation. Int J Radiat Oncol Biol Phys. 2010;78(5):1387–93.
59. Oshiro Y, et al. Stereotactic body radiotherapy for lung tumors at the pulmonary hilum. Strahlenther Onkol. 2010;186(5):274–9.
60. Trovo M, et al. Stereotactic body radiation therapy for re-irradiation of persistent or recurrent non-small cell lung cancer. Int J Radiat Oncol Biol Phys. 2014;88(5):1114–9.
61. Kilburn JM, et al. Thoracic re-irradiation using stereotactic body radiotherapy (SBRT) techniques as first or second course of treatment. Radiother Oncol. 2014;110(3):505–10.
62. Parks J, et al. Stereotactic body radiation therapy as salvage for intrathoracic recurrence in patients with previously irradiated locally advanced non-small cell lung cancer. Am J Clin Oncol. 2016;39(2):147–53.
63. Repka MC, et al. Five-fraction SBRT for ultra-central NSCLC in-field recurrences following high-dose conventional radiation. Radiat Oncol. 2017;12(1):162.
64. Sood S, et al. Ultra-central thoracic re-irradiation using 10-fraction stereotactic body radiotherapy for recurrent non-small-cell lung cancer tumors: preliminary toxicity and efficacy outcomes. Clin Lung Cancer. 2021;22(3):e301–12.
65. Owen D, et al. Safety and tolerability of SBRT after high-dose external beam radiation to the lung. Front Oncol. 2014;4:376.
66. Trakul N, et al. Stereotactic ablative radiotherapy for reirradiation of locally recurrent lung tumors. J Thorac Oncol. 2012;7(9):1462–5.

67. Sumita K, et al. Re-irradiation for locoregionally recurrent tumors of the thorax: a single-institution, retrospective study. Radiat Oncol. 2016;11:104.
68. Binkley MS, et al. Dosimetric factors and toxicity in highly conformal thoracic reirradiation. Int J Radiat Oncol Biol Phys. 2016;94(4):808–15.
69. Chen AM, et al. Tolerance of the brachial plexus to high-dose reirradiation. Int J Radiat Oncol Biol Phys. 2017;98(1):83–90.
70. Sahgal A, et al. Reirradiation human spinal cord tolerance for stereotactic body radiotherapy. Int J Radiat Oncol Biol Phys. 2012;82(1):107–16.
71. Iyengar P, et al. Consolidative radiotherapy for limited metastatic non-small-cell lung cancer: a phase 2 randomized clinical trial. JAMA Oncol. 2018;4(1):e173501.
72. Wang XS, et al. Randomized trial of first-line tyrosine kinase inhibitor with or without radiotherapy for synchronous oligometastatic EGFR-mutated NSCLC. J Natl Cancer Inst. 2023;115(6):742–8.
73. Xu Q, et al. Consolidative local ablative therapy improves the survival of patients with synchronous oligometastatic NSCLC harboring EGFR activating mutation treated with first-line EGFR-TKIs. J Thorac Oncol. 2018;13(9):1383–92.
74. Theelen W, et al. Pembrolizumab with or without radiotherapy for metastatic non-small-cell lung cancer: a pooled analysis of two randomised trials. Lancet Respir Med. 2021;9(5):467–75.
75. Welsh J, et al. Pembrolizumab with or without radiation therapy for metastatic non-small cell lung cancer: a randomized phase I/II trial. J Immunother Cancer. 2020;8(2):e001001.
76. Gadgeel S, et al. Updated analysis from KEYNOTE-189: pembrolizumab or placebo plus pemetrexed and platinum for previously untreated metastatic nonsquamous non-small-cell lung cancer. J Clin Oncol. 2020;38(14):1505–17.
77. Gomez DR, et al. Local consolidative therapy versus maintenance therapy or observation for patients with oligometastatic non-small-cell lung cancer without progression after first-line systemic therapy: a multicentre, randomised, controlled, phase 2 study. Lancet Oncol. 2016;17(12):1672–82.
78. Mitchell KG, et al. Improved overall survival with comprehensive local consolidative therapy in synchronous oligometastatic non-small-cell lung cancer. Clin Lung Cancer. 2020;21(1):37–46 e7.
79. Lababede O, Meziane MA. The eighth edition of TNM staging of lung cancer: reference chart and diagrams. Oncologist. 2018;23(7):844–8.
80. Brooks ED, et al. Association of long-term outcomes and survival with multidisciplinary salvage treatment for local and regional recurrence after stereotactic ablative radiotherapy for early-stage lung cancer. JAMA Netw Open. 2018;1(4):e181390.
81. Huo J, et al. Low rates of patient-reported physician-patient discussion about lung cancer screening among current smokers: Data from Health Information National Trends survey. Cancer Epidemiol Biomark Prev. 2019;28(5):963–73.
82. Lin Y, Mak KS. Racial and socioeconomic disparities in the use of stereotactic body radiotherapy for treating non-small cell lung cancer: a narrative review. J Thorac Dis. 2021;13(6):3764–71.
83. Timmerman R, et al. Extracranial stereotactic radioablation: results of a phase I study in medically inoperable stage I non-small cell lung cancer. Chest. 2003;124(5):1946–55.
84. Kopek N, et al. Co-morbidity index predicts for mortality after stereotactic body radiotherapy for medically inoperable early-stage non-small cell lung cancer. Radiother Oncol. 2009;93(3):402–7.
85. Videtic GMM, et al. Ten-year experience in implementing single-fraction lung SBRT for medically inoperable early-stage lung cancer. Int J Radiat Oncol Biol Phys. 2021;111(2):436–42.
86. Haasbeek CJ, et al. Outcomes of stereotactic ablative radiotherapy for centrally located early-stage lung cancer. J Thorac Oncol. 2011;6(12):2036–43.
87. Onishi H, et al. Stereotactic hypofractionated high-dose irradiation for stage I nonsmall cell lung carcinoma: clinical outcomes in 245 subjects in a Japanese multiinstitutional study. Cancer. 2004;101(7):1623–31.

88. Nyman J, Johansson KA, Hulten U. Stereotactic hypofractionated radiotherapy for stage I non-small cell lung cancer--mature results for medically inoperable patients. Lung Cancer. 2006;51(1):97–103.
89. Dunlap NE, et al. Chest wall volume receiving >30 Gy predicts risk of severe pain and/or rib fracture after lung stereotactic body radiotherapy. Int J Radiat Oncol Biol Phys. 2010;76(3):796–801.
90. Coon D, et al. Fractionated stereotactic body radiation therapy in the treatment of primary, recurrent, and metastatic lung tumors: the role of positron emission tomography/computed tomography-based treatment planning. Clin Lung Cancer. 2008;9(4):217–21.
91. Timmerman R, et al. Excessive toxicity when treating central tumors in a phase II study of stereotactic body radiation therapy for medically inoperable early-stage lung cancer. J Clin Oncol. 2006;24(30):4833–9.

Chapter 22
Continuous Airway Pressure for Hypofractionation and SBRT Planning and Treatment

Zvi Symon and Galia Jacobson

22.1 Introduction

- Respiration-induced tumor motion is a major challenge for hypofractionated radiation therapy (RT) of tumors in the thorax [1–4].
- The strategy of modeling tumor trajectory using 4D computed tomography (CT) and creating an internal target volume (ITV) that is expanded further for setup uncertainty allows the patient to breathe freely during treatment and is most comfortable for the patient [5, 6].
- Abdominal compression belts are commonly used to dampen diaphragmatic breathing and thus limit tumor trajectory, resulting in a smaller ITV [7]. However, in general, the ITV approach is associated with larger volumes of normal lung tissue receiving high doses of radiation compared with other motion management strategies such as the use of respiratory gating, real-time tumor tracking, and deep inspiratory breath hold (DIBH) [6] .
- These approaches have numerous disadvantages including prolonged in-room treatment times, risk of pneumothorax, the inability of many patients to perform adequate breath-hold, and the need for sophisticated and expensive equipment [8, 9]. In addition, the "holy grail" of true real-time tracking is challenged by latency times of image acquisition and processing to synchronize the beam [10, 11]. Continuous airway positive pressure (CPAP) has been studied as an alternative innovative strategy to reproduce the favorable anatomy and tumor motion reduction associated with the DIBH technique [12–15].

Z. Symon (✉)
Radiation Oncology, Sheba Medical Center Affiliated with Tel Aviv University, Ramat Gan, Israel
e-mail: Zvi.Symon@sheba.health.gov.il

G. Jacobson
Radiation Oncology, Sheba Medical Center Affiliated with Tel Aviv University, Ramat Gan, Israel

Radiation Oncology, MD Anderson Cancer Center, Houston, TX, USA

O. Kaidar-Person, R. Chen (eds.), *Hypofractionated and Stereotactic Radiation Therapy*, https://doi.org/10.1007/978-3-031-47701-0_22

- The administration of positive pressure to the airways during the entire respiratory cycle using non-invasive ventilation with a face mask and a simple respirator, as shown in Fig. 22.1, is associated with hyperinflation of the lung and mimics the geometry achieved with breath-hold, while the patient continues to breathe freely.
- CPAP machines have a motor that pressurizes room temperature air delivered through a hose at an adjustable constant pressure greater than 1 atmosphere to a mask worn by the patient. As shown in Fig. 22.2, the increased pressure facilitates the opening of lung tissue in collapse and thus recruits more alveoli for ventilation [16].

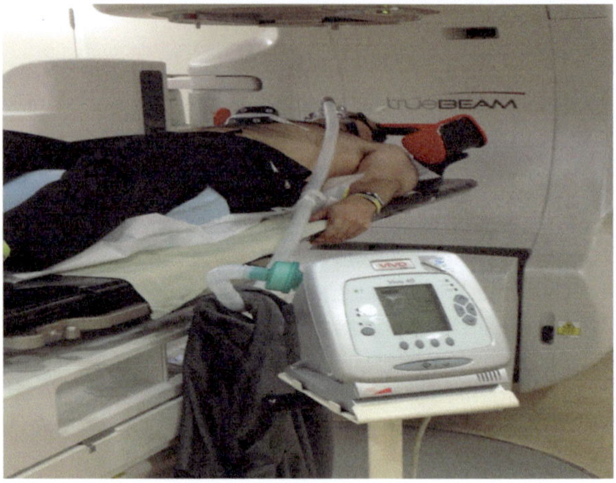

Fig. 22.1 Simulation and daily treatment are given with CPAP

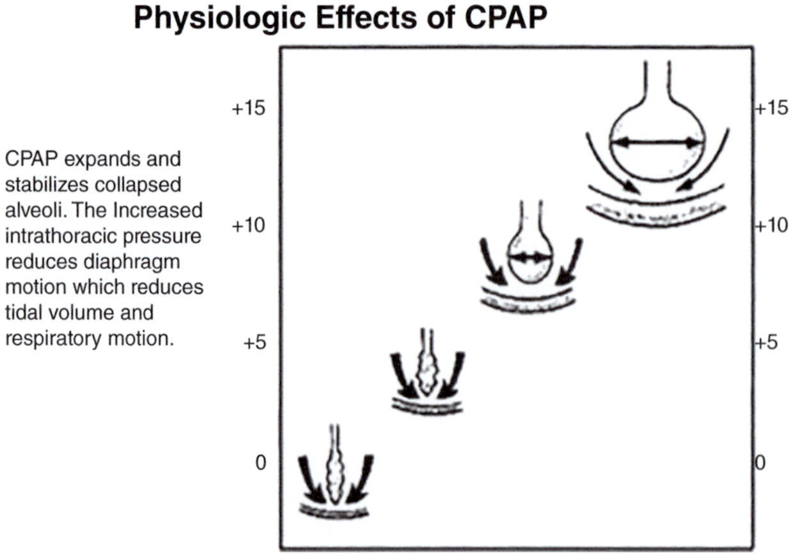

Fig. 22.2 Physiologic effect of CPAP

CPAP is commonly used as a treatment for obstructive sleep apnea as the positive pressure prevents upper airway collapse. It is also often employed and preferred to intubation, sedation, and invasive ventilation with positive end-expiratory pressure (PEEP) because it is non-invasive, and the risk of complications such as pneumothorax, infection, and subglottic stenosis is rare [17]. Patients connected to CPAP must initiate all their own breaths as CPAP mode ventilators do not cycle.

The utilization of CPAP for motion management in RT was first described in 2015 in a pilot study of 10 patients that demonstrated that, in most patients, CPAP increases lung volume by a third and hence displaces part of the healthy lung and the heart out of the treatment field. In some patients, CPAP also decreased the amplitude of respiration-induced tumor motion and thus reduced the planning target volume (PTV) [12].

In a larger follow-up study of 49 patients, lung volume was significantly augmented by the use of CPAP, with a mean absolute increase of 994 ± 768 cm^3, with a relative increase of 37% (95% CI 6–84%, $p < 0.001$) [13]. An example of maximal intensity projection is shown in Fig. 22.3. The lung volume elevation with the use of CPAP is independent of age, gender, BMI, smoking status, and chronic obstructive pulmonary disease (COPD) status. Patients with normal lung function derived the largest expansion of lung tissue on CPAP (mean ± SD, 1283 ± 1128 cm^3, $p = 0.0006$). Patients with restrictive patterns had moderate lung expansion (mean ± SD, 719 ± 341 cm^3, $p = 0.003$).

This study also attempted to estimate the potential of CPAP to reduce tumor motion according to tumor location in the lung. The use of CPAP was associated with a PTV reduction in the range of 7–42% for nine tumors located within 2 cm

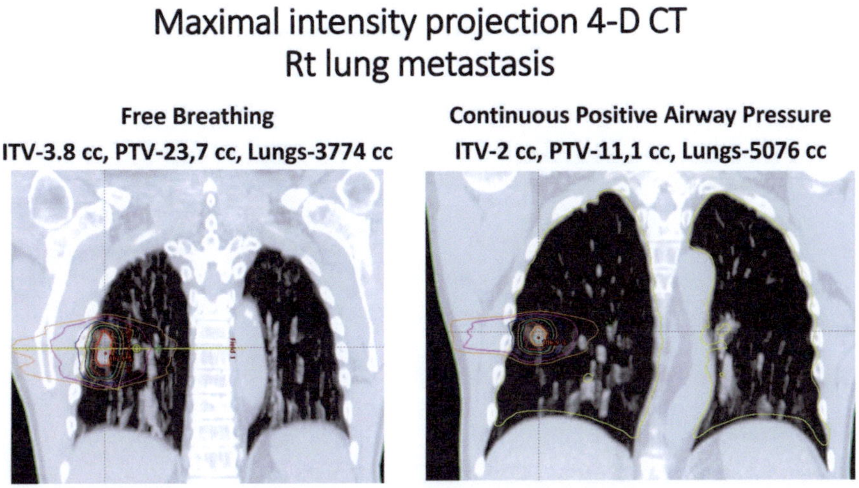

Fig. 22.3 Coronal CT images of maximal intensity projections of 4DCT in free breathing and CPAP demonstrate an increase in lung volume and decrease in ITV and PTV with CPAP versus free breathing, and as a result, lower dose to surrounding tissue. In addition, this image demonstrates better visualization of the tumor and surrounding organs' trajectory [13]. With permission from *International Journal of Radiation Oncology*Biology*Physic*

from the diaphragm; however, two tumors showed no reduction, and four tumors showed a greater trajectory of movement with a larger PTV. In the range of 2–4 cm above the dome of the diaphragm, there seems to be the most impact on tumor trajectory with a reduction in PTV of 34–69%. Between 4 and 6 cm, PTV reduction was modest in the range of 19–23%. Patients with tumors more than 6 cm above the diaphragm dome were under-represented in this study due to the observation that tumors higher in the chest tend to move less with respiration and rarely change their trajectory as a result of CPAP.

The use of CPAP was associated with a moderate dose reduction to both lung and heart as compared with free breathing.

Table 22.1 shows the difference in dosimetric values for plans generated using CPAP versus free breathing, with a statistically significant reduction in Lung V20, Lung V5, Mean Lung Dose, and Heart V5 [13]. Figure 22.4 shows a typical

Table 22.1 Relative reductions in critical organ radiation dose ($n = 24$)

	Free breathng	CPAP	Mean paired difference 95% CI	
Lungs V20 (%)	20.9 ± 14.4	16.1 ± 10.2	4.7 [2.2; 7.3]	$p < 0.01$
Lungs V5 (%)	46.8 ± 25.7	39.8 ± 20	7 [2.7; 11.3]	$p < 0.01$
Mean lung dose (Gy)	11 ± 6	9.2 ± 4.8	1.8 [0.98; 2.7]	$p < 0.01$
Heart V5 (%)	54.57 ± 30.1	45.6 ± 5.8	8.9 [3.6; 14.3]	$p < 0.01$
Mean heart dose (Gy)	10 ± 7.2	9 ± 7.5	1 [(−1);3]	$p = 0.3$

With permission from the *International Journal of Radiation Oncology*Biology*Physic* [13]

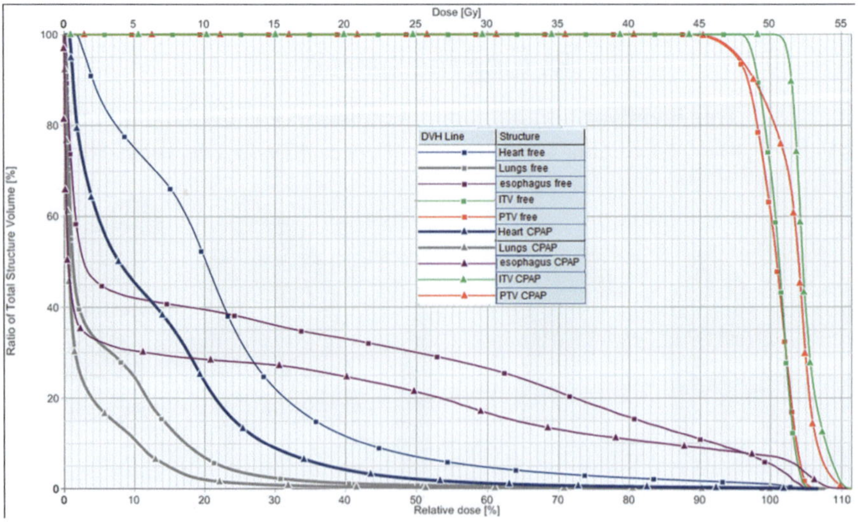

Fig. 22.4 Sample dose-volume histogram (DVH) comparison of Lung SBRT plans with and without showing improved dosimetry in lungs and heart with the use of CPAP. With permission from the *International Journal of Radiation Oncology*Biology*Physic* [13]

dose-volume histogram (DVH) comparing free breathing with CPAP Lung SBRT plans, demonstrating lower heart and lung doses with CPAP [13].

Reduction of dose to the lung may be due to either increased lung volume or reduced tumor motion; however, it is more substantial if both conditions are met.

Reduction of dose to the heart is due to an inferior and posterior displacement of the heart associated with the use of CPAP. The heart shape is thinner and more elongated and thus moves away from tumors located centrally.

22.2 Selection of Patients for CPAP

While the compliance of CPAP in obstructive sleep apnea is only around 50%, we have found that approximately 90% of all patients offered CPAP are motivated to reduce radiation exposure to the normal lung and, if appropriately coached, are fully compliant. Relative contraindication for CPAP includes trauma or burns involving the face, unstable cardiorespiratory status or respiratory arrest, and extremely anxious patients.

22.3 Workflow for SBRT with CPAP

Before RT planning CT (simulation) patients are fitted with a full-face mask (nose and mouth) suited to their size and checked to ensure that the mask is snugly fitted to ensure there are no leaks. Beginning with an initial CPAP pressure of 7.5 cm H_2O, patients undergo coaching to breathe calmly through the nose. Under nurse or respiratory therapist supervision, air pressure is increased from 7.5 cm H_2O to the maximal comfortably tolerated level up to a ceiling pressure of 15 cm H_2O. During the ramp-up, patients are monitored for blood pressure, O_2 saturation, and respiratory rate and are coached to breathe freely and relax. Once the maximal comfortable pressure is determined, the patient stays connected to CPAP for at least 30 min before undergoing a 4DCT simulation. It is important that the CPAP device can operate on a battery when disconnected to allow non-interrupted CPAP administration between the preparation room and the simulator or the linac. After the simulation, patients are discharged home with their masks, hoses, and filters and asked to bring them for daily treatment.

CPAP may be used in combination with DIBH for SBRT in patients who have inadequate lung expansion from DIBH alone or inadequate tumor motion reduction from the use of CPAP alone. A small pilot study showed that the combination of CPAP and DIBH improved lung volume by a further 600 cc over DIBH alone. The combination also distanced normal critical structures such as the heart and chest wall by an additional 5 mm [18].

22.4 Future Directions

Further work is needed to optimize the use of CPAP for the individual patient for hypofractionated radiotherapy and SBRT. New platforms such as the MRI Linac with planar MRI cinematography will facilitate the real-time effects of CPAP on the lung, heart, and tumor motion. The use of surface imaging to optimize CPAP pressure, to coach patients to reduce chest wall and diaphragmatic motion, and to monitor them during treatment is currently under investigation.

References

1. Keall PJ, et al. The management of respiratory motion in radiation oncology report of AAPM Task Group 76 a. Med Phys. 2006;33(10):3874–900.
2. Kwint M, et al. Intra thoracic anatomical changes in lung cancer patients during the course of radiotherapy. Radiother Oncol. 2014;113(3):392–7.
3. Kumagai M, Mori S. Movement of a small tumour in contact with the diaphragm: characterisation with four-dimensional CT. Japanese J Radiol. 2016;34(2):154–7.
4. Plathow C, et al. Analysis of intrathoracic tumor mobility during whole breathing cycle by dynamic MRI. Int J Radiat Oncol Biol Phys. 2004;59(4):952–9.
5. Ruben J, et al. Variation in lung tumour breathing motion between planning four-dimensional computed tomography and stereotactic ablative radiotherapy delivery and its dosimetric implications: any role for four-dimensional set-up verification? Clin Oncol. 2016;28(1):21–7.
6. Goossens S, et al. Assessment of tumor motion reproducibility with audio-visual coaching through successive 4D CT sessions. J Appl Clin Med Phys. 2014;15(1):47–56.
7. Langen KM, Jones DT. Organ motion and its management. Int J Radiat Oncol Biol Phys. 2001;50(1):265–78.
8. Mah D, et al. Technical aspects of the deep inspiration breath-hold technique in the treatment of thoracic cancer. Int J Radiat Oncol Biol Phys. 2000;48(4):1175–85.
9. Boda-Heggemann J, et al. Deep inspiration breath hold—based radiation therapy: a clinical review. Int J Radiat Oncol Biol Phys. 2016;94(3):478–92.
10. Chang Y, et al. Dosimetric effect of intrafraction tumor motion in lung stereotactic body radiotherapy using Cyberknife static tracking system. Technol Cancer Res Treatment. 2019;18:1533033819859448.
11. Menten MJ, et al. Lung stereotactic body radiotherapy with an MR-linac–quantifying the impact of the magnetic field and real-time tumor tracking. Radiother Oncol. 2016;119(3):461–6.
12. Goldstein JD, et al. Continuous positive airway pressure for motion management in stereotactic body radiation therapy to the lung: a controlled pilot study. Int J Radiat Oncol Biol Phys. 2015;93(2):391–9.
13. Jacobson G, et al. Benefits of continuous positive airway pressure (CPAP) during radiation therapy: a prospective trial. Int J Radiat Oncol Biol Phys. 2021;10(5):1466–72.
14. Allen AM, et al. CPAP (continuous positive airway pressure) is an effective and stable solution for heart sparing radiotherapy of left sided breast cancer. Radiat Oncol. 2020;15(1):1–6.
15. Di Perri D, et al. Effect of continuous positive airway pressure administration during lung stereotactic ablative radiotherapy: a comparative planning study. Strahlenther Onkol. 2018;194(6):591–9.
16. Corda L, et al. Short-and long-term effects of CPAP on upper airway anatomy and collapsibility in OSAH. Sleep Breath. 2009;13(2):187–93.
17. Mao J, et al. Spontaneous pneumothorax caused by excessive positive airway pressure therapy for obstructive sleep apnea, in D36. Pleural disease: case reports II. American Thoracic Society; 2018. p. A6682.
18. Reckhow J, et al. Continuous positive airway pressure with deep inspiration breath hold in left-sided breast radiation therapy. Med Dosim. 2021;46(2):127–31.

Part VI
Breast Cancer

Chapter 23
Breast Cancer

Kevin Pearlstein and Ellen Jones

23.1 Introduction

The benefit of post-lumpectomy and post-mastectomy radiation therapy (RT) in improving local control and overall survival has been demonstrated through multiple randomized trials. The classic fractionation scheme was typically 25 fractions (2 Gy/fraction) to the whole breast or chest wall with an additional RT boost to the lumpectomy cavity or mastectomy scar. However, multiple randomized studies have subsequently explored hypofractionated whole-breast RT in specific populations. There are also emerging data supporting the use of hypofractionated post-mastectomy RT. These alternative approaches to conventional whole-breast and post-mastectomy RT are viable options in certain patient populations.

23.2 Pearls

- Breast cancer is the most commonly diagnosed cancer, with 230,000 new cases in the United States annually.
- The median age at diagnosis is 62 years.
- There is a strong female predominance, and < 1% of new cases are in men.
- Risk factors include older age, estrogen exposure (high natural estrogen levels, hormone replacement), early menarche, late menopause, nulliparity, and obesity (in post-menopausal women).

K. Pearlstein · E. Jones (✉)
Department of Radiation Oncology, University of North Carolina at Chapel Hill, Chapel Hill, NC, USA
e-mail: Ellen_Jones@med.unc.edu

O. Kaidar-Person, R. Chen (eds.), *Hypofractionated and Stereotactic Radiation Therapy*, https://doi.org/10.1007/978-3-031-47701-0_23

- Known genetic risk factors include mutations in BRCA1/2, p53 (Li-Fraumeni syndrome), STK11 (Petuz-Jeghers Syndrome), PALB2, and PTEN (Cowden syndrome).
- An abnormal screening mammogram is the most common presentation in developed countries. The most common physical exam finding is a firm palpable mass, while more advanced findings include palpable axillary or supraclavicular lymphadenopathy. Indications of inflammatory breast cancer include breast erythema, skin thickening, nipple changes, and peau d'orange (skin dimpling).
- Core biopsy should be performed to confirm the diagnosis.
  - Proliferative lesions that are not necessarily precursors to invasive cancer, but do increase the risk of malignancy include lobular carcinoma in situ (LCIS) and atypical hyperplasia (AH).
  - Ductal carcinoma in situ (DCIS) is considered a precursor to invasive cancer. Higher nuclear grade and comedo subtype are associated with a higher risk of invasion and recurrence.
  - Invasive carcinomas include infiltrating ductal carcinoma (70–80% of invasive cancer) and infiltrating lobular carcinoma (more often bilateral and multicentric). More rare types (<5%) include mucinous, tubular, medullary, and papillary subtypes.
  - Invasive cancers can be classified according to ER, PR, and HER2 status.
- Historically, the breast tissue generally lies between the second and sixth ribs and extends from the edge of the sternum to the mid-axillary line. However, with the use of planning CT, the glandular tissue can be more precisely identified.
  - Axillary lymph nodes are divided into anatomic groups based on relation to pectoralis minor: level I (lateral), level II (posterior), level III (medial), and level IV (medial supraclavicular nodes). Internal mammary lymph nodes (IMN) are located in intercostal spaces near internal mammary vessels from the retroclavicular area to the fifth intercostal space.
- Lymph node drainage is predominantly to axillary lymph nodes, but also to IMN and level III and IV lymph nodes. The inner quadrant lesions are more likely to drain to IMN compared with outer quadrant lesions.
- The most common sites of distant spread include bone, lung, brain, and liver and are highly dependent on breast cancer molecular subtype.
- Diagnostic evaluation can include different imaging studies.
  - Diagnostic mammogram includes mediolateral oblique (MLO) and craniocaudal (CC) views.
  - Ultrasound of the breast can further characterize mass, is very sensitive for breast cancer, and can help identify targets for core needle biopsy.
  - Breast MRI is very sensitive (>90%) but has lower specificity (~70%). It can be used to evaluate young women with dense breast tissue and further evaluate inconclusive breast masses seen on mammograms or ultrasounds.
- Treatment options
  - Surgery is used as a treatment for both in situ and invasive breast cancer and can be lumpectomy or mastectomy. Axillary lymph node dissection can be performed in the clinically positive axilla, whereas sentinel lymph node biopsy is more commonly used in the clinically negative axilla.

The equivalency of lumpectomy followed by whole breast radiation therapy (RT) and mastectomy has been demonstrated in multiple clinical trials.
The omission of post-lumpectomy RT can be considered in older women (>65–70) with early-stage (T1–2, N0) hormone-positive breast cancers.
Post-mastectomy radiation may be recommended for those with high-risk clinical and/or pathologic features including T3 tumors and node-positive diseases.
RT alone and/or endocrine therapy if ER/PR positive can be considered for patients with poor performance status or who are otherwise unfit for surgical management (IBTR! Version 2.0 and MSKCC DCIS nomograms).

- 5–10 years of endocrine therapy (Tamoxifen or aromatase inhibitor) is generally recommended for ER/PR-positive patients.
- Primary systemic therapy may be appropriate in some situations including triple negative cancer, HER2 cancers, node-positive disease, and inoperable disease.
- Adjuvant systemic therapy can be used for those at high risk for locoregional or distant recurrence (triple negative, large tumors, positive lymph nodes). Genomic tests such as Oncotype DX can help guide decisions for node-negative, ER-positive cancers.

23.3 Tumor and Patient Selection

23.3.1 Hypofractionated Whole-Breast RT

- As part of the Choosing Wisely Campaign, ASTRO recommends against initiating post-lumpectomy RT in women ≥50 with early-stage invasive breast cancer without considering hypofractionation [1].
- 2018 ASTRO guidelines to assist in patient selection for the hypofractionated approach include: [2].
  - Any age.
  - Treated with breast-conserving surgery.
  - Any stage provided intent is to treat the whole breast without regional nodal coverage.
  - The volume of breast tissue receiving >105% of prescriptions should be minimized.

St. Gallen recommendations: [3].

Based on longer follow-ups from multiple randomized trials, the 2021 Panel strongly recommends moderately hypofractionated radiation treatment courses, consisting of 15 or 16 treatments, as standard therapy, irrespective of tumor subtype or patient age.

The Panel also strongly endorsed routine use of moderate hypofractionation in women receiving post-mastectomy radiation and/or regional nodal irradiation (RNI), irrespective of patient age or tumor subtype, and endorsed these hypofractionated radiation therapy schedules among patients with reconstructions after mastectomy.

European Society for Radiotherapy and Oncology (ESTRO) Advisory Committee in Radiation Oncology Practice: [4].

Moderately hypofractionated radiotherapy can be offered to any patient for whole breast, chest wall (with or without reconstruction), and nodal volumes. Ultrafractionation (five fractions) can also be offered for non-nodal breast or chest wall (without reconstruction) radiotherapy either as the standard of care or within a randomized trial or prospective cohort.

23.4 Treatment and Planning

Hypofractionated whole breast

Simulation instructions	• Patients placed in a supine position with an immobilization device. • Bilateral arms externally rotated with hands placed behind head using wingboard. • Head tilted to the opposite direction of the involved breast. • Prone positioning can be considered an alternative. This positioning can be particularly useful for women with large pendulous breasts. • Markers should be placed: over the scar, below the clavicle, 2 cm below palpable breast tissue, mid-sternum, and mid-axilla. • A single isocenter is generally placed below the bottom edge of the clavicle. • For left-sided cancers, deep inspiration breath hold can be used to minimize heart dose.
Image guidance	• At a minimum, weekly verification films should be obtained while the patient is under treatment. • For left-sided breast cancers, deep inspiratory breath hold or respiratory gating can be used with each fraction to minimize cardiac dose.
Tumor target/ margins	• Target is the whole breast treated using opposed tangents. – Whole-breast CTV: The superior border is variable but approximately level of second rib insertion, the inferior border is where CT apparent breast is lost, the medial border is sternal-rib junction, the lateral border is a mid-axillary line, the anterior border is skin, and the posterior border is pectoralis/chest wall muscles or ribs. • If used, tumor boost can be delivered with en-face electrons or photons (wedge pair or mini-tangent) to target lumpectomy cavity +1.5–2 cm margin. • Locoregional LN can be treated depending on the clinical scenario—usually with a single AP field but may need a PA field for deeper targets. In addition, a hybrid technique could be utilized with tangent fields for breast targets and partial arcs for lymph nodes. – The field borders are according to the delineated volumes (e.g., see ESTRO's nodal atlas).
Dosimetric considerations	• Keep max 3D point dose in breast <110% prescription. • Limit amount of breast receiving 105% prescription. V107–110% < 2 cc. • Homogeneity may be suboptimal for breast separation >25 cm. • Multiple field-in-field segments are used to improve homogeneity and reduce hot spots. Volumetric IMRT can be considered in selected patients.

Similar approaches to the design of tangent beams for chest wall hypofractionation would also apply. As the skin is not considered part of the clinical target volume post-mastectomy except in T4b, c, and d, not all chest wall irradiation mandates a bolus. A bolus may be applied to assure full coverage (0.5 cm daily) to allow for full coverage of the target volume, although, if there is a severe skin reaction, this may be discontinued to avoid treatment breaks. A custom bolus (i.e., not covering the whole chest wall) can be applied to allow full dose to volumes that are at high risk, e.g., in areas where the chest wall is very thin (Figs. 23.1 and 23.2).

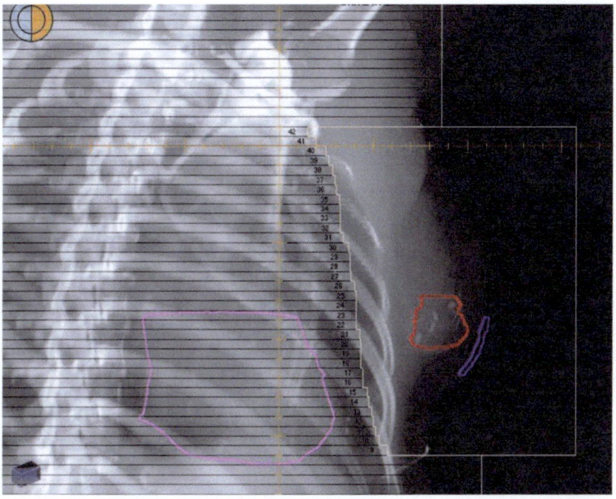

Fig. 23.1 DRR of L medial tangent field covering the whole breast using deep inspiratory breath hold technique. Lumpectomy cavity is contoured in red, surgical scar in purple, and heart in pink

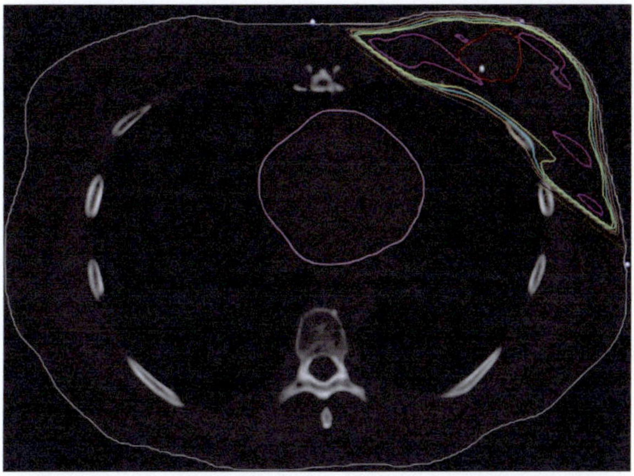

Fig. 23.2 Final treatment plan using the field-in-field technique to optimize plan homogeneity

23.5 Doses

23.5.1 Hypofractionated Whole-Breast RT

Multiple treatment regimens have been evaluated in prospective trials

- α/β estimated ~3–4 [5].

Dose/fx	# of fx	Total dose	Duration of treatment	Notes
3 Gy	13	39 Gy	5 Weeks, qod	Fractionation from START A [6], RMH/GOC [7]
2.66 Gy	15	40 Gy	3 Weeks, daily	Fractionation from START B [8]
3.2 Gy	13	41.6 Gy	5 Weeks, qod	Fractionation from START A [6]
2.66 Gy	16	42.5 Gy	3 Weeks, daily	Fractionation from OCOG [9]
3.3 Gy	13	42.9 Gy	5 Weeks, qod	Fractionation from RMH/GOC [7]
5.2 Gy	5	26 Gy	1 Week, daily	Fractionation from FAST-Forward [10]
5.7 Gy	5	28.5	Once weekly	Fractionation from FAST Trial (CRUKE/04/015) [11]
6.0 Gy	5	30	Once weekly	Fractionation from FAST Trial (CRUKE/04/015) [11]

Abbreviations: *START* UK Standardisation of Breast Radiotherapy, *RMH/GOC* Royal Marsden Hospital/Gloucestershire Oncology Centre, *OCOG* Ontario Clinical Oncology Group

- An ASTRO task force favored a dosing schedule of 42.5 Gy in 16 or 40 Gy in 15 fractions [2].
- A tumor bed boost was not consistently used in clinical trials evaluating hypofractionated whole breast RT:
  - A sequential boost is routinely incorporated at our institution, generally 10 Gy delivered in four fractions. Simultaneous integrated boost can also be used (RTOG 1005).

Moderately hypofractionated radiotherapy can be offered to any patient for whole breast, chest wall (with or without reconstruction), and nodal volumes (see ARCOP-ESTRO guidelines).

23.5.2 Hypofractionated Post-Mastectomy Radiation

There is emerging evidence for the safety and efficacy of hypofractionated RT in the post-mastectomy setting.

- Mastectomy was performed in a minority of patients on START A (15%), START B (8%), and FAST-Forward (6%).
- Hypofractionated PMRT has been specifically evaluated in prospective trials (see table below).
- Ongoing trials, including Alliance A221505 (RT CHARM) and FABREC, are further exploring this approach.

Dose/fx	# of fx	Total dose	Duration of treatment	Notes
2.9 Gy	15	43.5	3 weeks, daily	Fractionation from Wang et al. [12]
3.3 Gy	11	36.6	2.2 weeks, daily	Fractionation from Poppe et al. [13]
2.66 Gy	Chest wall: 16 LN: 15	Chest wall: 42.56 Gy LN: 39.9 Gy	3.4 weeks, daily	Fractionation from FABREC (NCT03422003)
2.66 Gy	16	42.56 Gy	3 weeks, daily	Fractionation from RT CHARM (NCT03414970)

23.6 Normal Tissue Constraints

23.6.1 Hypofractionated Whole Breast

ASTRO Taskforce noted that optimal dose-volume parameters for lung and heart when using the hypofractionated approach are not known [2].

Constraints used at our institution and in the RTOG 1005 (NCT01349322) hypofractionation trial include:

Structure	RTOG 1005 constraint	Our institutional practice
Heart	$V_{10\,Gy} < 30\%$ (L)	$V_{10\,Gy} < 35\%$
	$V_{10\,Gy} < 10\%$ (R)	$V_{20\,Gy} < 5\%$
	$V_{20\,Gy} < 5\%$ (L)	Mean < 4 Gy
	$V_{20\,Gy} = 0\%$ (R)	
	Mean < 4 Gy	
Ipsilateral lung	$V_{5\,Gy} < 50\%$	$V_{5\,Gy} < 50\%$
	$V_{10\,Gy} < 35\%$	$V_{20\,Gy} < 15\%$
	$V_{20\,Gy} < 15\%$	Mean < 16 Gy
Contralateral lung	$V_{5\,Gy} < 10\%$	–
Contralateral breast	$V_{1.86\,Gy} < 5\%$	–
	$D_{max} < 3.1$ Gy	
Thyroid	$D_{max} < 2\%$ prescription	–

There are no well-validated constraints to use when treating locoregional lymph nodes with hypofractionation. In currently accruing trials, the constraints are similar to those listed above except ipsilateral lung dose constraints are less restrictive ($V_{18} < 35\%$ in RT CHARM).

23.7 Patient Management

- **Acute toxicity**
  - Skin reaction: It is common and can range from mild skin erythema to more significant dry or wet desquamation. The rate appears similar or lower with hypofractionation as compared with conventional fractionated in most studies [14].

    Prevention: Various approaches have been explored for the prevention of acute skin reactions with mixed results. General precautions include avoidance of skin irritants (alcohol-based or fragrant lotions and soaps), use of moisturizing agents (Aquaphor, aloe, Calendula, etc.), and maintenance of a dry environment, particularly in the inframammary fold.

    Skin erythema: symptomatic management only.

    Folliculitis: consider the use of topical steroids (1% hydrocortisone cream).

    Dry desquamation: symptomatic management only.

    Moist desquamation: consider the use of a physical barrier (Mepilex) or 1% silvadene cream. These should be applied after RT treatments.
  - Pain: OTC pain medications are often adequate, but prescription pain medications may be needed.
- **Late toxicity**
  - Breast cosmesis: It can include fibrosis, edema, and telangiectasias. Mild changes were seen in the majority of patients. More significant late toxicity is uncommon (<5%).

    Late cosmetic outcomes appear similar (or slightly better) with hypofractionation compared with conventional fractionation.

    Use of Pentoxifylline (400 mg tid or 800 mg qd) and Vitamin E (300–1000 IU daily) for 6 months has been found to reduce the risk of fibrosis [15], as well as improve cosmetic outcomes in those who develop fibrosis [16].
  - If a patient has undergone breast reconstruction prior to RT, cosmetic issues such as asymmetry, hardness, or capsular contraction can occur in up to 40% following RT.
- **Rare late toxicities**
  - Cardiac toxicity: There does not appear to be a threshold dose. The absolute increase in the risk of a coronary event is small if the RT dose to heart is limited (likely <1% if mean heart dose <3 Gy) [17].
  - Radiation pneumonitis: The risk of clinically significant pneumonitis is <1% but depends on lung volume in the field.

If symptomatic, it can be treated with a course of steroids tapered over 6–12 weeks.
- Lymphedema: The risk is <5% with breast RT alone and 10–12% if locoregional LNs are treated as well. The rate is higher if axillary surgery is performed.
- Brachial plexopathy: <1% risk with conventional RT doses; similar rates are seen in hypofractionated trials [18].
- Rib fracture: <2% in hypofractionated trials [18].

23.8 Follow-Up

ASCO and NCCN Recommendations for breast cancer follow-up include [19, 20]:

- Clinical evaluation, including breast exam and assessment of acute/late toxicities:
  - Year 1–3 every 3–6 months.
  - Year 4–5 every 6–12 months.
  - Year >5 annually.
- First mammogram no earlier than 6 months following treatment completion. Subsequent mammograms every 6–12 months:
  - In certain high-risk patients (BRCA population), breast MRI may be appropriate for surveillance.
- Bone density evaluation is recommended for women receiving aromatase inhibitors at baseline and periodically thereafter.

23.9 Relevant Literature

23.9.1 Hypofractionated Whole-Breast RT

Study	Patients	Treatment	Median follow-up	Outcomes
Randomized trials				
OCOG [9]	*N* = 1234, pT1–2, pN0 following ALND. 75% >50 yo. 80% T1	**Arm 1:** 42.5 Gy/16 fx **Arm 2:** 50 Gy/25 fx No tumor bed boost	12 years	**Arm 1:** • 6.2% 10 year LR, 84.6% 10 year OS • 70% Good/excellent cosmesis • 2.5% G3 skin toxicity **Arm 2:** • 6.7% 10 year LR (NS), 84.4% 10 year OS (NS) • 71% good/excellent cosmesis (NS) • 2.7% G3 skin toxicity (NS)

Study	Patients	Treatment	Median follow-up	Outcomes
START A [6]	$N = 2236$, pT1–3, N0–1. 77% >50 yo. 29% N+, 70% G1/2. BCS (85%) or mastectomy (15%)	**Arm 1:** 39 Gy/13 fx **Arm 2:** 41.6 Gy/13 fx **Arm 3:** 50 Gy/25 fx Note: all tx delivered over 5 weeks 61% received boost	9 years	**Arm 1:** • 8.8% 10 year LRR, 10.7% 5 year all-cause mortality • 10 year cosmesis: 3% telangiectasia, 7% breast edema, 22% breast induration **Arm 2:** • 6.3% 10 year LRR, 11.3% 5 year all-cause mortality • 10 year cosmesis similar to arm 3 **Arm 3:** • 7.4% 10 year LRR (NS), 11.1% 5 year all-cause mortality (NS) • 10 year cosmesis: 7% telangiectasia ($p < 0.01$ vs. arm 1), 14% breast edema ($p < 0.01$), 27% breast induration ($p = 0.03$)
START B [8]	$N = 2215$, pT1–3, pN0–1 79% >50 yo. 23% N+, 75% G1/2. BCS (92%) or mastectomy (8%)	**Arm 1**: 40 Gy/15 fx **Arm 2**: 50 Gy/25 fx Note: Hypofx tx delivered over 3 weeks 43% received boost	10 years	**Arm 1:** • 4.3% 10 year LRR • 10 year cosmesis: 25% breast shrinkage, 4% telangiectasia, 5% breast edema **Arm 2:** • 5.5% 10 year LRR • 10 year cosmesis: 31% breast shrinkage ($p = 0.02$), 6% telangiectasias ($p = 0.03$), 9% breast edema ($p < 0.01$)

Study	Patients	Treatment	Median follow-up	Outcomes
RMH / GOC [7]	$N = 1410$, pT1–3, ≤1 pos LN. 70% >50 yo. 94% T1–2, 16% cN+, 33% pN+	**Arm 1:** 39 Gy/13 fx **Arm 2:** 42.9 Gy/13 fx **Arm 3:** 50 Gy/25 fx Note: All tx delivered over 5 weeks 75% received boost	10 years	**Arm 1:** • 15% 10 year IBTR • 5 year cosmesis: 43% breast shrinkage, 11% breast edema, 45% fair/poor cosmesis **Arm 2:** • 10% 10 year IBTR ($p = 0.03$ vs arm 1) • 5 year cosmesis: 53% breast shrinkage, 20% breast edema, 62% fair/poor cosmesis **Arm 3:** • 12% 10 year IBTR • 5 year cosmesis, 50% breast shrinkage ($p = 0.03$), 12% breast edema ($p < 0.01$), 56% fair/poor cosmesis ($p < 0.01$)
MD Anderson [14]	$N = 286$, DCIS or pT1–2, pN0-N1	**Arm 1**: 42.6 Gy/16 fx + boost (10–12.5 Gy/4–5 fx) **Arm 2**: 50 Gy/25 fx + boost (10–14 Gy/5–7 fx)	NA	**Arm 1:** • 73% good/excellent cosmesis at 3 years • 23% patient-reported fatigue at 6 months **Arm 2:** • 78% good/excellent cosmesis at 3 years (NS) • 39% patient-reported fatigue at 6 months ($p < 0.01$)
UK FAST [11]	$N = 915$, age > 50 years, tumor size <3 cm, pN0	**Arm 1**: 28.5 Gy/5 fx (weekly tx) **Arm 2**: 30 Gy/5 fx (weekly tx) **Arm 3**: 50 Gy/25 fx (daily tx)	37 months	3 year moderate/marked adverse cosmesis **Arm 1:** • 11% **Arm 2:** • 17% ($p < 0.01$) **Arm 3:** • 10% (NS vs. arm 1)

Study	Patients	Treatment	Median follow-up	Outcomes
UK FAST-Forward [10]	$N = 4096$, pT1–3, pN0–1 86% >50 yo 19% pN+ 79% pT1 94% BCS 6% mastectomy	**Arm 1:** 40 Gy/15 fx **Arm 2:** 27 Gy/5 fx **Arm 3:** 26 Gy/5 fx All daily treatments 25% received boost (10–16 Gy/5–8 fx)	6 years	**Arm 1** 2.1% 5 year IBTR 6% breast shrinkage, 2% breast edema, 11% any adverse event **Arm 2** 1.7% 5 year IBTR (NS vs. arm 1) 9% breast shrinkage, 3% breast edema, 16% any adverse event ($p < 0.01$ vs. arm 1) **Arm 3** 1.4% 5 year IBTR (NS vs. arm 1) 6% breast shrinkage, 2% breast edema, 12% any adverse event (NS vs. arm 1)
DBCG HYPO [21]	$N = 1882$ DCIS or pT1–2, pN0-N1mi 89% >50 yo 81% T1 10% pN1mi	**Arm 1:** 40 Gy/15 fx **Arm 2:** 50 Gy/25 fx 23% received boost	7 years	**Arm 1** 3.0% 9 year LRR 11% induration 91% Patients satisfied with cosmesis **Arm 2** 3.3% 9 year LRR (NS vs. arm 1) 13% induration 90% patients satisfied with cosmesis
Meta-analysis				
Cochrane review [22]	$N = 8228$,[a] early-stage breast cancer treated with breast-conserving surgery	Hypofractionated regimens vs. 50 Gy/25 fx	NA	• No difference in recurrence-free survival (HR 0.94, 0.77–1.15) • No difference in cosmetic outcome (RR 0.90, 0.81–1.01) • Less acute skin toxicity with hypofractionation (RR 0.32, 0.22–0.45)

Abbreviations: *START* UK Standardisation of Breast Radiotherapy, *RMH/GOC* Royal Marsden Hospital/Gloucestershire Oncology Centre, *OCOG* Ontario Clinical Oncology Group, *ALND* axillary lymph node dissection, *Gy* gray, *fx* fraction(s), *LR* local recurrence/relapse, *OS* overall survival, *BCS* breast-conserving surgery, *LRR* locoregional recurrence, *LN* lymph node(s), *IBTR* ipsilateral breast tumor recurrence, *DCIS* ductal carcinoma in situ

[a]>98% patients from OCOG, START A, START B, RMH/GOC, MD Anderson, and UK FAST trials

23.9.2 Hypofractionated Post-Mastectomy RT

Study	Patients	Treatment	Median follow-up	Outcomes
Wang et al. [12]	*N* = 820, pT3–4 or N2 s/p mastectomy and ALND No reconstruction	Arm 1: 50 Gy/25 fx Arm 2: 43.5 Gy/16 fx RT targeted chest wall and axillary LN (No IMN)	59 months	**Arm 1** 8.1% 5 year LRR 8% G3 acute skin toxicity 0% G3 late skin toxicity 1% lymphedema **Arm 2** 8.3% 5 year LRR 3% G3 acute skin toxicity ($p < 0.01$) <1% G3 late skin toxicity 1% lymphedema
Poppe et al. [13] (Phase 2 trial)	*N* = 69, T2–4, N1–3 Reconstruction allowed (46%)	36.63 Gy/11 fx RT targeted chest wall and regional LN (54% IMN coverage) 97% received scar boost (13.32 Gy/4 fx)	54 months	4.6% 5 year LRR 35% grade 3–4 reconstruction complications No non-reconstruction grade 3–4 late toxicities

Abbreviations: *ALND* axillary lymph node dissection, *Gy* gray, *fx* fraction(s), *LN* lymph node(s), *IMN* internal mammary nodes, *LRR* locoregional recurrence, *RT* radiotherapy

References

1. ASTRO. Choosing Wisely: Five things Physicians and Patients Should Question. 2014; http://www.choosingwisely.org/wp-content/uploads/2015/02/ASTRO-Choosing-Wisely-List.pdf. Accessed Nov 14, 2022.
2. Smith BD, Bellon JR, Blitzblau R, et al. Radiation therapy for the whole breast: executive summary of an American Society for Radiation Oncology (ASTRO) evidence-based guideline. Pract Radiat Oncol. 2018;8(3):145–52.
3. Burstein HJ, Curigliano G, Thurlimann B, et al. Customizing local and systemic therapies for women with early breast cancer: the St. Gallen International Consensus Guidelines for treatment of early breast cancer 2021. Ann Oncol. 2021;32(10):1216–35.
4. Meattini I, Becherini C, Boersma L, et al. European Society for Radiotherapy and Oncology Advisory Committee in Radiation Oncology Practice consensus recommendations on patient selection and dose and fractionation for external beam radiotherapy in early breast cancer. Lancet Oncol. 2022;23(1):e21–31.
5. Qi XS, White J, Li XA. Is alpha/beta for breast cancer really low? Radiother Oncol. 2011;100(2):282–8.
6. Bentzen SM, Agrawal RK, Aird EGA, et al. The UK Standardisation of Breast Radiotherapy (START) Trial A of radiotherapy hypofractionation for treatment of early breast cancer: a randomised trial. Lancet Oncol. 2008;9(4):331–41.

7. Owen JR, Ashton A, Bliss JM, et al. Effect of radiotherapy fraction size on tumour control in patients with early-stage breast cancer after local tumour excision: long-term results of a randomised trial. Lancet Oncol. 2006;7(6):467–71.
8. Bentzen SM, Agrawal RK, Aird EGA, et al. The UK Standardisation of Breast Radiotherapy (START) Trial B of radiotherapy hypofractionation for treatment of early breast cancer: a randomised trial. Lancet. 2008;371(9618):1098–107.
9. Whelan TJ, Pignol JP, Levine MN, et al. Long-term results of hypofractionated radiation therapy for breast cancer. N Engl J Med. 2010;362(6):513–20.
10. Murray Brunt A, Haviland JS, Wheatley DA. Hypofractionated breast radiotherapy for 1 week versus 3 weeks (FAST-Forward): 5-year efficacy and late normal tissue effects results from a multicentre, non-inferiority, randomised, phase 3 trial. Lancet. 2020;395(10237):1613–26.
11. Yarnold JR, Agrawal RK, Alhasso A, et al. First results of the randomised UK FAST Trial of radiotherapy hypofractionation for treatment of early breast cancer (CRUKE/04/015). Radiother Oncol. 2011;100(1):93–100.
12. Wang S, Fang H, Song Y, et al. Hypofractionated versus conventional fractionated postmastectomy radiotherapy for patients with high-risk breast cancer: a randomised, non-inferiority, open-label, phase 3 trial. Lancet Oncol. 2019;20(3):352–60.
13. Poppe MM, Yehia ZA, Baker C, et al. 5-year Update of a multi-institution, prospective phase 2 hypofractionated postmastectomy radiation therapy trial. Int J Radiat Oncol Biol Phys. 2020;107(4):694–700.
14. Shaitelman S, Schlembach P, Arzu I, et al. Acute and short-term toxic effects of conventionally fractionated vs hypofractionated whole-breast irradiation: a randomized clinical trial. JAMA Oncol. 2015;1(7):931–41.
15. Jacobson G, Bhatia S, Smith BJ, Button AM, Bodeker K, Buatti J. Randomized trial of pentoxifylline and vitamin E vs standard follow-up after breast irradiation to prevent breast fibrosis, evaluated by tissue compliance meter. Int J Radiat Oncol Biol Phys. 2013;85(3):604–8.
16. Delanian S, Porcher R, Balla-Mekias S, Lefaix JL. Randomized, placebo-controlled trial of combined pentoxifylline and tocopherol for regression of superficial radiation-induced fibrosis. J Clin Oncol. 2003;21(13):2545–50.
17. Darby SC, Ewertz M, McGale P, et al. Risk of ischemic heart disease in women after radiotherapy for breast cancer. N Engl J Med. 2013;368(11):987–98.
18. Haviland JS, Owen JR, Dewar JA, et al. The UK Standardisation of Breast Radiotherapy (START) trials of radiotherapy hypofractionation for treatment of early breast cancer: 10-year follow-up results of two randomised controlled trials. Lancet Oncol. 2013;14(11):1086–94.
19. Khatcheressian J, Hurley P, Bantug E, Esserman L, Grunfeld E, Halberg F, Hantel A, Henry NL, Muss HB. Breast cancer follow-up and management after primary treatment: American Society of Clinical Oncology clinical practice guideline update. J Clin Oncol. 2013;31(7):961–5.
20. NCCN Clinical Practice Guidelines in Oncology: Breast Cancer. V 2.2016. Available at: http://nccn.org. Accessed November 14, 2022.
21. Offersen BV, Alsner J, Nielsen HM. Hypofractionated versus standard fractionated radiotherapy in patients with early breast cancer or ductal carcinoma in situ in a randomized phase III trial: the DBCG HYPO trial. J Clin Oncol. 2020;38(31):3615–25.
22. James ML, Lehman M, Hider PN, Jeffery M, Hickey BE, Francis DP. Fraction size in radiation treatment for breast conservation in early breast cancer. Cochrane Database Syst Rev. 2010;(11):CD00386. https://doi.org/10.1002/14651858.CD003860.pub3.

Chapter 24
Partial Breast Irradiation

Icro Meattini, Daniel Keleti, and Philip Poortmans

24.1 Introduction

The benefit of post-lumpectomy and postmastectomy radiation therapy (RT) in improving local control and overall survival has been demonstrated through multiple randomized trials. Whole-breast irradiation (WBI) continues to be the most used standard of care, but there is increasing acceptance of a role for partial breast irradiation (PBI) targeting only the primary tumor bed in selected low-risk patients. Several phase 3 trials on external beam PBI versus WBI showed non-inferior local control and comparable rates of distant metastases, breast cancer-specific, and overall survival in patients at low risk of recurrence [1–4]. Reports on late normal tissue effects showed variable results, with higher fraction sizes, twice-daily fractionation, and larger irradiated volumes likely being related to higher risks for fibrosis and unfavorable cosmetic outcomes. Systematic reviews and meta-analyses comparing several PBI techniques with WBI for breast cancer patients demonstrated that the balance between benefits and risks of PBI appears best for well-selected women with low risk for local recurrence [5–7].

I. Meattini (✉)
Department of Experimental and Clinical Biomedical Sciences "M. Serio", University of Florence, Florence, Italy
e-mail: icro.meattini@unifi.it

D. Keleti
Department of Radiation Oncology, University of Kansas Medical Center, Kansas City, KS, USA
e-mail: dkeleti@kumc.edu

P. Poortmans
Department of Radiation Oncology, Iridium Netwerk, University of Antwerp, Faculty of Medicine and Health Sciences, Antwerp, Belgium

O. Kaidar-Person, R. Chen (eds.), *Hypofractionated and Stereotactic Radiation Therapy*, https://doi.org/10.1007/978-3-031-47701-0_24

24.2 Tumor and Patient Selection

Major published guidelines on patient selection criteria for PBI are summarized below (Table 24.1) [8]. A consensus-based update of ASTRO Society has been recently published [9] and further commented by the European Society [10]. The American Brachytherapy Society published the updated consensus statement on partial breast irradiation in 2022 [11]. The Groupe Européen de Curiethérapie-European Society for Radiotherapy and Oncology (GEC-ESTRO) Guideline was published in 2010 [12] and the ESTRO-Advisory Committee in Radiation Oncology Practice (ACROP) recommendations on patient selection and dose and fractionation for external beam radiotherapy in early breast cancer were published in 2022, including selection criteria for both invasive and non-invasive ductal carcinoma in situ (DCIS) [13, 14] (Table 24.2).

Table 24.1 ASTRO Guidelines (update 2016) [8]

Clinical characteristic		Suitable	Cautionary	Unsuitable
Patient factors	Age	≥50	40–49 (all other factors "suitable") ≥50 (with other "cautionary" factor	<40 40–49 with "cautionary" factor
	BRCA 1–2 mutation	Not present	–	Present
Pathologic factors	Tumor size	≤2 cm	2.1–3 cm	>3 cm
	T stage	T1, tis	T2	T3–4
	Histology	Invasive ductal, screen-detected DCIS ≤2.5 cm	Invasive lobular, DCIS ≤3 cm	DCIS >3 cm
	ER status	Positive	Negative	–
	Path margins	Invasive: Neg (≥2 mm), DCIS: Neg (≥3 mm)	Close (<2 mm)	Positive
	Grade	Invasive: Any, DCIS: low/intermediate	–	–
	N stage	pN0	–	pN1–3
	LVSI	No	Limited/focal	Extensive
	EIC	No	≤3 cm	>3 cm
	Multicentricity	Unicentric	–	Multicentric
	Multifocality	Unifocal	–	Multiple foci
	Associated LCIS	Allowed	–	–
Treatment factors	Neoadjuvant therapy	Not allowed	–	Yes
	Nodal surgery	SLN Bx, ALND	–	None performed

Note: 2016 ASTRO recommendations for intraoperative RT include:

- Limit treatment with electrons to women with invasive cancer and only "suitable" factors
- Low-energy X-ray IORT should not be used for treatment outside of registry or clinical trial

Table 24.2 Groupe Européen de Curiethérapie-European Society for Radiotherapy and Oncology (GEC-ESTRO) 2010 Guideline and ESTRO-ACROP 2021 recommendations [12, 13]

Clinical characteristic		GEC-ESTRO 2010 Suitable	GEC-ESTRO 2010 Cautionary	GEC-ESTRO 2010 Unsuitable	ESTRO-ACROP 2021 Recommendations
	ER/PR status	Any	–	–	Luminal-like subtypes (≤3 cm)
	Path margins	Negative (≥2 mm)	Close (<2 mm)	Positive	Negative (≥2 mm)
	Grade	Any	–	–	Grade 1–2
	N stage	pN0	pN1mi, pN1 (by ALND)	pNx, ≥pN2a	pN0 (including isolated tumor cells)
	LVI	Not present	–	Present	Not present
	EIC	Not present	–	Present	–
	Multicentricity	Unicentric	–	Multicentric	Unicentric
	Multifocality	Unifocal	Multifocal (limited to within 2 cm of index lesion)	Multifocal (>2 cm from index lesion)	Unifocal
	DCIS				Low-to-intermediate grade DCIS, sized ≤2.5 cm, clear surgical margins (≥3 mm)
	Associated LCIS	Allowed	–	–	–
Treatment factors	Neoadjuvant therapy	No	No	Yes	No

24.2.1 Second Breast-Conservative Treatment for Ipsilateral Tumor Recurrence

Women who experience local recurrence following BCS and wish to have repeat breast-conserving surgery can be considered for re-irradiation with PBI [15–19]. The ESTRO and European Organisation for Research and Treatment of Cancer consensus on re-irradiation focused on definition, reporting, and clinical decision-making was published in 2022 [20].

Studies have examined this approach, mainly in women with:

- Unicentric recurrence >1 year from initial treatment.
- Refusal of mastectomy.
- Repeat BCS with negative margins.

24.3 Treatment and Planning

There are multiple techniques for delivering PBI that are used in clinical practice following BCS including brachytherapy, IOeRT, and EBRT. There are two basic principles behind PBI: (1) to select low-risk breast cancer patients characterized by low postoperative ipsilateral breast tumor recurrence rates and (2) to apply an accurate tumoricidal RT dose to the target volume. If these two concepts are both respected, then outcomes after PBI will not be inferior to whole-breast RT, whatever PBI technique is used [21]. Delineation of target and OAR volumes is a critical part of modern radiation therapy planning and an essential step after deciding the indication, patient discussion, and image acquisition. The adoption of volume-based treatment planning for non-metastatic breast cancer has increased greatly along with the use of improved planning techniques, which are essential for modern therapy [22]. All techniques can be considered adequate, as long as they cover the entire target volume with the prescribed dose. The target volume size is a predictive factor of toxic effects and cosmesis outcomes; therefore, the target volume definition and contouring phases are crucial for successful planning to eradicate residual tumor cells while limiting side effects [23, 24].

The target volume is essentially independent of the technique that is used:

Target/ margins	• GTV: representing the site of the original tumor, defined by preoperative imaging and clinical examination, taking into account the surgical procedure and postoperative surgical clips, seroma, and pathology report • CTV: GTV + 2 cm (minus the tumor-free margin) expansion, followed by cropping to within the CTV_whole breast (thereby 5 mm inside skin and excluding chest wall and pectoralis major muscle) • PTV: CTV + 0–1 cm expansion, depending on the technique and the IGRT protocol Of note, the surgical cavity rarely coincides with the CTV, as the tumor is very rarely located exactly in the central part of the excision specimen. Therefore, it is of paramount importance to first delineate a "primary tumor bed," representing the (resected) GTV, using all available information including imaging and surgical effects

24.3.1 Brachytherapy

The GEC-ESTRO Breast Cancer Working Group published in 2018 main practical recommendations for implementing accelerated partial breast irradiation (APBI) with multi-catheter brachytherapy used as PBI alone or as a boost, focusing on treatment planning issues, catheter insertion, dosimetry, and quality assurance (see Table 24.3). Guidelines are mandatory to ensure precise catheter insertion for coverage of the target volume and to guarantee high-quality dosimetry [26].

Table 24.3 Brachytherapy

Technique	Multiple techniques exist for catheter placement around the lumpectomy cavity either at the time of lumpectomy or as a separate procedure: • Interstitial catheter brachytherapy (Fig. 24.1) • Intracavitary balloon brachytherapy using single or multiple catheters (e.g., MammoSite) • A combination of the two approaches (e.g., SAVI) Source location, number of positions, and dwell times determined by CT-based 3D treatment planning
Interstitial brachytherapy dosimetric considerations	≥90% PTV coverage by ≥90% prescription
	Dose homogeneity index $(1 - V_{150\%}/V_{100\%}) \geq 0.75$
	$V_{150\%} \leq 70$ cm^3
	$V_{200\%} \leq 20$ cm^3
	Skin $D_{max} \leq 100\%$
	Ipsilateral breast $V_{\geq 50\%} \leq 60\%$
Intracavitary brachytherapy dosimetric considerations Note: to be used with great caution because the surgical cavity is most often poorly representing the target volume, as described above	MammoSite, SAVI: ≥90% PTV coverage by ≥90% prescription
	Tissue-balloon conformance (volume of trapped air/PTV) <10%
	Balloon symmetry deviation of ≤2 mm from expected
	Balloon surface–skin distance: • Ideal: ≥7 mm • Acceptable: 5–7 mm if skin $D_{max} \leq 145\%$ for MammoSite And skin $D_{max} \leq 100\%$ for SAVI [25] for 10 fraction treatment
	MammoSite/SAVI: Ipsilateral breast $V_{150\%} \leq 50$ cm^3
	SAVI (Fig. 24.2): breast $V_{200\%} \leq 20$ cm^3 MammoSite: Ipsilateral breast $V_{200\%} \leq 10$ cm^3
	Ipsilateral breast $V_{\geq 50\%} \leq 60\%$

24.3.2 Intraoperative RT

ESTRO IORT Task Force/ACROP published in 2020 main recommendations on criteria for patient selection, technical details/requirements, physical aspects, and outcome data for intraoperative radiation therapy with electrons (IOERT) in breast cancer [27].

A single fraction of 21 Gy can be delivered with electrons at the time of surgery.

If an endocavitary balloon technique is used, fractionated RT is delivered in a couple of days immediately following surgery. For all techniques, appropriate shielding of the thoracic wall should be used to minimize heart, lung, and chest wall exposure (see Table 24.4).

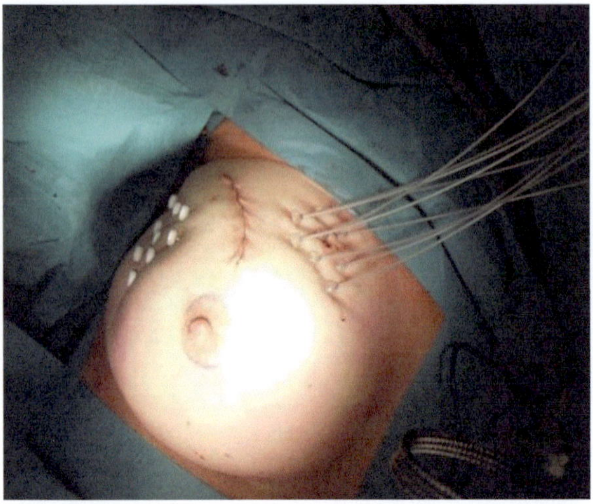

Fig. 24.1 Interstitial brachytherapy catheter placement [Kaidar-Person O, Oldenborg S, Poortmans P. Re-irradiation and hyperthermia in breast cancer. Clin Oncol R Coll Radiol. 2018;30(2):73–84]. Image used with permission of Elsevier Publishing

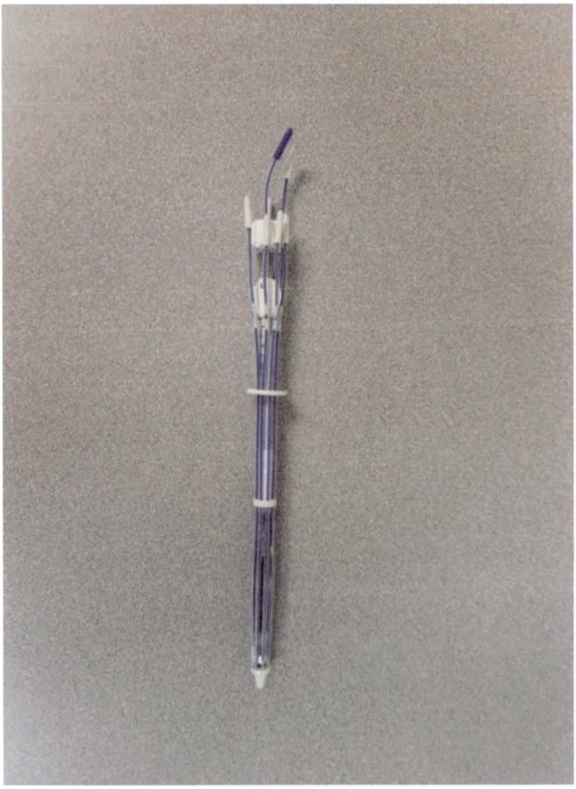

Fig. 24.2 SAVI intracavitary brachytherapy. Image used with permission of Daniel Keleti (Department of Radiation Oncology, University of Kansas Medical Center, Kansas City, Kansas, USA)Note: to be used with great caution because the surgical cavity is most often poorly representing the target volume, as described above

Table 24.4 Intraoperative RT

Technique	Multiple techniques exist for the intraoperative delivery of radiation therapy during lumpectomy surgery. • Intraoperative electron radiation therapy (Fig. 24.3) • HDR brachytherapy
Electrons	Appropriately sized applicator (1.5–2 cm larger than target) placed into lumpectomy cavity after resection (Fig. 24.3) Appropriate electron energy selected based on depth measurement to the chest wall (generally 8–12 MeV) If required, shield positioned deep from CTV to protect dose entering underlying non-target structures Dose delivered to 90% depth
Intermediate-energy photons delivered by brachytherapy device	Appropriately sized applicator placed into lumpectomy cavity after resection Ensure adequate separation of the applicator and skin RT delivered using photons emitted by Iridium-192 (average energy 0.355 MeV)
Low-energy photons delivered by an X-ray source	Appropriately sized applicator placed into lumpectomy cavity after resection Ensure adequate separation of the applicator and skin RT delivered using an X-ray of 50 kV

Note: to be used with great caution because the surgical cavity is most often poorly representing the target volume, as described above

24.3.3 External Beam RT

External beam RT represents the most diffuse technique for PBI delivery. Several techniques, dose, and fractionation schedules have been investigated. It is an easy-to-implement approach for PBI (see example of dosimetric constraints in Table 24.5). Recently, the ESTRO Guideline Committee, which focuses on breast cancer, published consensus recommendations on patient selection and dose and fractionation for external beam radiotherapy in early breast cancer [13].

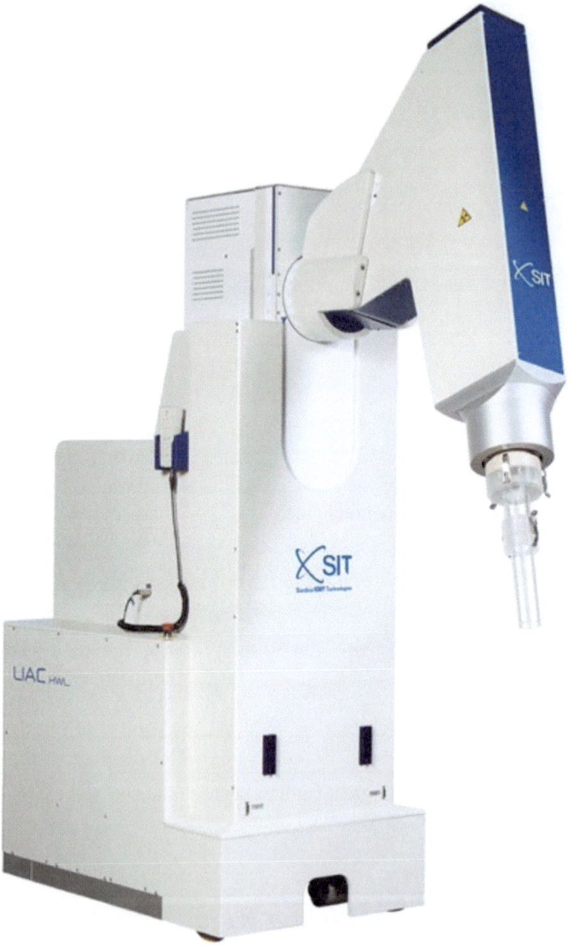

Fig. 24.3 LIAC HWL system for IOeRT treatment developed by SIT. Image used with permission of Sordina IORT Technologies

Table 24.5 Example of dosimetric constraints for external beam partial breast irradiation

Simulation	See the simulation section for hypofractionated whole-breast RT
Dosimetric constraints	• $\geq$ 95% of prescription dose covering $\geq$90% of PTV_EVAL • Maximum breast dose $\leq$120% prescription dose • Minimize dose delivered to uninvolved ipsilateral breast <35% of the breast should receive the prescribed dose <60% of the breast should receive >50% of the prescribed dose • Contralateral breast: $\leq$3% of the prescribed dose for the entire volume • Homolateral lung: >30% of the prescribed dose administered to <15% • Heart: 5% of the prescribed dose to <5% of the volume for lesions of the right breast 5% of the prescribed dose to <40% of the volume for lesions of the left breast • Thyroid: <5% of the prescribed dose to the entire volume

24.4 Doses

The most common dose and fractionation schedules investigated in main studies focused on partial breast irradiation are summarized in Table 24.6.

Table 24.6 Common fractionations used to deliver PBI

Treatment modality	Dose/fx	# of fx	Total dose	Duration of treatment	Notes
External beam RT	6 Gy	5	30 Gy	2 weeks, QOD	From Florence trial [4, 28] (Fig. 24.4)
	3.75 Gy	10	37.5 Gy	1 week, BID	From Barcelona trial [29]
	3.85 Gy	10	38.5 Gy	1 week, BID	From NSABP B39 [30], RAPID [2], RTOG 0319 [31]
	2 Gy	25	50 Gy	5 weeks, daily	From Hungary trial [32]
	2.67 Gy	15	40.05 Gy	3 weeks, daily	From IMPORT-LOW [1] and DBCG [33]
	5.2 Gy	5	26 Gy	1 week, daily	From FAST-FORWARD [34] and ESTRO-ACROP consensus [13]
Intra-RT (IOeRT)	20 Gy	1	20 Gy	Intra-op	20% also received EBRT (50 Gy equivalent delivered over 3–5 weeks). From TARGIT [15]
	21 Gy	1	21 Gy	Intra-op	From ELIOT [35]
Brachytherapy	5.2 Gy	7	36.4 Gy	4 days, BID	From Hungary trial [32]
	4 Gy	8	32 Gy	4 days, BID	From GEC-ESTRO trial [3]
	4.33 Gy	7	30.3 Gy	4 days, BID	From GEC-ESTRO trial [3]
	3.4 Gy	10	34 Gy	5 days, BID	From NSABP B39 [30], MammoSite study [36], RTOG 9517 [37]
	7.5 Gy	3	22.5 Gy	2–3 days, BID	From TRIUMPH T trial [38]

Abbreviations: *BID* 2 fractions per day, *QOD* fractions on alternate days

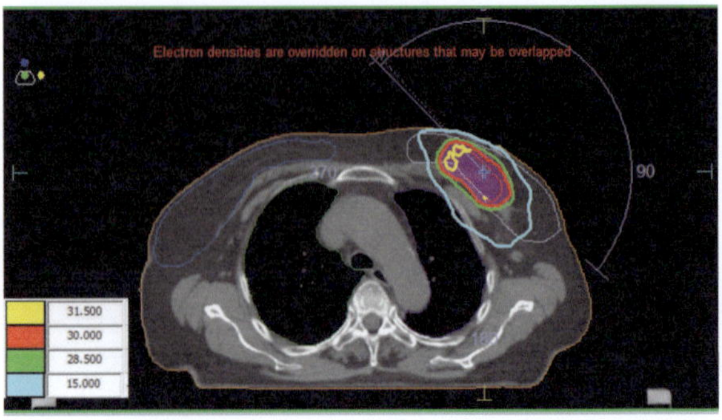

Fig. 24.4 Dose distribution of a VMAT treatment plan for PBI treatment (30 Gy in 5 fractions). In magenta color wash the PTV. Image used with permission of Livia Marrazzo (Medical Physics Unit, Radiation Oncology Department, Florence University Hospital, Florence, Italy)

24.5 Normal Tissue Constraints

Dose constraints vary by study and modality. ASTRO's most recent guidelines recommend following the dosimetric constraints in the NSABP B39/RTOG 0413 trial [30]. Especially for bis-in-day (BID) schedules (i.e., RAPID trial and IRMA trial) the tolerance of the ribs should not exceed suggested dose constraints to avoid rib fractures/pain (Table 24.7) [2]. However, BID schedules are not recommended by international guidelines [13] due to the reported worse toxic effects and cosmetic outcomes [2, 39]. Target and OAR dose constraints for plan optimization from the APBI-IMRT-Florence trial (30 Gy in 5 fractions) are reported in Table 24.8 [25].

Table 24.7 ASTRO guidelines

Technique	Normal tissue	Constraint
Brachytherapy	Skin	$D_{max} \leq 100\%$
	Ipsilateral breast	$V_{\geq 50\%} \leq 60\%$
MammoSite	Ipsilateral breast	$V_{150\%} \leq 50\ cm^3$
		$V_{200\%} \leq 10\ cm^3$
		$V_{\geq 50\%} \leq 60\%$
SAVI	Ipsilateral breast	*(3 fx)*$V_{150\%}$ *<40* cm^3 *(10 fx)* $V_{150\%} \leq 50\ cm^3$
		(3 fx)$V_{200\%}$ *<17*cm^3 *(10 fx)*$V_{200\%} \leq 20\ cm^3$
		$V_{\geq 50\%} \leq 60\%$
External beam	Ipsilateral breast	$V_{\geq 50\%} \leq 60\%$ $V_{100\%} \leq 35\%$
	Contralateral breast	$D_{max} \leq 3\%$
	Ipsilateral lung	$V_{30\%} < 15\%$
	Contralateral lung	$V_{5\%} < 15\%$
	Heart (R)	$V_{5\%} < 5\%$
	Heart (L)	$V_{5\%} < 40\%$
	Thyroid	$D_{max} \leq 3\%$

Table 24.8 Target and OARs dose constraints for plan optimization from the APBI-IMRT-Florence trial (30 Gy in 5 fx) [25]

Target and OARs	Original dose constraints for plan optimization	Updated dose constraints for plan optimization	
		Ideal	Minor deviation accepted
PTV	$V_{28.5\ Gy} = v100\%$	$V_{28.5\ Gy} \geq 98\%$	$V_{28.5\ Gy} \geq 95\%$
	$D_{max} \leq 105\%$	$V_{31.5\ Gy} \leq 5\%$	$V_{31.5\ Gy} \leq 10\%$
	$D_{min} \geq 28$ Gy	$D_{max} \leq 110\%$	
Ipsilateral uninvolved breast	$V_{15\ Gy} \leq 50\%$	$V_{15\ Gy} \leq 50\%$	
Ipsilateral lung	$V_{10\ Gy} \leq 20\%$	$V_{10\ Gy} \leq 20\%$	
Contralateral lung	$V_{5\ Gy} \leq 10\%$	$V_{5\ Gy} \leq 10\%$	
Contralateral breast	$D_{max} \leq 1$ Gy	$D_{max} \leq 1$ Gy	$D_{max} \leq 2$ Gy
Heart	$V_{3\ Gy} \leq 10\%$	$V_{3\ Gy} \leq 10\%$	

24.6 Patient Management

In general, as contemporary PBI applies very similar prescriptions compared with WBI, side effects, both acute and late, are significantly lower compared with WBI, as demonstrated in several trials, because of the lower size of the irradiated volumes. If care is taken to respect appropriate indications, prescriptions, and techniques, side effects are low both in frequency and in severity. Of course, they remain subject to specific circumstances such as a target volume close to the skin (especially if at the inframammary fold), individual patient's radiosensitivity, and, as a special case, re-irradiation with PBI as part of second breast-conserving therapy. The recent publication of the volume analysis of the DBCG-PBI trial nicely demonstrated a relation between breast induration grade 2–3 at 3 years after treatment and the irradiated breast volume, valid for PBI as well as for WBI. Grade 2–3 induration 5% and 10% risks were observed for ≥40 Gy delivered to breast volumes of 177 ml (95% CI, 94–260 ml) and 426 ml (95% CI, 286–567 ml), respectively, strongly favoring small volumes and PBI [33, 40].

24.6.1 Acute Toxicity

Skin reaction: It is common in case of WBI and commonly characterized by mild skin erythema; dry or wet desquamation represents exceptional cases, even more when using PBI. The rate depends on several technical factors, patient's anatomy (skin folds), and individual radiosensitivity. It appears similar or lower with hypofractionation as compared with conventional fractionated in most studies [41]. PBI reported improved outcomes in terms of acute toxic effects as compared with WBI usually delivered using 2 Gy per fraction schedules [1, 2, 4, 30, 35]. Fat necrosis usually appears as a palpable mass with or without pain, and it has been reported with various treatment modalities, especially brachytherapy [36].

- Prevention: Various approaches have been explored for the prevention of acute skin reactions with mixed results. General precautions include avoidance of skin irritants (alcohol-based or fragrant lotions and soaps), use of moisturizing agents (Aquaphor, aloe, Calendula, etc.), and maintenance of a dry environment, particularly in skin folds such as the inframammary fold.
- Skin erythema: symptomatic management only.
- Folliculitis: consider the use of topical steroids (1% hydrocortisone cream).
- Moist desquamation: consider the use of a physical barrier (Mepilex) or 1% Silvadene cream. These should be applied after RT treatments.

Pain: OTC pain medications are often adequate, but prescription pain medications may be needed.

24.6.2 Late Toxicity

Breast cosmesis: It can include fibrosis, edema, and telangiectasias. Mild changes are seen in the majority of patients. More significant late toxicity is less common (<5%). Late cosmetic outcomes appear similar (or slightly better) with hypofractionation compared with conventional fractionation.

The use of pentoxifylline (400 mg tid or 800 mg qd) and vitamin E (300–1000 IU daily) for 6 months has been found to reduce the risk of fibrosis [42]. If the patient has undergone breast reconstruction prior to RT, cosmetic issues such as asymmetry, hardness, or capsular contraction can occur following RT.

24.6.3 Rare Late Toxicities

Cardiac toxicity: There does not appear to be a threshold dose. The absolute increase in the risk of a coronary event is small if the RT dose to the heart is limited (likely <1% if the mean heart dose <3 Gy) [43].

Radiation pneumonitis: The risk of clinically significant pneumonitis is <1% but depends on lung volume in the field. If symptomatic, it can be treated with a course of steroids tapered over 6–12 weeks.

Rib fracture: <2% in hypofractionated trials [44]. Patients treated with brachytherapy or IOeRT PBI can experience additional side effects, at slightly higher rates compared with surgery alone, such as infection, in less than 10% of cases.

24.7 Follow-Up

ASCO and NCCN recommendations for breast cancer follow-up include [45]:

- Clinical evaluation, including breast exam and assessment of acute/late toxicities:
  - Year 1–3 every 3–6 months.
  - Year 4–5 every 6–12 months.
  - Year 5–10 annually.
- First mammogram no earlier than 6 months following treatment completion and then only if signs, symptoms, or if required per trial participation. Subsequent mammograms every 12 months.

Especially as PBI is given to low-risk patients, only basic imaging-based follow-up is required, with extra checks based on signs and symptoms. A first clinical evaluation after a couple of months and annual imaging with phone-based consultation can also give excellent patient satisfaction [46, 47]. In the case of re-irradiation, follow-up should be adapted [48].

24.8 Relevant Literature

24.8.1 Brachytherapy

Two randomized studies and several non-randomized studies have evaluated PBI delivered via brachytherapy following breast-conserving surgery (see Table 24.9). Few prospective and retrospective studies have evaluated APBI brachytherapy for

Table 24.9 Relevant literature: brachytherapy

Study	Patients	Treatment	Median follow-up	Outcomes
Randomized trials				
GEC-ESTRO [3]	$N = 1184$, age > 40, size ≤ 3 cm (89% T1), 95% pN0	**Arm 1:** APBI multicatheter interstitial HDR (32 Gy/8 fx or 30.3 Gy/7 fx, BID) or PDR (50 Gy, pulses 0.6–0.8 Gy/h) **Arm 2:** Whole breast 50 Gy/25 fx or 50.4 Gy/28 fx + 10 Gy boost	6.6 years	**Arm 1:** • 1.4% 5-year LR • 3.2% G2/3 Late side effects **Arm 2:** • 0.9% 5-year LR (NS) • 5.7% G2/3 Late side effects ($p = 0.08$)
National Institute of Oncology-Hungary [32]	$N = 258$, age > 40 (median 49), T1, pN0–N1mi, grade 1–2, no ILC, 68% received hormonal therapy (89% ER pos)	**Arm 1:** APBI multicatheter interstitial HDR (36.4 Gy/7 fx) or EBRT with electrons (see EBRT APBI) **Arm 2:** Whole breast 50 Gy/25 fx	10.2 years	**Arm 1:** • 5.9% LR rate • 81% with good/excellent cosmesis **Arm 2:** • 5.1% LR rate (NS) • 63% with good/excellent cosmesis ($p < 0.01$)

Abbreviations: *APBI* accelerated partial breast irradiation, *HDR* high dose rate, *PDR* pulsed dose rate, *Gy* gray, *fx* fraction(s), *LR* local recurrence/relapse, *ILC* invasive lobular carcinoma, *ER* estrogen receptor, *EBRT* external beam radiation therapy

individuals experiencing local recurrence following initial breast-conserving therapy who choose to have repeat lumpectomy (see Table 24.10). A relevant systematic review reported the main studies [17].

24.8.2 IeORT

There is a major phase 3 trial that assessed the use of IeORT to deliver accelerated PBI (Table 24.10).

24.8.3 External Beam RT

The use of external beam RT to deliver accelerated PBI has been examined in multiple randomized and non-randomized trials (Table 24.11).

Table 24.10 Relevant literature: IORT for the primary tumor

Study	Patients	Treatment	Median follow-up	Outcomes
ELIOT [35]	*N* = 1305, age 48–75, tumor size <2.5 cm, 74% N0	**Arm 1:** IORT 21 Gy to tumor bed with electrons **Arm 2:** Whole breast: 50 Gy/25 fx + 10 Gy boost	12.4 years	**Arm 1:** • 8.1% 10-year IBTR • 90.7% 10-year OS • 1% acute skin toxicity (5 years) • 1% late skin toxicity (5 years) **Arm 2:** • 1.1% 10-year IBTR ($p < 0.01$) • 92.7% 10-year OS (NS) • 7% acute skin toxicity ($p < 0.01$) (5 years) • 1% late skin toxicity (5 years)

Abbreviations: *IORT* intraoperative radiation therapy, *Gy* gray, *fx* fraction(s), *IBTR* ipsilateral breast tumor recurrence, *OS* overall survival

Table 24.11 Relevant literature: external beam RT

Study	Patients	Treatment	Median follow-up	Outcomes
Randomized trials				
National Institute of Oncology-Hungary [32]	*N* = 258, age > 40 (median 49), T1, pN0–N1mi, grade 1–2, no ILC, 68% received hormonal therapy (89% ER pos)	**Arm 1:** APBI multicatheter interstitial HDR (36.4 Gy/7 fx) or EBRT with electrons (see EBRT APBI) **Arm 2:** Whole breast 50 Gy/25 fx	10.2 years	**Arm 1:** • 5.9% LR rate • 81% with good/excellent cosmesis **Arm 2:** • 5.1% LR rate (NS) • 63% with good/excellent cosmesis ($p < 0.01$)
University of Florence [4]	*N* = 520, age > 40, size <2.5 cm, 86% pN0	**Arm 1:** APBI with IMRT 30 Gy/5 fx **Arm 2:** Whole breast: 50 Gy + 10 Gy boost	10.7 years	**Arm 1:** • 3.7% 10-year IBTR 94.7% with excellent cosmesis • 2% grade ≥ 2 acute toxicity **Arm 2:** • 2.5% 10-year IBTR (NS) • 72.7% with excellent cosmesis ($p = 0.05$) • 37.7% grade ≥ 2 acute toxicity ($p = 0.02$)

(continued)

Table 24.11 (continued)

Study	Patients	Treatment	Median follow-up	Outcomes
Barcelona [29]	$N = 102$, age ≥ 60, tumor size ≤ 3 cm (90% T1), pN0, grade 1 or 2	**Arm 1:** APBI: 37.5 Gy/10 fx (BID) **Arm 2:** Whole breast: 48 Gy/24 fx ±10 Gy boost	5 years	**Arm 1:** • No local failures • 18% acute grade ≥ 2 toxicity **Arm 2:** • No local failures • 75% acute grade ≥ 2 toxicity
RAPID [2]	$N = 2135$, 88% over age > 50, 18% DCIS, size ≤ 3 cm, pN0	**Arm 1:** APBI: 38.5 Gy/10 fx (BID) **Arm 2:** Whole breast: 42.5 Gy/16 fx or 50 Gy/25 fx ± boost	8.2 years	**Arm 1:** • 3% IBTR 8-year cumulative incidence • 28% acute grade ≥ 2 toxicity • 32% late grade ≥ 2 toxicity **Arm 2:** • 2.8% IBTR 8-year cumulative incidence • 45% acute grade ≥ 2 toxicity • 13% late grade ≥ 2 toxicity
Other prospective trials				
RTOG 0319 [49]	$N = 52$, size ≤ 3 cm, ≤ 3 Pos LN	APBI: 38.5 Gy/10 fx (BID over 5 days)	5.3 years	• 82% with patient-reported good/excellent cosmesis • 56% with G2/3 skin toxicity

Abbreviations: *ILC* invasive lobular carcinoma, *ER* estrogen receptor, *APBI* accelerated partial breast irradiation, *HDR* high dose rate, *EBRT* external beam radiation therapy, *Gy* gray, *fx* fraction(s), *LR* local recurrence/relapse, *IMRT* intensity-modulated radiotherapy, *IBTR* ipsilateral breast tumor recurrence, *DCIS* ductal carcinoma in situ

24.8.4 Summary

A reduction of irradiated breast volume is of utmost importance even in this era of 26 Gy in 5 fractions, introduced as WBI schedule, and cardiac toxicity prevention tools such as breath-hold and intensity-modulated techniques [50]. In selected patients, following the most recent international guidelines and recommendations, PBI should be preferred over WBI in order to obtain the best balance between treatment course length, disease control, and toxicity/cosmetic outcomes [40, 51]. We have probably reached a plateau in terms of the optimal number of fractions for PBI delivery, and in the future, new perspectives will be investigated, such as the preoperative intent of radiation, alone or integrated with systemic therapies [52].

References

1. Coles CE, Griffin CL, Kirby AM, et al. Partial-breast radiotherapy after breast conservation surgery for patients with early breast cancer (UK IMPORT LOW trial): 5-year results from a multicentre, randomised, controlled, phase 3, non-inferiority trial. Lancet. 2017;390:1048–60.
2. Whelan TJ, Julian JA, Berrang TS, et al. External beam accelerated partial breast irradiation versus whole breast irradiation after breast conserving surgery in women with ductal carcinoma in situ and node-negative breast cancer (RAPID): a randomised controlled trial. Lancet. 2019;394:2165–72.
3. Strnad V, Ott OJ, Hildebrandt G, et al. 5-year results of accelerated partial breast irradiation using sole interstitial multicatheter brachytherapy versus whole-breast irradiation with boost after breast-conserving surgery for low-risk invasive and in-situ carcinoma of the female breast: a randomised, phase 3, non-inferiority trial. Lancet. 2016;387:229–38.
4. Meattini I, Marrazzo L, Saieva C, et al. Accelerated partial-breast irradiation compared with whole-breast irradiation for early breast cancer: long-term results of the randomized phase III APBI-IMRT-Florence Trial. J Clin Oncol. 2020;38:4175–83.
5. Lv Y, He L, Wang C, et al. A systematic review of clinical outcomes and radiotherapy-associated toxicity in multicatheter accelerated partial breast irradiation. Medicine (Baltimore). 2019;98:e14407.
6. Marta GN, Barrett J, Porfirio GJM, et al. Effectiveness of different accelerated partial breast irradiation techniques for the treatment of breast cancer patients: Systematic review using indirect comparisons of randomized clinical trials. Rep Pract Oncol Radiother. 2019;24:165–74.
7. Viani GA, Arruda CV, Faustino AC, De Fendi LI. Partial-breast irradiation versus whole-breast radiotherapy for early breast cancer: A systematic review and update meta-analysis. Brachytherapy. 2020;19:491–8.
8. Correa C, Harris EE, Leonardi MC, et al. Accelerated partial breast irradiation: executive summary for the update of an ASTRO Evidence-Based Consensus Statement. Pract Radiat Oncol. 2017;7:73–9.
9. Shaitelman SF, Anderson BM, Arthur DW, et al. Partial Breast Irradiation for Patients With Early-Stage Invasive Breast Cancer or Ductal Carcinoma In Situ: An ASTRO Clinical Practice Guideline. Pract Radiat Oncol. 2023 Nov 14:S1879-8500(23)00296-5. doi: 10.1016/j.prro.2023.11.001. Epub ahead of print. PMID: 37977261.
10. Kaidar-Person O, et al. ESTRO addition to the publication of the American Society for Radiation Oncology clinical practice guideline for partial breast irradiation for patients with early-stage invasive breast cancer or ductal carcinoma in situ. Practical Radiation Oncology. 2024. In press.
11. Anderson B, Arthur D, Hannoun-Levi JM, et al. Partial breast irradiation: An updated consensus statement from the American brachytherapy society. Brachytherapy. 2022;21:726–47.
12. Polgar C, Van Limbergen E, Potter R, et al. Patient selection for accelerated partial-breast irradiation (APBI) after breast-conserving surgery: recommendations of the Groupe Europeen de Curietherapie-European Society for Therapeutic Radiology and Oncology (GEC-ESTRO) breast cancer working group based on clinical evidence (2009). Radiother Oncol. 2010;94:264–73.
13. Meattini I, Becherini C, Boersma L, et al. European Society for Radiotherapy and Oncology Advisory Committee in Radiation Oncology Practice consensus recommendations on patient selection and dose and fractionation for external beam radiotherapy in early breast cancer. Lancet Oncol. 2022;23:e21–31.
14. Meattini I, Poortmans P, Livi L, et al. Partial breast irradiation for ductal carcinoma in situ: The Goldilocks principle? Breast J. 2018;24:1118–9.
15. Hannoun-Levi JM, Gal J, Schiappa R, Chand ME. 10-Year oncological outcome report after second conservative treatment for ipsilateral breast tumor event. Clin Transl Radiat Oncol. 2023;38:71–6.
16. Hannoun-Levi JM, Gal J, Van Limbergen E, et al. Salvage mastectomy versus second conservative treatment for second ipsilateral breast tumor event: a propensity score-matched cohort

analysis of the GEC-ESTRO Breast Cancer Working Group Database. Int J Radiat Oncol Biol Phys. 2021;110:452–61.
17. Montagne L, Hannoun A, Hannoun-Levi JM. Second conservative treatment for second ipsilateral breast tumor event: A systematic review of the different re-irradiation techniques. Breast. 2020;49:274–80.
18. Montagne L, Gal J, Chand ME, et al. GEC-ESTRO APBI classification as a decision-making tool for the management of 2nd ipsilateral breast tumor event. Breast Cancer Res Treat. 2019;176:149–57.
19. Arthur DW, Winter KA, Kuerer HM, et al. Effectiveness of breast-conserving surgery and 3-dimensional conformal partial breast reirradiation for recurrence of breast cancer in the ipsilateral breast: the NRG Oncology/RTOG 1014 Phase 2 Clinical Trial. JAMA Oncol. 2020;6:75–82.
20. Andratschke N, Willmann J, Appelt AL, et al. European Society for Radiotherapy and Oncology and European Organisation for Research and Treatment of Cancer consensus on re-irradiation: definition, reporting, and clinical decision making. Lancet Oncol. 2022;23:e469–78.
21. Kaidar-Person O, Meattini I, Zippel D, Poortmans P. Apples and oranges: comparing partial breast irradiation techniques. Rep Pract Oncol Radiother. 2020;25:780–2.
22. Kaidar-Person O, Offersen BV, Boersma L, et al. Tricks and tips for target volume definition and delineation in breast cancer: lessons learned from ESTRO breast courses. Radiother Oncol. 2021;162:185–94.
23. Strnad V, Hannoun-Levi JM, Guinot JL, et al. Recommendations from GEC ESTRO Breast Cancer Working Group (I): Target definition and target delineation for accelerated or boost Partial Breast Irradiation using multicatheter interstitial brachytherapy after breast conserving closed cavity surgery. Radiother Oncol. 2015;115:342–8.
24. Major T, Gutierrez C, Guix B, et al. Recommendations from GEC ESTRO Breast Cancer Working Group (II): Target definition and target delineation for accelerated or boost partial breast irradiation using multicatheter interstitial brachytherapy after breast conserving open cavity surgery. Radiother Oncol. 2016;118:199–204.
25. Marrazzo L, Meattini I, Simontacchi G, et al. Updates on the APBI-IMRT-Florence Trial (NCT02104895) Technique: from the intensity modulated radiation therapy trial to the volumetric modulated arc therapy clinical practice. Pract Radiat Oncol. 2023;13(1):e28–234.
26. Strnad V, Major T, Polgar C, et al. ESTRO-ACROP guideline: Interstitial multi-catheter breast brachytherapy as Accelerated Partial Breast Irradiation alone or as boost—GEC-ESTRO Breast Cancer Working Group practical recommendations. Radiother Oncol. 2018;128:411–20.
27. Fastner G, Gaisberger C, Kaiser J, et al. ESTRO IORT Task Force/ACROP recommendations for intraoperative radiation therapy with electrons (IOERT) in breast cancer. Radiother Oncol. 2020;149:150–7.
28. Marrazzo L, Meattini I, Simontacchi G, et al. Updates on the APBI-IMRT-Florence Trial (NCT02104895) technique: from the intensity modulated radiation therapy trial to the volumetric modulated arc therapy clinical practice. Pract Radiat Oncol. 2023;13:e28–34.
29. Rodriguez N, Sanz X, Dengra J, et al. Five-year outcomes, cosmesis, and toxicity with 3-dimensional conformal external beam radiation therapy to deliver accelerated partial breast irradiation. Int J Radiat Oncol Biol Phys. 2013;87:1051–7.
30. Vicini FA, Cecchini RS, White JR, et al. Long-term primary results of accelerated partial breast irradiation after breast-conserving surgery for early-stage breast cancer: a randomised, phase 3, equivalence trial. Lancet. 2019;394:2155–64.
31. Rabinovitch R, Moughan J, Vicini F, et al. Long-Term Update of NRG Oncology RTOG 0319: a phase 1 and 2 trial to evaluate 3-dimensional Conformal radiation therapy confined to the region of the lumpectomy cavity for stage I and II breast carcinoma. Int J Radiat Oncol Biol Phys. 2016;96:1054–9.
32. Polgar C, Fodor J, Major T, et al. Breast-conserving therapy with partial or whole breast irradiation: ten-year results of the Budapest randomized trial. Radiother Oncol. 2013;108:197–202.

33. Offersen BV, Alsner J, Nielsen HM, et al. Partial breast irradiation versus whole breast irradiation for early breast cancer patients in a randomized phase III trial: the Danish Breast Cancer Group Partial Breast Irradiation Trial. J Clin Oncol. 2022;40:4189–97.
34. Murray Brunt A, Haviland JS, Wheatley DA, et al. Hypofractionated breast radiotherapy for 1 week versus 3 weeks (FAST-Forward): 5-year efficacy and late normal tissue effects results from a multicentre, non-inferiority, randomised, phase 3 trial. Lancet. 2020;395:1613–26.
35. Orecchia R, Veronesi U, Maisonneuve P, et al. Intraoperative irradiation for early breast cancer (ELIOT): long-term recurrence and survival outcomes from a single-centre, randomised, phase 3 equivalence trial. Lancet Oncol. 2021;22:597–608.
36. Shah C, Badiyan S, Ben Wilkinson J, et al. Treatment efficacy with accelerated partial breast irradiation (APBI): final analysis of the American Society of Breast Surgeons MammoSite((R)) breast brachytherapy registry trial. Ann Surg Oncol. 2013;20:3279–85.
37. Rabinovitch R, Winter K, Kuske R, et al. RTOG 95–17, a Phase II trial to evaluate brachytherapy as the sole method of radiation therapy for Stage I and II breast carcinoma--year-5 toxicity and cosmesis. Brachytherapy. 2014;13:17–22.
38. Khan AJ, Chen PY, Yashar C, et al. Three-fraction accelerated partial breast irradiation (APBI) delivered with brachytherapy applicators is feasible and safe: first results from the TRIUMPH-T trial. Int J Radiat Oncol Biol Phys. 2019;104:67–74.
39. Meduri B, Baldissera A, Iotti C, et al. Cosmetic results and side effects of accelerated partial-breast irradiation versus whole-breast irradiation for low-risk invasive carcinoma of the breast: the randomized phase III IRMA trial. J Clin Oncol. 2023;41(12):2201–10.
40. Thomsen MS, Alsner J, Nielsen HM, et al. Volume matters: breast induration is associated with irradiated breast volume in the Danish Breast Cancer Group phase III randomized Partial Breast Irradiation trial. Radiother Oncol. 2022;177:231–5.
41. Shaitelman SF, Schlembach PJ, Arzu I, et al. Acute and short-term toxic effects of conventionally fractionated vs hypofractionated whole-breast irradiation: a randomized clinical trial. JAMA Oncol. 2015;1:931–41.
42. Jacobson G, Bhatia S, Smith BJ, et al. Randomized trial of pentoxifylline and vitamin E vs standard follow-up after breast irradiation to prevent breast fibrosis, evaluated by tissue compliance meter. Int J Radiat Oncol Biol Phys. 2013;85:604–8.
43. Darby SC, Ewertz M, McGale P, et al. Risk of ischemic heart disease in women after radiotherapy for breast cancer. N Engl J Med. 2013;368:987–98.
44. Haviland JS, Owen JR, Dewar JA, et al. The UK Standardisation of Breast Radiotherapy (START) trials of radiotherapy hypofractionation for treatment of early breast cancer: 10-year follow-up results of two randomised controlled trials. Lancet Oncol. 2013;14:1086–94.
45. Runowicz CD, Leach CR, Henry NL, et al. American Cancer Society/American Society of Clinical Oncology Breast Cancer Survivorship Care Guideline. J Clin Oncol. 2016;34:611–35.
46. Kimman ML, Dirksen CD, Voogd AC, et al. Nurse-led telephone follow-up and an educational group programme after breast cancer treatment: results of a 2 × 2 randomised controlled trial. Eur J Cancer. 2011;47:1027–36.
47. Kimman ML, Bloebaum MM, Dirksen CD, et al. Patient satisfaction with nurse-led telephone follow-up after curative treatment for breast cancer. BMC Cancer. 2010;10:174.
48. De Rose F, Meduri B, De Santis MC, et al. Rethinking breast cancer follow-up based on individual risk and recurrence management. Cancer Treat Rev. 2022;109:102434.
49. Chafe S, Moughan J, McCormick B, et al. Late toxicity and patient self-assessment of breast appearance/satisfaction on RTOG 0319: a phase 2 trial of 3-dimensional conformal radiation therapy-accelerated partial breast irradiation following lumpectomy for stages I and II breast cancer. Int J Radiat Oncol Biol Phys. 2013;86:854–9.
50. Essers M, Osman SO, Hol S, et al. Accelerated partial breast irradiation (APBI): are breath-hold and volumetric radiation therapy techniques useful? Acta Oncol. 2014;53:788–94.
51. Kaidar-Person O, Gentilini O, Poortmans P. Not only volumes matter for breast radiation therapy. Radiother Oncol. 2022;177:236–7.
52. Montalvo SK, Collins B, Vicini F, Rahimi A. Stereotactic partial breast irradiation: what does the future hold? Am J Clin Oncol. 2023;46:20–4.

Part VII
Gastrointestinal Cancer

Chapter 25
Hepatobiliary Malignancies

Chiao-Ling Tsai, Jason Chia-Hsien Cheng, Kyle Wang, Andrew Z. Wang, and Joel E. Tepper

25.1 Introduction

The radiosensitivity of hepatocytes and risk for radiation-induced liver disease (RILD) precluded the use of radiotherapy (RT) for liver tumors using conventional techniques. CT-based planning, stereotactic body radiation therapy (SBRT), and intensity-modulated radiation therapy (IMRT) have generated renewed interest and the growing need in the treatment of liver malignancies due to the new ability to deliver high doses to tumors with good normal tissue sparing. Though surgery is the primary treatment modality for liver tumors, RT provides previously unavailable opportunities for durable local control in patients who are inoperable or not candidates for other ablative approaches. The growing evidence of large multi-center retrospective studies and few randomized trials supports the role of RT in small HCC with non-inferior control to radiofrequency ablation and combined RT and embolization in advanced HCC with superior survival outcomes to sorafenib. Here, we review hypofractionated RT (for tumors close to bowels) and SBRT (preferred option) for hepatocellular carcinoma (HCC), cholangiocarcinoma (predominantly

C.-L. Tsai · J. C.-H. Cheng (✉)
Division of Radiation Oncology, Department of Oncology, National Taiwan University Hospital, Taipei, Taiwan
e-mail: jasoncheng@ntu.edu.tw

K. Wang
Cincinnati, OH, USA

A. Z. Wang
UT Southwestern Medical Center, Dallas, TX, USA

J. E. Tepper
Department of Radiation Oncology, University of North Carolina Hospitals, Chapel Hill, NC, USA

O. Kaidar-Person, R. Chen (eds.), *Hypofractionated and Stereotactic Radiation Therapy*, https://doi.org/10.1007/978-3-031-47701-0_25

intrahepatic and perihilar types), and liver metastases. Though these are distinct clinical entities, the principles of SBRT delivery are similar. Patients with HCC may have comorbid cirrhosis which may impact treatment planning.

25.2 Pearls

Hepatocellular Carcinoma (HCC)

- In 2018, 8 new cases per 100,000 were reported in the United States. It is the second leading cause of cancer mortality worldwide and is more common in males. The median age of diagnosis is 65 years.
- The major risk factor is cirrhosis due to any cause, most commonly viral hepatitis, but also hemochromatosis, alcohol, and nonalcoholic steatohepatitis. Hepatitis C is the dominant factor in the United States, though hepatitis B is more common worldwide.
- Clinical presentation often reflects underlying liver disease and may include symptoms of portal hypertension and/or impaired metabolisms such as ascites, gastrointestinal (GI) variceal bleeding, and hepatic encephalopathy.
- HCC arises from hepatocytes and may be well, moderately, or poorly differentiated, with rarer subtypes including small cell, giant cell, and spindle cell variants.
- It may present anywhere in the liver as circumscribed solitary or multifocal nodules.
- It may spread regionally to portohepatic, peripancreatic, gastroduodenal, portocaval, and para-aortic nodes. The most common distant sites of spread are the lung and bone.
- Medical work-up: LFTs including tests of synthetic function such as PT-INR and albumin, total bilirubin, HBV/HCV viral serologies, CBC, chemistries, and AFP.
- Imaging work-up: Ultrasound is used for screening high-risk patients. Three-phase CT and MRI are used for definitive diagnosis and post-RT follow-up. Biopsy is not required if imaging is conclusive.
- Treatment: Options include surgery (transplant/partial hepatectomy), microwave/radiofrequency ablation, RT, embolization (bland−/chemo−/radio-), targeted drugs, immunotherapy, and chemotherapy.

Cholangiocarcinoma

- Includes intrahepatic, perihilar (Klatskin tumors), and distal types. Incidence is 1–2 per 100,000 in the United States and increases with age (median 60–70) and male sex, with roughly an equal distribution of intrahepatic and extrahepatic (including perihilar) varieties.
- Intrahepatic cholangiocarcinoma in the past was often thought to represent metastatic disease to the liver of unknown primary. With increasing recognition of its etiology as a distinct bile duct cancer, the reported incidence has risen in recent decades.

- Risk factors include primary sclerosing cholangitis, cystic liver disease, hepatolithiasis, and parasitic infections. There is some association with cirrhosis and hepatitis.
- Genetic predisposing conditions include Lynch syndrome and biliary papillomatosis.
- Presents with signs/symptoms of biliary obstruction, abdominal pain, and weight loss. Intrahepatic varieties are less likely to present with biliary obstruction.
- Most are adenocarcinomas and are divided into nodular, sclerosing, and papillary types.
- Intrahepatic cholangiocarcinomas are further subdivided into mass-forming, periductal invasion, and intraductal growth types.
- 30–40% of patients with intrahepatic cholangiocarcinoma have nodal involvement at the time of surgical treatment.
- Medical work-up: CA 19–9 (elevated in 75%), CEA (less sensitive and specific than CA 19–9), AFP (more likely mixed HCC if elevated), and LFTs.
- Imaging work-up: MRI is the most informative. Other modalities include CT, abdominal and endoscopic ultrasound, and biliary tract imaging including ERCP and MRCP. Therapeutic biliary stents may be deployed during work-up for distal tumors.
- Treatment: Surgery with postop chemotherapy ± RT if resectable; chemotherapy ± RT if unresectable.

Liver Metastases

- Common site of distant metastasis for many malignancies, especially colorectal cancer but also lung, breast, and others.
- Usually detected with staging scans or elevated tumor markers, though can present with symptoms of abdominal pain, jaundice, and laboratory abnormalities.
- Medical work-up: Liver synthetic function tests including PT-INR, albumin, and platelet count are helpful in assessing the ability of the patient to tolerate aggressive locoregional therapy.
- Imaging work-up: Includes contrast-enhanced CT, MRI, and PET scans.
- Treatment: For limited metastatic disease (usually from colorectal cancer), aggressive locoregional treatment such as surgery, ablation, and/or RT may be used.

25.3 Barcelona Clinic Liver Cancer (BCLC) [1] Staging Table: Hepatocellular Carcinoma

0: Very early	Solitary <2 cm tumor, Child-Pugh A, ECOG 0
A: Early	Single or ≤ 3 nodules <3 cm, Child-Pugh A-B, ECOG 0
B: Intermediate	Large multinodular, Child-Pugh A-B, ECOG 0
C: Advanced	Portal invasion, extrahepatic spread, Child-Pugh A-B, ECOG 1–2
D: Terminal	Child-Pugh C, ECOG 3–4

25.4 Tumor/Patient Selection

- SBRT is used in patients with limited disease, alone or in combination with surgery or RFA, for:
  - Inoperable patients (e.g., due to disease extent, surgically difficult sites, and/or comorbidities).
  - Lesions located in areas precluding the use of other ablation techniques, such as RFA (e.g., major vessels that act as a heat sink, bile ducts prone to heat injury, and liver capsule where RFA may cause pain).
  - Positive surgical margins.
  - Consolidative treatment following TACE/selective internal radiation therapy (SIRT) [2, 3].
  - As a bridge to liver transplant [4].
  - Neoadjuvant treatment before resection [5].
  - Salvage for patients with progression in isolated sites.
- In addition to the above patient selection criteria, the combination of tumor size and total liver volume must meet liver dose-volume constraints (see Toxicities).
- For patients with large tumors or compromised liver function, dosimetric studies suggest advantages of charged particle therapy such as carbon ions and protons in reducing the low-dose volume, which is of particular importance in a radiosensitive, "parallel" organ such as the liver [6, 7].
- Disease-specific considerations **(HCC)**:
  - For patients ineligible for other treatments, SBRT and other conformal hypofractionated RT techniques lead to impressive local control, even for large tumors with adverse features such as tumor vascular thrombi.
  - SBRT should not be used concurrently with sorafenib based on a recent Phase I study reporting unacceptably high rates of GI toxicity [8].
  - Both EBRT and SBRT are category 2 recommendations for locoregional treatment in the NCCN guidelines for inoperable HCC [9].
  - The frequent presence of cirrhosis reduces liver "reserve" and requires the use of more stringent dose-volume criteria during patient selection and radiation planning for patients with compromised liver function, e.g., Child-Pugh B patients (see Toxicities).
- Disease-specific considerations **(cholangiocarcinoma)**:
  - Similar to HCC, standard management is surgical resection, but many tumors/patients are inoperable.
  - The use of SBRT or hypofractionated conformal RT provides an opportunity for durable local control and potential cure.
- Disease-specific considerations **(liver metastases)**:
  - For patients with limited colorectal cancer liver metastases, aggressive locoregional therapy is warranted in the absence of extrahepatic disease.
  - The use of RT for patients ineligible for resection of liver metastases is a category 3 recommendation in the NCCN guidelines [10].

25.5 Treatment Planning Considerations (Fig. 25.1)

Simulation instructions	• Position: Supine with arms overhead (for CyberKnife, patients are simulated with arms at their side for comfort during long treatments) • Immobilization: Vac-Lok or similar device • 4D CT to assess tumor motion • Real-time Position Management (RPM) system with respiratory gating window or breath-hold system for beam delivery • Abdominal compression devices can be used to reduce respiratory variation if RPM or breath-hold system is not satisfactory • The authors usually administer IV contrast to aid triple-phase tumor delineation with arterial (for enhanced HCC), portal-venous (for biliary and hepatic anatomy), and delayed venous (for wash-out HCC), but obtaining proper timing can be difficult, especially for HCC (where diagnostic triphasic CT may be needed for proper visualization)
Image guidance	Linac: • Daily cone beam CT with lesions containing the embolized materials or ablated region close to the tumor for alignment • Fiducials are helpful for daily alignment given the difficulty of visualizing the actual tumor using CT • Respiratory gating or breath-hold techniques may help account for motion CyberKnife: • Fiducial markers for tumor tracking, typically placed by Interventional Radiology at least 7 days prior to simulation
Tumor delineation	• Qualified tri-phase contrast-enhanced simulation CT can be used for direct target delineations, with arterial (enhanced HCC), portal-venous (biliary and hepatic anatomy), and delayed venous (wash-out HCC) phases. • Alternatively, an MRI with contrast can be obtained • HCCs show enhancement on the immediate post-contrast MRI, with later sequences showing washout of the lesion compared with the rest of the liver. The authors select the series and sequence with the best subjective visualization of the tumor for fusion to the CT • Accurate image fusion is difficult and should be based on structures and liver contours close to the target and verified boundaries • The authors contour the GTV on the MRI and verify its accuracy (when possible) on the planning CT itself
Margins	Linac: • An ITV is generated by combining the GTVs at various respiratory phases (if 4D scan is obtained) • CTV, if used with the expansion of GTV by 3–5 mm, is trimmed to be within liver • Based on the degree of tumor motion and uncertainty, a total CTV + PTV margin of 5–10 mm is added around the ITV CyberKnife: • With tumor tracking using fiducials, the authors typically add a 5 mm radial and 8 mm superior/inferior total CTV + PTV margin around the GTV • In cases where motion is greater or MRI fusion is suboptimal, we use total CTV + PTV margins up to 1 cm
Dosimetric considerations	• Goal: 95% of PTV receives 100% prescription dose • To meet constraints of critical nearby structures, especially small bowel, decreased coverage may be accepted, and/or CTV/PTV margins selectively reduced

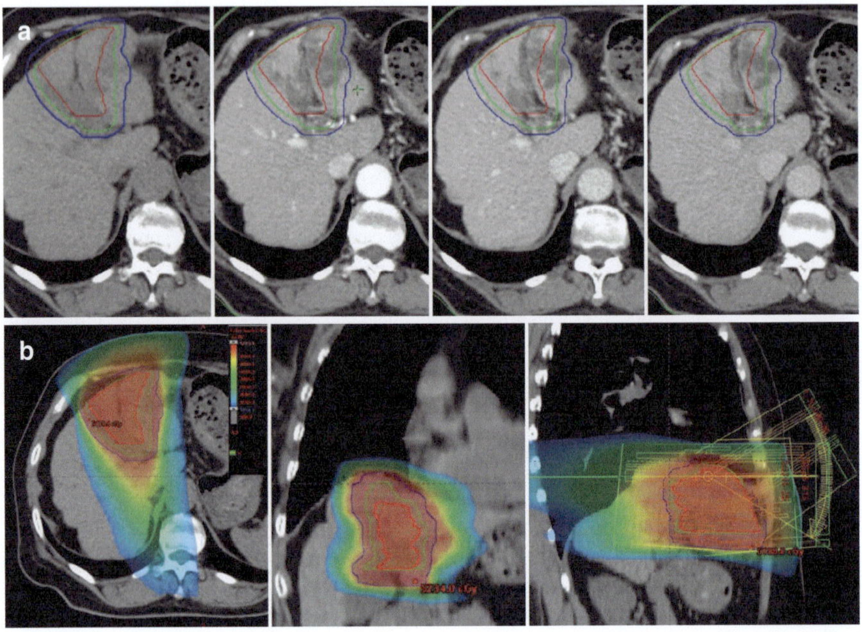

Fig. 25.1 A patient with infiltrative HCCs in the left hepatic lobe refractory to RFA, with left portal vein tumor thrombosis. Contouring and planning considerations for linac-based liver SBRT with 48 Gy in six fractions. (**a**) Selected slices from triphasic contrast-enhanced CT simulation (from left to right: no contrast, arterial, portal-venous, and delayed venous phases), acquired by using a breath-hold system for immobilization. (**b**) The GTV is shown in red, the CTV in green, and the PTV in blue. The treatment plan combined coplanar and non-coplanar VMAT for right-lobe liver sparing

25.6 Commonly Used Dose/Fractionation Schemes

Dose/fx	# of fx	Total dose	Notes
15–20 Gy	3	45–60 Gy	HCC (typically Child-Pugh A) and metastases, typically 1–5 cm [11–16]
7–8 Gy	5	35–40 Gy	HCC, Child-Pugh A or B, typically 1–5 cm [17, 18]
10–15 Gy	3	30–45 Gy	Cholangiocarcinoma, size variable [19, 20]
10–12 Gy	4	48 Gy	HCC (typically Child-Pugh A) and metastases, typically 1–5 cm [15, 21]
6–7 Gy	6	36–42 Gy	HCC (Child-Pugh A), cholangiocarcinoma, and metastases, up to ≈15 cm [22–24]
4.5 Gy	15	67.5 Gy	Cholangiocarcinoma, up to ≈15 cm [25]

Authors' Recommendations

- At the University of North Carolina Hospitals, three-fraction treatments for liver SBRT are generally used
- For patients who meet liver constraints, we typically use 15–20 Gy × 3 fx
- For liver metastases, we typically use slightly higher doses, e.g., 18–20 Gy × 3 fx
- Great care must be taken when deciding to treat Child-Pugh B patients. We only treat patients in the lowest echelon of Child-Pugh B (Child-Pugh 7) with adequate liver volume. Dose/fractionation is variable but ranges between 15 Gy × 3 fx and 7 Gy × 5 fx to more aggressively meet constraints and minimize toxicity
- Deliver SBRT treatments every other day
- Highly recommended: $BED_{10} \geq 100$ Gy for liver SBRT [26]

25.7 Normal Tissue Tolerances

TG101 [27]		Other(s)	Our institutional practice
Liver (minus GTV) Endpoint: grade 3 toxicity			
1 fx	≥700 cc ≤ 9.1 Gy	QUANTEC [28]: Endpoint: 5% RILD (3–5 fx) ≥ 700 cc ≤ 15 Gy **Liver cancer (Child-Pugh A):** (3 fx) mean < 13 Gy (6 fx) mean < 18 Gy **Liver cancer (Child-Pugh B):** (4–6 Gy/fx) mean < 6 Gy **Metastases:** (3 fx) mean < 15 Gy (6 fx) mean < 20 Gy	(3 fx) Mean < 15 Gy ≥700 cc ≤ 15 Gy (Child-Pugh A) ≥700 cc ≤ 13 Gy (Child-Pugh B)
3 fx	≥700 cc ≤ 19.2 Gy		
5 fx	≥700 cc ≤ 21 Gy		
Small bowel (duodenum) Endpoint: Ulceration			
1 fx	*V* 11.2 Gy < 5 cc Dmax ≤ 12.4 Gy	Goldsmith et al. [29] Endpoint: 5% Grade 3 hemorrhage/stricture (1 fx) D 5 cc < 11.2 Gy (3 fx) D 5 cc < 21 Gy (5 fx) D 5 cc < 25.8 Gy (1 fx) D 0.035 cc < 16 Gy (3 fx) D 0.035 cc < 30 Gy (5 fx) D 0.035 cc < 32 Gy	(3 fx) < 1 cc > 30 Gy (5 fx) < 1 cc > 32 Gy
3 fx	*V* 16.5 Gy < 5 cc Dmax ≤ 22.2 Gy		
5 fx	*V* 18 Gy < 5 cc Dmax ≤ 32 Gy		
Stomach Endpoint: Ulceration/fistula			
1 fx	*V* 11.2 Gy < 10 cc Dmax ≤ 12.4 Gy		(3 fx) < 1 cc > 30 Gy
3 fx	*V* 16.5 Gy < 10 cc Dmax ≤ 22.2 Gy		
5 fx	*V* 18 Gy < 10 cc Dmax ≤ 32 Gy		
Esophagus Endpoint: Stenosis/fistula			
1 fx	*V* 11.9 Gy < 5 cc Dmax ≤ 15.4 Gy		(3 fx) < 1 cc > 30 Gy
3 fx	*V* 17.7 Gy < 5 cc Dmax ≤ 25.2 Gy		
5 fx	*V* 19.5 Gy < 5 cc Dmax ≤ 35 Gy		

TG101 [27]		Other(s)	Our institutional practice
Kidney (bilateral) Endpoint: grade 3 toxicity			
1 fx	≥200 cc ≤ 8.4 Gy		We do not have strict unilateral kidney guidelines provided that the patient has adequate bilateral renal function
3 fx	≥200 cc ≤ 16 Gy		
5 fx	≥200 cc ≤ 17.5 Gy		
Colon Endpoint: Colitis/fistula			
1 fx	*V* 14.3 Gy < 20 cc Dmax ≤ 18.4 Gy		
3 fx	*V* 24 Gy < 20 cc Dmax ≤ 28.2 Gy		
5 fx	*V* 25 Gy < 20 cc Dmax ≤ 38 Gy		
Lungs (total) Endpoint: Grade 3 pneumonitis			
1 fx	≥1000 cc ≤ 7.4 Gy		
3 fx	≥1000 cc ≤ 12.4 Gy		
5 fx	≥1000 cc ≤ 13.5 Gy		
Rib Endpoint: Pain/fracture			
1 fx	*V* 22 Gy < 1 cc Dmax ≤ 30 Gy		
3 fx	*V* 28.8 Gy < 1 cc *V* 30 Gy < 30 cc Dmax ≤ 36.9 Gy		
5 fx	*V* 35 Gy < 1 cc Dmax ≤ 43 Gy		

25.8 Patient Management Considerations

- Premedications are optional and the data behind their use are lacking.
  - Dexamethasone (4 mg, once prior to treatment) to reduce acute edema.
  - Antiemetics (e.g., ondansetron 8 mg once prior to treatment) to prevent nausea.
  - For patients who may have difficulty tolerating long treatments, we consider administering a single small dose of a benzodiazepine (e.g., lorazepam, 0.5–1 mg) 30 min prior to treatment.

- Toxicities: Nausea, abdominal pain, and fatigue may occur acutely but are rare. Other acute toxicities include transient thrombocytopenia and elevation in transaminases, as well as RILD, which can also be a late toxicity. Overall, grade 3 toxicities are higher in patients with HCC and worse baseline liver function (typically 10–15%) [16, 21, 22, 30] vs. liver metastases (typically <5%) [31, 32].
- "Classic" RILD occurs within 4 months of RT and is manifested by anicteric hepatomegaly, ascites, and elevated LFTs (especially alkaline phosphatase) often leading to liver failure and death. The pathophysiology is thought to be inflammation leading to venous congestion, which may worsen portal hypertension. Reports are rare in modern series utilizing highly conformal RT.
- "Nonclassic" RILD includes a decline in liver function or transient LFT elevation in the absence of classic RILD; it was originally found with the pathogenesis of viral hepatitis from HBV reactivation [33, 34]. Although many patients have progression of pre-existing liver disease after treatment, RT may accelerate this process and lead to a worsening of Child-Pugh score and/or class, which is observed in 10–20% of HCC patients according to recent SBRT series [13, 17, 18, 22].
- Biliary stenosis in the absence of disease progression is rare (<5%), even after treatment for centrally located tumors [25, 35]. Patients with signs of biliary obstruction should undergo ERCP.
- Patients with tumors located near the esophagus and bowel are at risk for ulceration, stenosis, and bleeding, though reports of severe non-hepatic toxicities are rare.
- A prospective assessment of QOL in 222 patients treated with SBRT for liver tumors showed an acute worsening of appetite and fatigue at 1 month post-treatment but recovery by 3 months. Overall QOL appeared to be stable at 3 and 12 months post treatment [36].
- Management of toxicity is usually supportive to the decompensated liver and/or directed at the underlying liver disease, with close monitoring of LFTs. Early diagnosis of HBV reactivation and/or preventive prescription of anti-viral agents are key to managing non-classic RILD. Patients with GI bleeding or disproportionate pain after treatment should receive an urgent upper endoscopy.

25.9 Follow-Up

- Abdominal MRI for surveillance every 3 months post-treatment, along with blood work (including complete blood counts, PT/INR, bilirubin, transaminases, alkaline phosphatase, and albumin).
- For patients with HCC, a decline of a pretreatment elevated AFP may have prognostic significance.

25.10 Relevant Literature: Toxicity

- **Classic RILD**: The University of Michigan and others have published guidelines using the Lyman NTCP model for classic RILD with twice-a-day fraction sizes of 1.5–1.6 Gy. The mean liver dose in patients experiencing RILD was ≈25 Gy, leading to QUANTEC's recommendation of mean liver dose <13–18 Gy when using SBRT-level hypofractionation [28, 37–39]. The incidence of RILD in these series was much higher among Child-Pugh B patients, and several authors recommended limiting the mean liver dose to as low as 6 Gy for these higher-risk patients [28, 39]. Clinical signs of classic RILD include hepatomegaly, ascites, weight gain, fatigue, and elevation of alkaline phosphatase. These signs can appear as early as 2 weeks and may happen up to 6 months following RT [40].
- **Nonclassic RILD**: National Taiwan University Hospital and others reported the different presentations of liver toxicity in hepatitis B patients and defined them as non-classic RILD [41]. A parallel dosimetric guideline seeks to prevent non-classic RILD (e.g., worsening of liver function) by ensuring that a minimum volume of effective "functional" liver remains after RT. Based on the partial hepatectomy series, the most common recommendation is that ≥700 cc of normal liver receives less than a certain threshold dose (usually 15 Gy) for Child-Pugh class A patients [28]. A more ambitious criterion is likely prudent for Child-Pugh B patients, though no common volumetric guidelines exist.
- **Biliary Toxicity**: There is a concern for increased biliary toxicity with centrally located tumors. However, in an analysis of 50 patients receiving significant central biliary system dose (≥20 Gy, prescription dose 35–50 Gy in 5 fx), there were only two cases of bile duct stenosis (both asymptomatic), and no patient experienced cholangitis or obstructive jaundice [35]. This has also been confirmed in unpublished data from our institution. SBRT to these doses therefore appears to be safe for tumors adjacent to the central biliary system. For cholangiocarcinoma (especially perihilar variants), many studies used either prophylactic or therapeutic pre-RT biliary stents and appeared to have higher biliary complications after RT. However, it is unclear whether complications were due to RT or tumor progression or issues related to the stent itself [20, 25, 42, 43].

25.11 Relevant Literature: Hepatocellular Carcinoma

- Studies for hepatocellular carcinoma have been highly variable. Doses range from 24 to 60 Gy in 3–6 fractions. The size of treated tumors has also varied greatly. Most have included patients with small (2–3 cm) tumors, with results indicating excellent control and acceptable toxicity.
- The study by Bujold et al. [22] was unique in that it included very large (10 cm) tumors, half of which were associated with tumor vascular thrombosis. With a

median dose of 36 Gy in six fractions, control was excellent, though there were seven deaths (7%) potentially attributed to treatment. Overall results appeared favorable given the tumor burden and poor prognosis of these patients.

- The report by Wahl et al. [30] retrospectively compared SBRT with RFA and found comparable rates of control and toxicity, establishing SBRT as an acceptable first-line modality treatment for inoperable HCC.
- The phase III randomized trial by Kim et al. [44] compared hypofractionated proton RT to 66 Gy equivalent (GyE) in 10 fractions vs. RFA in patients with small HCC (size <3 cm, number ≤ 2). The local progression-free survival with RT was non-inferior to RFA.
- The phase III randomized trial by Yoon et al. [45] demonstrated superior survival from combined hypofractionated RT and TACE vs. sorafenib in HCC patients with major vascular invasion.
- Most patients in the following series have received extensive prior treatment (surgery, RFA, and/or chemotherapy).

Study	Patients	Treatments	Median follow-up	Outcomes
Prospective trials				
Takeda 2016 [17] Phase II	• 90 pts • 90% size ≤2 cm • 91% Child-Pugh A	89%: 40 Gy in 5 fx 11%: 35 Gy in 5 fx	41.7 months (55.9 months in survivors)	• 96% 3-year LC • 67% 3-year OS • 9% had a 2-point worsening of Child-Pugh score
Bujold 2013 [22] Phase I/II	• 102 pts • 55% with tumor vascular thrombosis • Median size 10 cm • Median GTV 117 cc • All Child-Pugh A	24–54 Gy in 6 fx (median 36 Gy)	31.4 months	• 87% 1-year LC • 17 mo median OS • 29% had worsened Child-Pugh class at 3 months • 7 deaths at least partially related to treatment (5 due to liver failure)
Kang 2012 [13] Phase II	• 47 pts • Median size 2.9 cm • Median GTV 15 cc • 87% Child-Pugh A	42–60 Gy in 3 fx	17 months (22 months in survivors)	• 95% 2-year LC • 69% 2-year OS • 2 pts with gastric ulcer perforation • 13% had worsened Child-Pugh class at 3 months
Kim 2021 [44] Phase III	• 144 pts with recurrent/residual HCC (size <3 cm, number ≤ 2) • >50% Child-Pugh A	RFA vs. Proton 66 GyE in 10 fx	51.6 months (67 months in survivors)	RFA • 84% 2-year LC • 93%2-year OS Proton • 95% 2-year LC ($p < 0.001$) • 89% 2-year OS ($p = 0.6$)

Study	Patients	Treatments	Median follow-up	Outcomes
Yoon 2018 [45] Phase III	• 90 pts with liver-confined HCC with macroscopic vascular invasion • Median size 9.7 cm • 90% Child-Pugh A	Sorafenib 400 mg twice daily vs. TACE plus RT 45 Gy (15–18 fx)	13.8 months (35 months in survivors)	Sorafenib • 34% 12-week LC • 14% 96-week OS TACE plus RT • 87% 12-week LC ($p < 0.01$) • 30% 96-week OS ($p = 0.04$)
Wei 2019 [5] Phase III	• 164 pts with resectable HCC and PVTT • > 95% Child-Pugh A	Hepatectomy alone vs. RT followed by hepatectomy	15 months	Hepatectomy alone • 15% 1-year LC • 43% 1-year OS RT followed by hepatectomy • 33% 1-year LC ($p < 0.001$) • 75% 1-year OS ($p < 0.001$)
Retrospective studies				
Kim 2021 [26]	• 510 pts, 619 lesions • Median size 3 cm • Median GTV 22.5 cc • 85% Child-Pugh A	Median: • $BED_{10} \geq 100$ Gy: 55 Gy in 5 fx • $BED_{10} < 100$ Gy: 40 Gy in 4 fx	22 months	**$BED_{10} \geq 100$ Gy** • 89% 2-year LC • 80% 2-year OS **$BED_{10} < 100$ Gy** • 69% 2-year LC • 67% 2-year OS
Wahl 2016 [30]	• RFA (161 pts, 249 lesions, median 1.8 cm) vs. SBRT (63 pts, 83 lesions, median 2.2 cm) • RFA pts had worse baseline liver function	SBRT 27–60 Gy in 3 or 5 fx	**RFA** 20 months (50.9 months in survivors) **SBRT** 13 months (27 months in survivors)	**RFA** • 84% 1-year LC • 80% 2-year LC • 11% acute grade 3 toxicity **SBRT** • 97% 1-year LC • 84% 2-year LC • 5% acute grade 3 toxicity
Huertas 2015 [12]	• 77 pts • Median size 2.4 cm • Median GTV 12 cc • 85% Child-Pugh A	45 Gy in 3 fx	12 months	• 99% 2-year LC • 57% 2-year OS • 23% 2-year hepatic toxicity (any grade)
Kimura 2015 [21]	• 64 pts • Median size 1.6 cm • 86% Child-Pugh A	48 Gy in 4 fx	26 months	• 100% 2-year LC • 76% 2-year OS • 23% 1-year grade ≥ 3 hepatic toxicity

Study	Patients	Treatments	Median follow-up	Outcomes
Yoon 2013 [16]	• 93 pts • Median size 2 cm • 74% Child-Pugh A	30–60 Gy in 3–4 fx	25.6 months	• 92% 3-year LC • 54% 3-year OS • 7% had grade ≥ 3 hepatic toxicity

Abbreviations: *BED_{10}* biological effective dose with the alpha/beta ratio of 10, *fx* fraction(s), *GTV* gross tumor volume, *Gy* gray, *GyE* gray equivalent, *LC* local control, *OS* overall survival, *pts* patients, *PVTT* portal vein tumor thrombus, *RFA* radiofrequency ablation, *SBRT* stereotactic body radiotherapy, *TACE* transarterial chemoembolization

25.12 Relevant Literature: Cholangiocarcinoma

- Given the rarity of cholangiocarcinoma, most published studies are very small. Studies included a mix of small to large tumors, but most showed moderate to good local control with acceptable toxicity with RT.
- The study by Tao et al. [25] was unique in that patients had very large tumors (median 8 cm). In these patients, high doses were delivered using hypofractionated conformal RT, with doses further escalated in the geometric "center" of tumors. This approach produced impressive outcomes, with excellent local control and survival despite the size of these tumors, with no documented cases of RILD.

Study	Patients	Treatments	Median follow-up	Outcomes
Prospective trials				
Tse 2008 [24] Phase I	• 10 pts • Intrahepatic • Median GTV 172 cc	• 24–54 Gy (median 36 Gy) in 6 fx	17.6 months	• 65% 1-year LC • 57% 1-year OS • 2 pts transient biliary stenosis; 2 pts worsened Child-Pugh class; 1 pt small bowel obstruction
Retrospective studies				
Tao 2016 [25]	• 79 pts • Intrahepatic • Median size 8 cm • median GTV 198 cc • 89% had pre-RT chemo	• 35–100 Gy in 3–30 fx • Most common regimens: 58.05 Gy in 15 fx, 67.5 Gy in 15 fx, 75 Gy in 25 fx	24 months (33 months in survivors)	• 44% 3-year OS • Higher OS and LC if BED >80.5 Gy • No case of RILD despite large tumors • 9% biliary stenosis (most also had tumor progression)

Study	Patients	Treatments	Median follow-up	Outcomes
Mahadevan 2015 [20]	• 34 pts • Intrahepatic • Median GTV 64 cc	• 30 Gy in 3 fx • 62% had biliary stent	38 months	• 88% 1-year LC • 58% 1-year OS • 12% grade 3 toxicity (duodenal ulcer, cholangitis, abscess)
Welling 2014 [43]	• 12 pts • Perihilar, unresectable • Mean size 1.4 cm	• 50–60 Gy in 3–5 fx • Xeloda post-RT until transplant	14 months	• 6 pts received liver transplant: 1-year OS 83% in these pts • 6 pts (50%) had cholangitis, attributed to stent dysfunction
Barney 2012 [46]	• 10 pts (12 lesions) • 6 intrahepatic, 3 perihilar • Median PTV 79 cc	• 45–60 Gy in 3–5 fx	14 months in survivors	• 100% LC • 73% 1-year OS • 1 pt grade 3 biliary stenosis; 1 pt grade 5 liver failure
Polistina 2011 [42]	• 10 pts • Perihilar, unresectable	• 30 Gy in 3 fx • Weekly gemcitabine • All pts had biliary stent	35.5 months	• 30 months median TTP • 80% 2-year OS • No grade ≥ 3 acute or late toxicities
Kopek 2010 [19]	• 27 pts • Perihilar • Median CTV 32 cc	• 45 Gy in 3 fx • All pts had biliary stent	5.4 years	• 84% 1-year LC • 11 months median OS • 6 pts duodenal ulceration; 3 pts duodenal stenosis • Mean duodenum D1cc was 37 Gy in pts with grade ≥ 2 ulceration or stenosis

Abbreviations: *BED_{10}* biological effective dose with the alpha/beta ratio of 10, *duodenum D1cc* minimum doses to highest irradiated 1 cc area of duodenum, *fx* fraction(s), *GTV* gross tumor volume, *Gy* gray, *LC* local control, *OS* overall survival, *RILD* radiation-induced liver disease, *TTP* time to progression

25.13 Relevant Literature: Liver Metastases

- There is substantial variation in published studies in dose, size, and number of treated metastases.
- Patients with liver metastases are often “healthier” with better baseline liver function than patients with HCC who often have comorbid cirrhosis. This is reflected in the higher allowable dose constraints published in QUANTEC [28]

and also by the higher doses prescribed. Though 45 Gy in three fractions is perhaps the most common, several studies have also delivered 60–75 Gy in three fractions, reporting greater than 90% 2-year LC [14, 47]. There is a suggestion that patients with liver metastases require higher doses for local control than HCC.

- Two significant studies are pooled analyses, one with patients from Stanford University, Princess Margaret Hospital, and the University of Colorado; and the other from Case Western University, University of Rochester, Memorial Sloan Kettering, and Cleveland Clinic [31, 32]. The Chang et al. study appeared to show improved local control with doses ≥42 Gy, which may justify dose escalation in these patients.
- Most patients in the following series received extensive prior treatment (surgery, RFA, and/or chemotherapy).

Study	Patients	Treatments	Median follow-up	Outcomes
Prospective trials				
Scorsetti 2015 [47] Phase II	• 42 pts, 52 lesions • Colorectal primary • Median size 3.5 cm • Median CTV 19 cc	75 Gy in 3 fx	24 months	• 91% 2-year LC • 65% 2-year OS • No grade ≥ 3 toxicity
Rusthoven 2009 [14] Phase I/II	• 47 pts, 63 lesions • 32% colorectal • Median size 2.7 cm • Median GTV 15 cc	36–60 Gy in 3 fx (60 Gy most common)	16 months	• 92% 2-year LC • 30% 2-year OS • 2% grade ≥ 3 toxicity
Lee 2009 [23] Phase I	• 68 pts • 59% colorectal • Median GTV 75 cc	27.7–60 Gy (median 41.4 Gy) in 6 fx	10.8 months	• 71% 1-year LC • 47% 18-month OS • 3 pts late grade ≥ 4 GI toxicity (duodenal bleed, bowel obstruction) • 6% had worsened Child-Pugh class at 3 months
Hoyer 2006 [11] Phase II	• 64 pts (44 liver), 141 lesions • Colorectal • Median size 3.5 cm	45 Gy in 3 fx	4.3 years	• 86% 2-year LC (per lesion) • 19% 2-year PFS • 38% 2-year OS • 4 pts had grade ≥ 3 GI toxicity
Retrospective studies				
[a]Berber 2013 [31]	• 153 pts, 363 lesions • 56% colorectal • Mean GTV 139 cc	Mean 37.5 Gy in 2–8 fx	25.2 months	• 62% LC • 51% 1-year OS • 3% grade ≥ 3 toxicity

Study	Patients	Treatments	Median follow-up	Outcomes
[b]Chang 2011 [32]	• 65 pts, 102 lesions • Colorectal • Median GTV 30 cc	22–60 Gy in 1–6 fx (Median 42 Gy in 3 fx)	1.2 years (1.4 years in survivors)	• 55% 2-year LC (per lesion) • 38% 2-year OS • Higher LC with ≥42 Gy (84%) vs. <42 Gy (43%) • 6% grade ≥ 2 late GI toxicity
Vautravers-Dewas [15]	• 42 pts, 62 lesions • 67% colorectal • Median size 2.5 cm • Median GTV 13 cc	64%: 40 Gy in 4 fx 36%: 45 Gy in 3 fx	14.3 months	• 86% 2-year LC • 48% 2-year OS • 1 pt liver failure; 1 pt gastric ulceration
Katz 2007 [48]	• 69 pts, 174 lesions • 29% colorectal • Median size 2.7 cm	"Preferred" 50 Gy in 10 fx	14.5 months	• 57% 20-month LC • 37% 20-month OS • No grade ≥ 3 toxicity

Abbreviations: *CTV* clinical tumor volume, *fx* fraction(s), *GI* gastrointestinal, *GTV* gross tumor volume, *Gy* gray, *LC* local control, *OS* overall survival, *PFS* progression-free survival, *RILD* radiation-induced liver disease

[a]Pooled results from Case Western, Rochester, Memorial Sloan Kettering, and Cleveland Clinic

[b]Pooled results from Stanford, Princess Margaret, and Colorado

References

1. Llovet JM, Burroughs A, Bruix J. Hepatocellular carcinoma. Lancet. 2003;362(9399):1907–17.
2. Jacob R, et al. Adjuvant stereotactic body radiotherapy following transarterial chemoembolization in patients with non-resectable hepatocellular carcinoma tumours of ≥3 cm. HPB (Oxford). 2015;17(2):140–9.
3. Wang TH, et al. Combined Yttrium-90 microsphere selective internal radiation therapy and external beam radiotherapy in patients with hepatocellular carcinoma: from clinical aspects to dosimetry. PLoS One. 2018;13(1):e0190098.
4. Nugent FW, et al. A randomized phase II feasibility study of individualized stereotactic body radiation therapy (SBRT) versus transarterial chemoembolization (TACE) with DEBDOX beads as a bridge to transplant in hepatocellular carcinoma (HCC). J Clin Oncol. 2020;38(Suppl. 15):4586.
5. Wei X, et al. Neoadjuvant three-dimensional conformal radiotherapy for resectable hepatocellular carcinoma with portal vein tumor thrombus: a randomized, open-label, multicenter controlled study. J Clin Oncol. 2019;37(24):2141–51.
6. Abe T, et al. Dosimetric comparison of carbon ion radiotherapy and stereotactic body radiotherapy with photon beams for the treatment of hepatocellular carcinoma. Radiat Oncol. 2015;10:187.
7. Gandhi SJ, et al. Clinical decision tool for optimal delivery of liver stereotactic body radiation therapy: photons versus protons. Pract Radiat Oncol. 2015;5(4):209–18.

8. Brade AM, et al. Phase 1 trial of sorafenib and stereotactic body radiation therapy for hepatocellular carcinoma. Int J Radiat Oncol Biol Phys. 2016;94(3):580–7.
9. Hepatobiliary, N., Hepatobiliary Cancers (Version 4.2021). https://www.nccn.org/professionals/physician_gls/pdf/hepatobiliary.pdf. Accessed 17 Sep 2021.
10. Colon, N., Colon cancer (version 3.2021). https://www.nccn.org/professionals/physician_gls/pdf/colon.pdf. Accessed 17 Sep 2021.
11. Hoyer M, et al. Phase II study on stereotactic body radiotherapy of colorectal metastases. Acta Oncol. 2006;45(7):823–30.
12. Huertas A, et al. Stereotactic body radiation therapy as an ablative treatment for inoperable hepatocellular carcinoma. Radiother Oncol. 2015;115(2):211–6.
13. Kang JK, et al. Stereotactic body radiation therapy for inoperable hepatocellular carcinoma as a local salvage treatment after incomplete transarterial chemoembolization. Cancer. 2012;118(21):5424–31.
14. Rusthoven KE, et al. Multi-institutional phase I/II trial of stereotactic body radiation therapy for liver metastases. J Clin Oncol. 2009;27(10):1572–8.
15. Vautravers-Dewas C, et al. Image-guided robotic stereotactic body radiation therapy for liver metastases: is there a dose response relationship? Int J Radiat Oncol Biol Phys. 2011;81(3):e39–47.
16. Yoon SM, et al. Stereotactic body radiation therapy as an alternative treatment for small hepatocellular carcinoma. PLoS One. 2013;8(11):e79854.
17. Takeda A, et al. Phase 2 study of stereotactic body radiotherapy and optional transarterial chemoembolization for solitary hepatocellular carcinoma not amenable to resection and radiofrequency ablation. Cancer. 2016;122(13):2041–9.
18. Andolino DL, et al. Stereotactic body radiotherapy for primary hepatocellular carcinoma. Int J Radiat Oncol Biol Phys. 2011;81(4):e447–53.
19. Kopek N, et al. Stereotactic body radiotherapy for unresectable cholangiocarcinoma. Radiother Oncol. 2010;94(1):47–52.
20. Mahadevan A, et al. Stereotactic body radiotherapy (SBRT) for intrahepatic and hilar cholangiocarcinoma. J Cancer. 2015;6(11):1099–104.
21. Kimura T, et al. Stereotactic body radiotherapy for patients with small hepatocellular carcinoma ineligible for resection or ablation therapies. Hepatol Res. 2015;45(4):378–86.
22. Bujold A, et al. Sequential phase I and II trials of stereotactic body radiotherapy for locally advanced hepatocellular carcinoma. J Clin Oncol. 2013;31(13):1631–9.
23. Lee MT, et al. Phase I study of individualized stereotactic body radiotherapy of liver metastases. J Clin Oncol. 2009;27(10):1585–91.
24. Tse RV, et al. Phase I study of individualized stereotactic body radiotherapy for hepatocellular carcinoma and intrahepatic cholangiocarcinoma. J Clin Oncol. 2008;26(4):657–64.
25. Tao R, et al. Ablative radiotherapy doses lead to a substantial prolongation of survival in patients with inoperable intrahepatic cholangiocarcinoma: a retrospective dose response analysis. J Clin Oncol. 2016;34(3):219–26.
26. Kim N, et al. Dose-response relationship in stereotactic body radiation therapy for hepatocellular carcinoma: a pooled analysis of an Asian Liver Radiation Therapy Group Study. Int J Radiat Oncol Biol Phys. 2021;109(2):464–73.
27. Benedict SH, et al. Stereotactic body radiation therapy: the report of AAPM Task Group 101. Med Phys. 2010;37(8):4078–101.
28. Pan CC, et al. Radiation-associated liver injury. Int J Radiat Oncol Biol Phys. 2010;76(Suppl. 3):S94–100.
29. Goldsmith C, et al. Dose-volume histogram analysis of stereotactic body radiotherapy treatment of pancreatic cancer: a focus on duodenal dose constraints. Semin Radiat Oncol. 2016;26(2):149–56.
30. Wahl DR, et al. Outcomes after stereotactic body radiotherapy or radiofrequency ablation for hepatocellular carcinoma. J Clin Oncol. 2016;34(5):452–9.

31. Berber B, et al. Multicentre results of stereotactic body radiotherapy for secondary liver tumours. HPB (Oxford). 2013;15(11):851–7.
32. Chang DT, et al. Stereotactic body radiotherapy for colorectal liver metastases: a pooled analysis. Cancer. 2011;117(17):4060–9.
33. Cheng JC, et al. Biologic susceptibility of hepatocellular carcinoma patients treated with radiotherapy to radiation-induced liver disease. Int J Radiat Oncol Biol Phys. 2004;60(5):1502–9.
34. Chou CH, et al. Radiation-induced hepatitis B virus reactivation in liver mediated by the bystander effect from irradiated endothelial cells. Clin Cancer Res. 2007;13(3):851–7.
35. Eriguchi T, et al. Acceptable toxicity after stereotactic body radiation therapy for liver tumors adjacent to the central biliary system. Int J Radiat Oncol Biol Phys. 2013;85(4):1006–11.
36. Klein J, et al. Prospective longitudinal assessment of quality of life for liver cancer patients treated with stereotactic body radiation therapy. Int J Radiat Oncol Biol Phys. 2015;93(1):16–25.
37. Dawson LA, et al. Analysis of radiation-induced liver disease using the Lyman NTCP model. Int J Radiat Oncol Biol Phys. 2002;53(4):810–21.
38. Kim TH, et al. Dose-volumetric parameters predicting radiation-induced hepatic toxicity in unresectable hepatocellular carcinoma patients treated with three-dimensional conformal radiotherapy. Int J Radiat Oncol Biol Phys. 2007;67(1):225–31.
39. Xu ZY, et al. Prediction of radiation-induced liver disease by Lyman normal-tissue complication probability model in three-dimensional conformal radiation therapy for primary liver carcinoma. Int J Radiat Oncol Biol Phys. 2006;65(1):189–95.
40. Toesca DAS, et al. Strategies for prediction and mitigation of radiation-induced liver toxicity. J Radiat Res. 2018;59(Suppl. 1):i40–9.
41. Cheng JC, et al. Radiation-induced liver disease after radiotherapy for hepatocellular carcinoma: clinical manifestation and dosimetric description. Radiother Oncol. 2002;63(1):41–5.
42. Polistina FA, et al. Chemoradiation treatment with gemcitabine plus stereotactic body radiotherapy for unresectable, non-metastatic, locally advanced hilar cholangiocarcinoma. Results of a five year experience. Radiother Oncol. 2011;99(2):120–3.
43. Welling TH, et al. Neoadjuvant stereotactic body radiation therapy, capecitabine, and liver transplantation for unresectable hilar cholangiocarcinoma. Liver Transpl. 2014;20(1):81–8.
44. Kim TH, et al. Proton beam radiotherapy vs. radiofrequency ablation for recurrent hepatocellular carcinoma: a randomized phase III trial. J Hepatol. 2021;74(3):603–12.
45. Yoon SM, et al. Efficacy and safety of transarterial chemoembolization plus external beam radiotherapy vs sorafenib in hepatocellular carcinoma with macroscopic vascular invasion: a randomized clinical trial. JAMA Oncol. 2018;4(5):661–9.
46. Barney BM, et al. Clinical outcomes and toxicity using stereotactic body radiotherapy (SBRT) for advanced cholangiocarcinoma. Radiat Oncol. 2012;7:67.
47. Scorsetti M, et al. Final results of a phase II trial for stereotactic body radiation therapy for patients with inoperable liver metastases from colorectal cancer. J Cancer Res Clin Oncol. 2015;141(3):543–53.
48. Katz AW, et al. Hypofractionated stereotactic body radiation therapy (SBRT) for limited hepatic metastases. Int J Radiat Oncol Biol Phys. 2007;67(3):793–8.

Chapter 26
Pancreas Cancer

Morgan M. Bailey, Andrew Z. Wang, Joel E. Tepper, and Kyle Wang

26.1 Introduction

The use of radiation therapy (RT) for pancreatic cancer was historically controversial. Randomized trials of conventionally fractionated chemoradiation in the postoperative and definitive settings have shown improvements in local control but not overall survival. However, treatment for all patients with nonmetastatic pancreatic cancer is shifting toward total neoadjuvant therapy, and the PREOPANC randomized trial recently showed an overall survival benefit for preoperative chemoradiation [1]. In addition, technological advances now allow the delivery of high, potentially ablative radiation doses while maintaining safe bowel limits. In this chapter, we will discuss the use of hypofractionated RT (including SBRT) for pancreatic cancer.

26.2 Pearls

- Over 60,000 cases per year in the United States, median age 70 years, and the third leading cause of cancer mortality. Only 15–20% are candidates for surgery at diagnosis.

M. M. Bailey
Department of Radiation Oncology, University of Cincinnati, Cincinnati, OH, USA

A. Z. Wang
UT Southwestern Medical Center, Dallas, TX, USA

J. E. Tepper
Department of Radiation Oncology, University of North Carolina Hospitals, Chapel Hill, NC, USA

K. Wang (✉)
Cincinnati, OH, USA

O. Kaidar-Person, R. Chen (eds.), *Hypofractionated and Stereotactic Radiation Therapy*, https://doi.org/10.1007/978-3-031-47701-0_26

- Risk factors include chronic pancreatitis, pancreatic cysts, cigarette smoking, obesity, alcohol, and genetic causes.
- Up to 10% of cases have hereditary causes, and risk is increased with some inherited syndromes including BRCA, Peutz-Jeghers syndrome, and hereditary pancreatitis.
- Patients typically present with weight loss, abdominal pain, nausea, new onset of type 2 diabetes, and signs of biliary obstruction including jaundice and dark urine.
- The majority is exocrine pancreatic adenocarcinoma originating in the ductal epithelium.
- Most commonly located in the pancreatic head. Resectability is determined by the degree of involvement of the superior mesenteric and celiac arteries and, to a lesser extent, by the involvement of the superior mesenteric and portal veins.
- Commonly spreads to regional lymph nodes around the common hepatic, celiac, and splenic arteries. Distant spread is very common, especially to the liver and peritoneum.
- CA 19–9 has a relatively high sensitivity for pancreatic cancer and may be used to monitor the response to treatment and as a marker for recurrence (10% of the population lacks the Lewis antigen and does not express CA 19–9).
- Imaging: Ultrasound, pancreatic protocol "triple-phase" CT, MRI, and PET are all employed. Endoscopic biopsy may be used for obtaining tissue, and ERCP may be employed for therapeutic biliary stenting.
- Treatment:
  - For patients with clearly resectable disease, surgery with adjuvant chemotherapy has been the historical standard, but total neoadjuvant therapy is increasingly favored given the high risk of metastatic disease. Though preoperative RT is usually not used for resectable disease, patients with resectable disease comprised 55% of the PREOPANC trial cohort which demonstrated an overall survival benefit from total neoadjuvant therapy [1].
  - Patients with borderline resectable or locally advanced disease receive upfront chemotherapy with periodic re-evaluations of response and resectability. If an attempted resection is planned, preoperative RT can be considered and may be delivered with conventional fractionation or moderate hypofractionation using 3D or IMRT with concurrent chemotherapy, or with 3–5 fractions of SBRT without chemotherapy.
  - Off-bowel ablative RT to higher doses may be considered to improve local control in certain scenarios, including anatomic and medical inoperability, or as a preoperative boost for areas at high risk of residual disease (e.g., tumor–vessel interface). This can be achieved with dose-escalated moderate hypofractionation or SBRT but is much higher risk and provider/institutional expertise is needed.
  - Based on limited and mostly historical evidence, postoperative (conventionally fractionated) RT can be considered for adverse features (e.g., positive margins) after surgery. The role of postoperative RT may be influenced by the upcoming results of RTOG 0848. However, total neoadjuvant approaches incorporating chemotherapy with or without additional preoperative RT are now preferred.

26.3 Tumor/Patient Selection

- A discussion on hypofractionated RT for pancreatic cancer must consider the roles of surgery and chemotherapy, treatment intent (preoperative for borderline resectable disease vs. ablative for locally advanced disease), and patients' unique bowel, tumor, and vascular anatomy. In general, most patients who are candidates for curative treatment should be strongly considered for neoadjuvant/initial chemotherapy, which both locoregionally downstages while addressing potentially microscopic distant metastases. The roles of RT and surgery should be discussed in close conjunction during periodic evaluations of chemotherapy response.
- **Surgical considerations:** The key consideration for patients with nonmetastatic pancreatic cancer is resectability, and RT intent must therefore consider surgical intent. If surgery is planned, preoperative RT may be delivered to moderate doses (e.g., bowel-safe doses biologically equivalent to 45–54 Gy delivered with conventional fractionation). If surgery is not planned, ablative RT doses may be considered for durable control/cure in appropriate patients. However, the radiographic distinction between borderline vs. unresectable disease may be unclear, especially with neoadjuvant chemotherapy. Indeed, one study of total neoadjuvant chemotherapy and radiotherapy led to a 61% R0 resection rate in patients with locally advanced disease [2]. Thus, resection may be reasonably attempted or aborted based on intraoperative findings even in very borderline cases, and ablative RT doses with careful bowel prioritization can also be delivered preoperatively if surgical exploration is planned, but resection is uncertain.
- **Preoperative RT:** Patients considered for preoperative RT typically have at least borderline resectable disease, e.g., with arterial involvement <90° and/or venous involvement 90–270° as defined by the PREOPANC trial [3]. Coordination between the surgeon and radiation oncologist is important to determine specific areas of vessel abutment at risk for positive margins and/or residual disease. Preoperative RT may be delivered with moderate hypofractionation to relatively low total doses with concurrent gemcitabine or 5-FU based chemotherapy, based on the PREOPANC trial (36 Gy at 2.4 Gy/fx) or MD Anderson practice (30 Gy at 3 Gy/fx) [3, 4]. Alternatively, five-fraction preoperative RT regimens (typically to 25–30 Gy) without concurrent chemotherapy are reasonable using IMRT or SBRT.
- **Ablative RT:** Ablative intent RT is the concept of delivering very high doses (variably defined as BED 70–100 Gy with α/β 10 Gy) using IMRT or SBRT and may be accomplished with various fractionation schemes utilizing $\geq$3 Gy/fx (e.g., 75 Gy in 25 fx, 67.5 Gy in 15 fx, and 40–50 Gy in 5 fx). Concurrent fluoropyrimidine-based chemotherapy may be used with fractionated ablative RT per the MSKCC paradigm. Concurrent chemotherapy is not used with SBRT. However, promising phase I/II results have been reported for concurrent SBRT and GC4419 (a selective superoxide dismutase mimetic hypothesized to both protect normal tissue and sensitize tumor), and a randomized Phase II trial

is ongoing [5, 6]. The feasibility and safety of ablative RT depend on the proximity of the small bowel and stomach to gross disease (or vascular abutment if ablative RT is delivered preoperatively) and institutional experience. Ablative RT is delivered with complex, heterogeneous, two- to three-level simultaneous-integrated boost plans that prioritize limiting a sensitive bowel volume to a selected "safe" dose (e.g., Dmax ≤ 30–35 Gy in 5 fractions). The remainder of the tumor and/or high-risk target volume is boosted to very high doses. It is generally presumed that there is clinical benefit even if only a portion of the tumor can safely be treated to the highest dose. Careful patient instructions, simulation, treatment planning, image guidance, and motion management are critical (see Sect. 26.4).

- Tumors with direct bowel or stomach invasion may not be suitable for aggressive fractionation regimens due to concern for perforation, fistula, and/or hemorrhage with rapid tumor regression.
- **Guidelines:** The 2016 ASCO guideline for locally advanced, unresectable pancreatic cancer [7] recommends consideration of conventional chemoradiation or SBRT in patients with ECOG PS ≤ 2, adequate comorbidity profile, no distant metastasis, and with either local progression after chemotherapy or stable disease but poor chemotherapy tolerance. The 2019 ASTRO guideline similarly recommends (conditional or strong recommendation) chemoradiation to doses ranging from 45 to 56 Gy in 25–30 fx for neoadjuvant or definitive treatment. SBRT delivered in 30–40 Gy in 5 fx is also recommended. Ablative doses are not discussed in current guidelines. Representative bowel dose/volume guidelines are shown below (Sect. 26.6, Table) [8, 9].

26.4 Treatment Planning Considerations (Fig. 26.1)

Simulation instructions	• To minimize stomach distension and maximize reproducibility, patients should be instructed to fast 4–6 h before simulation and treatment and to generally avoid carbonated beverages. • A small amount of oral contrast may be given 10–20 min before simulation to slightly improve bowel visualization, though it is the authors' preference to avoid oral contrast to maximize reproducibility. • Patients are simulated supine with arms overhead. (For CyberKnife, patients are simulated with arms at their side for comfort during long treatments.) Immobilization using a Vac-Lok or similar device. • IV contrast is an important aid in both gross tumor volume (GTV) delineation and accurately delineating critical vasculature. • When delivering ablative doses in 3–5 fx, treatment every other day is the authors' preference as this has been shown to decrease toxicity in many SBRT contexts and is generally more forgiving.

Motion management	• With ablative RT, motion management is important, accounting for *both* bowel and target motion. Motion management is generally less critical with bowel-safe dose regimens. • A breath-hold approach is optimal for its ability to minimize motion and avoids the need for a large bowel planning risk volume (PRV) or tumor/target internal target volume (ITV) but is highly dependent on technology, expertise, and patient ability/participation. Various systems exist, including volumetric inhalation monitoring (e.g., SDX®) and surface-guided visual monitoring (e.g., VisionRT). • If a breath-hold approach is not feasible, abdominal compression may be considered to reduce respiratory variation. However, abdominal compression may also variably displace the bowel and should be used with caution. • Without breath hold, 4D simulation (e.g., with simulation CT slices taken throughout the respiratory cycle) with or without abdominal compression should be used to assess bowel, stomach, and tumor/vasculature motion.
Image guidance	• Fiducial markers may be considered for Linac SBRT for target localization and are required with CyberKnife for both localization and motion tracking. Usefulness is highly dependent on accurate placement. With CyberKnife, fiducials accurately placed in the pancreatic head may approximate both tumor and C-loop duodenum motion, but 4D assessment should still be used to address other at-risk bowel motion that may not necessarily correlate with fiducial motion. It may be preferable to omit fiducials in preoperative cases to avoid unnecessary delays, especially if moderate doses are planned. • In the authors' experience, localization is feasible by aligning to the great vessels and major trunks (e.g., celiac and superior mesenteric artery) with careful window leveling on cone beam CTs, including 4D CBCTs to assess motion at the time of RT delivery (if breath hold is not used). • MRI linacs allow accurate daily localization due to superior visualization (compared with cone beam CT) of both the tumor and neighboring bowel. • Surface-guided breath-hold techniques perform image guidance by monitoring and aligning to the chest's spatial position (reconstructed as a 3D model), using an array of mounted cameras. Volumetric breath-hold techniques rely on patients visually monitoring the degree of deep inspiration, with a visual "target" at the correct threshold.

Target/bowel delineation	• Contrast CT scan is adequate in most cases to delineate bowel, tumor, and vasculature. Delineation may be further aided by the fusion of a diagnostic CT, MRI, or PET. Typically, the tumors themselves are *hypo*-enhancing. Given motion inaccuracies, scan fusions should prioritize the aorta, celiac trunk, and superior mesenteric artery in most cases. • With ablative RT, the most important contour is the bowel. Once the bowel is confidently delineated, the remainder of the target volume may be safely dose-escalated. The stomach, duodenum, and small bowel may be combined into one high-risk PRV, as they have similar dose tolerances. Nearby large bowel may be combined into a separate intermediate-risk PRV and given a slightly higher dose tolerance. Without breath hold, bowel motion should be assessed and included in the PRV, along with a final bowel safety margin (3–5 mm). • Given the daily variation in bowel position/volume, adaptive re-planning prior to each fraction (of SBRT) may improve accuracy and safety, though it is resource intensive. Adaptive planning has been best described in the context of MRI linacs [10, 11]. • Many earlier SBRT studies treated the tumor only. However, it is increasingly evident that optimal pancreatic clinical tumor volume delineation includes a homogeneously-dosed elective region that includes surrounding vascular and nodal anatomy, especially with modern conformal techniques that can maintain safe dose limits [12–14]. Gross tumor volume is often vague (even more so with neoadjuvant chemotherapy); vasculature is high-risk due to perineural spread and risk of residual disease after surgery, and nodal spread is common. A recent Stanford study reported a locoregional failure rate of 23% vs. 45% in patients treated with vs. without elective nodal irradiation, respectively [13]. • An ITV should be generated for each clinical target volume accounting for motion (unless CyberKnife or breath hold is used). A small PTV can then be added.
Dosimetric considerations	• Selection of both target prescription dose and bowel dose limits (see Sect. 26.6. Normal Tissue Tolerances) depends on treatment intent, clinical context, and practical factors. With ablative doses, protracted fractionation may be advantageous if there is a greater degree of bowel abutment or uncertainty. On the contrary, shorter treatment courses minimize treatment delays (e.g., between chemotherapy and surgery) and patient burden. • With ablative RT, traditional dosimetric goals of homogeneity and target coverage are mostly irrelevant. It is common to accept very low target coverage (e.g., 50–70%) in order to ensure safety.

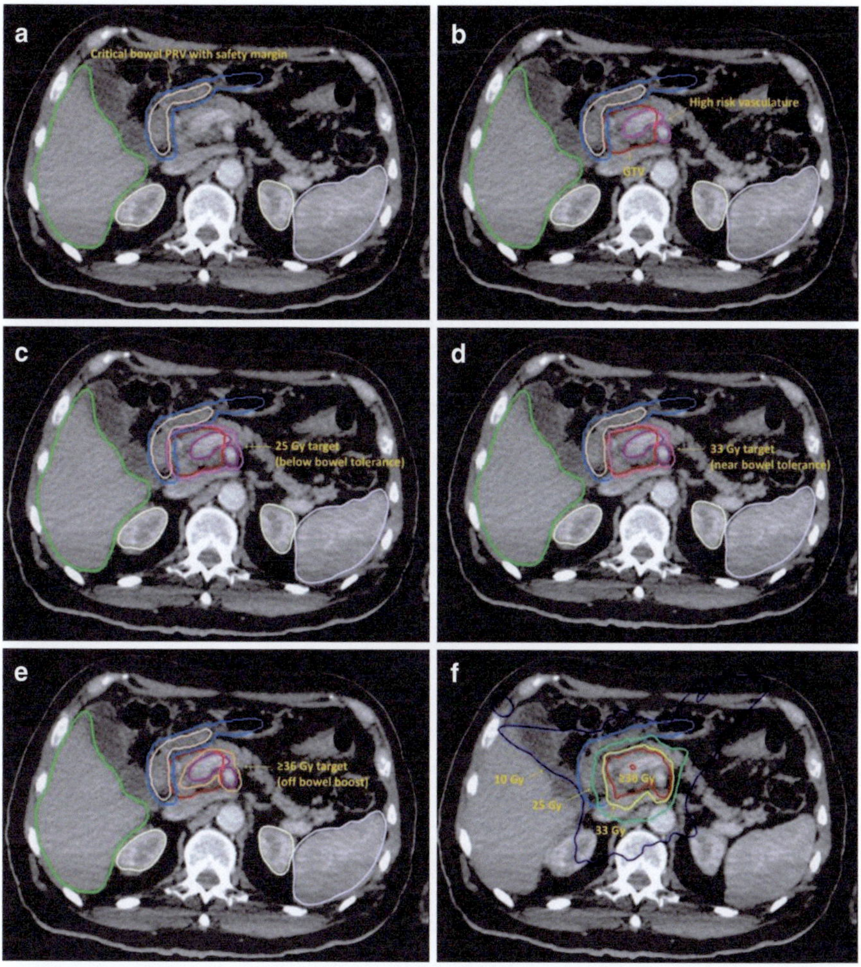

Fig. 26.1 Example of treatment planning for a patient with borderline resectable pancreatic adenocarcinoma treated with SBRT with preoperative intent. (**a**) Delineation of the high-risk bowel with an arbitrary safety margin accounting for motion. Note: The stomach in this case was not included in the critical bowel PRV but delineated separately. (**b**) Delineation of the GTV and high-risk target regions including the tumor–vessel interface. (**c**) Creation of a bowel-safe, "low risk" target volume that may include bowel near tumor. Though elective nodal/vascular radiation was not used in this example, it would also be reasonable to include a larger volume if care is taken to minimize dose heterogeneity near the bowel. (**d**) Creation of an "intermediate risk" target volume near bowel tolerance that includes the entire tumor and nearby vasculature. (**e**) Creation of a high-risk target volume that may receive ablative doses. In this example, only the tumor–vessel interface was included in this boost volume, but it would be reasonable to include the entire GTV. (**f**) Final treatment plan with doses displayed

26.5 Commonly Used Dose/Fractionation Schemes

Dose/fx	# of fx	Total dose	Notes
2.4–3 Gy	10–15	30–36 Gy	Doses in these ranges (e.g., 30 Gy/10 fx or 36 Gy/15 fx) are typically delivered preoperatively and may be used with concurrent chemotherapy. These doses are bowel-safe, and target volumes should generally include elective nodes and vasculature in addition to tumor
10–12 Gy	3	30–36 Gy	HyTEC review estimates 79–86% 1-year LC without surgery for 30–36 Gy/3 fx. Three-fraction regimens are typically used for unresectable diseases with minimal bowel abutment [9]
5–7 Gy	5	25–35 Gy	HyTEC review estimates 77% 1-year LC without surgery for 33 Gy/5 fx [9]. These 5-fx regimens are typically preoperative or a conservative approach to unresectable disease, equivalent to approximately 50 Gy delivered with conventional fractionation
8–10 Gy	5	40–50 Gy	These "ablative" 5-fx SBRT regimens are delivered without concurrent chemotherapy and may improve local control and be considered for unresectable tumors or select regions of borderline resectable tumors but require rigorous bowel safety assessment
4.5 Gy	15	67.5 Gy	The Memorial Sloan Kettering fractionated ablative regimens, which are more forgiving to the bowel while maintaining ablative potential, may be delivered with concurrent fluoropyrimidine
3 Gy	25	75 Gy	

1. It is the authors' general practice to use 5-fraction approaches. For either of the 5-fraction regimens above, it is reasonable to include an elective volume delivering up to 25 Gy in 5 fractions, but, with heterogeneous plans, it is important to incorporate a bowel safety margin and minimize the overall volume of bowel receiving 20–25 Gy.
2. Two to three clinical target volumes may be used with a 5-fraction approach that may or may not incorporate elective and/or ablative target volumes:
    - Low risk: Low-dose, bowel-safe elective volume (e.g., homogeneously dose-painted 20–25 Gy/5 fx) including nodal regions and vasculature distant from the tumor.
    - Intermediate risk: Moderate-dose volume at bowel tolerance (e.g., 30–35 Gy/5 fx) including GTV and nearby vasculature.
    - High risk: Ablative-dose volume above bowel tolerance (e.g., ≥40–50 Gy/5 fx) including GTV with or without nearby vasculature.
3. Early pancreas SBRT studies utilized one fraction, but this is no longer advised given concerns regarding single-fraction bowel tolerance.

26.6 Normal Tissue Tolerances

The principal organs at risk with hypofractionated pancreas RT delivered using modern conformal techniques are the stomach, duodenum, and remainder of the small bowel. As discussed above, it is reasonable to combine these gastrointestinal luminal organs into one high-risk PRV, given their nearly identical dose tolerances, with any nearby large bowel given a higher dose limit. Areas of bowel directly abutting the tumor (as is often the case with the duodenum) are sometimes contoured separately to allow a higher dose limit (depending on the degree of acceptable risk) and increase tumor coverage. The liver and kidneys should also be delineated but rarely reach clinically significant doses and are not discussed in this section.

	Seminars review [8]	Stanford [13][a]	MSKCC [15, 16][b]	Authors' practice[c]
Stomach				
3 fx				
5 fx		V33 Gy < 1 cc V30 Gy < 5 cc Dmax < 40 Gy		Dmax < 33–38 Gy V30–33 Gy < 5 cc Minimize V25 Gy
15 fx			Dmax < 45 Gy	
25 fx			Dmax < 60 Gy	
Duodenum				
3 fx	D_{1cc} < 30 Gy			
5 fx	D_{1cc} < 35 Gy	V33 Gy < 1 cc V30 Gy < 5 cc Dmax < 40 Gy		Dmax < 33–38 Gy V30–33 Gy < 5 cc Minimize V25 Gy
15 fx			Dmax < 45 Gy	
25 fx			Dmax < 60 Gy	
Small bowel				
3 fx	D_{2cc} < 24.5 Gy D_{5cc} < 21 Gy			
5 fx	D_{2cc} < 30 Gy D_{5cc} < 25 Gy	V33 Gy < 1 cc V30 Gy < 5 cc Dmax < 40 Gy		Dmax < 33–38 Gy V30–33 Gy < 5 cc Minimize V25 Gy
15 fx			Dmax < 40 Gy	
25 fx			Dmax < 55 Gy	
Large bowel				
3 fx				
5 fx				Dmax < 35–40 Gy
15 fx			Dmax < 50 Gy	
25 fx			Dmax < 65 Gy	

[a]Stomach, duodenum, and small bowel are considered separate structures. Efforts were made to limit V25 Gy < 30 cc for each of these organs

[b]Stomach is combined with the first two segments of the duodenum

[c]Stomach, duodenum, and small bowel in the general vicinity of the target are combined into one high-risk PRV

26.7 Patient Management Considerations

- Acute nausea is common and usually manageable with prophylactic antiemetics before treatment.
- Acute gastritis can be managed with antacids, H2-antagonists, and proton pump inhibitors. Most acute toxicities are minor and self-limiting [17–19]. It is the authors' practice to initiate or increase the dose of a proton pump inhibitor (e.g., pantoprazole 40–80 mg daily) for at least 3–6 months to both address the symptoms of acute acid-related disease and as prophylaxis against late ulceration [20].
- Patients should be closely followed for signs of late gastrointestinal toxicity, with a low threshold to re-initiate antacids and/or proton pump inhibitors. Those with severe symptoms or GI bleeding should receive an urgent evaluation with consideration of upper endoscopy. Patients who require anticoagulation for other reasons may be at higher risk of GI bleeding [16]. The rate of grade 3 events has been reported to be 3–8% in modern series using ablative doses at experienced institutions.
- Other possible late toxicities of pancreatic RT include radiation enteritis, nutritional deficiencies, bile salt malabsorption, and pancreatic endocrine/exocrine insufficiency that may require enzyme/nutritional replacement. Rarely, an uncontrolled late ulceration can progress to a bowel obstruction or perforation, though many such cases are due in part to tumor.

26.8 Follow-Up

- The authors generally obtain a contrast CT of the chest, abdomen, and pelvis; CA 19–9; and evaluate patients for adverse events (particularly GI toxicity) every 3 months.

26.9 Relevant Literature

Study	Patients	Treatments	Median follow-up	Outcomes
Preoperative intent				
Moffit Chuong 2013 [21] Mellon 2015 [19] (Retrospective)	$N = 159$ (110 BRPC, 49 LAPC)	• PTV: 30 Gy in 5 fx • Plus simultaneous integrated boost for a total of 30–50 Gy in 5 fx • Chemo: 100%, given pre-RT	14 months	• BRPC: 19-month median OS, 49% R0 resection • LAPC: 15-month median OS, 10% R0 resection • 7% grade ≥ 3 toxicity (6 pts GI bleeding)

Study	Patients	Treatments	Median follow-up	Outcomes
MDACC Cloyd 2016 [4] (Retrospective)	*N* = 224 in hypofx CRT cohort (202 resectable,17 BRPC, 5 LAPC)	• 30 Gy in 10 fx • Chemo: 100% concurrent with RT, 43% preop, 21% postop	49.1 months	• 22% LR • 31% 5-year RFS • 34 month median OS
PREOPANC Versteijne 2020 [3] and 2022 [1] (Phase 3)	**Preop CRT vs. Immediate surgery** *N* = 246 (133 resectable, 113 BRPC)	**Arm 1:** 36 Gy in 15 fx concurrent with second of three cycles preop gemcitabine, surgery, four cycles postop gemcitabine. **Arm 2:** Immediate surgery, six cycles postop gemcitabine	59 months	**Arm 1:** • Median locoregional failure-free interval (LFFI) not reached • 20.5% 5-year OS • 71% R0 resection • 7% grade 5 toxicity **Arm 2:** • 13.4-month median LFFI ($p = 0.003$) • 6.5% 5-year OS ($p = 0.025$) • 40% R0 resection • 7% grade 5 toxicity
Definitive intent				
Johns Hopkins Herman 2015 [22] (Phase 2)	• *N* = 49 • LAPC • Median PTV 71 cc	• 33 Gy in 5 fx • Chemo: Pre and post-RT gemcitabine, no concurrent	13.9 months in survivors	• 78% 1-year LC • 18% 2-year OS • 4 pts had R0 resection • 6% late grade ≥ 3 toxicity (1 fistula, 2 GI blccd) • Improvement in pain-related QoL
Milano, Italy Comito 2016 [23] (Phase 2)	• *N* = 45 • LAPC • Median PTV 65 cc	• 45 Gy in 6 fx • Chemo: 78% pre-RT, 48% post-RT, no concurrent	13.5 months (23.5 months in survivors)	• 87% 2-year LC • 18% 2-year OS • No late grade 3 toxicity
Sinai Baltimore Didolkar 2010 [24] (Retrospective)	• *N* = 85 • Unresectable • Re-irradiation in 34% • Median GTV 60 cc	• 15–30 Gy in 1–4 fx (Median 26 Gy, 3 fx) • Chemo: 56% pre-RT, 100% post-RT, no concurrent	NA	• 92% LC • 19-month median OS • 22% acute or late grade ≥ 3 GI toxicity (duodenitis, gastritis, and diarrhea)

Study	Patients	Treatments	Median follow-up	Outcomes
Beth Israel Deaconess Mahadevan 2011 [17] (Retrospective)	• *N* = 39 • Unresectable • Median PTV 64 cc	• 24–36 Gy in 3 fx • Chemo: Pre- and post-RT gemcitabine, no concurrent	9.1 months (21 months in survivors)	• 85% LC • 20-month median OS • 9% late grade ≥ 3 toxicity (GI bleed, bowel obstruction) • Significant improvement in pain-related QoL
Stanford Pollom 2014 [25] (Retrospective)	• *N* = 167 • Unresectable • Median PTV 50 cc	• 25 Gy in 1 fx, *n* = 76 • 25–45 Gy in 5 fx, *n* = 91	7.9 months	• 90% 1-year LC • 33% 1-year OS • More grade 2 GI toxicity with a single fraction: 26% (1 fx), 8% (5 fx)
MSKCC Reyngold 2021 [16] (Retrospective)	• *N* = 119 • LAPC or unresectable	• 75 Gy in 25 fx, *n* = 96 • 67.5 Gy in 15 fx, *n* = 23 • Chemo: 97.5% pre-RT (103 pts mFOLFIRINOX or gemcitabine/ nab-paclitaxel)	18.4 months	• 67% 2-year LC • 38% 2-year OS • 8% grade 3 toxicity
Miami Chuong 2021 [10] (Retrospective)	• *N* = 35 (28 LAPC, 3 BRPC, 4 resectable) • Stereotactic MR-guided adaptive RT	• 50 Gy in 5 fx • 20 pts (57%) received elective nodal RT • Chemo: 91.4% pre-RT (28 pts FOLFIRINOX or gemcitabine/ nab-paclitaxel)	10.3 months	• 88% 1-year LC • 59% 1-year OS • 1 pt late grade 2 GI bleed; 1 pt late grade 3 biliary stenosis
Washington University Hassanzadeh 2021 [11] (Retrospective)	• *N* = 44 (28 LAPC, 6 BRPC, 10 resectable) • Stereotactic MR-guided adaptive RT	• 50 Gy in 5 fx • Chemo: 82% pre-RT (31 pts FOLFIRINOX or gemcitabine/ nab-paclitaxel)	16 months	• 59% 2-year LC • 38% 2-year OS • 3 pts late grade 2 toxicity (1 duodenal perforation, 2 ulceration); 2 late grade 3 ulceration

Study	Patients	Treatments	Median follow-up	Outcomes
Stanford Miller 2022 [13] (Retrospective)	• $N = 150$ (79 LAPC, 42 BRPC, 29 resectable) • Propensity matched 2:1 SBRT alone vs. SBRT + elective nodal irradiation (ENI)	• 33–40 Gy in 5 fx SBRT alone, $n = 100$ • 40 Gy in 5 fx SBRT with 25 Gy in 5 fx ENI, $n = 50$ • Chemo: 91% pre-RT	28 months	**SBRT alone:** • 55% 2-year LC • 77% 1-year OS • 20% acute grade 1–2 GI toxicity • 2% late grade 3 toxicity **SBRT + ENI:** • 77% 2-year LC ($p = 0.01$) • 80% 2-year OS (NS) • 60% acute grade 1–2 toxicity (mostly nausea, $p < 0.001$) • 5% late grade 3 toxicity (NS)
Re-irradiation				
Georgetown Lominska 2012 [26] (Retrospective)	• $N = 28$ • Most had prior CRT to 50.4 Gy • Median GTV 44 cc	• 20–30 Gy in 3–5 fx	5.9 months	• 86% LC • 18% 1-year OS • 2 pts grade ≥ 3 late GI toxicity (obstruction, perforation)
Beth Israel Deaconess Dagoglu 2016 [27] (Retrospective)	• $N = 30$ • Prior SBRT or CRT • Median 18 months from prior RT • Median GTV 41 cc	• 24–36 Gy in 3–5 fx	11 months	• 78% 2-year LC • 50% 1-year OS • 1 pt grade 3 GI bleed; 1 pt grade 3 pain; 2 pts grade 3 bowel obstruction
Stanford Koong 2017 [28] (Retrospective)	• $N = 23$ • Prior CRT	• 25 Gy in 1 fx, $n = 9$ • 20–33 Gy in 5 fx, $n = 14$	28 months	• 81% 1-year LC • 30% 1-year OS • More grade ≥ 2 GI toxicity with a single fraction: 44% (1 fx), 14% (5 fx)

Abbreviations: *BRPC* borderline resectable pancreatic cancer, *LAPC* locally advanced pancreatic cancer, *CRT* chemoradiotherapy, *LR* local recurrence, *RFS* recurrence-free survival, *OS* overall survival, *LC* local control, *pts* patients, *ENI* elective nodal irradiation

References

1. Versteijne E, van Dam JL, Suker M, et al. Neoadjuvant chemoradiotherapy versus upfront surgery for resectable and borderline resectable pancreatic cancer: long-term results of the Dutch randomized PREOPANC trial. J Clin Oncol. 2022;40(11):1220–30.
2. Murphy JE, Wo JY, Ryan DP, et al. Total neoadjuvant therapy with FOLFIRINOX followed by individualized chemoradiotherapy for borderline resectable pancreatic adenocarcinoma: a phase 2 clinical trial. JAMA Oncol. 2018;4(7):963–9.
3. Versteijne E, Suker M, Groothuis K, et al. Preoperative chemoradiotherapy versus immediate surgery for resectable and borderline resectable pancreatic cancer: results of the Dutch Randomized Phase III PREOPANC Trial. J Clin Oncol. 2020;38(16):1763–73.
4. Cloyd JM, Crane CH, Koay EJ, et al. Impact of hypofractionated and standard fractionated chemoradiation before pancreatoduodenectomy for pancreatic ductal adenocarcinoma. Cancer. 2016;122(17):2671–9.
5. Hoffe SE, Kim DW, Costello J, et al. GRECO-2: a randomized, phase 2 study of stereotactic body radiation therapy (SBRT) in combination with GC4711 in the treatment of unresectable or borderline resectable nonmetastatic pancreatic cancer (PC). J Clin Oncol. 2021;39(Suppl. 15):TPS4175.
6. Holmlund J, Brookes M, Colbert LE, et al. Adaptive dose escalation trial of stereotactic body radiation therapy (SBRT) in combination with GC4419 in pancreatic cancer. J Clin Oncol. 2019;37(Suppl. 15):TPS4164.
7. Balaban EP, Mangu PB, Khorana AA, et al. Locally advanced, unresectable pancreatic cancer: American Society of Clinical Oncology clinical practice guideline. J Clin Oncol. 2016;34(22):2654–68.
8. Pollom EL, Chin AL, Diehn M, Loo BW, Chang DT. Normal tissue constraints for abdominal and thoracic stereotactic body radiotherapy. Semin Radiat Oncol. 2017;27(3):197–208.
9. Mahadevan A, Moningi S, Grimm J, et al. Maximizing tumor control and limiting complications with stereotactic body radiation therapy for pancreatic cancer. Int J Radiat Oncol Biol Phys. 2021;110(1):206–16.
10. Chuong MD, Bryant J, Mittauer KE, et al. Ablative 5-fraction stereotactic magnetic resonance-guided radiation therapy with on-table adaptive replanning and elective nodal irradiation for inoperable pancreas cancer. Pract Radiat Oncol. 2021;11(2):134–47.
11. Hassanzadeh C, Rudra S, Bommireddy A, et al. Ablative five-fraction stereotactic body radiation therapy for inoperable pancreatic cancer using online MR-guided adaptation. Adv Radiat Oncol. 2021;6(1):100506.
12. Kharofa J, Mierzwa M, Olowokure O, et al. Pattern of marginal local failure in a phase II trial of neoadjuvant chemotherapy and stereotactic body radiation therapy for resectable and borderline resectable pancreas cancer. Am J Clin Oncol. 2019;42(3):247–52.
13. Miller JA, Toesca DAS, Baclay JRM, et al. Pancreatic stereotactic body radiation therapy with or without hypofractionated elective nodal irradiation. Int J Radiat Oncol Biol Phys. 2022;112(1):131–42.
14. Zhu X, Ju X, Cao Y, et al. Patterns of local failure after stereotactic body radiation therapy and sequential chemotherapy as initial treatment for pancreatic cancer: implications of target volume design. Int J Radiat Oncol Biol Phys. 2019;104(1):101–10.
15. Reyngold M, Parikh P, Crane CH. Ablative radiation therapy for locally advanced pancreatic cancer: techniques and results. Radiat Oncol. 2019;14(1):95.
16. Reyngold M, O'Reilly EM, Varghese AM, et al. Association of ablative radiation therapy with survival among patients with inoperable pancreatic cancer. JAMA Oncol. 2021;7(5):735–8.
17. Mahadevan A, Miksad R, Goldstein M, et al. Induction gemcitabine and stereotactic body radiotherapy for locally advanced nonmetastatic pancreas cancer. Int J Radiat Oncol Biol Phys. 2011;81(4):e615–22.
18. Rwigema JC, Parikh SD, Heron DE, et al. Stereotactic body radiotherapy in the treatment of advanced adenocarcinoma of the pancreas. Am J Clin Oncol. 2011;34(1):63–9.

19. Mellon EA, Hoffe SE, Springett GM, et al. Long-term outcomes of induction chemotherapy and neoadjuvant stereotactic body radiotherapy for borderline resectable and locally advanced pancreatic adenocarcinoma. Acta Oncol. 2015;54(7):979–85.
20. Augustyn A, Reed VI, Ahmad N, et al. Implementation of a stereotactic body radiotherapy program for unresectable pancreatic cancer in an integrated community academic radiation oncology satellite network. Clin Transl Radiat Oncol. 2021;27:147–51.
21. Chuong MD, Springett GM, Freilich JM, et al. Stereotactic body radiation therapy for locally advanced and borderline resectable pancreatic cancer is effective and well tolerated. Int J Radiat Oncol Biol Phys. 2013;86(3):516–22.
22. Herman JM, Chang DT, Goodman KA, et al. Phase 2 multi-institutional trial evaluating gemcitabine and stereotactic body radiotherapy for patients with locally advanced unresectable pancreatic adenocarcinoma. Cancer. 2015;121(7):1128–37.
23. Comito T, Cozzi L, Clerici E, et al. Can stereotactic body radiation therapy be a viable and efficient therapeutic option for unresectable locally advanced pancreatic adenocarcinoma? Results of a phase 2 study. Technol Cancer Res Treat. 2017;16(3):295–301.
24. Didolkar MS, Coleman CW, Brenner MJ, et al. Image-guided stereotactic radiosurgery for locally advanced pancreatic adenocarcinoma results of first 85 patients. J Gastrointest Surg. 2010;14(10):1547–59.
25. Pollom EL, Alagappan M, von Eyben R, et al. Single- versus multifraction stereotactic body radiation therapy for pancreatic adenocarcinoma: outcomes and toxicity. Int J Radiat Oncol Biol Phys. 2014;90(4):918–25.
26. Lominska CE, Unger K, Nasr NM, Haddad N, Gagnon G. Stereotactic body radiation therapy for reirradiation of localized adenocarcinoma of the pancreas. Radiat Oncol. 2012;7:74.
27. Dagoglu N, Callery M, Moser J, et al. Stereotactic body radiotherapy (SBRT) reirradiation for recurrent pancreas cancer. J Cancer. 2016;7(3):283–8.
28. Koong AJ, Toesca DAS, von Eyben R, Pollom EL, Chang DT. Reirradiation with stereotactic body radiation therapy after prior conventional fractionation radiation for locally recurrent pancreatic adenocarcinoma. Adv Radiat Oncol. 2017;2(1):27–36.

Chapter 27
Rectal Cancer

Morgan M. Bailey, Andrew Z. Wang, Joel E. Tepper, and Kyle Wang

27.1 Introduction

Preoperative radiation therapy (RT) is utilized for locally advanced (e.g., T3 or N+) rectal cancer and may be delivered with either conventional fractionation over 5–6 weeks with concurrent chemotherapy, or "short-course" hypofractionated RT alone delivering 25 Gy in 5 fractions with or without additional sequential preoperative chemotherapy. Randomized trials have established general equivalence between these two approaches in the preoperative setting. However, questions remain regarding optimal patient selection and the role of short-course RT with the modern paradigms of total neoadjuvant treatment and nonoperative management. In contrast to the other chapters of this section, neither IMRT nor SBRT has well-defined roles in the treatment of rectal cancer; short-course RT is delivered to typical pelvic volumes usually with 3D-CRT.

27.2 Pearls

- There are approximately 150,000 cases of colorectal cancer in the United States per year (median age 67 years). Around 45,000 of these are rectal cancers.

M. M. Bailey
Department of Radiation Oncology, University of Cincinnati, Cincinnati, OH, USA

A. Z. Wang
UT Southwestern Medical Center, Dallas, TX, USA

J. E. Tepper
Department of Radiation Oncology, University of North Carolina Hospitals, Chapel Hill, NC, USA

K. Wang (✉)
Cincinnati, OH, USA

O. Kaidar-Person, R. Chen (eds.), *Hypofractionated and Stereotactic Radiation Therapy*, https://doi.org/10.1007/978-3-031-47701-0_27

- Most cases are sporadic rather than familial, and general risk factors include obesity, diabetes, tobacco, and alcohol use.
- Several genetic disorders increase risk, including familial adenomatous polyposis and Lynch syndrome (hereditary nonpolyposis colorectal cancer). Risk is substantially increased in patients with long-standing inflammatory bowel disease, particularly ulcerative colitis.
- Rectal cancers (vs. colon cancer) more frequently present with symptoms including hematochezia, rectal pain, tenesmus, and decreased stool caliber.
- Most are adenocarcinomas and similar in appearance to colonic adenocarcinomas. The dentate line forms an anatomic boundary below which squamous epithelium predominates (characteristic of anal cancer).
- Lymphatic spread is common. Beyond the immediate perirectal nodes, lower rectal tumors commonly spread to internal iliac nodes via the middle and inferior rectal vasculature, and upper rectal tumors commonly spread to inferior mesenteric nodes via the inferior mesenteric vasculature. Tumors below the dentate line (usually anal squamous cell carcinoma) often spread to inguinal and external iliac nodes.
- The liver and lung are the most common sites of distant metastasis. Similar to colon cancer, some patients with a limited number of metastases (usually liver-only) may be cured with aggressive locoregional therapy.
- Workup:
  - Colonoscopy to diagnose the local tumor and to look for synchronous tumors.
  - MRI and endoscopic ultrasound to evaluate for the involvement of the circumferential resection margin (CRM) and tumor stage, respectively.
  - Total body CT for staging.
  - Baseline CEA for prognostic purposes and to use during follow-up.
- Treatment:
  - Surgery is integral for the treatment of most patients with M0 disease and ideally involves a total mesorectal excision (TME). The location within the rectum is specified based on distance from the anal verge or dentate line and has important implications on whether anal sphincter-sparing low anterior resection (LAR) is possible, vs. abdominoperineal resection (APR).
  - Neoadjuvant RT is recommended in patients with Stage T3–4 or N+ disease. Conventionally fractionated RT may be given postoperatively (e.g., for unexpected pathologic findings).
  - Chemotherapy has usually been delivered postoperatively (extrapolating from colon cancer data) but is increasingly delivered preoperatively (either after or before RT) as part of total neoadjuvant treatment (TNT).
  - Select patients (e.g., those who would require an APR or a low LAR) with a clinical complete response to neoadjuvant treatment may be offered nonoperative management with aggressive locoregional surveillance.
  - Patients presenting with clinical symptoms of bowel obstruction (not endoscopic "obstruction") due to tumor should receive a palliative diverting ostomy if planned for neoadjuvant treatment including RT.

27.3 Tumor/Patient Selection

- Though short-course fractionation has become the standard of care in many European countries, there has been slowly increasing adoption in the United States. With further emerging evidence (including the RAPIDO trial), longer follow-up, and the increasing emphasis on value-based care, there is likely to be increased uptake of this approach.
- Ideal patients for short-course preoperative RT were traditionally thought to be those with proximal tumors and minimal concern for sphincter preservation and/or mesorectal fascia involvement, though these limitations appear to be mitigated by additional preoperative chemotherapy in the setting of total neoadjuvant therapy.
- Conventionally fractionated CRT may be better suited for patients with very low-lying tumors in whom nonoperative management may be desired.
- In patients with low-volume metastatic disease, definitive treatment of all sites of disease may be curative. Short-course RT is preferable when there are competing priorities of isolated distant metastases and symptomatic locoregional disease to minimize time to surgery and/or chemotherapy.
- **Surgical considerations:** A key question for all rectal cancer patients is whether patients can retain a functional anal sphincter and avoid permanent colostomy. In cases borderline for sphincter preservation, a more protracted preoperative course (e.g., conventional CRT) has generally been preferred due to increased downstaging and pathologic complete response (pCR) compared with a short course. However, the RAPIDO and Stockholm III trials have challenged this notion through the additional downstaging seen with the incorporation of neoadjuvant chemotherapy and delay to surgery, respectively [1–3].
- **Patient selection:** Historical short-course RT trials (see Relevant Literature) included many patients with Stage I–II disease or tumors >5 cm from the anal verge. For patients with high-risk rectal cancer (T4, extramural vascular invasion, or mesorectal fascia involvement), the RAPIDO trial suggests that neoadjuvant short-course RT with sequential chemotherapy is associated with higher locoregional failure compared with neoadjuvant conventional concurrent chemoradiotherapy [1].
- **Chemotherapy (and total neoadjuvant therapy):** Chemotherapy is not delivered concurrently with short-course RT, though chemotherapy increases downstaging and local control when given concurrently with conventionally fractionated preoperative RT. [4] The importance of concurrent chemotherapy is likely declining given the increased emphasis on sequential chemotherapy, which was traditionally delivered postoperatively based on colon cancer data. Many institutions have moved to "total neoadjuvant therapy" (TNT) where sequential chemotherapy is delivered preoperatively (before or after preoperative RT). TNT has the advantages of better patient compliance and downstaging (potentially reducing surgical morbidity or allowing for nonoperative management) and may be superior to preoperative RT with adjuvant chemotherapy [1, 5].

- **Nonoperative management:** Increasing data suggest that patients with a complete response to neoadjuvant therapy may be offered nonoperative management (the "watch and wait" strategy), especially if surgery would consist of an APR. These patients have an increased risk of local failure and require aggressive surveillance in order to detect and salvage early local tumor regrowth; further studies are needed to confirm that OS is not compromised [6]. A greater number of preoperative chemotherapy cycles is associated with a higher pCR rate [7]; thus, TNT may facilitate nonoperative management. Most watch-and-wait studies include patients treated only with conventional chemoRT. Emerging data, however, suggest that short-course RT may produce similar results in the context of TNT [8], but further follow-up and comparisons with conventional chemoRT are needed to establish equivalence when the goal is nonoperative management.
- **Toxicity:** Randomized trials have *not* shown an increased rate of toxicity using the short course regimen when compared to conventional fractionation [9, 10]. The Stockholm III trial showed that short-course RT with surgery within 1 week led to more postoperative complications (50%) compared with both short-course RT with a 4- to 8-week delay to surgery (38%) and conventional preoperative RT (without chemo, 39%) [2].
- **Guidelines:** The use of neoadjuvant short-course RT is included in the 2023 NCCN and 2020 ASTRO guidelines as an acceptable neoadjuvant treatment where surgery is planned. However, short-course RT is noted to be associated with increased locoregional failure compared with conventional concurrent chemoradiotherapy for high-risk rectal cancer [1]. In addition, the NCCN guidelines state a preference for short courses in patients with resectable metastases [11]. The ASTRO guidelines recommend conventional fractionation if nonoperative management is pursued [12].

27.4 Treatment Planning Considerations (Figs. 27.1 and 27.2)

Simulation instructions	• Depending on body habitus, the patient may be simulated either prone or supine. Patients with a larger girth may benefit from prone simulation with a belly board to displace the bowel from the field • An anal marker may be helpful to localize the tumor with the distance from the anal verge to the tumor determined on the exam • Simulations should also be performed with a full bladder to displace the small bowel superiorly, especially in short-course RT given the potential for high doses per fraction to cause bowel toxicity
Image guidance	For conventional 3D-CRT, weekly portal films are typically adequate. However, daily cone-beam CT is reasonable with short-course RT given the higher dose per fraction, and if intensity-modulated radiation therapy (IMRT) is used

Treatment planning	• The fields and targets for short-course fractionation for rectal cancer are typically similar or identical to those used for conventional fractionation • The most important target volumes are the mesorectum and mesorectal fascia. In addition, target volumes include presacral, mesorectal, obturator, and internal iliac lymph nodes with a superior field border at the lower edge of L5 [13] • The anal canal should be included for very low tumors, but, otherwise, anal sphincter dose should be minimized while maintaining mesorectal coverage
Dosimetric considerations	Similar to conventional fractionation, the major dosimetric consideration with short-course RT is the minimization of small bowel dose and volume. Though 25 Gy in 5 fx is below bowel tolerance for late toxicity, earlier short-course RT studies using older (e.g., two-field) techniques and larger fields resulted in a higher frequency of late bowel obstruction. These concerns are mitigated by the use of modern techniques

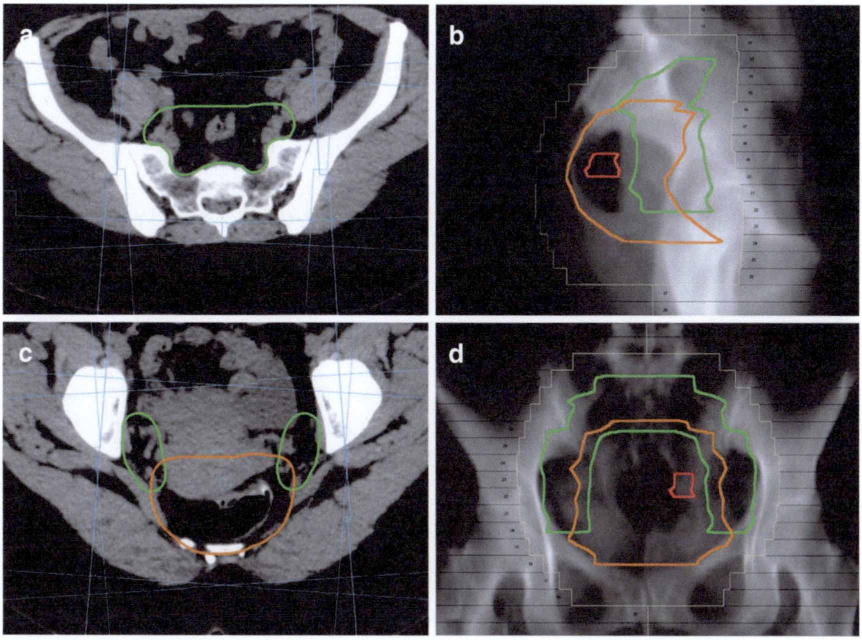

Fig. 27.1 Example of standard rectal cancer treatment planning using 3D-CRT in a patient receiving short-course RT. Four opposed fields are shown, though a three-field technique using wedged opposed laterals and a single posterior–anterior beam may reduce dose to anterior structures including bladder and bowel. This patient had limited metastatic disease and received initial chemotherapy with a good local response. The GTV is red, the mesorectum is orange, and the nodal region is green. (**a**) Coverage of presacral and high internal iliac nodes with inclusion of the rectosigmoid. (**b**) Coverage of mesorectum and low internal iliac nodes. (**c**) Lateral field view showing a generous posterior field edge to ensure coverage of the presacral space, superior field edge at the inferior border of L5, and limited anterior field edge to spare bowel. (**d**) Anterior field view. The anal canal was not covered due to the proximal location of the tumor

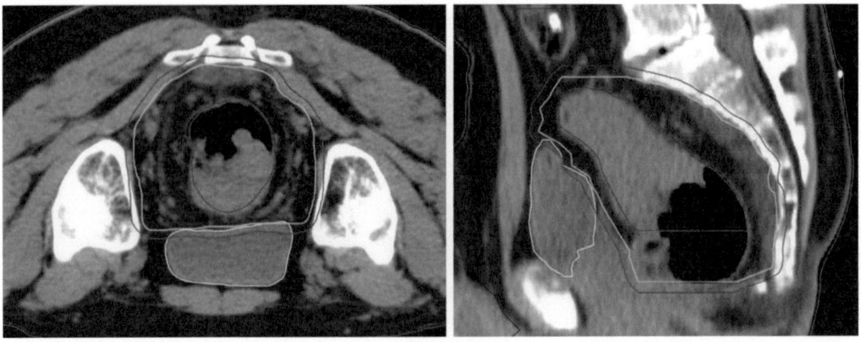

Fig. 27.2 Example of treatment volumes for an IMRT plan in a patient receiving short-course RT in the prone position. The GTV is red, the CTV encompassing the mesorectum and regional nodes is green, the PTV (3–7 mm) is violet, and the bladder is yellow. Treatment planning with IMRT may facilitate avoidance of low-lying small bowel and integration of a simultaneous boost in certain clinical situations, e.g., for gross nodal disease outside of the anticipated surgical field or even to the primary tumor if the goal is nonoperative management

27.5 Commonly Used Dose/Fractionation Schemes

Dose/fx	# of fx	Total dose	Notes
5 Gy	5	25 Gy	Standard short-course preop RT fractionation delivered daily using either 3D-CRT or IMRT. No concurrent chemotherapy

27.6 Normal Tissue Tolerances

- Though dose-volume tolerances of pelvic organs are well-described with conventional fractionation, relatively little data exist for hypofractionation and short-course RT. Generally, a dose of 25 Gy in 5 fractions is well tolerated by most pelvic organs, but the volume of small bowel receiving this dose should be minimized and hot spots avoided.
- Given that short-course rectal RT is delivered in 5 fractions, abdominal and pelvic organ tolerances generally used for SBRT may have applicability especially if doses exceeding 25 Gy are planned. For instance, a simultaneous boost (e.g., 30–40 Gy) may be used for gross nodal disease outside of the planned surgical field while prioritizing bowel tolerance.
- The rectum itself has not typically been considered an organ at risk given that it is usually removed at the time of surgery. However, irradiated distal rectum (and anal canal) are not removed with a low anterior resection and it is the combination of surgery and irradiation that determines postoperative anorectal function. With nonoperative management where the entire rectum remains intact, further research is needed to determine rectal dose tolerances to both short-course and conventionally fractionated RT.

	Washington University [8]	Comments
Small bowel	Dmax <25 Gy	Small bowel doses can be minimized through careful dosimetry, treatment with bladder full, and in some cases with prone positioning. If excess small bowel falls within the field, conventional fractionation could be considered. Based on pancreatic SBRT studies, the risks of severe toxicity rise with doses ≥30 Gy [14]
Colon		The colon and rectum are considered slightly more resistant to radiation toxicity compared with the small bowel, but it is prudent to avoid hot spots in any bowel when possible
Bladder	Dmax <38 Gy	The bladder can tolerate doses in excess of 25 Gy in 5 fx based on prostate SBRT studies [5]. Acute genitourinary symptoms may result from the dose to both bladder and urethra. The volume of the bladder receiving 20–25 Gy should thus be minimized without compromising target coverage
Vagina		In women, treatment of anorectal malignancies may lead to sexual dysfunction from vaginal stenosis and fibrosis. For patients where this is a priority, the dose to the anterior vagina can be lowered with the use of a vaginal dilator at simulation and each treatment (with daily image guidance) [15]
Femoral heads	V30 Gy < 10 cc	With standard rectal 3D-CRT, the femoral head dose is impacted by the weighting of the lateral fields and lateral margin of the anterior/posterior fields

27.7 Patient Management Considerations

- Because of the short duration of treatment, the rates of reported acute toxicity from short-course RT are low, perhaps manifesting after completion of RT or during the perioperative period. Patients nonetheless may develop acute enteritis requiring antidiarrheals, radiation dermatitis requiring emollients, and cystitis that may mimic a urinary tract infection.
- Rates of late toxicity appear comparable with patients receiving conventional fractionation and usually involve gastrointestinal changes including increased frequency of bowel movements and incontinence. Late grade 3 gastrointestinal toxicities have been reported to occur in around 5–10% [9, 10], though low-grade toxicities may occur in up to 50% [16]. Though challenging to manage, these late symptoms can be reduced by alteration of diet and the use of anti-motility agents.

27.8 Follow-Up

- Patients receiving preoperative short-course RT proceed to surgery within 1 week of completing RT (immediate) or 4–10 weeks post-RT (delayed).
- Following surgery, patients should be evaluated every 3–6 months with rectal examination and CEA. Patients should also receive a colonoscopy at 1 year and annual CT scans.
- Follow-up of patients achieving a clinical complete response undergoing nonoperative management includes the above evaluations but also more frequent and sensitive monitoring for local regrowth with pelvic MRI and/or direct endoscopic examination every 3 months.

27.9 Relevant Literature

- **Toxicity:** Late gastrointestinal toxicity has been reported to be higher than surgery alone in the Swedish and Dutch short-course trials. Though some patients developed very late (e.g., 5 years post-RT) bowel obstructions, the use of older techniques (often with opposed anterior–posterior fields) likely resulted in high bowel doses and are not applicable today [16, 17]. Studies randomizing patients to short course vs. conventional RT using modern techniques have generally shown similar rates of acute and late toxicity. Late small bowel toxicity can be minimized through careful treatment planning and patient instructions [9, 10, 18]. With the addition of chemotherapy in a total neoadjuvant approach, more patients experience toxicity during the preop period. In the RAPIDO trial, short-course RT with additional preoperative chemotherapy led to 48% preoperative grade 3 toxicity vs. only 25% in patients receiving standard fractionation preop chemoradiation. The rates of grade 3 diarrhea in these arms were 18% and 9%, respectively [1].
- The trials summarized in this section (Table) are organized by clinical question and roughly by chronologic order. The first three trials (Swedish, Dutch, UK) compared short-course preop RT vs. surgery alone in rectal cancer patients of all stages. The initial Swedish short-course trial [19] demonstrated the feasibility and effectiveness of short-course RT. The Dutch [20] and UK [21] trials confirmed this benefit when standardizing surgery to TME.
- The next two trials (Polish I and TROG) compared short-course preop RT with conventional preop chemoradiotherapy and included only advanced tumors. These trials showed comparable survival and cancer control outcomes, similar late toxicities, but significantly greater rates of pathologic complete response and possibly sphincter preservation in the conventionally treated patients [9, 10].
- The next two trials (Polish II and RAPIDO) intensified preop treatment through a total neoadjuvant strategy for advanced tumors, comparing standard conventional preop chemoradiotherapy with sequential short-course preop RT with

additional preop chemotherapy (3 cycles in Polish II and 6–9 cycles in RAPIDO). In the Polish II trial, the short-course total neoadjuvant approach demonstrated comparable cancer control, overall survival, and rates of acute grade 3 toxicities and late toxicities, along with similar rates of pathologic complete response and sphincter preservation [18, 22]. The RAPIDO trial demonstrated better pCR rate and decreased metastasis, but increased locoregional recurrence, with total neoadjuvant therapy using short-course preop RT and additional preop chemotherapy as compared with conventional fractionation preop chemoradiation with optional adjuvant chemotherapy. Furthermore, more toxicities were noted during the more extended regimen of preoperative chemotherapy in the total neoadjuvant arm [1].

- The final listed study (Stockholm III) was initially a three-arm randomization comparing short-course RT with immediate surgery, short-course RT with delayed surgery, and conventional preop RT (without concurrent chemo) and delayed surgery. A protocol amendment then allowed institutions to randomize between the short-course arms alone. In the three-arm randomization analysis, there was no difference in local control or overall survival. In the two-arm randomization analysis, postoperative complications appeared to be increased in patients receiving short-course RT and immediate surgery (vs. short-course RT and delayed surgery) [2]. In a subsequent analysis, the pathologic complete response rate was highest with short-course RT and delayed surgery (10.4%), vs. conventional preop RT and delayed surgery (2.2%) and short-course RT and immediate surgery (0.3%) [3].

Study	Patients	Treatments	Median follow-up	Outcomes
Randomized trials				
Trial that compared surgery vs. short-course RT followed by surgery				
Swedish 1997 [19]	• $N = 908$ • Dukes' stage A (30%), B (33%), C (37%)	**Arm 1**: 25 Gy (5 fx, daily), surgery within one week **Arm 2:** Surgery alone (TME not reported)	6.25 years in survivors	**Arm 1:** • 11% 5-year LR • 58% 5-year OS **Arm 2:** • 27% 5-year LR ($p < 0.001$) • 48% 5-year OS ($p = 0.004$)
Dutch Kapiteijn 2001 [20] Peeters 2007 (long-term follow-up) [23]	• $N = 1805$ • Stage I (28%), II (29%), III (35%) • 28% ≤5 cm from anal verge	**Arm 1**: 25 Gy (5 fx, daily), surgery **Arm 2:** Surgery alone (TME both arms)	6.1 years in survivors	**Arm 1:** • 6% 5-year LR • 64% 5-year OS **Arm 2:** • 11% 5-year LR ($p < 0.001$) • 64% 5-year OS (NS)

UK Sebag-Montefiore 2009 [21]	• $N = 1350$ • Stage I (26%), II (30%), III (40%) • 34% ≤5 cm from anal verge	**Arm 1**: 25 Gy (5 fx, daily), surgery 1 week post-RT **Arm 2:** Surgery (10% received conventional postop chemoradiotherapy) (TME both arms)	4 years in survivors	**Arm 1**: • 5% 5-year LR • 70% 5-year OS **Arm 2:** • 12% 5-year LR ($p < 0.001$) • 68% 5-year OS (NS)
Trials that compared preop short-course RT vs. preop conventional chemoradiation				
Polish I Bujko 2006 [9]	• $N = 312$ • T3/4	**Arm 1**: 25 Gy (5 fx, daily), surgery 1 week post-RT **Arm 2:** 50.4 Gy (28 fx), concurrent 5-FU, surgery 4–6 weeks post-RT (TME for low-lying tumors, both arms)	4 years in survivors	**Arm 1**: • 11% 4-year LR • 67% 4-year OS • 1% pCR, 13% positive CRM • Toxicity: 3% grade ≥3 acute, 10% severe late **Arm 2:** • 16% 4-year LR (NS) • 66% 4-year OS (NS) • 16% pCR, 4% positive CRM • Toxicity: 18% grade ≥3 acute, 7% severe late
TROG Ngan 2012 [10]	• $N = 323$ • T3 • 37% node positive • 24% ≤5 cm from anal verge	**Arm 1**: 25 Gy (5 fx, daily), surgery 1 week post-RT **Arm 2:** 50.4 Gy (28 fx), concurrent 5-FU, surgery 4–6 weeks post-RT (TME both arms)	5.9 years	**Arm 1**: • 8% 5-year LR • 74% 5-year OS • 1% pCR, 37% APR • 6% late grade 3/4 toxicity **Arm 2:** • 6% 5-year LR (NS) • 70% 5-year OS (NS) • 15% pCR, 31% APR • 8% late grade 3/4 toxicity

Trials that compared preop sequential short-course RT with chemotherapy vs. preop conventional chemoradiation				
Polish II Bujko 2016 [18] (long-term follow-up) [22]	• $N = 515$ • Fixed T3/4 • 56% ≤5 cm from anal verge	**Arm 1**: 25 Gy (5 fx, daily), sequential FOLFOX4 x3 cycles, surgery 6 weeks post-chemo **Arm 2:** 50.4 Gy (28 fx), concurrent 5-FU + weekly oxaliplatin, surgery 6 weeks post-RT (TME both arms)	7.0 years	**Arm 1**: • 22% 3-year LR • 43% 8-year DFS • 49% 8-year OS • 16% pCR, 37% APR • 11% late grade ≥3 complications **Arm 2:** • 21% 3-year LR (NS) • 41% 8-year DFS (NS) • 49% 8-year OS (NS) • 12% pCR, 41% APR • 9% late grade ≥3 complications
RAPIDO Bahadoer 2021 [24], 2023 [25] Dijkstra 2023 [1]	• $N = 912$ • T4a/T4b, N2, EMVI, mesorectal fascia involvement, and/or involved lateral nodes • 24% <5 cm from anal verge	**Arm 1:** 25 Gy (5 fx over ≤8 days), sequential CAPOX ×6 cycles or FOLFOX4 ×9 cycles, surgery 2–4 weeks post-chemo **Arm 2:** 50–50.4 (25–28 fx), concurrent capecitabine, surgery 6–10 weeks post-RT, optional adjuvant chemo (TME both arms)	5.6 years	**Arm 1:** • 10% 3-year LRR • 23% 5-year DM • 89% 3-year OS • 28% pCR • 38% serious adverse events • 18% acute grade 3 diarrhea **Arm 2:** • 6% 3-year LRR ($p = 0.027$) • 30% 5-year DM ($p = 0.011$) • 89% 3-year OS (NS) • 14% pCR ($p < 0.001$) • 34% serious adverse events • 9% acute grade 3 diarrhea

Trial that compared different timing between short-course and long-course preop RT to surgery				
Stockholm III Erlandsson 2017 [2], 2019 [3]	• $N = 385$ (3-arm randomization) • Any clinical stage • 36% ≤5 cm from anal verge	**Arm 1:** 25 Gy (5 fx, daily), surgery 1-week post-RT **Arm 2:** 25 Gy (5 fx, daily), surgery 4–8 weeks post-RT **Arm 3:** 50 Gy (25 fx, daily), surgery 4–8 weeks post-RT (TME all arms)	5.7 years	**Arm 1:** • 0.3% pCR • 2% 5-year LR • 74% 5-year OS **Arm 2:** • 10.4% pCR ($p < 0.001$) • 3% 5-year LR (NS) • 76% 5-year OS (NS) **Arm 3:** • 2.2% pCR • 5% 5-year LR (NS) • 78% 5-year OS (NS) * Pooled analysis of arm 1 vs. arm 2: Higher operative complications with immediate (53%) vs. delayed surgery (41%) after short-course RT

Abbreviations: *CRM* circumferential resection margin, *EMVI* extramural venous invasion, *LR* local recurrence, *OS* overall survival, *PFS* progression-free survival, *pCR* pathologic complete response, *fx* fractions, *RT* radiotherapy, *APR* abdominoperineal resection, *chemo* chemotherapy, *LRR* locoregional recurrence

References

1. Dijkstra EA, Nilsson PJ, Hospers GA, et al. Locoregional failure during and after short-course radiotherapy follwoed by chemotehrapy and surgery compared to long-course chemoradiotherapy and surgery— a five-year follow-up of the RAPIDO trial. Ann Surg. 2023;278:e766; Epub ahead of print.
2. Erlandsson J, Holm T, Pettersson D, et al. Optimal fractionation of preoperative radiotherapy and timing to surgery for rectal cancer (Stockholm III): a multicentre, randomised, non-blinded, phase 3, non-inferiority trial. Lancet Oncol. 2017;18(3):336–46.
3. Erlandsson J, Lörinc E, Ahlberg M, et al. Tumour regression after radiotherapy for rectal cancer—results from the randomised Stockholm III trial. Radiother Oncol. 2019;135:178–86.
4. Bosset JF, Collette L, Calais G, et al. Chemotherapy with preoperative radiotherapy in rectal cancer. N Engl J Med. 2006;355(11):1114–23.
5. Wang K, Mavroidis P, Royce TJ, et al. Prostate stereotactic body radiation therapy: an overview of toxicity and dose response. Int J Radiat Oncol Biol Phys. 2021;110(1):237–48.

6. Dossa F, Chesney TR, Acuna SA, Baxter NN. A watch-and-wait approach for locally advanced rectal cancer after a clinical complete response following neoadjuvant chemoradiation: a systematic review and meta-analysis. Lancet Gastroenterol Hepatol. 2017;2(7):501–13.
7. Garcia-Aguilar J, Chow OS, Smith DD, et al. Effect of adding mFOLFOX6 after neoadjuvant chemoradiation in locally advanced rectal cancer: a multicentre, phase 2 trial. Lancet Oncol. 2015;16(8):957–66.
8. Chin RI, Roy A, Pedersen KS, et al. Clinical complete response in patients with rectal adenocarcinoma treated with short-course radiation therapy and nonoperative management. Int J Radiat Oncol Biol Phys. 2022;112(3):715–25.
9. Bujko K, Nowacki MP, Nasierowska-Guttmejer A, Michalski W, Bebenek M, Kryj M. Long-term results of a randomized trial comparing preoperative short-course radiotherapy with preoperative conventionally fractionated chemoradiation for rectal cancer. Br J Surg. 2006;93(10):1215–23.
10. Ngan SY, Burmeister B, Fisher RJ, et al. Randomized trial of short-course radiotherapy versus long-course chemoradiation comparing rates of local recurrence in patients with T3 rectal cancer: Trans-Tasman Radiation Oncology Group trial 01.04. J Clin Oncol. 2012;30(31):3827–33.
11. NCCN. Rectal cancer version 3.2023. National Comprehensive Cancer Network. 2023.
12. Wo JY, Anker CJ, Ashman JB, et al. Radiation therapy for rectal cancer: executive summary of an ASTRO clinical practice guideline. Pract Radiat Oncol. 2021;11(1):13–25.
13. Myerson RJ, Garofalo MC, El Naqa I, et al. Elective clinical target volumes for conformal therapy in anorectal cancer: a radiation therapy oncology group consensus panel contouring atlas. Int J Radiat Oncol Biol Phys. 2009;74(3):824–30.
14. Mahadevan A, Moningi S, Grimm J, et al. Maximizing tumor control and limiting complications with stereotactic body radiation therapy for pancreatic cancer. Int J Radiat Oncol Biol Phys. 2021;110(1):206–16.
15. Briere TM, Crane CH, Beddar S, et al. Reproducibility and genital sparing with a vaginal dilator used for female anal cancer patients. Radiother Oncol. 2012;104(2):161–6.
16. Peeters KC, van de Velde CJ, Leer JW, et al. Late side effects of short-course preoperative radiotherapy combined with total mesorectal excision for rectal cancer: increased bowel dysfunction in irradiated patients—a Dutch colorectal cancer group study. J Clin Oncol. 2005;23(25):6199–206.
17. Birgisson H, Pahlman L, Gunnarsson U, Glimelius B, Swedish Rectal Cancer Trial Group. Adverse effects of preoperative radiation therapy for rectal cancer: long-term follow-up of the Swedish Rectal Cancer Trial. J Clin Oncol. 2005;23(34):8697–705.
18. Bujko K, Wyrwicz L, Rutkowski A, et al. Long-course oxaliplatin-based preoperative chemoradiation versus 5 x 5 Gy and consolidation chemotherapy for cT4 or fixed cT3 rectal cancer: results of a randomized phase III study. Ann Oncol. 2016;27(5):834–42.
19. Swedish Rectal Cancer Trial. Improved survival with preoperative radiotherapy in resectable rectal cancer. Swedish Rectal Cancer Trial. N Engl J Med. 1997;336(14):980–7.
20. Kapitcijn E, Marijnen CA, Nagtegaal ID, et al. Preoperative radiotherapy combined with total mesorectal excision for resectable rectal cancer. N Engl J Med. 2001;345(9):638–46.
21. Sebag-Montefiore D, Stephens RJ, Steele R, et al. Preoperative radiotherapy versus selective postoperative chemoradiotherapy in patients with rectal cancer (MRC CR07 and NCIC-CTG C016): a multicentre, randomised trial. Lancet. 2009;373(9666):811–20.
22. Cisel B, Pietrzak L, Michalski W, et al. Long-course preoperative chemoradiation versus 5 x 5 Gy and consolidation chemotherapy for clinical T4 and fixed clinical T3 rectal cancer: long-term results of the randomized Polish II study. Ann Oncol. 2019;30(8):1298–303.
23. Peeters KC, Marijnen CA, Nagtegaal ID, et al. The TME trial after a median follow-up of 6 years: increased local control but no survival benefit in irradiated patients with resectable rectal carcinoma. Ann Surg. 2007;246(5):693–701.

24. Bahadoer RR, Dijkstra EA, van Etten B, et al. Short-course radiotherapy followed by chemotherapy before total mesorectal excision (TME) versus preoperative chemoradiotherapy, TME, and optional adjuvant chemotherapy in locally advanced rectal cancer (RAPIDO): a randomised, open-label, phase 3 trial. Lancet Oncol. 2021;22(1):29–42.
25. Bahadoer RR, Hospers GAP, Marijnen CAM, et al. Risk and location of distant metastases in patients with locally advanced rectal cancer after total neoadjvant treatment or chemoradiotherapy in the RAPIDO trial. Eur J Cancer. 2023;185:139–49.

Part VIII
Genitourinary Cancer

Chapter 28
Prostate Cancer

Samantha L. Freije, Ronald C. Chen, and Jordan A. Holmes

28.1 Introduction

Prostate cancer is the most common malignancy diagnosed in men in the United States. Prostate cancer is hypothesized to have an alpha/beta ratio of <2 offering a potential therapeutic benefit for hypofractionation. In addition to biological reasons, the frequency of prostate cancer and the high health care cost of treatment have led to significant interest in shortening radiation treatment time. For intact prostate cancer, moderate hypofractionation is now considered the standard of care supported by several large randomized trials providing level I evidence for the safety and efficacy of moderate hypofractionation. There has been a more recent interest in stereotactic body radiation therapy (SBRT) for prostate cancer with many single- and multi-institutional studies reporting safety and efficacy for low- and intermediate-risk disease, as well as a recently published phase III randomized trial. SBRT for high-risk patients is an active area of ongoing research. Post-radical-prostatectomy hypofractionation is supported by promising results from NRG GU003 but remains an area of active investigation.

S. L. Freije
Department of Radiation Oncology, Indiana University School of Medicine, Indianapolis, IN, USA

R. C. Chen
Department of Radiation Oncology, KU Medical Center, The University of Kansas, Kansas City, USA

J. A. Holmes (✉)
Department of Radiation Oncology, Indiana University School of Medicine, Indianapolis, IN, USA

Indiana University Simon Comprehensive Cancer Center, Indianapolis, IN, USA
e-mail: jorholmes@iu.edu

O. Kaidar-Person, R. Chen (eds.), *Hypofractionated and Stereotactic Radiation Therapy*, https://doi.org/10.1007/978-3-031-47701-0_28

28.2 Pearls

- Prostate cancer is the most common non-cutaneous malignancy in men and the second leading cause of cancer mortality in men in the United States. An estimated 248,000 men will be diagnosed with prostate cancer in 2021 [1].
- The median age at diagnosis is 67 years. African American men are more likely to be diagnosed with prostate cancer than Caucasian men. There has been no clear causal relationship determined between a risk factor and the development of prostate cancer. Diet (high-fat diet), tobacco use, and higher BMI have been correlated with an increased risk of prostate cancer.
- Most prostate cancers are diagnosed while asymptomatic due to PSA screening. However, more advanced diseases can present with urinary obstruction and/or hematuria, and metastatic patients can present with bone pain.
- Prostate cancer is graded using the Gleason grading system. Grade groupings ranging from 1 to 5 (Group 1 = Gleason 6; Group 2 = Gleason 3 + 4; Group 3 = Gleason 4 + 3; Group 4 = Gleason 8; Group 5 = Gleason 9–10) are now commonly used.
- Over 95% of prostate cancers are adenocarcinoma. Uncommon variants include small cell, mucinous, and ductal prostate cancers. These rare variants are almost always found in the background of adenocarcinoma.
- The peripheral zone of the prostate makes up about 70% of the glandular tissue in an adult and contains almost all prostate cancers. The central zone makes up most of the remaining glandular tissue; the transitional zone surrounding the urethra (the site of BPH) and the anterior fibromuscular stroma are rare sites of cancer.
- The apex of the prostate is involved in over half of cancers, and because the prostatic capsule is not well defined at this level, extracapsular spread can be difficult to identify. Extracapsular extension is most frequently identified in the posterior and lateral portions of the gland along the neurovascular bundle.
- The seminal vesicles are superior to the prostate and can be involved in cancers involving the base of the gland by local extension.
- Prostate cancer typically follows a stepwise pattern of spread first to the internal iliac or obturator nodes and then to the common iliac and para-aortic nodes. Less commonly, pre-sacral and perirectal nodes can be involved (<20% of node-positive patients). When the seminal vesicles are involved, the risk of spread to the external iliac chain is increased.
- The risk of nodal spread is related to tumor volume, PSA, and Gleason score. The risk of adverse pathology (i.e., node-positive, extracapsular extension, and seminal vesicle invasion) can be estimated using prediction tools:
  - Roach Formula for risk of LN: $2/3 \times \text{PSA} + ([\text{Gleason-6}] \times 10)$.
  - Partin Nomograms: https://www.hopkinsmedicine.org/brady-urology-institute/conditions_and_treatments/prostate_cancer/risk_assessment_tools/partin-nomograms.html
  - MSKCC Nomograms: https://www.mskcc.org/nomograms/prostate/pre-op

- The overwhelming majority of prostate cancer metastases are to bone (>80%). Metastatic diseases to the lung and liver are more common in the later stages of the disease.
- Medical workup should include PSA, prostate biopsy (Gleason grade group), and digital rectal exam (to assess clinical T stage) to complete risk stratification. Basic labs including a CBC and basic chemistry panel should be obtained for any patient considering surgical intervention, and LFTs should be obtained for patients who are being considered for ADT.
- Imaging workup (per NCCN guidelines):
  - Bone scan if any of the following: T1 and PSA >20, T2 and PSA >10, Gleason ≥8, T3/4, or symptomatic.
  - CT/MRI pelvis if any of the following: T3/4 disease, T1/2 disease with nomogram predicted probability of lymph node involvement >10%.
  - A prostate-specific PET scan can be used instead of CT, MRI, and bone scan.
  - For patients with low and favorable intermediate-risk disease, no staging imaging is recommended.
- Treatment options
  - Low risk: Active surveillance is usually preferred especially for patients with low-volume, low-risk disease. For others, brachytherapy, SBRT, conventional fractionated or moderately hypofractionated external beam RT, or radical prostatectomy.
  - Favorable intermediate risk: External beam RT, brachytherapy, SBRT, or radical prostatectomy, usually without ADT.
  - Unfavorable intermediate risk: External beam RT ± brachytherapy usually with short-term ADT, or radical prostatectomy.
  - High risk: External beam RT ± brachytherapy + long-term ADT, or radical prostatectomy.
  - Low-volume metastatic prostate cancer: External beam RT to the prostate ± RT to metastatic sites.
  - Limited life expectancy (<5 years): Watchful waiting.

28.3 Tumor/Patient Selection

- Intact prostate hypofractionation
  - No history of proctitis, diverticulitis, or inflammatory bowel conditions
- Post-radical prostatectomy hypofractionation
  - No history of proctitis, diverticulitis, or inflammatory bowel conditions
- SBRT:
  - Low-risk or favorable intermediate-risk disease
  - No history of proctitis, diverticulitis, or inflammatory bowel conditions
  - Prostate volume <100 cc

28.4 Treatment Planning Considerations (Fig. 28.1)

Simulation instructions	• Intact prostate moderate hypofractionation: **Per RTOG 0415:** A urethrogram is encouraged to establish the inferior portion of the prostate. Patients should be simulated supine with CT slice thickness ≤5 mm. Extreme bladder or rectal filling should not be present at the time of the planning CT scan **Indiana University (IU) Practice:** Patients simulated supine. 3-mm CT slices are obtained from the mid-abdomen through the mid-thigh. Comfortably full bladder and empty rectum. We do not routinely fuse MRI images for prostate delineation • Intact prostate SBRT: **Per NRG-GU005:** One enema before simulation and each treatment and use of a hollow (Rob-Nel) catheter to evacuate the flatus are highly recommended to allow for a narrow posterior PTV margin. The use of rectal manipulation is allowed and based on institutional standards (e.g., rectal balloon, hydrogel spacer, or no manipulation). A full bladder for CT simulation and daily treatment is strongly recommended. Consistent bladder filling procedures should be used for an individual patient for simulation and for each treatment. CT scan of the pelvis should start at or above the iliac crest down to the perineum. CT scan thickness should be <2 mm throughout the area of the prostate. This will be fused with MRI in the treatment planning software **IU Practice:** Patients are recommended to undergo hydrogel spacer and fiducial marker placement prior to simulation. They are then instructed to perform a Fleets enema at home 2 h before simulation and each treatment. Simulate patients supine with a comfortably full bladder and empty rectum. 1.5-mm CT slices are obtained from the iliac crests through the mid-thigh. MRI is fused for treatment planning • Post-radical prostatectomy hypofractionation: **Per NRG-GU003:** Patients are simulated supine with the empty rectum (<3 cm in anterior–posterior dimension ideal, can achieve with enema 1–2 h prior to stimulation or red-rubber catheter for flatus evacuation) and comfortably full bladder. CT scan thickness <3 mm through the region that contains target volumes. Retrograde urethrogram or MRI is recommended for fusion in order to identify the most inferior portion of the prostate fossa
Image guidance	• Intact prostate moderate hypofractionation: Daily image guidance with either real-time tracking (Calypso® transponders, ultrasound), daily 3D imaging (KV-CBCT), or alignment to fiducials • Intact prostate SBRT: Daily image guidance with either real-time tracking (Calypso® transponders, ultrasound) or daily 3D imaging with intrafraction verification (KV-CBCT, real-time KV fiducial tracking) • Post-radical prostatectomy: Daily image guidance with 3D imaging (KV-CBCT)

Margins	• Intact prostate moderate hypofractionation: **RTOG 0415:** Prostate = CTV, CTV+ at least 4 mm for PTV. Sup/Inf PTV margin of 4–10 mm **IU Practice:** Prostate = CTV, CTV+ 5–8 mm = PTV. We do not routinely plan pelvic radiation for patients treated with hypofractionation • Intact prostate SBRT: **NRG-GU005:** Prostate = GTV. Prostate ± 1 cm of SV = CTV; CTV + 5 mm sup/inf/laterally + 3 mm ant/posteriorly = PTV • Post-radical prostatectomy hypofractionation (NRG-GU003): *Prostatic bed:* Superior: Beginning at the level of the caudal vas deferens remnant, should include seminal vesicle remnants (if present) if pathologic evidence of involvement Inferior: 8–12 mm inferior to the vesicourethral anastomosis Anterior: posterior aspect of the pubic symphysis; above the symphysis include 1–2 cm of the posterior bladder wall Posterior: anterior rectal wall Prostatic bed = CTV; CTV + 7–10 mm = PTV
Dosimetric considerations	• Intact prostate moderate hypofractionation (RTOG 0415): – Prostate PTV V100% prescription ≥98% – Prostate PTV D95% prescription = 100% – Dmax ≤107% • Intact prostate SBRT (NRG-GU005): – Prostate PTV V100% prescription ≥98% – Prostate PTV D95% prescription >99% – D0.03 cc [Gy] < 107% • Post-radical prostatectomy hypofractionation (NRG-GU003): – Prostatic bed PTV V100% prescription ≥95% – 0DMax <115%

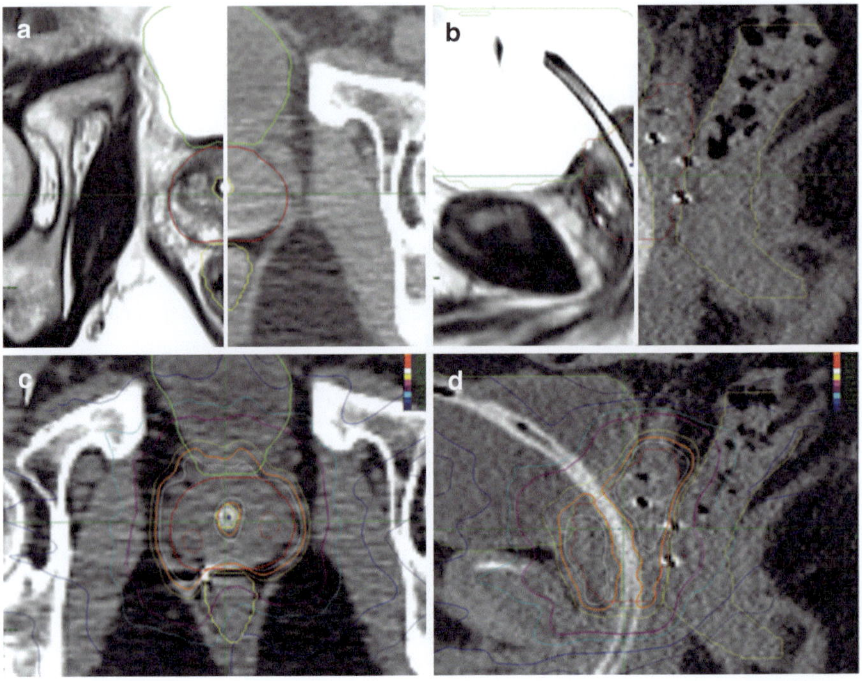

Fig. 28.1 Representative axial (**a**) and sagittal (**b**) sections of the prostate, rectum, and bladder with CT (right half of the image) and T2-weighted MRI (left half of the image) in a patient planned to receive CyberKnife SBRT. The same axial (**c**) and sagittal (**d**) slices showing the final radiation plan

28.5 Commonly Used Dose/Fractionation

Dose/fx	# of fx	Total dose	Frequency	Notes
Intact Prostate				
Hypofractionation				
2.5 Gy	28	70 Gy	Daily	RTOG 0415 [2]
3 Gy	20	60 Gy	Daily	CHHiP [3] and PROFIT [4]
3.4 Gy	19	64.6 Gy	Every other day	HYPRO [5]
Ultra-hypofractionation				
6.1 Gy	7	42.7 Gy	3×/week	HYPO-RT-PC [6]
SBRT				
9.5 Gy	4	38 Gy	Daily	Fuller [7]
7.25 Gy	5	36.25 Gy	2–3 fx per week	NRG-GU005, PACE-B [8]
8 Gy	5	40 Gy	Every other day	
Post-operative hypofractionation				
2.5 Gy	25–26	62.5–65 Gy	Daily	Lewis [9], NRG-GU003

28.6 Normal Tissue Tolerances*

Organ	TG101	Other
Bladder		
SBRT		
• 3 fx	DMax: 28.2 Gy V16.8 <15 cc	
• 5 fx	DMax: 38 Gy V18.3 <15 cc	NRG-GU005 D0.03 cc [Gy] <39 D50% [Gy] <15 PACE-B [8] V18.1 < 40% V37 < 10 cc V37 < 5 cc (optimal)
Limiting toxicity	≥Grade 3 cystitis	
Intact hypofractionation		
• 70 Gy/28 fx		RTOG 0415 [2] V79 <15% V74 <25% V69 <35%
Post-op hypofractionation		
• 65 Gy/26 fx		Lewis et al. 2016 [9] V43 <50% V62.4 <25%
• 62.5 Gy/25 fx		NRG-GU003 V35 <70% V57 <50%
Rectum		
SBRT		
• 3 fx	DMax: 28.2 Gy V24 <20 cc	
• 5 fx	DMax: 38 Gy V25 <20 cc	NRG-GU005 D0.03 cc [Gy] <38 D3 cc [Gy] <35 D10% [Gy] <32 D20% [Gy] <25 D50% [Gy] <18 PACE-B [8] V18.1 < 50% V29 < 20% V36 < 1 cc

Organ	TG101	Other
Limiting toxicity	≥Grade 3 proctitis	
Intact hypofractionation		
• 70 Gy/28 fx		RTOG 0415 [2] V74 <15% V69 <25% V64 <35%
Post-op hypofractionation		
• 65 Gy/26 fx		Lewis et al. 2016 [9] V53.8 <50% V66.8 <25%
• 62.5 Gy/25 fx		NRG-GU003 V36 <55% V59 <35%
Urethra		
SBRT		
• 5 fx		NRG-GU005 D0.03 cc [Gy] <38.78 (107%) PACE-B [8] V42 < 50% (optional)
Penile bulb		
SBRT		
• 5 fx		NRG-GU005 (recommended constraints) D0.03 cc [%] <100 D3 cc [%] <55 PACE-B [8] V29.5 < 50%
Intact hypofractionation		
• 70 Gy/28 fx		RTOG 0415 [2] Mean ≤51 Gy

*Our institution follows GU005 guidelines for all organs at risk

28.7 Patient Management Considerations

- Pre-medication:
  - Moderate hypofractionation: None
  - SBRT:

Patients are started on a prophylactic alpha blocker (0.4 mg tamsulosin QD) at the time of simulation. Therapy is continued through at least the first follow-up at 1 month after treatment.
Dexamethasone 4 mg can be given before each fraction of SBRT.

- Common acute and late toxicity
  - Obstructive urinary symptoms (frequency, incomplete emptying, and poor flow) occur in 7–54% of patients [10, 11].

    Start with tamsulosin 0.4 mg once a day, which can increase to twice a day if inadequate response.
    Second-tier symptom management with silodosin 8 mg (Rapaflo)

  - Incontinence/urgency ≥grade 3 occurs in ~11% of patients [11].

    Start with oxybutynin 10 mg QD, which can increase to 5 mg TID if inadequate response.
    Second-line mirabegron 25 mg QD, which can increase to 50 mg QD.

  - Macroscopic/gross hematuria is rare (<2%) [11]: Referral to urology for workup including cystoscopy.
  - Rectal bleeding is uncommon [11]: Referral to gastroenterology for workup including endoscopy.
  - Fecal incontinence is very rare (~2%): Referral to gastroenterology.
  - Erectile dysfunction is a common side effect after any treatment for prostate cancer. Medical management includes sildenafil (Viagra) 50–100 mg or tadalafil (Cialis) 10–20 mg. If medical management fails, additional options include a penile pump, injectable medications, and surgery (prosthesis). Referral to a specialist is often necessary beyond medical management.

28.8 Follow-Up for Both Intact and Post-prostatectomy (NCCN Guidelines): [12]

- Frequency: every 6–12 months PSA for years 1–5, then yearly. Every 3–4 months monitoring may be appropriate for patients at high risk of recurrence.
- Tests needed: PSA and DRE (optional if PSA is undetectable).

28.9 Relevant Literature

Guidelines: NCCN 2021 Guidelines for Intact Prostate [13]:

- Moderately hypofractionated image-guided IMRT regimens (2.4–4 Gy per fraction over 4–6 weeks) are preferred over conventional fractionation for all non-metastatic disease.

- Extremely hypofractionated image-guided SBRT regimens (6.5 Gy per fraction or greater) can be considered an alternative to conventional or hypofractionated regimens at clinics with appropriate technology, physics, and clinical expertise for low-, intermediate-, and high-risk disease.

Study	Patients	Treatment	Median follow-up	Outcomes
Intact prostate moderate hypofractionation				
Randomized trials				
Low risk				
RTOG 0415 [2, 13] Non-inferiority study	$n = 1115$ T1b–T2c (78% T1c) PSA <10 Gleason 2–6 PS 0–1	73.8 Gy/41 fx 70 Gy/28 fx ADT not allowed	5.8 years	5-year disease-free survival 73.8 Gy: 85.3% 70 Gy: 86.3% (non-inferior) No difference in overall survival No difference in early GI or GU toxicity Increased late grade 2 GI (18.3% vs. 11.4%, $p = 0.005$) and late grade 2 GU (26.2% vs. 20.5%) toxicity in the hypofractionation arm No difference in patient-reported QOL in any domain (bowel, urinary, sexual, hormonal) between the two arms
Intermediate risk				
Pollack [14, 15]	$n = 307$ Intermediate- (66%) and high-risk (34%) patients	76 Gy/38 fx 70.2 Gy/27 fx 0–4 months ADT intermediate risk, 24 months high risk	5.6 years	10-year biochemical/clinical disease failure: 76 Gy: 25.9% 70.2 Gy: 30.6% ($p = 0.25$) No difference in overall survival No difference in acute or late GI/GU toxicity On multivariable analysis hypofractionated patients with baseline IPSS >12 more likely to develop late GU toxicity

Study	Patients	Treatment	Median follow-up	Outcomes
CHHiP [3, 16, 17] Non-inferiority study	$n = 3216$ T1b–T3a PS 0–1 73% intermediate risk	74 Gy/37 fx 60 Gy/20 fx 57 Gy/19 fx 3–6 months ADT	5.2 years	5-year DFS 74 Gy: 88.3% 60 Gy: 90.6% (non-inferior to 74 Gy) 57 Gy: 85.9% (inferior to 74 Gy) No difference in overall survival More acute grade ≥2 bowel toxicity in hypofractionated groups (38% combined 57/60 Gy vs. 25% for 74 Gy), resolved by 2 years No difference in QOL scores through 5 years
PROFIT [4] Non-inferiority study	$n = 1206$ T1a–T2c PSA ≤20 Gleason ≤7 Intermediate risk by Canadian consensus criteria	78 Gy/39 fx 60 Gy/20 fx Allowed pre-randomization ADT up to 90 days; no post-randomization ADT	6 years	5-year biochemical-clinical disease-free survival 85% in both arms (HR 0.96, 90% CI 0.77–1.2), hypofractionated arm non-inferior. No difference in OS No difference in acute grade ≥3 GI or GU toxicity No difference in late grade ≥3 GI or GU toxicity No difference in QOL scores at 48 months
Hoffman [18]	$n = 206$ T1b-T3b PSA <20 Majority intermediate-risk disease (71%) 28% low risk 1% high risk	75.6 Gy/42 fx 72 Gy/30 fx 24% received ADT	8.5 years	8-year failure rate: 15.4% conventional 10.7% hypofractionated ($p = 0.036$) Conclusion: Superior cancer control with dose-escalated hypofractionation No difference OS ($p = 0.39$) Toxicity: • Trend toward increased late grade 2–3 GI toxicity at 8 years with hypofractionation (5% vs. 12.6%, $p = 0.08$) • GI toxicity decreased to 8.6% for hypofractionated arm when rectal volume receiving 65 Gy <15%

Study	Patients	Treatment	Median follow-up	Outcomes
High risk				
HYPRO [5, 11, 19, 20]	$n = 820$ T1b–T4a PSA <60 PS 0–2 26% intermediate risk, 74% high risk	78 Gy/39 fx 64.6 Gy/19 fx ADT at physician discretion (67%)	5 years	7-year relapse-free survival 78 Gy: 67.6% 64.6 Gy: 71.7% ($p = 0.52$) No difference in cumulative incidence of acute (<120 days) ≥ grade 2 GU toxicity (57.8% vs. 60.5% hypofractionated) Increase in cumulative incidence of acute (<120 days) ≥ grade 2 GI toxicity (31.2% vs. 42.0% hypofractioanted) Increase in cumulative incidence of late ≥ grade 2 GI toxicity at 5 years (12.9% vs. 19.0% hypofractionated) No difference in cumulative incidence of late ≥ grade 2 GU toxicity at 5 years (2.6% vs. 3.3% hypofractionated)
Intact prostate SBRT				
Prospective phase I–II				
Fuller 2022 [21] Multi-institutional All patients treated with CyberKnife SBRT	$N = 259$ 43% low risk 57% intermediate risk	38 Gy/4 fx Daily treatment No ADT	5.5 years	10-year freedom from biochemical recurrence • Low risk: 100% • Favorable intermediate risk: 84.3% • Unfavorable intermediate risk: 68.4% Acute grade 3 GU toxicity (≤90 days): 1.1% Acute grade 3 GI toxicity: 0 10-year grade 3+ GU toxicity: 2.6% 10-year grade 3+ GI toxicity: 0

Study	Patients	Treatment	Median follow-up	Outcomes
King 2013 [22] Multi-institutional, combined data of several prospective phase II studies. All patients treated with CyberKnife SBRT	$n = 1100$ 58% low risk 30% intermediate risk 11% high risk	35–40 Gy/5 fx Daily treatment for >95% of patients	36 months	5-year biochemical relapse-free survival: 93% • Low risk: 95% • Intermediate risk: 83% • High risk: 81%
King 2013 [23] Multi-institutional, combined data of several prospective phase II studies. All patients treated with CyberKnife SBRT	$n = 864$	36.25 Gy/5 fx 39 Gy/4 fx	36 months	Decrease in GU quality of life at 3 months, return to baseline at 6–9 months Decrease in GI quality of life at 3 months, return to baseline at 6–9 months
RTOG 0938 [24] Randomized phase II trial	$n = 246$	36.25 Gy/5 fx 51.6 Gy/12 fx	3.8 years	Worsening of EPIC bowel score at 1 year: 5 fx 30%; 12 fx 28% Worsening of EPIC urinary score at 1 year: 5 fx 46%; 12 fx 42% Worsening of EPIC sexual score at 1 year: 5 fx: 33%, 12 fx 31% No grade 4–5 toxicity
Katz 2014 [25] All patients treated with CyberKnife SBRT	$n = 515$	35–36.25 Gy/5 fx	72 months	7-year actuarial freedom from biochemical failure: • Low risk: 95.8% • Intermediate risk: 89.3% • High risk: 68.5% No acute grade 3 or 4 toxicity Late grade 2 rectal toxicity 4%, late grade 2 GU toxicity 9.1% Mean EPIC urinary and bowel QOL declined at 1 month, returned to baseline by 2 years

Study	Patients	Treatment	Median follow-up	Outcomes
Boike 2011 [26] Phase I	$n = 45$	Dose escalation study 45 Gy/5 fx 47.5 Gy/5 fx 50 Gy/5 fx	30 months 18 months 12 months	97% biochemical control overall Toxicity: • No grade ≥ 3 toxicity in 45 Gy dose level. One patient with grade 2 GU toxicity • One patient with grade ≥ 3 toxicity in 47.5 Gy dose level • Two patients with ≥ 3 toxicity in 50 Gy dose level
Zelefesky 2019 [27] Phase I	$n = 136$	Dose escalation study 32.5 Gy/5 fx 35 Gy/5 fx 37.5 Gy/5 fx 40 Gy/5 fx	5.9 years 5.4 years 4.1 years 3.5 years	5-year PSA failure: 15%, 6%, 0%, 0% at the four dose levels 2-year positive biopsy: 48%, 19%, 18%, 8% Toxicity by dose level: • Acute grade 2 rectal: 0%, 3%, 2.8%, 11.4% No acute grade 3–4 • Acute grade 2 GU: 16.7%, 23%, 8.3%, 17% No acute grade 3–4 • Late grade 2 rectal: none • Late grade 2+ GU: 23%, 26%, 28%, 31% (all grade 2 except 1 pt grade 3 in 40 Gy arm)

Study	Patients	Treatment	Median follow-up	Outcomes
Prospective phase III				
HYPO-RT-PC [6, 28] Non-inferiority study	$n = 1200$	78 Gy/39 fx 42.7 Gy/7 fx	5 years	5-year failure-free survival 84% in both arms Ultra-hypofractionated regimen non-inferior to conventional Toxicity: • 1 year late grade 2+ GU toxicity 2% vs. 6%, $p = 0.004$ (worse in ultra-hypofractionated arm) • No difference in late grade 2+ GU at 5 years • No difference in grade 2+ GI at any point Patient-reported QOL: • Acute clinically-relevant GI toxicity higher in ultra-hypofractionated arm by end of therapy • No difference in acute GU or sexual QOL • No difference in GI QOL at 6 years
PACE-B [8] Non-inferiority study	$n = 874$ 8% low-risk 92% intermediate-risk	78 Gy/39 fx or 62 Gy/20 fx 36.25 Gy/5 fx No ADT	Not reported	2 year: grade 2+ GU toxicity: 2% vs. 3% SBRT ($p = 0.39$) grade 2+ GI toxicity: 3% vs. 2% SBRT ($p = 0.32$)
Meta-analysis				
Jackson 2019 [29] Pooled analysis of 38 prospective trials for low-, intermediate-, and high-risk prostate cancer	$n = 6116$	Median dose per fraction 7.25 Gy (5–10 Gy) Median 5 fx (4–9)	39 months	5-year biochemical-PFS: 95.3% 7-year biochemical-PFS: 93.7% Toxicity: Late grade 3+ GU: 2.7% Late grade 3+ GI: 3% (Higher dose associated with greater acute GU toxicity, but this normalized by 2 years)
Post-radical prostatectomy hypofractionation				
Prospective phase I–II				
Cozzarini 2008 [30]	$n = 50$ T3 or positive margins and N0	58 Gy/20 fx	2.2 years	Acute grade ≥ 2 toxicity GI 4%; GU 10%

Study	Patients	Treatment	Median follow-up	Outcomes
Massaccesi 2013 [31]	*n* = 49 Positive margins or ECE or SVI AND >7% risk of nodal involvement (Roach), OR positive pelvic nodes, OR PSA failure after RP	62.5 Gy/25 fx using simultaneous integrated boost Pelvic nodes treated to 45 Gy in 25 fx	Not reported	Acute grade ≥ 2 toxicity GI 32.6%; GU 11.5%
Katayama 2014 [32]	*n* = 39 T3 or positive margins or PSA recurrence	54 Gy/18 fx	Not reported	Acute grade ≥ 2 toxicity GI 18%; GU 0%
Gladwish 2015 [33]	*n* = 30 T3 or positive margins or PSA recurrence	51 Gy/17 fx	2 years	Acute grade ≥ 2 toxicity GI 0%; GU 6%
Prospective phase III				
NRG-GU003 [34]	*n* = 296	66.6 Gy/37 fx (COPORT) 62.5 Gy/25 fx (HYPORT)	2.1 years	No difference in GU EPIC change scores at end RT, 6, 12, 24 months EPIC GI change scores significantly different at end RT (−15.0 HYPORT vs. −6.8 COPRT, *P* < 0.01). No difference in EPIC GI change scores at 6, 12, 24 months
Retrospective series				
Kruser 2011 [35]	*n* = 108 Biochemical recurrence after RP 87% pathologic Gleason ≤7	65 Gy/26 fx	2.7 years	4-year actuarial freedom from biochemical progression: 67% Acute grade ≥ 2 toxicity GI 14%; GU 7% Late grade ≥ 2 toxicity GI 4%; GU15%
Lewis 2016 [9]	*n* = 56	57.5–65 Gy/23–26 fx	4 years	4-year biochemical progression-free survival: 75% Acute grade ≥ 2 toxicity GI 3.6%; GU 16% Late grade ≥ 3 toxicity GI 12.5%; GU 27%

Abbreviations: *Gy* Gray, *PSA* prostate-specific antigen, *PS* performance status, *fx* fractions, *ADT* androgen deprivation therapy, *GI* gastrointestinal, *GU* genitourinary, *QOL* quality of life, *ECE* extracapsular extension, *RP* radical prostatectomy, *SVI* seminal vesicle invasion

28.10 Summary

- Intact prostate moderate hypofractionation: Moderate hypofractionation is now considered the preferred standard of care for men with localized prostate cancer based on level 1 evidence from multiple randomized controlled trials. Hypofractionation is non-inferior to conventional dose-escalated radiation for disease control.
- Intact prostate SBRT: SBRT can be considered as a treatment option for low- and intermediate-risk prostate cancer patients based on multiple prospective phase II trials and preliminary results from two phase III trials. Results from these studies have shown favorable disease control and long-term toxicity outcomes. SBRT for high-risk patients is an active area of ongoing research.
- Post-radical-prostatectomy hypofractionation: NRG GU003 provides promising results for moderate hypofractionation in terms of 2-year QOL outcomes. There is a relative lack of long-term data on the safety and efficacy of post-prostatectomy SBRT. This is an area of continued active investigation.

References

1. Siegel RL, Miller KD, Fuchs HE, Jemal A. Cancer statistics, 2021. CA Cancer J Clin. 2021;71(1):7–33. https://doi.org/10.3322/caac.21654.
2. Lee WR, Dignam JJ, Amin MB, et al. Randomized phase III noninferiority study comparing two radiotherapy fractionation schedules in patients with low-risk prostate cancer. J Clin Oncol. 2016;34(20):2325–32. https://doi.org/10.1200/jco.2016.67.0448.
3. Dearnaley D, Syndikus I, Mossop H, et al. Conventional versus hypofractionated high-dose intensity-modulated radiotherapy for prostate cancer: 5-year outcomes of the randomised, non-inferiority, phase 3 CHHiP trial. Lancet Oncol. 2016;17(8):1047–60. https://doi.org/10.1016/s1470-2045(16)30102-4.
4. Catton CN, Lukka H, Gu CS, et al. Randomized trial of a hypofractionated radiation regimen for the treatment of localized prostate cancer. J Clin Oncol. 2017;35(17):1884–90. https://doi.org/10.1200/jco.2016.71.7397.
5. Incrocci L, Wortel RC, Alemayehu WG, et al. Hypofractionated versus conventionally fractionated radiotherapy for patients with localised prostate cancer (HYPRO): final efficacy results from a randomised, multicentre, open-label, phase 3 trial. Lancet Oncol. 2016;17(8):1061–9. https://doi.org/10.1016/s1470-2045(16)30070-5.
6. Widmark A, Gunnlaugsson A, Beckman L, et al. Ultra-hypofractionated versus conventionally fractionated radiotherapy for prostate cancer: 5-year outcomes of the HYPO-RT-PC randomised, non-inferiority, phase 3 trial. Lancet. 2019;394(10196):385–95. https://doi.org/10.1016/s0140-6736(19)31131-6.
7. Fuller DB, Falchook AD, Crabtree T, et al. Phase 2 multicenter trial of heterogeneous-dosing stereotactic body radiotherapy for low- and intermediate-risk prostate cancer: 5-year outcomes. Eur Urol Oncol. 2018;1(6):540–7. https://doi.org/10.1016/j.euo.2018.06.013.
8. Tree AC, Ostler P, van der Voet H, et al. Intensity-modulated radiotherapy versus stereotactic body radiotherapy for prostate cancer (PACE-B): 2-year toxicity results from an open-label, randomized, phase 3, non-inferiority trial. Lancet Oncol. 2022;23(10):1308–20. https://doi.org/10.1016/s1470-2045(22)00517-4.

9. Lewis SL, Patel P, Song H, et al. Image guided hypofractionated postprostatectomy intensity modulated radiation therapy for prostate cancer. Int J Radiat Oncol Biol Phys. 2016;94(3):605–11. https://doi.org/10.1016/j.ijrobp.2015.11.025.
10. Pollack A, Hanlon AL, Horwitz EM, et al. Dosimetry and preliminary acute toxicity in the first 100 men treated for prostate cancer on a randomized hypofractionation dose escalation trial. Int J Radiat Oncol Biol Phys. 2006;64(2):518–26. https://doi.org/10.1016/j.ijrobp.2005.07.970.
11. Aluwini S, Pos F, Schimmel E, et al. Hypofractionated versus conventionally fractionated radiotherapy for patients with prostate cancer (HYPRO): acute toxicity results from a randomised non-inferiority phase 3 trial. Lancet Oncol. 2015;16(3):274–83. https://doi.org/10.1016/s1470-2045(14)70482-6.
12. Prostate cancer. National Comprehensive Cancer Network. https://www.nccn.org/professionals/physician_gls/pdf/prostate.pdf. Accessed 10 Dec 2021.
13. Bruner DW, Pugh SL, Lee WR, et al. Quality of life in patients with low-risk prostate cancer treated with hypofractionated vs conventional radiotherapy: a phase 3 randomized clinical trial. JAMA Oncol. 2019;5(5):664–70. https://doi.org/10.1001/jamaoncol.2018.6752.
14. Pollack A, Walker G, Horwitz EM, et al. Randomized trial of hypofractionated external-beam radiotherapy for prostate cancer. J Clin Oncol. 2013;31(31):3860–8. https://doi.org/10.1200/jco.2013.51.1972.
15. Avkshtol V, Ruth KJ, Ross EA, et al. Ten-year update of a randomized, prospective trial of conventional fractionated versus moderate hypofractionated radiation therapy for localized prostate cancer. J Clin Oncol. 2020;38(15):1676–84. https://doi.org/10.1200/jco.19.01485.
16. Dearnaley D, Syndikus I, Sumo G, et al. Conventional versus hypofractionated high-dose intensity-modulated radiotherapy for prostate cancer: preliminary safety results from the CHHiP randomised controlled trial. Lancet Oncol. 2012;13(1):43–54. https://doi.org/10.1016/s1470-2045(11)70293-5.
17. Wilkins A, Mossop H, Syndikus I, et al. Hypofractionated radiotherapy versus conventionally fractionated radiotherapy for patients with intermediate-risk localised prostate cancer: 2-year patient-reported outcomes of the randomised, non-inferiority, phase 3 CHHiP trial. Lancet Oncol. 2015;16(16):1605–16. https://doi.org/10.1016/s1470-2045(15)00280-6.
18. Hoffman KE, Voong KR, Levy LB, et al. Randomized trial of hypofractionated, dose-escalated, intensity-modulated radiation therapy (IMRT) versus conventionally fractionated IMRT for localized prostate cancer. J Clin Oncol. 2018;36(29):2943–9. https://doi.org/10.1200/jco.2018.77.9868.
19. Aluwini S, Pos F, Schimmel E, et al. Hypofractionated versus conventionally fractionated radiotherapy for patients with prostate cancer (HYPRO): late toxicity results from a randomised, non-inferiority, phase 3 trial. Lancet Oncol. 2016;17(4):464–74. https://doi.org/10.1016/s1470-2045(15)00567-7.
20. de Vries KC, Wortel RC, Oomen-de Hoop E, Heemsbergen WD, Pos FJ, Incrocci L. Hyprofractionated versus conventionally fractionated radiation therapy for patients with intermediate- or high-risk, localized, prostate cancer: 7-year outcomes from the randomized, multicenter, open-label, phase 3 HYPRO trial. Int J Radiat Oncol Biol Phys. 2020;106(1):108–15. https://doi.org/10.1016/j.ijrobp.2019.09.007.
21. Fuller DB, Crabtree T, Lane BL, et al. High dose "HDR-like" prostate SBRT: PSA 10-year results from a mature, multi-institutional clinical trial. Front Oncol. 2022;12:935310.
22. King CR, Collins S, Fuller D, et al. Health-related quality of life after stereotactic body radiation therapy for localized prostate cancer: results from a multi-institutional consortium of prospective trials. Int J Radiat Oncol Biol Phys. 2013;87(5):939–45. https://doi.org/10.1016/j.ijrobp.2013.08.019.
23. King CR, Freeman D, Kaplan I, et al. Stereotactic body radiotherapy for localized prostate cancer: pooled analysis from a multi-institutional consortium of prospective phase II trials. Radiother Oncol. 2013;109(2):217–21. https://doi.org/10.1016/j.radonc.2013.08.030.

24. Lukka HR, Pugh SL, Bruner DW, et al. Patient reported outcomes in NRG oncology RTOG 0938, evaluating two ultrahypofractionated regimens for prostate cancer. Int J Radiat Oncol Biol Phys. 2018;102(2):287–95. https://doi.org/10.1016/j.ijrobp.2018.06.008.
25. Katz AJ, Kang J. Quality of life and toxicity after SBRT for organ-confined prostate cancer, a 7-year study. Front Oncol. 2014;4:301. https://doi.org/10.3389/fonc.2014.00301.
26. Boike TP, Lotan Y, Cho LC, et al. Phase I dose-escalation study of stereotactic body radiation therapy for low- and intermediate-risk prostate cancer. J Clin Oncol. 2011;29(15):2020–6. https://doi.org/10.1200/jco.2010.31.4377.
27. Zelefsky MJ, Kollmeier M, McBride S, et al. Five-year outcomes of a phase 1 dose-escalation study using stereotactic body radiosurgery for patients with low-risk and intermediate-risk prostate cancer. Int J Radiat Oncol Biol Phys. 2019;104(1):42–9. https://doi.org/10.1016/j.ijrobp.2018.12.045.
28. Fransson P, Nilsson P, Gunnlaugsson A, et al. Ultra-hypofractionated versus conventionally fractionated radiotherapy for prostate cancer (HYPO-RT-PC): patient-reported quality-of-life outcomes of a randomised, controlled, non-inferiority, phase 3 trial. Lancet Oncol. 2021;22(2):235–45. https://doi.org/10.1016/s1470-2045(20)30581-7.
29. Jackson WC, Silva J, Hartman HE, et al. Stereotactic body radiation therapy for localized prostate cancer: a systematic review and meta-analysis of over 6,000 patients treated on prospective studies. Int J Radiat Oncol Biol Phys. 2019;104(4):778–89. https://doi.org/10.1016/j.ijrobp.2019.03.051.
30. Cozzarini C, Fiorino C, Di Muzio N, et al. Hypofractionated adjuvant radiotherapy with helical tomotherapy after radical prostatectomy: planning data and toxicity results of a phase I-II study. Radiother Oncol. 2008;88(1):26–33. https://doi.org/10.1016/j.radonc.2008.03.021.
31. Massaccesi M, Cilla S, Deodato F, et al. Hypofractionated intensity-modulated radiotherapy with simultaneous integrated boost after radical prostatectomy: preliminary results of a phase II trial. Anticancer Res. 2013;33(6):2785–9.
32. Katayama S, Striecker T, Kessel K, et al. Hypofractionated IMRT of the prostate bed after radical prostatectomy: acute toxicity in the PRIAMOS-1 trial. Int J Radiat Oncol Biol Phys. 2014;90(4):926–33. https://doi.org/10.1016/j.ijrobp.2014.07.015.
33. Gladwish A, Loblaw A, Cheung P, et al. Accelerated hypofractioned postoperative radiotherapy for prostate cancer: a prospective phase I/II study. Clin Oncol (R Coll Radiol). 2015;27(3):145–52. https://doi.org/10.1016/j.clon.2014.12.003.
34. Buyyounouski MK, Pugh S, Chen RC, et al. Primary endpoint analysis of a randomized phase III trial of hypofractionated vs. conventional post-prostatectomy radiotherapy: NRG oncology GU003. Int J Radiat Oncol Biol Phys. 2021;111(3 Suppl):S2–3.
35. Kruser TJ, Jarrard DF, Graf AK, et al. Early hypofractionated salvage radiotherapy for postprostatectomy biochemical recurrence. Cancer. 2011;117(12):2629–36. https://doi.org/10.1002/cncr.25824.

Chapter 29
Kidney Cancers

May Elbanna, Ronald C. Chen, and Jordan A. Holmes

29.1 Introduction

Surgery remains the standard of care for patients with primary renal cell carcinoma, which has classically been considered radio-resistant; however, there is growing evidence that stereotactic body radiation therapy (SBRT) with high dose per fraction can likely overcome the previously described radio-resistance [1]. To date, clinical experience is limited to mostly retrospective series that have demonstrated promising outcomes. Published series have used many different dosing regimens but suggest that high doses per fraction using SBRT can provide excellent local control for appropriately selected patients who cannot undergo surgery.

M. Elbanna
Department of Radiation Oncology, Indiana University School of Medicine, Indianapolis, IN, USA
e-mail: melbanna@iupui.edu

R. C. Chen
Department of Radiation Oncology, KU Medical Center, The University of Kansas, Kansas City, USA
e-mail: rchen2@kumc.edu

J. A. Holmes (✉)
Department of Radiation Oncology, Indiana University School of Medicine, Indianapolis, IN, USA
Indiana University Simon Comprehensive Cancer Center, Indianapolis, IN, USA
e-mail: jorholme@iu.edu

O. Kaidar-Person, R. Chen (eds.), *Hypofractionated and Stereotactic Radiation Therapy*, https://doi.org/10.1007/978-3-031-47701-0_29

29.2 Pearls

- Renal cell carcinoma (RCC) is one of the 10 most common malignancies in the developed world, comprising approximately 4% of new cancer diagnoses each year. An estimated 13,780 deaths are expected in 2021 from RCC. The incidence of RCC has been increasing in the United States at a rate of 2–3% per year mostly due to incidental early detection on abdominal imaging.
- RCC incidence is the highest in North America and Scandinavia, and African Americans and Whites have the highest rates of diagnosis.
- The median age at diagnosis is 64 years, and men are twice as likely to develop RCC as women.
- Smoking and obesity have both been suggested as risk factors for developing RCC.
- Inherited forms of RCC have been linked to VHL, TSC1, TSC2, and Met1 gene alterations, but in cases with a family history and no identifiable mutations, the risk of developing RCC can still be increased by as much as twofold.
- Most early-stage RCCs are diagnosed incidentally on abdominal imaging. However, more advanced diseases can present with abdominal pain, hematuria, or a palpable abdominal mass. Rarely male patients can present with a varicocele from impaired testicular drainage. Paraneoplastic symptoms can include fevers, hypercalcemia, hypertension, and liver dysfunction.
- Greater than 90% of all primary kidney cancers are renal cell carcinoma, and of these >80% are clear cell carcinoma. The remaining RCCs are classified as chromophobe, papillary, or collecting duct types. Clear cell tumors have a worse prognosis than the other subtypes.
- Direct extension of RCCs can include invasion into the perinephric fat, adrenal gland, or inferior vena cava.
- Nodal drainage and metastasis can spread to the renal hilar, paracaval, aortic, and retroperitoneal lymph nodes. Bloodborne metastatic disease has a predilection for the lungs, brain, and bone.
- Medical workup should include basic labs to establish renal function and surgical suitability (CBC, metabolic panel), LDH, and urinalysis. Imaging should include chest staging (X-ray or CT) and contrasted imaging of the abdomen and pelvis (CT or MRI). Imaging of the brain for neurologic symptoms (MRI) and bones for pain (bone scan, PET/CT) is appropriate.
- Surgical resection remains the primary treatment option for non-metastatic RCC. For patients who refuse or cannot undergo surgery, SBRT or other local ablative treatments (cryotherapy, HIFU) are also recommended options in NCCN guidelines.

29.3 Tumor/Patient Selection

- For patients who refuse or are not candidates for surgery, published data have shown that SBRT is safe and effective. NCCN guidelines recommend SBRT as an option for Stage I–III RCC.

29.4 Treatment Planning Considerations (Fig. 29.1)

Simulation instructions	• Patients are simulated supine, immobilized in a Vac-Lok, with 3-mm CT slices • CT should include non-contrast and contrast-enhanced phases • 4D imaging should be obtained to assess tumor motion • Consider MRI for difficult-to-visualize tumors
Image guidance	Linac: • Daily image guidance with either real-time tracking (Calypso® transponders, US, or fiducial tracking) or daily 3D imaging (KV-CBCT) CyberKnife: • Fiducial markers, need at least 3 for translational and rotational tracking
Tumor movement	Because renal tumors can potentially move significantly with respiration [2], real-time tracking, breath hold, and/or abdominal compression is preferred [3, 4].
Margins	• GTV = CTV • CTV+ 3 mm = PTV • PTV margins may need to be larger depending on the image guidance technique
Dosimetric considerations	• 100% of prescription to 95% of PTV • 95% of prescription to 100% of PTV • DMax <107% of prescription (<120% for CyberKnife) • CI: <1.5

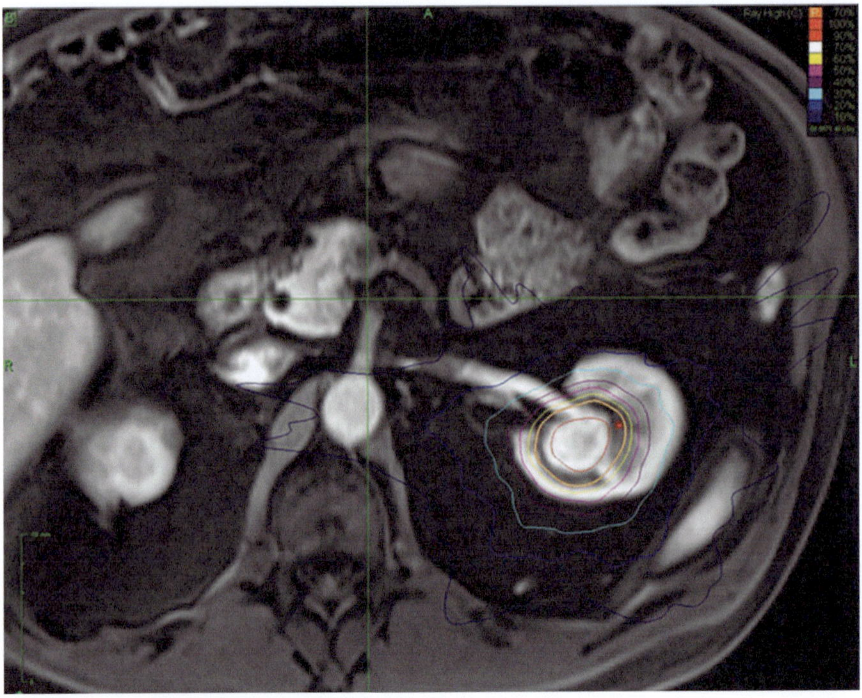

Fig. 29.1 Representative axial T2-weighted MRI of a CyberKnife SBRT plan for a primary renal cell carcinoma). The total dose delivered was 13 Gy × 3 fractions.

29.5 Commonly Used Dose/Fractionation

Small series have been published using many dosing regimens. Some of these regimens are summarized below:

Dose/fx	# of fx	Total dose	Frequency
13 Gy	3	39	Every day
16 Gy	3	48 Gy	Every other day
12 Gy	4	48 Gy	Every other day
8 Gy	5	40 Gy	Every other day
25–26 Gy	1	25–26 Gy	Once

29.6 Normal Tissue Tolerances*

Organ	TG101 [5]	IROCK consortium [6]	Other
Stomach			
• 1 fx	DMax: 12.4 Gy V11.2 < 10 cc	V11 < 10 cc V22.5 < 5 cc	
• 3 fx	DMax: 22.2 Gy V16.5 < 10 cc	DMax: 30 Gy V16.5 < 10 cc V22.5 < 5 cc	
• 4 fx			Ponsky 2015 [7] ≤1 cc at 22 Gy
• 5 fx	DMax: 32 Gy V18 < 10 cc	DMax: 30 Gy V18 < 5 cc	
Limiting toxicity	≥Grade 3 Ulceration/ fistula		
Duodenum			
• 1 fx	DMax: 12.4 Gy V11.2 < 10 cc		
• 3 fx	DMax: 22.2 Gy V16.5 < 10 cc		
• 5 fx	DMax: 32 Gy V18 < 10 cc		Chang 2016 [8] DMax: 32 Gy V18 < 5 cc
Limiting toxicity	≥Grade 3 ulceration		
Small bowel			
• 1 fx	DMax: 15.4 Gy V11.9 < 5 cc	V14 < 20 cc Full circumference < 12.5 Gy	Pham 2014 30 cc < 12.5 Gy
• 3 fx	DMax: 25.2 Gy V17.7 < 5 cc	DMax: 30 Gy V11.4 < 10 cc V24 < 1 cc	Pham 2014 [9] DMax: 30 Gy Svedman 2008 [10] DMax: 21 Gy
• 4 fx			Ponsky 2015 [7] ≤1 cc at 24 Gy Svedman 2008 [10] DMax: 28 Gy
• 5 fx	DMax: 35 Gy V19.5 < 5 cc	DMax: 30 Gy V20 < 5 cc	Chang 2016 [8] DMax: 35 Gy V19.5 < 5 cc
Limiting toxicity	≥Grade 3 Enteritis/ Obstruction		

Organ	TG101 [5]	IROCK consortium [6]	Other
Colon			
• 1 fx	DMax: 18.4 Gy V14.3 < 20 cc	ALARA	
• 3 fx	DMax: 28.2 Gy V24 < 20 cc	ALARA, minimize volume receiving >30 Gy	
• 4 fx			Ponsky 2015 [7] ≤1 cc at 24 Gy
• 5 fx	DMax: 38 Gy V25 < 20 cc	Dmax: 38 Gy V25 < 20 cc	Chang 2016 [8] DMax: 38 Gy V25 < 20 cc
Limiting toxicity	≥Grade 3 colitis/ fistula		
Liver			
• 1 fx	700 cc < 9.1 Gy		Pham 2014 [9] 700 cc ≤ 15 Gy
• 3 fx	700 cc < 19.2 Gy	700 cc < 15 Gy V17 < 66%	Pham 2014 [9] 700 cc ≤ 15 Gy
• 4 fx			Ponsky 2015 [7] ≤2/3 of liver <17 Gy ≥800 cc at ≤15 Gy
• 5 fx	700 cc <21 Gy	700 cc <15 Gy	
Limiting toxicity	Decline in liver function		
Skin			
• 1 fx	DMax: 26 Gy V23 < 10 cc	Dmax: 24 Gy	Pham 2014 [9] DMax: 18 Gy
• 3 fx	DMax: 33 Gy V30 < 10 cc	V30 < 10 cc	Pham 2014 [9] DMax: 24 Gy
• 5 fx	DMax: 39.5 Gy V36.5 < 10 cc	V15 < 10 cc V30 < 0.03 cc	Chang 2016 [8] DMax: 39.5 Gy V36.5 < 10 cc
Limiting toxicity	≥Grade 3 ulceration		
Spinal cord			
• 1 fx	DMax: 14 Gy	V8 < 1 cc V12 < 0.03 cc	Pham 2014 [9] DMax: 12 Gy
• 3 fx	DMax: 21.9 Gy	DMax: 22.2 Gy V18 < 0.03 cc	Pham 2014 [9] DMax: 18 Gy
• 4 fx			Ponsky 2015 [7] <0.3 cc at 24 Gy
• 5 fx	DMax: 30 Gy	V23 < 0.5 cc V27.5 < 0.03 cc	Chang 2016 [8] DMax: 25.3 Gy
Limiting toxicity	Myelitis		

Organ	TG101 [5]	IROCK consortium [6]	Other
Chest wall			
• 3 fx		V30 < 700 cc	
• 5 fx		V37 < 70 cc	
Heart			
• 1 fx		15 cc to <16 Gy	
• 3 fx		Dmax 27.9 Gy	
• 5 fx		Dmax 38 Gy <15 cc to 32 Gy	
Contralateral kidney			
• 1 fx		ALARA	
• 3 fx		V10 < 33% V5 < 14 Gy	

* Our institution follows TG101 guidelines for all organs at risk

29.7 Patient Management Considerations

- Pre-medication: Dexamethasone 4 mg may be given before each fraction of SBRT.
- Common acute and late toxicity
  - Most patients do not experience significant acute toxicity.
  - The most common acute side effects are fatigue, nausea, and enteritis.
  - Patients with baseline chronic kidney disease may experience a worsening in kidney function after treatment in 5–10% of cases [7, 11].

29.8 Follow-Up (Per NCCN Guidelines) [12]

- H&P annually
- Imaging:
  - Abdominal CT or MRI with and without IV contrast at 1–6 months after treatment, then CT or MRI (preferred) or US annually for 5 years or longer as clinically indicated. If the patient is unable to receive contrast, MRI is the preferred modality. If there is concern for recurrence, then more frequent imaging and/or renal mass biopsy as indicated.
  - CT chest or CXR once a year for 5 years.

- Lab tests: Comprehensive metabolic panel with every follow-up to assess kidney function and electrolyte balance (i.e., annually and as clinically indicated)

29.9 Relevant Literature

Study	Patients	Treatment	Median follow-up	Outcomes
Prospective studies				
Svedman 2006 [13] Phase I trial	$n = 5$ Medically inoperable	8 Gy × 4 every other day 10 Gy × 4 every other day 15 Gy × 2 every other day 15 Gy × 3 every other day	52 months	Crude LC 80% Estimated 2 years LC: 91%
Kaplan 2009, McBride 2013 [14, 15] Phase I trial	$n = 15$ Medically inoperable Stage IA/B Median age 75 Biopsy not mandatory Lesion ≤5 cm (mean 3.4 cm) KPS ≥70 60% with baseline CKD	7 Gy × 3 every other day 9 Gy × 3 every other day 11 Gy × 3 every other day 13 Gy × 3 every other day 16 Gy × 3 every other day	37 months	Crude LC: 87% (both failures in low dose arms 7–9 ×3, both failures at 31 months) No dose-limiting toxicity 1 pt with worsening CKD
Ponsky 2015 [7] Phase I trial	$n = 19$ Medically inoperable KPS ≥60 Median age 78 Median tumor volume 58 cc	6 Gy × 4 every other day 8 Gy × 4 every other day 10 Gy × 4 every other day 12 Gy × 4 every other day	14 months	6-month crude local control 95% No dose-limiting toxicity 1 pt with grade 4 duodenal ulcer 3 pts with worsening CKD
Staehler 2015 [16] Phase I trial	$n = 40$ (30 RCC, 10 urothelial carcinoma) Medically inoperable Median age 64 Median tumor volume 33.7 cc ECOG 0–1	25 Gy ×1	28.1 months	9-month local control 98% Remission per RECIST in 39/45 lesions: 19 CR, 13 reduced >30%, 6 reduced <30% and 7 SD Median decrease in creatinine clearance 6.5 mL/min/1.73 m^2 Median PFS and OS not reached 13% grade 1–2 toxicity

Siva 2017 [11] Phase I trial	$n = 37$ Median PTV: • Fractionated ($n = 17$): 172 cc • Single fraction ($n = 17$): 77.2 cc Median age 78	14 Gy × 3 (≥5 cm) every other day 26 Gy × 1 (<5 cm)	24 months	100% freedom from local progression at 2 years Mean decrease in GFR at 1 year of 11 mL/min 3% grade 3 toxicity (fatigue) No grade ≥ 4 toxicity
Correa 2018 [17] Phase I trial	$n = 12$ Medically inoperable Stage IV Median age 67 Median KPS 70 Median tumor size 87 mm	5 Gy × 5 every other day 6 Gy × 5 every other day 7 Gy × 5 every other day	22 months	Two DLT events were reported in the 35 Gy cohort (MTD reached, no recruits to higher dose cohorts) Median tumor size reduction of 17.3% (range: +5.3 to −54.4) at 5.3 months 3 grade 3 events, no grade 4–5 events Median OS 6.7 months (all patients progressed systemically)
Retrospective series				
Qian 2003 [18]	$n = 27$ Mean age 62 Mean tumor volume 367 cc	8 Gy × 5	12 months	Crude control rate 93%
Beitler 2004 [19]	$n = 9$ Median tumor volume 97 cc	8 Gy × 5 every other day	27 months	Crude local control 100%
Wersall 2005 [20]	$n = 8$ Medically inoperable KPS ≥ 60	8 Gy × 5 (>4 cm) every other day 10 Gy × 3 (≤4 cm) every other day	37 months	Crude local control 100%
Gilson 2006 [21]	$n = 14$ Mean 62 years Mean tumor volume 356 cc	40–50 Gy/5 fx	17 months	Crude local control 88%

Teh 2007 [22]	$n = 2$ Medically inoperable	24–48 Gy/3–6 fx	9 months	Crude local control 100% Pain improved in both patients No change in kidney function
Nomiya 2008 [23]	$n = 10$ Carbon ion therapy Median diameter 43 mm	Median 4.5 Gy × 16 every day	58 months	5-year local control 100% 5-year progression-free survival 100% 1 pt with late grade 4 skin toxicity No change in kidney function in patients with normal baseline function
Svedman 2008 [10]	$n = 7$ Only patients with one kidney Mean age 64	10 Gy × 3 every other day 10 Gy × 4 every other day	49 months	Crude local control 86% No change in kidney function
Chang 2016 [8]	$n = 16$ Medically inoperable Median age 73 Median diameter 40 mm	8 Gy × 5 every other day 7 Gy × 5 every other day 6.5 Gy × 5 every other day 6 Gy × 5 every other day	19 months	Crude local control 100% 1 pt with change in CKD
Kaidar-Person 2017 [2]	$n = 6$ Tumors ≥4 cm	13 Gy × 3 every day	29.5 months	No clinical evidence of disease progression 2 patients with acute grade 1 nausea 1 patient with acute grade 2 colitis No worsening of renal function No late toxicity

Pooled analysis (IROCK)				
Siva 2022 [24]	$N = 190$ Median age 73.6, 73% men Median diameter 4.0 cm 75% medically inoperable, 29% with one kidney Median GFR pre-SBRT 60.0 mL/min	Single fraction (43% of patients): median dose 25 Gy Fractionated (57%): median dose 42 Gy in 2–10 fx	5.0 years	Local failure: 5.5% (5 years), 8.4% (7 years) Cancer-specific survival: 92.0% (5 years), 92.0% (7 years) Dominant pattern of progression was distant 1% acute grade 4 duodenal ulcer and late grade 4 gastritis 4% required post-SBRT dialysis
Correa 2019 [25]	$n = 81$ Only patients with one kidney Mean age 67.3 KPS ≥70 Median diameter 37 mm Mean GFR 67 mL/min	25 Gy × 1 (71% of patients)	2.6 years	2-year LC, CSS, PFS, and OS 98%, 98.2%, 77.5%, 81.5% eGFR decreased by 5.8 ± 10.8 mL/min Tumor ≥4 cm was associated with eGFR decrease of ≥15 mL/min (OR 4.2, $p = 0.029$). No patient with solitary kidney required dialysis
Siva 2020 [26]	$n = 49$ Mean age 76 Median diameter 49 mm, ≥T1b KPS ≥70 (81%) Mean eGFR 57 mL/min (30% <45 mL/min) Patients with one kidney 30% ($n = 28$) Medically inoperable 78%	Median 26 Gy × 1	2.7 years	2-year CSS, PFS, OS 96%, 81%, 84% 4-year CSS, PFS, OS 91%, 65%, 69% 4-year local, distant, any failure 2.9%, 11.1%, 12.1% Grade ½ toxicity 40% No grade 3+ toxicity reported eGFR decreased by 7.9 mL/min 3.2% ($n = 3$) required dialysis

Abbreviations: *CKD* chronic kidney disease, *CR* complete response, *CSS* cause-specific survival, *eGFR* estimated glomerular filtration rate, *Gy* gray, *GFR* glomerular filtration rate, *KPS* Karnofsky Performance Status, *LC* local control, *MTD* maximal tolerated dose, *OS* overall survival, *PFS* progression-free survival, *PTV* planning target volume, *RCC* renal cell carcinoma

29.10 Summary

SBRT for primary RCC is an emerging treatment option, with increasing published studies that have demonstrated promising outcomes. Studies have used many different dosing regimens, but have consistently shown that high doses per fraction using SBRT can overcome the relative radio-resistance of RCC.

References

1. Siva S, Kothari G, Muacevic A, et al. Radiotherapy for renal cell carcinoma: renaissance of an overlooked approach. Nat Rev Urol. 2017;14(9):549–63.
2. Kaidar-Person O, Price A, Schreiber E, Zagar TM, Chen RC. Stereotactic body radiotherapy for large primary renal cell carcinoma. Clin Genitourin Cancer. 2017;15(5):e851–4. https://doi.org/10.1016/j.clgc.2017.03.012.
3. Pham D, Kron T, Bressel M, et al. Image guidance and stabilization for stereotactic ablative body radiation therapy (SABR) treatment of primary kidney cancer. Pract Radiat Oncol. 2015;5(6):e597–605. https://doi.org/10.1016/j.prro.2015.08.002.
4. Pham D, Kron T, Styles C, et al. The use of dual vacuum stabilization device to reduce kidney motion for stereotactic radiotherapy planning. Technol Cancer Res Treat. 2015;14(2):149–57. https://doi.org/10.7785/tcrt.2012.500410.
5. Benedict SH, Yenice KM, Followill D, et al. Stereotactic body radiation therapy: the report of AAPM Task Group 101. Med Phys. 2010;37(8):4078–101. https://doi.org/10.1118/1.3438081.
6. Siva S, Ellis RJ, Ponsky L, et al. Consensus statement from the international radiosurgery oncology consortium for kidney for primary renal cell carcinoma. Future Oncol. 2016;12(5):637–45.
7. Ponsky L, Lo SS, Zhang Y, et al. Phase I dose-escalation study of stereotactic body radiotherapy (SBRT) for poor surgical candidates with localized renal cell carcinoma. Radiother Oncol. 2015;117(1):183–7. https://doi.org/10.1016/j.radonc.2015.08.030.
8. Chang JH, Cheung P, Erler D, Sonier M, Korol R, Chu W. Stereotactic ablative body radiotherapy for primary renal cell carcinoma in non-surgical candidates: initial clinical experience. Clin Oncol (R Coll Radiol). 2016;28(9):e109–14. https://doi.org/10.1016/j.clon.2016.04.002.
9. Pham D, Thompson A, Kron T, et al. Stereotactic ablative body radiation therapy for primary kidney cancer: a 3-dimensional conformal technique associated with low rates of early toxicity. Int J Radiat Oncol Biol Phys. 2014;90(5):1061–8. https://doi.org/10.1016/j.ijrobp.2014.07.043.
10. Svedman C, Karlsson K, Rutkowska E, et al. Stereotactic body radiotherapy of primary and metastatic renal lesions for patients with only one functioning kidney. Acta Oncol. 2008;47(8):1578–83. https://doi.org/10.1080/02841860802123196.
11. Siva S, Pham D, Kron T, et al. Stereotactic ablative body radiotherapy for inoperable primary kidney cancer: a prospective clinical trial. BJU Int. 2017;120(5):623–30. https://doi.org/10.1111/bju.13811.
12. Motzer RJ, Jonasch E, Boyle S, et al. NCCN guidelines insights: kidney cancer, version 1.2021: featured updates to the NCCN guidelines. J Natl Compr Cancer Netw. 2020;18(9):1160–70.
13. Svedman C, Sandstrom P, Pisa P, et al. A prospective phase II trial of using extracranial stereotactic radiotherapy in primary and metastatic renal cell carcinoma. Acta Oncol. 2006;45(7):870–5. https://doi.org/10.1080/02841860600954875.
14. Kaplan I, Redrosa I, Martin C, Collins C, Wagner A. Results of a phase I dose escalation study of stereotactic radiosurgery for primary renal tumors. Int J Radiat Oncol Biol Phys. 2009;78:s191.

15. McBride SM, Wagner A, Kaplan ID. A phase 1 dose escalation study of robotic radiosurgery in inoperable primary renal cell carcinoma. Int J Radiat Oncol Biol Phys. 2013;87:s84.
16. Staehler M, Bader M, Schlenker B, et al. Single fraction radiosurgery for the treatment of renal tumors. J Urol. 2015;193(3):771–5.
17. Correa RJ, Ahmad B, Warner A, et al. A prospective phase I dose-escalation trial of stereotactic ablative radiotherapy (SABR) as an alternative to cytoreductive nephrectomy for inoperable patients with metastatic renal cell carcinoma. Radiat Oncol. 2018;13(1):1–8.
18. Qian G, Lowry J, Silverman P, Grossman I, Makara D, Lederman G. Stereotactic extra-cranial radiosurgery for renal cell carcinoma. Int J Radiat Oncol Biol Phys. 2003;57:s283.
19. Beitler JJ, Makara D, Silverman P, Lederman G. Definitive, high-dose-per-fraction, conformal, stereotactic external radiation for renal cell carcinoma. Am J Clin Oncol. 2004;27(6):646–8.
20. Wersall PJ, Blomgren H, Lax I, et al. Extracranial stereotactic radiotherapy for primary and metastatic renal cell carcinoma. Radiother Oncol. 2005;77(1):88–95. https://doi.org/10.1016/j.radonc.2005.03.022.
21. Gilson B, Lederman G, Qian G, Fastaia M, Cangiane L. Hypo-fractionated stereotactic extra-cranial radiosurgery (HFSR) for primary and metastatic renal cell carcinoma. Int J Radiat Oncol Biol Phys. 2006;66:s349.
22. Teh B, Bloch C, Galli-Guevara M, et al. The treatment of primary and metastatic renal cell carcinoma (RCC) with image-guided stereotactic body radiation therapy (SBRT). Biomed Imaging Interv J. 2007;3(1):e6. https://doi.org/10.2349/biij.3.1.e6.
23. Nomiya T, Tsuji H, Hirasawa N, et al. Carbon ion radiation therapy for primary renal cell carcinoma: initial clinical experience. Int J Radiat Oncol Biol Phys. 2008;72(3):828–33. https://doi.org/10.1016/j.ijrobp.2008.01.043.
24. Siva S, Ali M, Correa RJM, et al. 5-year outcomes after stereotactic ablative body radiotherapy for primary renal cell carcinoma: an individual patient data meta-analysis from IROCK (the international radiosurgery consortium of the kidney). Lancet Oncol. 2022;23(12):1508–16.
25. Correa RJ, Louie AV, Staehler M, et al. Stereotactic radiotherapy as a treatment option for renal tumors in the solitary kidney: a multicenter analysis from the IROCK. J Urol. 2019;201(6):1097–104.
26. Siva S, Correa RJ, Warner A, et al. Stereotactic ablative radiotherapy for ≥T1b primary renal cell carcinoma: a report from the international radiosurgery oncology consortium for kidney (IROCK). Int J Radiat Oncol Biol Phys. 2020;108(4):941–9.

Part IX
Musculoskeletal

Chapter 30
Spine Tumors

Simon S. Lo, Arthur S. Yeh, Yolanda Tseng, Stephanie Schaub, Lia M. Halasz, and Edward Y. Kim

30.1 Introduction

Spine tumors is a broad term including primary and metastatic tumors. Only a minority of spine tumors are primary tumors. They include vertebral column (bone) tumors, intradural-extramedullary tumors, and intramedullary tumors.

For most primary spine tumors, the mainstay of treatment is maximal safe resection followed by conventional radiotherapy (RT). For intramedullary tumors, hypofractionated RT is seldom used as the target volume is located within the spinal cord, rendering delivery of a tumoricidal dose to the tumor more difficult without resulting in a higher risk for radiation myelopathy (RM). For intradural-extramedullary and vertebral column primary tumors, there are scarce data on the use of hypofractionated RT, most in the form of stereotactic body radiotherapy (SBRT).

The spine bone/vertebra is a common site of involvement in patients with bone metastases. Left untreated, progressive spinal metastases can lead to severe pain, hypercalcemia, pathologic fracture, and spinal cord compression. The standard treatment, depending upon patient and disease factors, is RT with or without surgical intervention. Factors determining the need for consideration for surgery include the histology (radiosensitive vs. radioresistant), Bilsky grade for metastatic epidural spinal cord compression (MESCC), neurologic status, spinal instability neoplastic score (SINS), and presence/absence of mechanical instability. The traditional RT

S. S. Lo (✉) · Y. Tseng · S. Schaub · L. M. Halasz · E. Y. Kim
Department of Radiation Oncology, University of Washington School of Medicine, Seattle, WA, USA

A. S. Yeh
Carmel High School, Carmel, IN, USA

O. Kaidar-Person, R. Chen (eds.), *Hypofractionated and Stereotactic Radiation Therapy*, https://doi.org/10.1007/978-3-031-47701-0_30

utilizes conventional or moderately hypofractionated regimens, but the amount of radiation that can be delivered is limited by the spinal cord tolerance. With the sophistication of radiation technology, stereotactic body radiotherapy (SBRT) has emerged as a means to deliver higher biologically effective doses to the metastatic tumors and one of the standard treatments for spine bone metastases in the setting of newly diagnosed disease, recurrent or progressive disease after prior RT, postoperative situation, and MESCC (rare). Recently, CCTG SC.24/TROG 17.06 randomized phase II/III trial showed that SBRT (24 Gy in 2 fractions) is superior to conventional radiotherapy (20 Gy in 5 fractions) in terms of complete pain response with no increased toxicities [1].

This chapter will focus on the use of SBRT for intradural-extramedullary and vertebral column primary tumors and vertebral (spine bone) metastatic tumors. Moderately hypofractionated RT delivering low doses of radiation has been the standard of care for spine bone metastatic tumors and is beyond the scope of this chapter.

30.2 Pearls

- Types of primary spine tumors based on location:
  - Vertebral column—Osteogenic sarcoma (malignant), hemangioma (benign), giant cell tumor (benign in most cases), chordoma (malignant), and chondrosarcoma (malignant).
  - Intradural-extramedullary—Meningioma (benign in most cases), nerve sheath tumors including schwannoma and neurofibroma (benign), and ependymoma.
  - Intramedullary—Astrocytoma and ependymoma.
- Benign tumors of the spine represent a wide variety of histologies that occur within the intradural space, and epidural, paraspinal, and vertebral body locations.
- Common benign tumors include meningiomas, schwannomas, and neurofibromas.
- Malignant tumors include malignant nerve sheath tumors, osteogenic sarcomas, chondrosarcomas, and chordomas.
- Symptoms include back pain, extremity weakness, and loss of bladder or bowel function.
- Pathology workup:
  - Biopsy to confirm pathologic diagnosis when a radiographic diagnosis cannot be confidently made.
  - Tissue can be obtained when surgery is done for tumor resection or debulking.
- Medical workup:
  - H&P, focusing on the assessment of pain symptoms and neurologic function. Physical examination requires thorough neurological examination to detect any motor and sensory deficits in the upper and lower extremities or any sensory level in the torso.

- Imaging workup: Crucial to determine the extent of tumor invasion, pathologic fracture, and tumor compression of the spinal cord, cauda equina, and nerve roots.
  - MRI of the spine w/wo contrast: Sagittal T1 and STIR to evaluate marrow replacement, axial T2 to evaluate epidural disease, volumetric T1 with gadolinium, and T2 for treatment planning.
- Treatment strategies:
  - Surgical resection is the mainstay of treatment for primary spine tumors.
  - Observation can be offered in patients with benign primary spine tumors if a gross total resection is achieved.
  - Observation or postoperative conventional RT or SBRT can be offered to patients with subtotally resected benign primary spine tumors (excluding intramedullary tumors).
  - Postoperative RT ± systemic therapy is offered to patients with malignant primary spine tumors regardless of the extent of resection. Postoperative SBRT is offered in rare situations.

30.3 Pearls

- Spinal metastases are diagnosed in approximately 40% of cancer patients during their disease course and are the most common spinal tumors.
- In post-mortem studies, up to 90% of cancer patients may have microscopic spinal metastases.
- The most common presenting symptom is back pain. Other symptoms can include upper or lower extremity weakness or numbness, sensory level in the torso, and loss of bladder or bowel control.
- Local anatomy:
  - Based on the International Spine Radiosurgery Consortium anatomic classification system, each vertebra is divided into six sectors: Sector 1, vertebral body; Sector 2, left pedicle; Sector 3, left transverse process and lamina; Sector 4, spinous process; Sector 5, right transverse process and lamina; and Sector 6, right pedicle [2] (Fig. 30.1). The anatomic classification system for the sacrum is a modification of the system for the cervical, thoracic, and lumbar spine [3] (Fig. 30.2).
- Progressive metastatic spine tumors can lead to spinal cord or nerve compression.
- Medical workup:
  - H&P, focusing on the assessment of pain symptoms and neurologic function. Physical examination requires thorough neurological examination to detect any motor and sensory deficits in the upper and lower extremities or any sensory level in the torso.

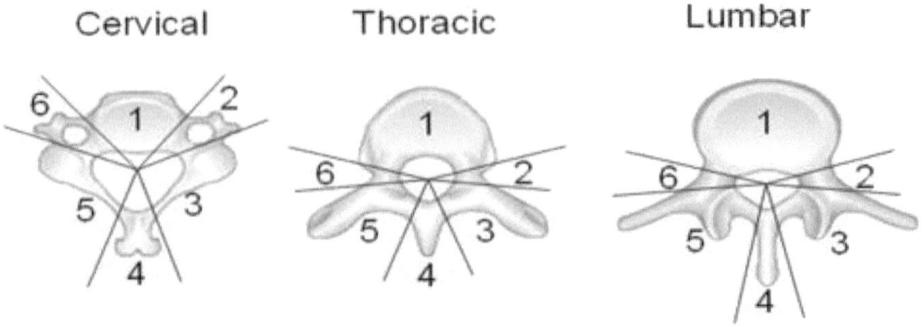

Fig. 30.1 International Spine Radiosurgery Consortium anatomic classification system for consensus target volumes for spine radiosurgery. (Reprinted from Int J Radiation Oncol Biol Phys, Vol. 83, No. 5, Cox et al., International Spine Radiosurgery Consortium Consensus Guidelines for Target Volume Definition in Spinal Stereotactic Radiosurgery, pp. e597–e605, Copyright (2012), with permission from Elsevier [2])

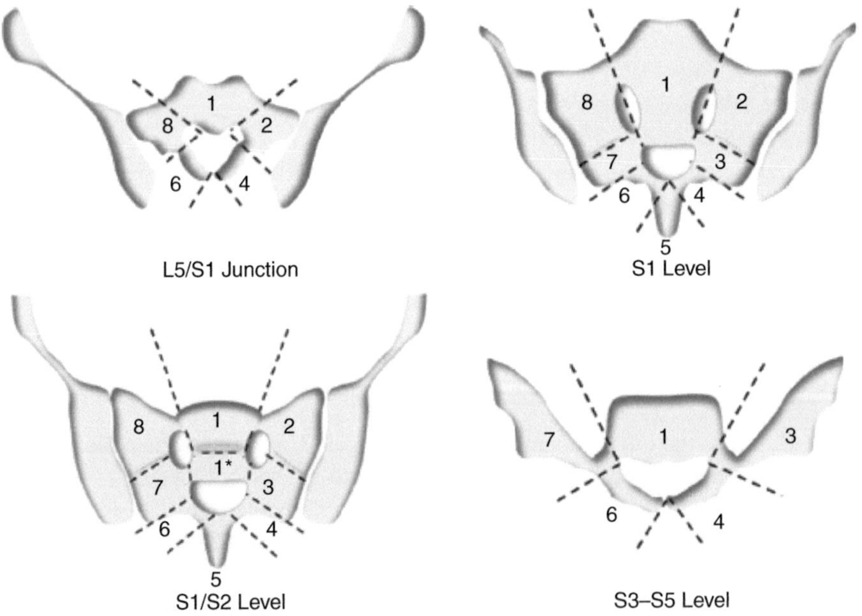

Fig. 30.2 Stereotactic Radiosurgery Sacral Classification System. (1) Vertebral body [1* represents the subsequent caudal vertebral body (S2 in this illustration)]; (2) left anterior ala; (3) left posterior ala; (4) left lamina; (5) spinous process; (6) right lamina; (7) right posterior ala; (8) right anterior ala. (Reprinted from Radiother Oncol., Vol. 145, Dunne et al., International consensus recommendations for target volume delineation specific to sacral metastases and spinal stereotactic body radiation therapy (SBRT), pp. 21–29, Copyright (2020), with permission from Elsevier [3])

- Imaging workup: Crucial to determine the extent of tumor invasion, bone retropulsion, and tumor compression of the spinal cord, cauda equina, and nerve roots.
  - MRI of the spine w/wo contrast and/or CT myelogram.
- MRI: Sagittal T1 and STIR to evaluate marrow replacement, axial T2 to evaluate epidural disease, volumetric T1 and T2 for treatment planning, and gadolinium-enhanced MRI to evaluate leptomeningeal disease.
- CT myelogram: To evaluate epidural disease, especially in postoperative patients with metallic hardware.
  - Pathology workup:
  - Biopsy to confirm metastatic disease if no prior pathologic diagnosis.
  - Tissue can be obtained when surgical decompression for the spinal cord compression is performed.
  - Radioresistant histologies including renal cell carcinoma, melanoma and sarcoma may benefit from utilizing SBRT to improve local control.

Treatment Strategies

- Conventional fractionation or moderately hypofractionated RT or SBRT for uncomplicated spinal and sacral metastases.
- Surgery plus conventional fractionation or moderately hypofractionated RT or SBRT for patients with bony retropulsion, high-grade MESCC, or mechanical instability.
- For very radiosensitive histologies such as myeloma or lymphoma, if there is no mechanical instability, conventional fractionation or moderately hypofractionated RT can be offered.

30.4 Staging

For spine bone metastases, there are two commonly used systems that objectively evaluate patients with regard to the extent of MESCC (Bilsky grade) and spinal stability (spinal instability neoplastic score), respectively. These tools are being used to evaluate the need for surgical intervention and the suitability for SBRT for spinal metastases.

Bilsky grading system for epidural disease [4]

Bilsky grade	Details
0	Absence of epidural disease
1a	Impingement but no deformation of thecal sac
1b	Impingement and deformation of thecal sac
1c	Deformation of thecal sac and abutment of spinal cord
2	Epidural spinal cord compression with visible CSF
3	Epidural spinal cord compression without visible CSF

The *Spinal Instability Neoplastic Score (SINS)* was developed by the Spine Oncology Study Group and was validated in terms of interobserver and intraobserver reliability among spine oncologic surgeons and radiation oncologists [5].

There are six parameters in the system (see table below). Patients with 0–6 points, 7–12 points, and 13–18 points are designated to have stable, potentially unstable, and unstable spine, respectively. In a patient with an unstable spine, surgical stabilization should be considered before RT.

Spinal Instability Neoplastic Score (SINS)

Component	0 points	1 point	2 points	3 points	4 points
Location	Rigid spine S2–S5	Semirigid spine T3–T10	Mobile spine C3–C6, L2–L4	Junctional spine Occiput–C2, C7–T2, T11–L1, L5–S1	–
Pain	Absence of pain	Occasional non-mechanical pain	Non-mechanical pain	Mechanical pain: Pain relief with recumbency and/or pain with movement/ loading of the spine	–
Bone lesion characteristic	Blastic	Mixed lytic/ blastic	Lytic lesion		–
Radiographic spinal alignment	Normal alignment	–	De novo deformity (kyphosis/ scoliosis)	–	Subluxation/ translation
Vertebral body collapse	None of the following	No collapse but with greater than 50% body involved	Less than 50% collapse	Greater than 50% collapse	–
Posterolateral involvement of the spinal elements (facet, pedicle, or costovertebral joint fracture or replacement)	None	Unilateral	–	Bilateral	–

30.5 Patient Selection for SBRT

- For primary spine tumors:
  - Benign spine tumors: Postoperative radiographically residual tumors or medically inoperable spine tumors, ideally at least 1–2 mm from the spinal cord.
  - Malignant spine tumors: The standard postoperative treatment is conventional RT or proton therapy. If SBRT is offered postoperatively or medically inoperable, there should ideally be a gap of at least 1–2 mm from the CTV to the spinal cord.
  - Reirradiation: Ideally, the last course of RT should be at least 5–6 months earlier, and there should be at least 1–2 mm from the CTV to the spinal cord (can be achieved by reoperation upon recurrence).
- For spinal metastases:
  - The American Society of Radiation Oncology (ASTRO) (see the table below) and American College of Radiology guidelines have detailed appropriate inclusion and exclusion criteria for spine SBRT [6, 7].
  - In broad terms, the inclusion criteria include spinal or paraspinal metastatic non-radiosensitive solid tumor histology in 3 or less contiguous segments, a reasonably stable spinal column, low-grade epidural disease based on Bilsky grading system, a life expectancy of 3 months or longer, and relatively limited extraspinal systemic disease.

Suggested inclusion and exclusion criteria for patients enrolled in trials to evaluate stereotactic body radiotherapy for spinal bone metastases from ASTRO guidelines [7]

Characteristic	Inclusion	Exclusion
Radiographic	1. Spinal or paraspinal metastasis by MRI 2. No more than two consecutive or three noncontiguous spine segments involved	1. Spinal MRI cannot be completed for any reason 2. Epidural compression of spinal cord or cauda equina 3. Spinal canal compromise >25% 4. Unstable spine requiring surgical stabilization 5. Tumor location within 5 mm of spinal cord or cauda equina (relative contraindication[a])
Patient	1. Age ≥18 years 2. KPS of ≥40–50 3. Medically inoperable (or patient refused surgery)	1. Active connective tissue disease 2. Worsening or progressive neurologic deficit 3. Inability to lie flat on table for SBRT 4. Patient in hospice or with <3-month life expectancy

Characteristic	Inclusion	Exclusion
Tumor	1. Histologic proof of malignancy 2. Biopsy of spine lesion recommended if first suspected metastasis 3. Oligometastatic or bone-only metastatic disease	1. Radiosensitive histology such as multiple myeloma 2. Extraspinal disease not eligible for further treatment
Previous treatment	Any of the following: 1. Previous EBRT <45-Gy total dose 2. Failure of previous surgery to that spinal level 3. Presence of gross residual disease after surgery	1. Previous SBRT to the same level 2. Systemic radionuclide delivery within 30 days before SBRT 3. EBRT within 90 days before SBRT 4. Chemotherapy within 30 days of SBRT

Abbreviations: *MRI* magnetic resonance imaging, *KPS* Karnofsky performance status, *SBRT* stereotactic body radiotherapy, *EBRT* external beam radiotherapy

Reprinted from Int J Radiation Oncol Biol Phys, Vol. 79, No. 4, Lutz et al. Palliative radiotherapy for bone metastases: an ASTRO evidence-based guideline, pp. 965–76, Copyright (2011), with permission from Elsevier [6]

[a] Relative indication that optimally tumor >5 mm from spinal cord; if this distance is closer, case-by-case discussion is required because published data suggest that the risk of failure is greater

30.6 Treatment Planning

Simulation instructions	SBRT • Immobilization using a long head and neck thermoplastic mask for lesions above T4 • Immobilization using a dual vacuum system (Body FIX) for LINAC-based system or a vacuum cushion for CyberKnife system for lesions T4 or below • Arms must be down for CyberKnife to avoid possible collision of robotically mounted LINAC with the arms • Repeat diagnostic volumetric MRI T1 w/wo contrast and T2 ± CT myelogram (if metallic hardware hinders visualization of the spinal cord) • Planning CT performed without IV contrast, if possible, 1.0–1.25 mm slices • Fuse the treatment planning CT to the new MRI and preoperative MRI (for postoperative cases) ± CT myelogram at the index spinal segments for target delineation Reirradiation • Same as radiation naïve cases • Fusion of the previous RT plan with the treatment planning CT will allow estimation of prior radiation dose to OARs and hence the determination of dose constraints to different OARs

Target delineation	• Primary benign spinal tumors: Contrast-enhanced tumor defined as GTV = CTV • Primary malignant spinal tumors: Contrast-enhanced tumor defined as GTV in intact cases; tumor bed + contrast-enhanced tumor defined as GTV in postoperative setting; for intact cases, CTV is defined based on Fig. 30.3; for postoperative case, CTV is defined based on Fig. 30.4 • Spinal metastases: CTV is defined as the whole vertebral body ± pedicles ± posterior elements except for metastases located mainly in the posterior elements; need to include all epidural (3.0–5.0 mm margin superiorly and inferiorly) and paraspinal (3.0–5.0 mm expansion from GTV) involvement; for postoperative case, need to take into account the preoperative extent of involvement; interested readers are advised to go to the consensus guidelines for contouring by Cox et al. (Fig. 30.3) and Redmond et al. (Fig. 30.4) published in IJROBP • Sacral metastases: Please refer to Fig. 30.5
Delineation of spinal cord, cauda equina, and plexuses	• Spinal cord: Typically, the T2 sequence of a volumetric MRI is used; in the postoperative case, a metallic artifact reduction technique on a lower Tesla MRI unit or a CT myelogram can be used; a PRV expansion is done (see below) • Cauda equina: The thecal sac is used as a surrogate for cauda equina and the contours should extend at least one level above and one level below the PTV. The bony canal below the thecal sac should be contoured down to the inferior aspect of S5. T2 sequence of a volumetric MRI should be used for contouring [9] • Brachial and lumbar plexuses: Please refer to Truong et al. [10] and Yi et al. [11]
Image guidance	• CyberKnife: Spine tracking • Linac: Daily pretreatment, post-shift, and midway CBCTs
Margins	PTV = CTV + 2.0–3.0 mm minus PRV cord or thecal sac at levels without cord PRV cord = Spinal cord + 1.5–3.0 mm (Typically 2.0 mm) (Thecal sac can also be used as PRV cord)
Dosimetric considerations	Dose prescribed to PTV. Goal = ≥80–90% of PTV and ≥80–90% of CTV covered by the prescribed IDL (typically 67–85%). In cases where there is a higher-grade epidural disease, the coverage of CTV may be worse than that for PTV (the subtracted PRV cord may contain epidural disease that is part of the CTV). The maximum hotspot allowed is 50% as per the SC24 trial [1] RTOG 0631: At least 90% of the CTV covered by 100% of the prescribed dose (acceptable variation: <90% but ≥80% coverage) SC24 trial [1]: At least 80% of CTV covered by 100% of the prescribed dose

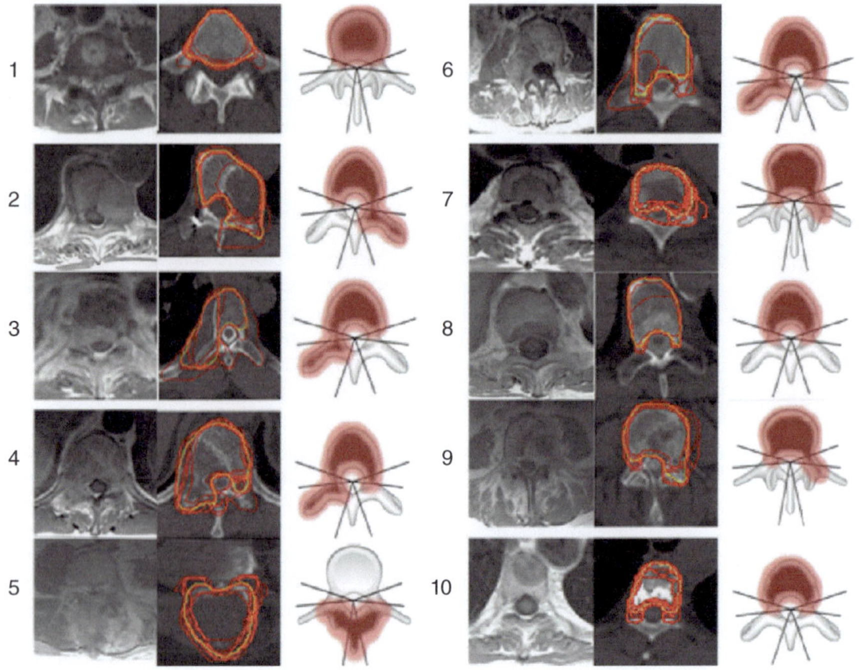

Fig. 30.3 Consensus clinical target volume contours for spine stereotactic radiosurgery for primary malignant spinal tumors or spinal metastasis. Red indicates individual contours, and orange indicates consensus contours. (Reprinted from Int J Radiation Oncol Biol Phys, Vol. 83, No. 5, Cox et al., International Spine Radiosurgery Consortium Consensus Guidelines for Target Volume Definition in Spinal Stereotactic Radiosurgery, pp. e597–e605, Copyright (2012), with permission from Elsevier [2])

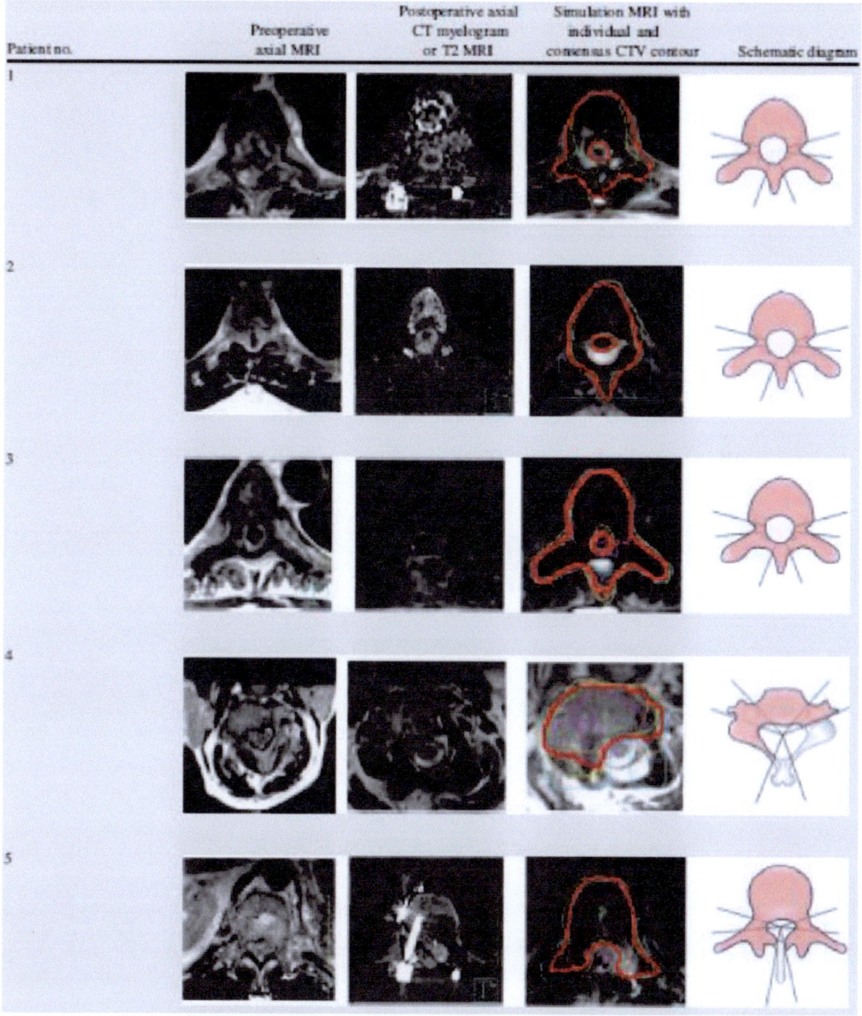

Fig. 30.4 Consensus CTV contours for postoperative SBRT for primary malignant spinal tumors or spine metastases. (Reprinted from Int J Radiation Oncol Biol Phys, Vol. 97, No. 1, Redmond et al., Consensus Contouring Guidelines for Postoperative Stereotactic Body Radiation Therapy for Metastatic Solid Tumor Malignancies to the Spine, pp. 64–77, Copyright (2017), with permission from Elsevier [8])

Patient no.	Preoperative axial MRI	Postoperative axial CT myelogram or T2 MRI	Simulation MRI with individual and consensus CTV contour	Schematic diagram
6	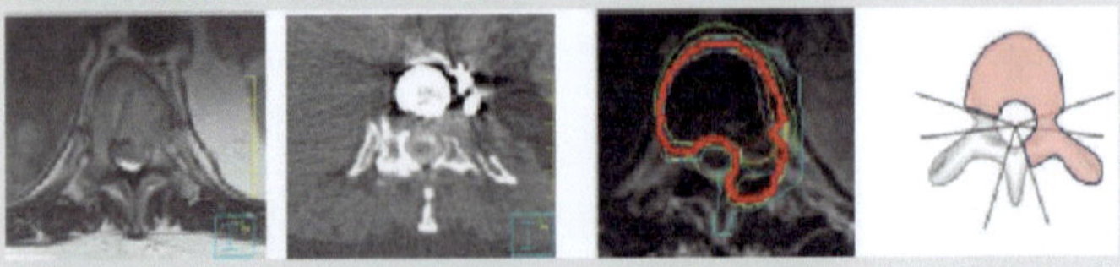			
7	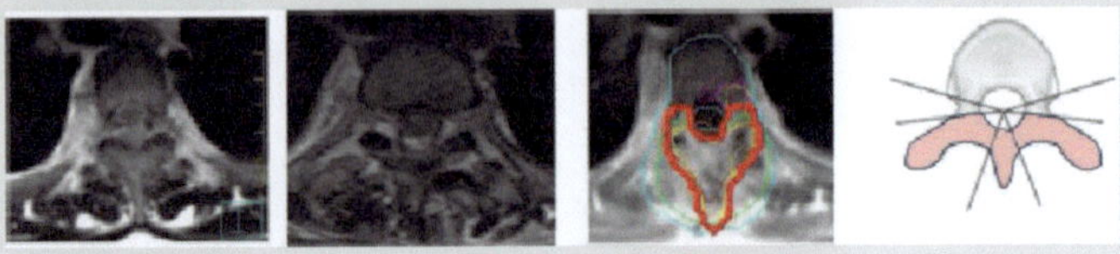			
8	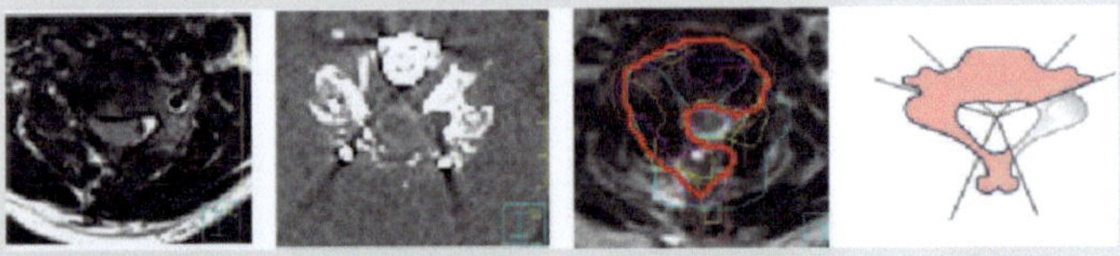			
9	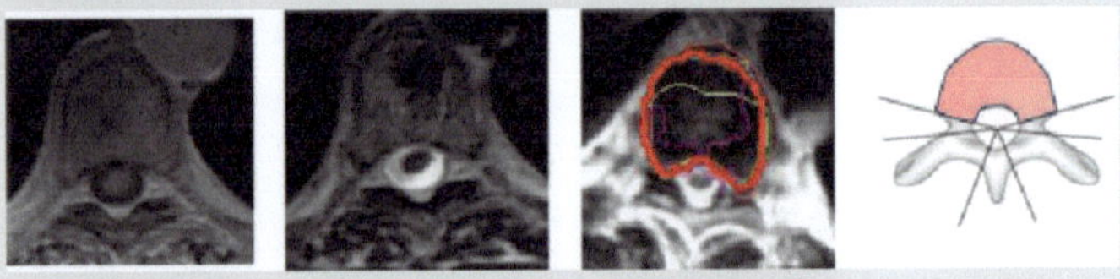			
10	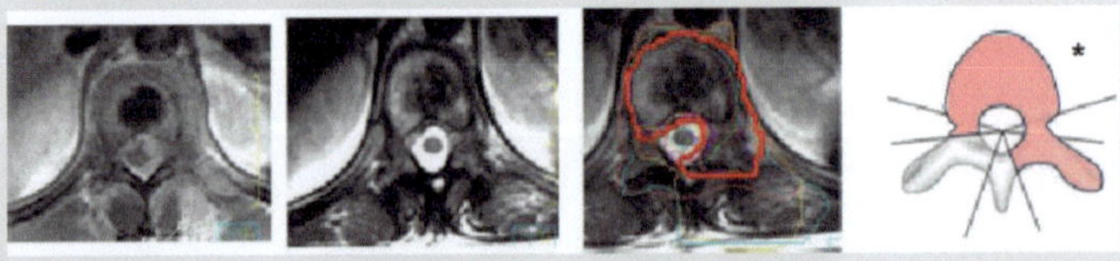			

Consensus contours are shown in bold red and individual contours are shown in unique colors. *As indicated in the recommendations, the entire pre-operative extent of paraspinal disease should at minimum be encompassed in the CTV. (A color version of this table is available at www.redjournal.org.)

Fig. 30.4 (continued)

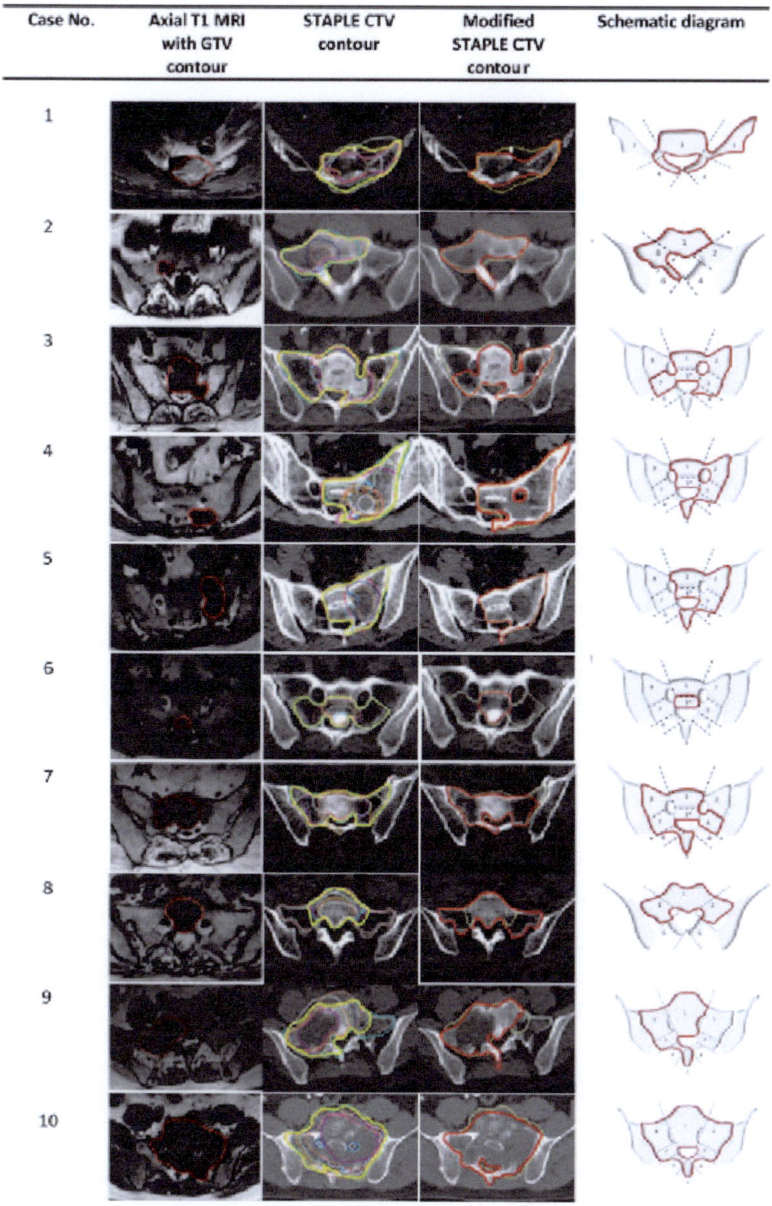

Fig. 30.5 Consensus contours for target volume definition of the sacrum. Simultaneous Truth and Performance Level Estimation (STAPLE) contours (yellow line). An expectation–maximization algorithm is used for the probabilistic determination of the true volume of a structure based on several input volumes generated by trained experts. A variety of colors represent the contours by individual experts' individual clinical target volume contours (variety of colors), modified STAPLE contours (red line). Abbreviations: CTV, clinical target volume. MRI, magnetic resonance imaging. (Reprinted from Radiother Oncol., Vol. 145, Dunne et al., International consensus recommendations for target volume delineation specific to sacral metastases and spinal SBRT, pp. 21–29, Copyright (2020), with permission from Elsevier [3])

30.6.1 Treatment Planning with Linear Accelerator

- 4–8 MV photons.
- Utilize 7–9 static, coplanar beams (IMRT) or 2–4 rotational arcs (VMAT).
- When the index vertebra(e) to be treated is located at a spinal region where there is a significant curvature, the use of multiple static beam IMRT or VMAT allows for the adjustment of the collimator angle of each beam to align with the long axis of the spinal cord, resulting in a steeper dose gradient.
- In patients with metallic hardware, the use of multiple static beam IMRT allows for the choice of beam angles where there is less metal along the beam paths.
- Beams shaped using multi-leaf collimators.

30.6.2 Treatment Planning with CyberKnife

- Composed of hundreds of pencil beams.
- For thoracic spine tumors, use Monte Carlo instead of Ray Tracing for treatment planning as Okoye et al. discovered that, when Ray Tracing was used for thoracic spine lesions, the coverage of the PTV is overestimated and the doses to the critical structures such as the spinal cord might be underestimated [12].
- Beams shaped using collimators of various sizes.
- Dosimetry:
- The prescription dose is typically prescribed to 75–85% IDL.
- Limit dose outside of the PTV to ≥105% of the prescription dose to a volume of less than or equal to 2.0 cc and dose of ≥105% of the prescription dose to a region within 1.0 cm from the edge of the PTV.

30.7 Common Dose/Fractionation Schemes (Figs. 30.6, 30.7, and 30.8)

Primary spine tumors

Dose/fx	# of fx	Total dose	Notes
Benign: 12–15 Gy Malignant: 16–24 Gy	1	Benign: 12–15 Gy Malignant: 16–24 Gy	Dose schemes for benign spine tumors are based on the literature on meningiomas, schwannomas, and neurofibromas, whereas those for malignant spine tumors are based on the literature on chordomas
Benign: 6–8 Gy Malignant: 9–12 Gy	3	Benign: 18–24 Gy Malignant: 27–36 Gy	Dose schemes for benign spine tumors are based on the literature on meningiomas, schwannomas, and neurofibromas, whereas those for malignant spine tumors are based on the literature on chordomas

Dose/fx	# of fx	Total dose	Notes
Benign: 5–6 Gy Malignant: 6–8 Gy	5	Benign: 25–30 Gy Malignant: 30–40 Gy	Dose schemes for benign spine tumors are based on the literature on meningiomas, schwannomas, and neurofibromas, whereas those for malignant spine tumors are based on the literature on chordomas

Spinal metastases

Dose/fx	# of fx	Total dose	Notes
16–24 Gy	1	16–24 Gy	Based on data from high-volume institutions [13, 14]
10–12 Gy	2	20–24 Gy	Based on data from high volume institutions [13, 14] and SC24 trial [1]
9 Gy	3	27 Gy	Based on data from high volume institutions [13, 14]
6 Gy	5	30 Gy	Based on data from high volume institutions [13, 14]

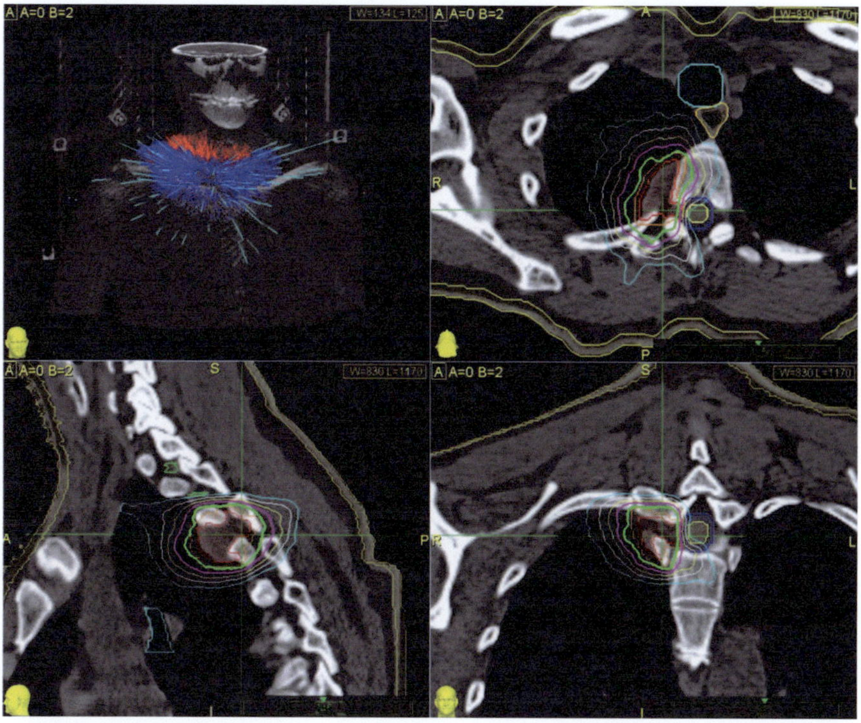

Fig. 30.6 A patient with a right T3 schwannoma treated with SBRT to a dose of 21 Gy in 3 fractions prescribed to the 80% isodose line (green)

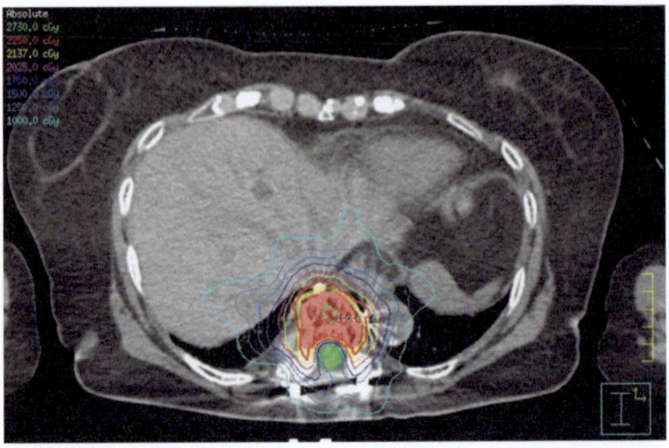

Fig. 30.7 A patient with a T9 hemangioma treated with SBRT to a dose of 22.5 Gy in 3 fractions after surgical decompression of spinal cord compression. The residual tumor regressed and there was no evidence of recurrence 4 years after treatment

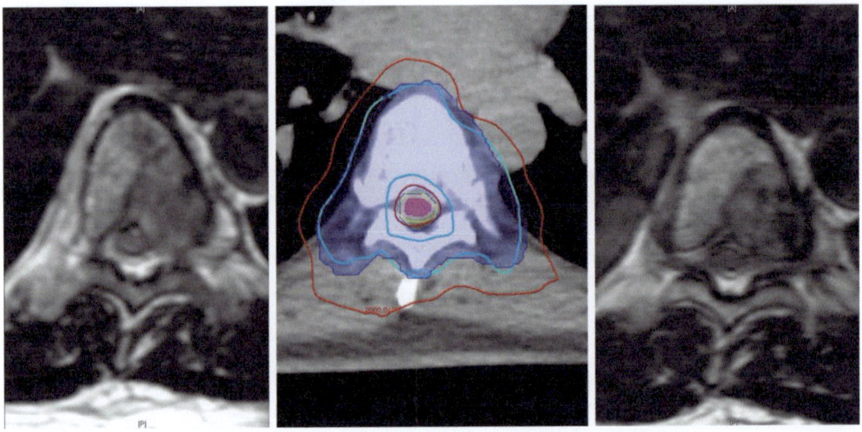

Fig. 30.8 A 61-year-old gentleman with metastatic thyroid cancer to T7 with Bilsky grade 2 metastatic spinal cord compression (left panel); he received SBRT delivering 27 Gy in 3 fractions (cyan) with PRV cord limited to 20.3 Gy (based on Sahgal et al. data) (middle panel); MRI after 3 months showed regression of epidural disease (Bilsky grade 1a disease)

30.8 Normal Tissue Tolerances

Organs-at-risk	Dmax	Volumetric	Notes
Brachial plexus			
• 1 fx	17.5 Gy 14 Gy	Maximum point <3 cc	RTOG 0631
• 2 fx (for sacral nerves only)	26 Gy	Maximum point	SC24 trial [1]
• 3 fx	24 Gy 20.4 Gy	Maximum point <3 cc	RTOG 1021
• 5 fx	32 Gy 30 Gy	Maximum point <3 cc	RTOG 0813

Organs-at-risk	Dmax	Volumetric	Notes
• DLT	Brachial plexopathy		
Cauda equina			
• 1 fx	16 Gy 14 Gy	Maximum point <3 cc	RTOG 0631
• 2 fx (for thecal sac at levels without spinal cord)	17 Gy	Maximum point	SC24 trial [1]
• 3 fx	24 Gy 20.4 Gy	Maximum point <3 cc	Extrapolation from brachial plexus constraints (Based on RTOG 1021)
• 5 fx	32 Gy 30 Gy	Maximum point <3 cc	Extrapolation from brachial plexus constraints (Based on RTOG 0813)
• DLT	Neuropathy		
Spinal cord surrogate (thecal sac or PRV cord with 1.5–2.0 mm expansion from spinal cord) for patients with no prior RT[a]			
• 1 fx	12.2 Gy	Maximum point	Based on a study by Sahgal et al. [15]
• 2 fx	17 Gy	Maximum point	SC24 trial [1]
• 3 fx	20.3 Gy	Maximum point	Based on a study by Sahgal et al. [15]
• 5 fx	25.3 Gy	Maximum point	Based on a study by Sahgal et al. [15]
• DLT	Radiation myelopathy		
Esophagus			
• 1 fx	16 Gy 11.9 Gy	Maximum point <5 cc	RTOG 0631
• 2 fx	20 Gy	Maximum point	SC24 trial [1]
• 3 fx	25.2 Gy 17.7 Gy	Maximum point <5 cc	RTOG 1021
• 5 fx	105% of PTV prescription 27.5 Gy	Maximum point <5 cc	RTOG 0813
• DLT	Esophageal injury		

[a] The spinal cord surrogate (thecal sac or PRV cord with 1.5–2.0 mm expansion from spinal cord) constraints from the study by Sahgal et al. were based on real patient data. RTOG constraints for spinal cord for 3 and 5 fx should not be applied to spine SBRT as those constraints were for non-spine SBRT trials where the spinal canal was used as the surrogate for spinal cord

Prior conventional RT	1 fx: SBRT dose to PRV cord or thecal sac (maximum point dose)	2 fx: SBRT dose to PRV cord or thecal sac (maximum point dose)	3 fx: SBRT dose to PRV cord or thecal sac (maximum point dose)	4 fx: SBRT dose to PRV cord or thecal sac (maximum point dose	5 fx: SBRT dose to PRV cord or thecal sac (maximum point dose)
20 Gy/5 fx, 30 Gy/10 fx, or 37.5 Gy/15 fx	9 Gy	12.2 Gy	14.5 Gy	16.2 Gy	18 Gy
40 Gy/20 fx or 45 Gy/25 fx	No information	12.2 Gy	14.5 Gy	16.2 Gy	18 Gy
50 Gy/25 fx	No information	11 Gy	12.5 Gy	14 Gy	15.5 Gy

Recommended dose constraints for reirradiation with SBRT from Sahgal et al. Int. J. Radiation Oncology Biol. Phys., Vol. 82, No. 1, pp. 107–116, 2012 [16]. SBRT must be at least 5 months after prior conventional RT with a reirradiation PRV cord or thecal sac nBED of 20–25 $Gy_{2/2}$ or less

30.9 Patient Management

1. Premedicate patients with antiemetic medication if the CTV is close to the stomach (e.g., ondansetron 4 mg PO 30 min before treatment).
2. For patients with severe back pain, premedicate with narcotic medication.
3. Consider premedication with Medrol Dosepak or dexamethasone 4 mg during and up to 4 days after completion of SBRT (or slower taper) for prophylaxis against pain flare.
4. Toxicity

   (a) Acute:

   - Skin/esophagus (dermatitis, odynophagia)
     - Emollients (Aquaphor, calendula). Remove 4 h prior to SBRT.
     - Oral solutions (first BLM, magic mouthwash). Use TID prior to meals.
     - Pain medication (Fentanyl patch 25–100 mcg q72 h, Oxycodone 5–20 mg q4–6 h).
   - Nausea/vomiting
     - Start with ondansetron 4 mg q8 h. Can increase to 8 mg q8 h.
     - Phenergan 12.5 mg q4–6 h. Can increase to 25 mg q4–6 h.
     - Compazine 5 mg q6 h. Can increase to 10 mg q6 h.

- Pain flare
  - Medrol Dosepak or dexamethasone 4 mg (up to 4 days after SBRT or slower taper)

(b) Subacute/late:

- Skin/soft tissue (discoloration, fibrosis)
- Vertebral compression fracture (fraction size dependent, higher risk if ≥20 Gy/fraction, peak incidence 2–3 months after SBRT)
  - Pain medication
  - Refer to a spine surgeon
- Radiation myelopathy (permanent, very rare <1%)
- Radiation plexopathy (rare)
- Esophageal stricture/stenosis (rare)
  - Recommend follow-up 1 month post-treatment completion to assess acute toxicity
  - Systemic therapy

(c) There is minimal data addressing the use of concurrent chemotherapy/systemic therapy with spine SBRT. Limited data suggest that concurrent tyrosine kinase inhibitors with SBRT for spine metastases appeared to be safe and improve local control [17].

30.10 Follow-Up [18]

- H&P, neurologic examination every 2–3 months for first 2 years, q6 months years 3–5, then annually.
- Spine MRI every 2–3 months after SBRT for the first 1–2 years, and every 3–6 months thereafter.

30.11 Relevant Literature

- There are a range of dose regimens used for SBRT for primary spine tumors and radiation naïve, previously irradiated and postoperative spine metastases and promising results have been demonstrated.

SBRT for primary spinal tumors

Series	Study type/ tumor type	# of patients/ tumors	Prescribed dose	Follow-up	Local control (%)
Gerszten et al. [19]	Retrospective Benign spine tumors	Meningiomas: 8/8 Schwannomas: 15/15 Neurofibromas: 7/7	18–21 Gy/3 fx	26 months	100%
Gerszten et al. [20]	Retrospective Benign spine tumors	Meningiomas: 13/13 Schwannomas: 35/35 Neurofibromas: 25/25	17.31 Gy/1 fx	37 months	100%
Yamada et al. [21]	Retrospective Chordoma of spine and sacrum	21 primary and 3 metastatic	24 Gy/1 fx	24 months	95%
Lockney et al. [22]	Retrospective Chordoma of mobile spine	12/12	24 Gy/1 fx, 24–36 Gy/3 fx	Postoperative: 65.9 months Salvage: 10.7 months	Postoperative: 80% Salvage: 57.1%

SBRT for spinal metastases

Series	Study type/patient population/tumor type	# of patients/tumors	Prescribed dose	Follow-up	Local control (%)	Pain control (%)
Sahgal et al. [1]	Phase II/III randomized trial (SC24) Intact de novo spine metastasis	SBRT: 114 Conventional RT: 115	SBRT (24 Gy/2 fx) vs. conventional RT (20 Gy/5 fx)	6.7 months	6-month local progression SBRT: 3% Conventional RT: 10%	3-month CR SBRT: 35% Conventional RT:14% 6-month CR SBRT: 32% Conventional RT:16%
Wang et al. [23]	Prospective Mixed intact de novo, previously irradiated and/ or surgically treated spinal metastases	149 (79 with prior RT ± surgery)/166	27–30 Gy/3 fx	15.9 months	1 year: 80.5% 2 years: 72.4%	BPI: 26% (baseline) to 54% (6 months)
Garg et al. [24]	Prospective RT naïve	61 (16 had prior surgery)/63	16–24 Gy/1 fx	20 months (mean)	18 months: 88%	18 patients pain-free at 3 and 6 months compared with 13 at baseline
Yamada et al. [25]	Retrospective RT naïve	93/103	18–24 Gy/1 fx	15 months	15 months: 90%	N/A
Guckeberger et al. [26]	Retrospective Intact de novo spine metastases	301/387	Median 24 Gy (10–60 Gy)/median 3 fx (1–20 fx)	11.8 months	1 year: 89.9% 2 years: 83.9%	N/A
Sahgal et al. [27]	Retrospective RT naïve	14/23	Median 24 Gy (7–40 Gy)/median 3 fx (1–5 fx)	9 months	1 year: 85% 2 years: 69%	N/A
Gerszten et al. [28]	Retrospective Postoperative	26/26	16–20 Gy/1 fx	16 months	N/A	92%

Series	Study type/patient population/tumor type	# of patients/tumors	Prescribed dose	Follow-up	Local control (%)	Pain control (%)
Laufer et al. [29]	Retrospective Postoperative	186/186	24 Gy/1 fx, or 24–30 Gy/3 fx, or 18–36 Gy/5–6 fx	7.6 months	1 year: 83.6%	N/A
Al-Omair et al. [30]	Retrospective Postoperative	80/80	Median 24 Gy (18–40 Gy)/median 2 fx (1–5)	8.3 months	1 year: 84%	N/A
Bate et al. [31]	Retrospective Postoperative	21/21	16–22 Gy/1 fx, or 20–30 Gy/2–5 fx	13.7 months	1 year: 90.5%	N/A

Abbreviations: *Gy* gray, *fx* fraction(s), *SBRT* stereotactic body radiotherapy, *RT* radiotherapy, *CR* complete response, *BPI* brachial plexus injury

30.12 Summary

There is wide variation in these studies with regard to dose, fraction size, and prescribed IDL. Overall, the results were promising with a very low incidence of radiation myelopathy for both primary spine tumors and spinal metastases, and high rates of local control.

References

1. Sahgal A, Myrehaug SD, Siva S, Masucci L, Foote MC, Brundage M, Butler J, Chow E, Fehlings MG, Gabos Z, Greenspoon J, Kerba M, Lee YK, Liu MC, Maralani P, Thibault I, Wong R, Hum M, Ding K, Prulekar W. CCTG SC.24/TROG 17.06: a randomized phase II/III study comparing 24Gy in 2 stereotactic body radiotherapy (SBRT) fractions versus 20Gy in 5 conventional palliative radiotherapy (CRT) fractions for patients with painful spinal metastases. Int J Radiat Oncol Biol Phys. 2020;108(5):1397–8. https://doi.org/10.1016/j.ijrobp.2020.09.019. Epub 2020 Nov 18.
2. Cox BW, Spratt DE, Lovelock M, Bilsky MH, Lis E, Ryu S, Sheehan J, Gerszten PC, Chang E, Gibbs I, Soltys S, Sahgal A, Deasy J, Flickinger J, Quader M, Mindea S, Yamada Y. International Spine Radiosurgery Consortium consensus guidelines for target volume definition in spinal stereotactic radiosurgery. Int J Radiat Oncol Biol Phys. 2012;83(5):e597–605. https://doi.org/10.1016/j.ijrobp.2012.03.009. Epub 2012 May 19. PMID:22608954.
3. Dunne EM, Sahgal A, Lo SS, Bergman A, Kosztyla R, Dea N, Chang EL, Chang UK, Chao ST, Faruqi S, Ghia AJ, Redmond KJ, Soltys SG, Liu MC. International consensus recommendations for target volume delineation specific to sacral metastases and spinal stereotactic body radiation therapy (SBRT). Radiother Oncol. 2020;145:21–9. https://doi.org/10.1016/j.radonc.2019.11.026. Epub 2019 Dec 23.
4. Bilsky MH, Laufer I, Fourney DR, Groff M, Schmidt MH, Varga PP, Vrionis FD, Yamada Y, Gerszten PC, Kuklo TR. Reliability analysis of the epidural spinal cord compression scale. J Neurosurg Spine. 2010;13(3):324–8. https://doi.org/10.3171/2010.3.SPINE09459. PMID: 20809724.
5. Fisher CG, DiPaola CP, Ryken TC, Bilsky MH, Shaffrey CI, Berven SH, Harrop JS, Fehlings MG, Boriani S, Chou D, Schmidt MH, Polly DW, Biagini R, Burch S, Dekutoski MB, Ganju A, Gerszten PC, Gokaslan ZL, Groff MW, Liebsch NJ, Mendel E, Okuno SH, Patel S, Rhines LD, Rose PS, Sciubba DM, Sundaresan N, Tomita K, Varga PP, Vialle LR, Vrionis FD, Yamada Y, Fourney DR. Reliability analysis of the epidural spinal cord compression scale. J Neurosurg Spine. 2010;13(3):324–8. https://doi.org/10.3171/2010.3.SPINE09459. PMID: 208097248.
6. Expert Panel on Radiation Oncology-Bone Metastases, Lo SS, Lutz ST, Chang EL, Galanopoulos N, Howell DD, Kim EY, Konski AA, Pandit-Taskar ND, Rose PS, Ryu S, Silverman LN, Sloan AE, Van Poznak C. ACR Appropriateness Criteria® spinal bone metastases. J Palliat Med. 2013;16(1):9–19. https://doi.org/10.1089/jpm.2012.0376. Epub 2012 Nov 20. PMID: 23167547.
7. Lutz S, Berk L, Chang E, Chow E, Hahn C, Hoskin P, Howell D, Konski A, Kachnic L, Lo S, Sahgal A, Silverman L, von Gunten C, Mendel E, Vassil A, Bruner DW, Hartsell W, American Society for Radiation Oncology (ASTRO). Palliative radiotherapy for bone metastases: an ASTRO evidence-based guideline. Int J Radiat Oncol Biol Phys. 2011;79(4):965–76. https://doi.org/10.1016/j.ijrobp.2010.11.026. Epub 2011 Jan 27. Review.
8. Redmond KJ, Robertson S, Lo SS, Soltys SG, Ryu S, McNutt T, Chao ST, Yamada Y, Ghia A, Chang EL, Sheehan J, Sahgal A. Consensus contouring guidelines for postoperative stereotactic body radiation therapy for metastatic solid tumor malignancies to the spine. Int J

Radiat Oncol Biol Phys. 2017;97(1):64–74. https://doi.org/10.1016/j.ijrobp.2016.09.014. Epub 2016 Sep 17.
9. Dunne EM, Lo SS, Liu MC, Bergman A, Kosztyla R, Chang EL, Chang UK, Chao ST, Dea N, Faruqi S, Ghia AJ, Redmond KJ, Soltys SG, Sahgal A. Thecal sac contouring as a surrogate for the cauda equina and intracanal spinal nerve roots for spine stereotactic body radiation therapy (SBRT): contour variability and recommendations for safe practice. Int J Radiat Oncol Biol Phys. 2022;112(1):114–20. https://doi.org/10.1016/j.ijrobp.2021.08.023. Epub 2021 Aug 25.PMID: 34454046.
10. Truong MT, Nadgir RN, Hirsch AE, Subramaniam RM, Wang JW, Wu R, Khandekar M, Nawaz AO, Sakai O. Brachial plexus contouring with CT and MR imaging in radiation therapy planning for head and neck cancer. Radiographics. 2010;30(4):1095–103. https://doi.org/10.1148/rg.304095105. PMID: 20631370.
11. Yi SK, Mak W, Yang CC, Liu T, Cui J, Chen AM, Purdy JA, Monjazeb AM, Do L. Development of a standardized method for contouring the lumbosacral plexus: a preliminary dosimetric analysis of this organ at risk among 15 patients treated with intensity-modulated radiotherapy for lower gastrointestinal cancers and the incidence of radiation-induced lumbosacral plexopathy. Int J Radiat Oncol Biol Phys. 2012;84(2):376–82. https://doi.org/10.1016/j.ijrobp.2011.11.074. Epub 2012 Feb 17.PMID: 22342301.
12. Okoye CC, Patel RB, Hasan S, Podder T, Khouri A, Fabien J, Zhang Y, Dobbins D, Sohn JW, Yuan J, Yao M, Machtay M, Sloan AE, Miller J, Lo SS. Comparison of ray tracing and Monte Carlo calculation algorithms for thoracic spine lesions treated with CyberKnife-based stereotactic body radiation therapy. Technol Cancer Res Treat. 2016;15(1):196–202. https://doi.org/10.1177/1533034614568026. Epub 2015 Jan 28.
13. Jabbari S, Gerszten PC, Ruschin M, Larson DA, Lo SS, Sahgal A. Stereotactic body radiotherapy for spinal metastases: practice guidelines, outcomes, and risks. Cancer J. 2016;22(4):280–9. https://doi.org/10.1097/PPO.0000000000000205.
14. Sahgal A, Larson DA, Chang EL. Stereotactic body radiosurgery for spinal metastases: a critical review. Int J Radiat Oncol Biol Phys. 2008;71(3):652–65. https://doi.org/10.1016/j.ijrobp.2008.02.060. Review. Erratum in: Int J Radiat Oncol Biol Phys. 2009 May 1;74(1):323.
15. Sahgal A, Weinberg V, Ma L, Chang E, Chao S, Muacevic A, Gorgulho A, Soltys S, Gerszten PC, Ryu S, Angelov L, Gibbs I, Wong CS, Larson DA. Probabilities of radiation myelopathy specific to stereotactic body radiation therapy to guide safe practice. Int J Radiat Oncol Biol Phys. 2013;85(2):341–7. https://doi.org/10.1016/j.ijrobp.2012.05.007. Epub 2012 Jun 17. PMID: 22713832.
16. Sahgal A, Ma L, Weinberg V, Gibbs IC, Chao S, Chang UK, Werner-Wasik M, Angelov L, Chang EL, Sohn MJ, Soltys SG, Létourneau D, Ryu S, Gerszten PC, Fowler J, Wong CS, Larson DA. Reirradiation human spinal cord tolerance for stereotactic body radiotherapy. Int J Radiat Oncol Biol Phys. 2012;82(1):107–16. https://doi.org/10.1016/j.ijrobp.2010.08.021. Epub 2010 Oct 15. PMID: 20951503.
17. Miller JA, Balagamwala EH, Angelov L, Suh JH, Rini B, Garcia JA, Ahluwalia M, Chao ST. Spine stereotactic radiosurgery with concurrent tyrosine kinase inhibitors for metastatic renal cell carcinoma. J Neurosurg Spine. 2016;25(6):766–74. Epub 2016 Jul 8.
18. Thibault I, Chang EL, Sheehan J, Ahluwalia MS, Guckenberger M, Sohn MJ, Ryu S, Foote M, Lo SS, Muacevic A, Soltys SG, Chao S, Gerszten P, Lis E, Yu E, Bilsky M, Fisher C, Schiff D, Fehlings MG, Ma L, Chang S, Chow E, Parelukar WR, Vogelbaum MA, Sahgal A. Response assessment after stereotactic body radiotherapy for spinal metastasis: a report from the SPIne response assessment in Neuro-Oncology (SPINO) Group. Lancet Oncol. 2015;16(16):e595–603. https://doi.org/10.1016/S1470-2045(15)00166-7. Review. PMID: 26678212.
19. Gerszten PC, Quader M, Novotny J Jr, Flickinger JC. Radiosurgery for benign tumors of the spine: clinical experience and current trends. Technol Cancer Res Treat. 2012;11(2):133–9. PMID: 22335407.

20. Gerszten PC, Burton SA, Ozhasoglu C, McCue KJ, Quinn AE. Radiosurgery for benign intradural spinal tumors. Neurosurgery. 2008;62(4):887–95; discussion 895–6. PMID: 18496194. https://doi.org/10.1227/01.neu.0000318174.28461.fc.
21. Yamada Y, Laufer I, Cox BW, Lovelock DM, Maki RG, Zatcky JM, Boland PJ, Bilsky MH. Preliminary results of high-dose single-fraction radiotherapy for the management of chordomas of the spine and sacrum. Neurosurgery. 2013;73(4):673–80; discussion 680. PMID: 23842548. https://doi.org/10.1227/NEU.0000000000000083.
22. Lockney DT, Shub T, Hopkins B, Lockney NA, Moussazadeh N, Lis E, Yamada Y, Schmitt AM, Higginson DS, Laufer I, Bilsky M. Spinal stereotactic body radiotherapy following intralesional curettage with separation surgery for initial or salvage chordoma treatment. Neurosurg Focus. 2017;42(1):E4. https://doi.org/10.3171/2016.9.FOCUS16373.
23. Wang XS, Rhines LD, Shiu AS, Yang JN, Selek U, Gning I, Liu P, Allen PK, Azeem SS, Brown PD, Sharp HJ, Weksberg DC, Cleeland CS, Chang EL. Stereotactic body radiation therapy for management of spinal metastases in patients without spinal cord compression: a phase 1-2 trial. Lancet Oncol. 2012;13(4):395–402. https://doi.org/10.1016/S1470-2045(11)70384-9. Epub 2012 Jan 27. PMID: 22285199.
24. Garg AK, Shiu AS, Yang J, Wang XS, Allen P, Brown BW, Grossman P, Frija EK, McAleer MF, Azeem S, Brown PD, Rhines LD, Chang EL. Phase 1/2 trial of single-session stereotactic body radiotherapy for previously unirradiated spinal metastases. Cancer. 2012;118(20):5069–77. https://doi.org/10.1002/cncr.27530. Epub 2012 Apr 17. PMID: 22511344.
25. Yamada Y, Bilsky MH, Lovelock DM, Venkatraman ES, Toner S, Johnson J, Zatcky J, Zelefsky MJ, Fuks Z. High-dose, single-fraction image-guided intensity-modulated radiotherapy for metastatic spinal lesions. Int J Radiat Oncol Biol Phys. 2008;71(2):484–90. https://doi.org/10.1016/j.ijrobp.2007.11.046. Epub 2008 Jan 30. PMID: 18234445.
26. Guckenberger M, Mantel F, Gerszten PC, Flickinger JC, Sahgal A, Létourneau D, Grills IS, Jawad M, Fahim DK, Shin JH, Winey B, Sheehan J, Kersh R. Safety and efficacy of stereotactic body radiotherapy as primary treatment for vertebral metastases: a multi-institutional analysis. Radiat Oncol. 2014;9:226. https://doi.org/10.1186/s13014-014-0226-2. PMID: 25319530.
27. Sahgal A, Ames C, Chou D, Ma L, Huang K, Xu W, Chin C, Weinberg V, Chuang C, Weinstein P, Larson DA. Stereotactic body radiotherapy is effective salvage therapy for patients with prior radiation of spinal metastases. Int J Radiat Oncol Biol Phys. 2009;74(3):723–31. https://doi.org/10.1016/j.ijrobp.2008.09.020. Epub 2008 Dec 25. PMID: 19095374.
28. Gerszten PC, Germanwala A, Burton SA, Welch WC, Ozhasoglu C, Vogel WJ. Combination kyphoplasty and spinal radiosurgery: a new treatment paradigm for pathological fractures. J Neurosurg Spine. 2005;3(4):296–301. PMID: 16266071.
29. Laufer I, Iorgulescu JB, Chapman T, Lis E, Shi W, Zhang Z, Cox BW, Yamada Y, Bilsky MH. Local disease control for spinal metastases following "separation surgery" and adjuvant hypofractionated or high-dose single-fraction stereotactic radiosurgery: outcome analysis in 186 patients. J Neurosurg Spine. 2013;18(3):207–14. https://doi.org/10.3171/2012.11.SPINE12111. Epub 2013 Jan 22. PMID: 23339593.
30. Al-Omair A, Masucci L, Masson-Cote L, Campbell M, Atenafu EG, Parent A, Letourneau D, Yu E, Rampersaud R, Massicotte E, Lewis S, Yee A, Thibault I, Fehlings MG, Sahgal A. Surgical resection of epidural disease improves local control following postoperative spine stereotactic body radiotherapy. Neuro Oncol. 2013;15(10):1413–9. https://doi.org/10.1093/neuonc/not101.
31. Bate BG, Khan NR, Kimball BY, Gabrick K, Weaver J. Stereotactic radiosurgery for spinal metastases with or without separation surgery. J Neurosurg Spine. 2015;22(4):409–15. https://doi.org/10.3171/2014.10.SPINE14252. Epub 2015 Jan 30.

Chapter 31
Non-spine Bone Metastases

Simon S. Lo, Arthur S. Yeh, Yolanda Tseng, Stephanie Schaub, Lia M. Halasz, and Edward Y. Kim

31.1 Introduction

Bone metastases are a common occurrence and can cause severe pain and pathologic fracture. Conventional radiotherapy using hypofractionated regimens with or without prophylactic fixation is the standard treatment. In patients with bone oligometastases or progressive bone metastases after prior conventional radiotherapy, stereotactic body radiation therapy (SBRT) may be considered. Data on SBRT for limited non-spine bone metastases are emerging, showing promising results. This chapter will focus on SBRT for non-spine bone metastases.

31.2 Pearls

- Bone metastases can cause severe pain and pathologic fractures. The treatment options for painful uncomplicated bone metastases include analgesics, bisphosphonates, surgical intervention, and radiotherapy.
- Patients with metastases in weight-bearing bone with significant cortical erosion are at higher risk for pathologic fractures and should be evaluated by an orthopedic surgeon for the consideration of prophylactic fixation.
- Medical workup:
  - H&P: Physical exam requires assessment of painful sites and associated soft tissue mass.

S. S. Lo (✉) · Y. Tseng · S. Schaub · L. M. Halasz · E. Y. Kim
Department of Radiation Oncology, University of Washington School of Medicine, Seattle, WA, USA

A. S. Yeh
Carmel High School, Carmel, IN, USA

O. Kaidar-Person, R. Chen (eds.), *Hypofractionated and Stereotactic Radiation Therapy*, https://doi.org/10.1007/978-3-031-47701-0_31

- Imaging workup:
  - Plain X-rays and CT w/w/o contrast for evaluation of soft tissue mass.
  - MRI if CT cannot show the lesion well.
  - Additionally may consider PET/CT for the determination of the extent of disease systemically and in the involved bone.
- Treatment strategies: Radiation therapy alone ± prophylactic fixation [1–3]. Stereotactic body radiation therapy (SBRT) may be considered in limited non-spine bone metastases or re-irradiation. For patients with metastases occurring in weight-bearing long bones, orthopedic consultation is recommended to assess the risk of a pathologic fracture.

31.3 AJCC Staging (AJCC 7th ed., 2010)

- All patients with bone metastases are designated as having M1 and stage IV disease.

31.4 Patient Selection for Hypofractionation Treatment

- Oligometastatic disease in the bone
- Progressive bone metastases after prior conventional radiotherapy to the same site

31.5 Treatment Planning

Simulation instructions	• Supine, immobilized with a body cradle. Arms must be down for CyberKnife to avoid possible collision of robotically mounted LINAC with the arms • Planning CT performed without IV contrast, if possible, 1.0–1.25 mm slices • Fuse diagnostic MRI T1 with and without contrast and/or PET with treatment planning CT • IMRT or VMAT planning for LINAC-based SBRT • CyberKnife SBRT-Multiplan
Target delineation and margins	• GTV-contrast-enhanced tumor on T1 with gadolinium ± PET uptake • CTV = GTV + 5–10 mm • PTV = CTV + 2–3 mm • Recent international consensus guidelines provide the following guidance [4] (Figs. 31.1 and 31.2): An intraosseous CTV margin of 5–10 mm within contiguous bone should be strongly considered An extraosseous CTV margin of 5–10 mm should be strongly considered in cases of associated soft tissue disease and/or significant cortical bone disruption All CTVs should be manually cropped to respect natural anatomic barriers to spread
Image guidance	Daily CBCT or stereoscopic X-rays are recommended
Dosimetric considerations	• Goals—95% of PTV covered by the prescribed IDL (typically 75–85%)

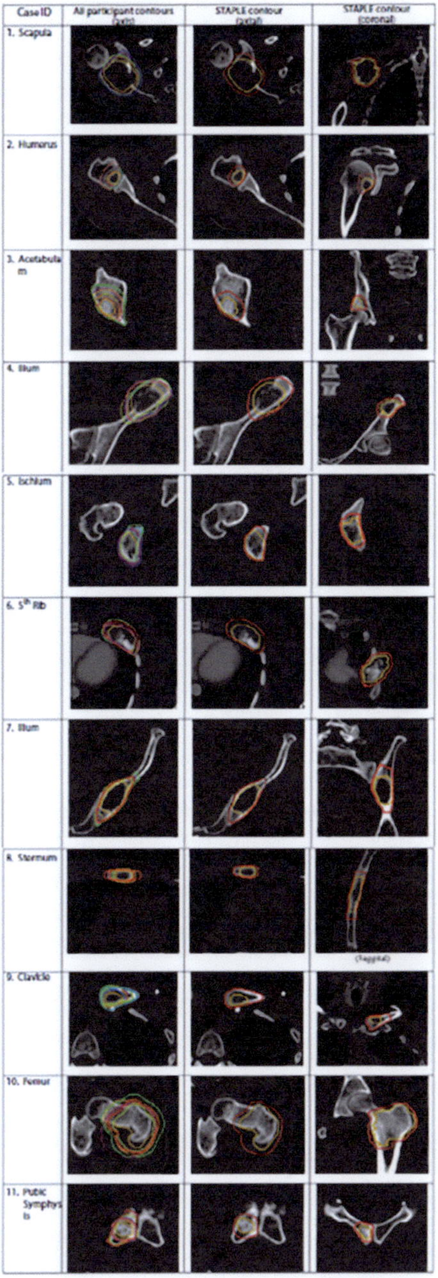

Fig. 31.1 Representative computed tomography images displaying all participant contours and simultaneous truth and performance level estimation contours for each case. Gross tumor volume is represented by the orange contour in each image. Simultaneous truth and performance level estimation (STAPLE): An Algorithm for the Validation of Image Segmentation. (Reprinted from Int J Radiation Oncol Biol Phys, Vol. 112(2), Nguyen et al., International Multi-institutional Patterns of Contouring Practice and Clinical Target Volume Recommendations for Stereotactic Body Radiation Therapy for Non-Spine Bone Metastases., pp. 351–360, Copyright (2022), with permission from Elsevier [4])

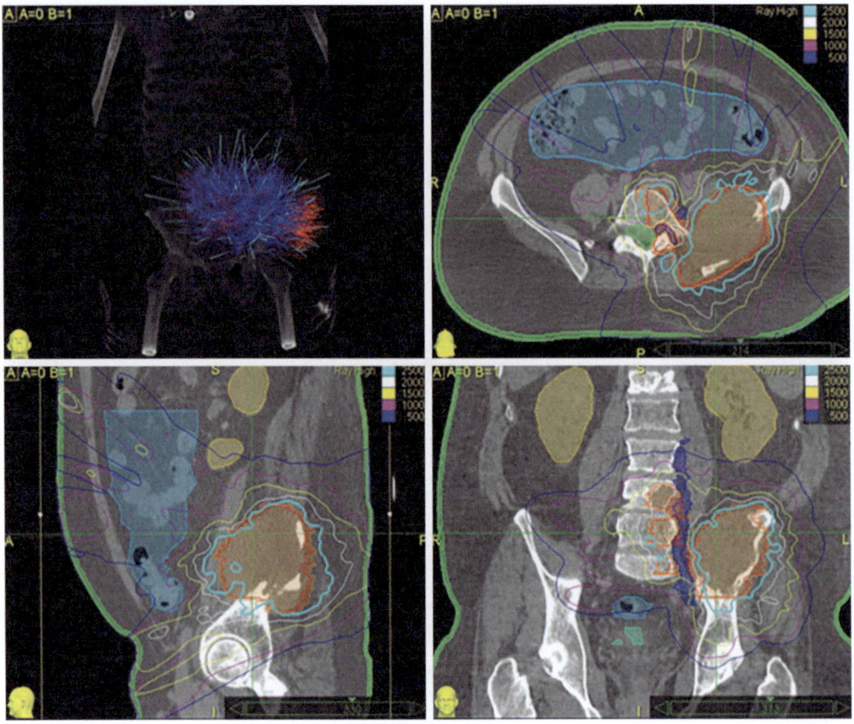

Fig. 31.2 42-year-old male with malignant fibrous histiocytoma, status post external beam radiotherapy to the left ilium (37.5 Gy/15 fractions). He developed progressive disease in the left iliac metastasis. A course of SBRT delivering 25 Gy in 5 fractions was given to the left iliac metastasis. The pain score decreased from 10 to 1 based on Brief Pain Inventory. The small bowel dose was limited to 15 Gy

Treatment planning with linear accelerator

- 4–8 MV photons
- Utilize 7–9 static, coplanar beams (IMRT) or 2–4 rotational arcs (VMAT)
- Beams shaped using multi-leaf collimators

Treatment planning with CyberKnife

- Composed of hundreds of pencil beams

31.6 Common Dose/Fractionation Schemes

Dose/fx	# of fx	Total dose	Notes
15–24 Gy	1	15–24 Gy (Authors' preference: 15–18 Gy) MD Anderson Cancer Center trial [5]: 12 Gy for metastasis >4 cm and 16 Gy for metastasis ≤4 cm	Based on limited literature [6]; normal tissue constraint permitting
6–12 Gy	3	18–36 Gy (Authors' preference: 24–27 Gy)	Based on limited literature [6]; normal tissue constraints permitting
5–10 Gy	5	25–50 Gy (Authors' preference: 25–35 Gy)	Based on limited literature [6]; normal tissue constraints permitting

31.7 Normal Tissue Tolerances

- For non-spine bone metastases, which organs at risk to consider depend on the:
- location of the bone treated.
- The normal tissue constraints of various organs at risk for hypofractionated radiotherapy are covered in other chapters.
- For re-irradiated cases, the prior radiation dose delivered and the prior radiation dose exposure to OARs have to be factored in when setting the dose constraints.

31.8 Patient Management

1. Pre-medicate patients with antiemetic medication if the CTV is close to the stomach (e.g., ondansetron 4 mg PO 30 min before treatment).
2. For patients with severe bone pain, premedicate with narcotic medication.
3. Consider premedication with Medrol Dosepak or dexamethasone 4 mg during and up to 4 days after completion of SBRT (or slower taper) for prophylaxis against pain flare.
4. Toxicity

   (a) Acute:

   - Skin/soft tissue/bone (dermatitis, pain flare)

     – Emollients (Aquaphor, calendula). Remove 4 h prior to RT treatment.
     – Medrol dose pak or dexamethasone 4 mg QD until 4 days after completion of SBRT
     – Pain medication (Fentanyl patch 25–100 mcg q72 h, Oxycodone 5–20 mg q4–6 h).

(b) Late:

- Skin/soft tissue (discoloration, fibrosis)
- Pathologic fracture
- Chronic chest wall pain after SBRT for rib metastases

31.9 Follow-Up

Should be per National/Institutional guidelines. Consider

- Repeat CT or MRI every 3 months; and/ or
- PET-CT every 3 months; and/ or
- Bone scan every 3 months.

31.10 Relevant Literature

Study	Study type/patient population	Prescribed dose	Median follow-up	Outcome
Nguyen 2019 [5]	Randomized phase II trial (intent-to-treat) SBRT: 81 Conventional RT: 79	SBRT: 12 Gy/1 fx if tumor >4 cm and 16 Gy if tumor ≤4 cm Conventional RT: 30 Gy/10 fx	N/A	CR + PR rate SBRT vs. conventional RT 1 month: 44% vs. 30% ($p = 0.18$) 3 months: 38% vs. 21% ($p = 0.05$) Local progression-free survival at 2 years SBRT vs. conventional RT: 100% vs. 75.6% ($p = 0.01$)
Owen 2014 [7]	Retrospective 74 patients with 85 bone metastases	18–24 Gy/1 fx, or 30 Gy/3 fx	7.6 years	1-year LC 91.8% Median OS: 9.5 months Median PFS: 9.7 months Toxicity: 1 grade 3 pain flare
Jhaveri 2012 [8]	Retrospective 18 patients with 24 renal cell carcinoma bone metastases	18–40 Gy/ 3–5 fx	38 weeks	78% symptomatic relief toxicity: No grade 2 or higher

Abbreviations: *CR* complete response, *PR* partial response, *LC* local control

31.11 Summary

SBRT for non-spine bone metastases is an emerging area of practice and preliminary research showed promising results. More research will be helpful to better define the role of SBRT for non-spine bone metastases.

References

1. Lutz S, Berk L, Chang E, Chow E, Hahn C, Hoskin P, Howell D, Konski A, Kachnic L, Lo S, Sahgal A, Silverman L, von Gunten C, Mendel E, Vassil A, Bruner DW, Hartsell W, American Society for Radiation Oncology (ASTRO). Palliative radiotherapy for bone metastases: an ASTRO evidence-based guideline. Int J Radiat Oncol Biol Phys. 2011;79(4):965–76. https://doi.org/10.1016/j.ijrobp.2010.11.026. Epub 2011 Jan 27. Review.
2. Lutz S, Balboni T, Jones J, Lo S, Petit J, Rich SE, Wong R, Hahn C. Palliative radiation therapy for bone metastases: update of an ASTRO evidence-based guideline. Pract Radiat Oncol. 2017;7(1):4–12. https://doi.org/10.1016/j.prro.2016.08.001. Epub 2016 Aug 5.
3. Kim EY, Chapman TR, Ryu S, Chang EL, Galanopoulos N, Jones J, Kubicky CD, Lee CP, Teh BS, Traughber BJ, Van Poznak C, Vassil AD, Weber K, Lo SS. ACR appropriateness criteria(®) non-spine bone metastases. J Palliat Med. 2015;18(1):11–7. https://doi.org/10.1089/jpm.2014.9395.
4. Nguyen TK, Chin L, Sahgal A, Dagan R, Eppinga W, Guckenberger M, Kim JH, Lo SS, Redmond KJ, Siva S, Stish BJ, Chan R, Lawrence L, Lau A, Tseng CL. International multi-institutional patterns of contouring practice and clinical target volume recommendations for stereotactic body radiation therapy for non-spine bone metastases. Int J Radiat Oncol Biol Phys. 2022;112(2):351–60. https://doi.org/10.1016/j.ijrobp.2021.09.004. Epub 2021 Sep 9. PMID: 34509549.
5. Nguyen QN, Chun SG, Chow E, Komaki R, Liao Z, Zacharia R, Szeto BK, Welsh JW, Hahn SM, Fuller CD, Moon BS, Bird JE, Satcher R, Lin PP, Jeter M, O'Reilly MS, Lewis VO. Single-fraction stereotactic vs conventional multifraction radiotherapy for pain relief in patients with predominantly non spine bone metastases: a randomized phase 2 trial. JAMA Oncol. 2019;5(6):872–8. https://doi.org/10.1001/jamaoncol.2019.0192. PMID: 31021390.
6. Bedard G, McDonald R, Poon I, Erler D, Soliman H, Cheung P, Chung H, Chu W, Loblaw A, Chow E, Sahgal A. Stereotactic body radiation therapy for non-spine bone metastases—a review of the literature. Ann Palliat Med. 2016;5(1):58–66. https://doi.org/10.3978/j.issn.2224-5820.2015.07.01. Review.
7. Owen D, Laack NN, Mayo CS, Garces YI, Park SS, Bauer HJ, Nelson K, Miller RW, Brown PD, Olivier KR. Outcomes and toxicities of stereotactic body radiation therapy for non-spine bone oligometastases. Pract Radiat Oncol. 2014;4(2):e143–9. https://doi.org/10.1016/j.prro.2013.05.006. Epub 2013 Jun 29.
8. Jhaveri PM, Teh BS, Paulino AC, Blanco AI, Lo SS, Butler EB, Amato RJ. A dose-response relationship for time to bone pain resolution after stereotactic body radiotherapy (SBRT) for renal cell carcinoma (RCC) bony metastases. Acta Oncol. 2012;51(5):584–8. https://doi.org/10.3109/0284186X.2011.652741. Epub 2012 Jan 17.

Part X
Gynecologic Malignancies

Chapter 32
Uterine Cervix Cancer

Brittaney-Belle E. Gordon, Mahesh Varia, and Ashley A. Weiner

32.1 Introduction

Hypofractionation has a select and important role in the radiotherapeutic management of gynecological cancers, primarily in the use of high-dose-rate (HDR) brachytherapy. Brachytherapy (in combination with external beam radiotherapy) is an integral component in the curative management of advanced cervical cancer. External beam radiation techniques (intensity-modulated radiotherapy or stereotactic body radiotherapy) alone are associated with poorer survival rates when utilized instead of brachytherapy [1, 2]. Intracavitary brachytherapy is the most common brachytherapy technique used for cervical cancer treatment, although interstitial or hybrid intracavitary/interstitial brachytherapy is typically used in more loco-regionally advanced cases. This chapter details the best practices for the use of hypofractionated radiotherapy, in particular brachytherapy, in cervical cancer treatment.

B.-B. E. Gordon
University of Pittsburgh Medical Center, Pittsburgh, PA, USA

Hillman Comprehensive Cancer Center, Pittsburgh, PA, USA

M. Varia · A. A. Weiner (✉)
University of North Carolina, School of Medicine, Chapel Hill, NC, USA

Department of Radiation Oncology, University of North Carolina, School of Medicine, Chapel Hill, NC, USA
e-mail: ashley_weiner@med.unc.edu

O. Kaidar-Person, R. Chen (eds.), *Hypofractionated and Stereotactic Radiation Therapy*, https://doi.org/10.1007/978-3-031-47701-0_32

32.2 Pearls

- In 2021, it is estimated that 14,480 women were diagnosed with cervical cancer in the United States, while 4290 women died from the disease [1].
- In the past 40 years, the incidence and mortality from cervical cancer have decreased significantly in the United States due to screening programs and more recently, vaccination against human papillomavirus (HPV).
- Cervical cancer remains the third most common gynecologic malignancy and the fourth leading cause of cancer-related death in women worldwide. Notably, 85% of cervical cancer diagnoses occur in developing countries and are commonly diagnosed in advanced stages.
- In the United States, the mean age of diagnosis is 48 years; however, cervical cancer has a bimodal disease distribution with peaks at ages 35–39 and 60–64 years.
- HPV infection is the greatest risk factor (mostly types 16 and 18) and is detected in more than 95% of cervical cancers.
- Other risk factors include young age at first intercourse, multiple sexual partners (>4), high-risk sexual partners, history of other STDs (e.g., chlamydia trachomatis, genital herpes), high parity, smoking, history of precancerous lesions or cancer, and prenatal DES exposure (clear cell carcinoma) and immunosuppression (immunodeficiency syndrome, chronic steroid usage, organ transplantation). Cervical cancer is an AIDS-defining malignancy in patients with HIV.
- Currently, there are no known genetic abnormalities/germline mutations that are associated with a higher risk for cervical cancer.
- The most common presenting symptoms are irregular vaginal bleeding/discharge or post-coital bleeding. Pelvic pain, back pain, bowel/bladder symptoms, and lower extremity lymphedema are symptoms of advanced disease.
- The two most common histologic types are squamous cell carcinoma (69%) and adenocarcinoma (25%). Other uncommon histologic types (6%) include clear cell carcinoma, small cell carcinoma (neuroendocrine), melanoma, or lymphoma.
- Over the past three decades, the incidence of adenocarcinoma has increased secondary to increased exposure to estrogen. Some cervical adenocarcinomas are HPV-related, whereas others are neither estrogen-driven nor HPV associated (such as gastric-type cervical adenocarcinoma).

- **Local anatomy and patterns of spread:**
  - The uterine cervix is located at the junction between the lower uterus and apical vagina. It consists of the endocervix and ectocervix, which are lined by stratified squamous and glandular epithelium, respectively. HPV infection causes malignant transformation at the transition zone between the two types of epithelia.
  - Cervical cancer progresses by direct contiguous spread to adjacent structures; most frequently to the parametria, upper vagina, or uterine corpus. More advanced disease may extend to the pelvic sidewall or lower vagina, or invade the peritoneal cavity, bladder, and/or rectum.

- There is an increasing frequency of lymph node involvement with advancing stage: <5% of patients with stage IA disease will have pelvic LN involvement. This increased to 15% of Stage IB patients, 30% of Stage II patients, 50% of Stage III patients, and 60% for Stage IV. Roughly, one-third of the patients with pelvic LN involvement will also have involved para-aortic LN.
- In early-stage patients, the depth of invasion below the basement membrane is also related to the risk of LN involvement: for <3 mm invasion, there is <1% risk of pelvic LN involvement. With invasion ≥3 mm or LVI (Stage IA2), the risk of LN spread increases to 2–8%.
- Lymphatic dissemination typically occurs in a predictable manner with initial pelvic LN involvement followed by dissemination to the para-aortic and finally left supraclavicular lymph nodes.
- Hematogenous dissemination is less common, though it may occur in the bone, liver, and/or lung.

- **Medical workup:**
  - H&P includes examination of vagina, vulva, and anal regions to exclude other HPV-associated malignancies. A full gynecologic examination (including speculum, bimanual, and rectovaginal examination) is essential for staging and for choosing the appropriate brachytherapy applicator for a patient's anatomy.
  - Laboratory tests include: CBC, LFTs, and BUN/creatinine (renal function important for cisplatin); urine pregnancy test is needed in women of reproductive age. Consider HIV testing. CBC is important to assess for anemia as many cervical cancer patients have several months' history of vaginal bleeding, and correction of anemia is important for treatment with surgery, chemotherapy, and optimizing radiation treatment outcomes.
  - Fertility consultation should be considered for patients of childbearing age.
  - Smoking cessation and counseling intervention.
- **Imaging workup:**
  - Optional for patients with ≤ stage IB1 and recommended for more advanced disease.
  - Pelvic MRI with contrast is a sensitive method for the detection of parametrial involvement, estimation of tumor size, and delineating uterine and cervical anatomy.
  - CT and ultrasound can be used if MRI is not available.
  - PET-CT is recommended for the detection of LN metastasis. CT of chest, abdomen, and pelvis with IV contrast can be used if PET-CT is unavailable.
  - Examination under anesthesia including cystoscopy/proctoscopy can be performed if bladder or rectum involvement is suspected.
  - If hydronephrosis is noted on imaging studies, stenting is recommended prior to initiation of therapy.
- Treatment strategies depend on the stage of disease and desire for fertility/ovarian hormonal function preservation.

- Surgery is the preferred choice for patients with early-stage disease.

  Cold-knife cone with negative margins.
  Radical trachelectomy with pelvic LN dissection or sentinel lymph node (SLN) biopsy.
  Modified radical hysterectomy with pelvic LN dissection.

- Chemoradiotherapy is the preferred treatment for patients with more advanced-stage disease. This treatment is composed of external beam radiotherapy to the pelvis ± para-aortics with weekly radiosensitizing cisplatin, plus brachytherapy.

  Brachytherapy is an integral part of primary radiation treatment and has been shown to increase local control and overall survival in comparison with external beam radiotherapy alone [2, 3].
  Brachytherapy should be incorporated into treatment as early as the tumor shrinks to a size that allows adequate applicator placement, to allow completion of all radiation treatments within 8 weeks. Prolonged treatment duration leads to a decrease in local control and survival of approximately 1% per day [4].

- Patients with distant metastatic disease are treated with combinations of chemotherapy and radiation therapy based on the extent of the disease and symptoms.

32.3 International Federation of Gynecology and Obstetrics Staging of Cancer of the Cervix (2018) [5]

FIGO staging	Definition
I	The carcinoma is strictly confined to the cervix uteri (extension to corpus should be disregarded)
IA	Invasive carcinoma that can be diagnosed only by microscopy, with maximum depth of invasion <5.0 mm[a]
IA1	Measured stromal invasion <3.0 mm in depth
IA2	Measured stromal invasion ≥3.0 mm and <5.0 mm in depth
IB	Invasive carcinoma with measured deepest invasion ≥5 mm (greater than IA); lesion limited to the cervix uteri[b]
IB1	Invasive carcinoma ≥5 mm depth of stromal invasion and <2 cm in greatest dimension
IB2	Invasive carcinoma ≥2 cm and <4 cm in greatest dimension
IB3	Invasive carcinoma ≥4 cm in greatest dimension
II	The carcinoma invades beyond the uterus but has not extended onto the lower third of the vagina or the pelvic wall

FIGO staging	Definition
IIA	Involvement limited to the upper two-thirds of the vagina without parametrial invasion
IIA1	Invasive carcinoma <4 cm in greatest dimension
IIA2	Invasive carcinoma ≥4 cm in greatest dimension
IIB	With parametrial invasion but not up to the pelvic wall
III	The carcinoma involves the lower third of the vagina and/or extends to the pelvic wall and/or causes hydronephrosis or non-functioning kidney and/or involves pelvic and/or para-aortic lymph nodes[c]
IIIA	Carcinoma involves the lower third of the vagina, with no extension to the pelvic wall
IIIB	Extension to the pelvic wall and/or causes hydronephrosis or non-functioning kidney (unless known to be due to another cause)
IIIC	Involvement of the pelvic and/or para-aortic lymph nodes, irrespective of tumor size and extent (with *r* and *p* notations)[c]
IIIC1	Pelvic lymph node metastasis only
IIIC2	Para-aortic lymph node metastasis
IV	The carcinoma has extended beyond the true pelvis or has involved (biopsy-proven) the mucosa of the bladder or rectum. A bullous edema, as such, does not permit a case to be allotted to Stage IV
IVA	Spread of the growth to adjacent organs
IVB	Spread to distant organs

[a] Imaging and pathology can be used, when available, to supplement clinical findings with respect to tumor size and extent, in all stages

[b] The involvement of vascular/lymphatic spaces does not change the staging. The lateral extent of the lesion is no longer considered

[c] Adding notation of *r* (radiographic imaging) and *p* (pathology) to indicate the findings that are used to allocate the case to stage IIIC. For example, if imaging indicates pelvic lymph node metastasis, the stage allocation would be stage IIIC1*r* and, if confirmed by pathological findings, it would be Stage IIIc1*p*. The type of imaging modality or pathology technique used should always be documented. When in doubt, the lower staging should be assigned

32.4 Patient Selection for Hypofractionated Radiation

- Brachytherapy alone may be considered as primary treatment for patients with very early-stage disease (IA) who are not candidates for surgical therapy [6, 7].
- For patients undergoing definitive radiation, brachytherapy is indicated in conjunction with EBRT for locally advanced disease (Stages IB2–IVA).
- Patients with Stage IB1/IB2 disease who are not suitable for brachytherapy should be evaluated for interval hysterectomy after EBRT.
- HDR brachytherapy is hypofractionated (3–6 high-dose fractions). Pulsed-dose rate (PDR) and low-dose rate (LDR) brachytherapy are alternative brachytherapy regimens and are beyond the scope of this chapter.

32.5 Treatment Planning Considerations

32.5.1 External Beam Radiotherapy with Weekly Cisplatin

In patients with locally advanced cervical cancer (by tumor size, tumor extent out of the cervix, or nodal involvement), curative intent treatment includes external beam radiotherapy (EBRT), weekly radiosensitizing cisplatin, and brachytherapy using an intracavitary and/or an interstitial approach. The EBRT portion may be delivered with either 3D conformal radiotherapy (3D-CRT) or intensity-modulated radiotherapy (IMRT), and treatment volumes include the gross disease and areas at risk of microscopic disease including the cervix, uterus, upper vagina, parametria, uterosacral ligament, pelvic nodal basins (external iliac, internal iliac, obturator, and presacral), and potentially the common iliac, para-aortic, or inguinal nodal regions depending on disease extent.

EBRT is typically conventionally fractionated (45 Gy in 25 fractions of 1.8 Gy). A parametrial boost of 5–10 Gy can be considered. When IMRT is used, involved lymph nodes may be treated with a hypofractionated simultaneous integrated boost (SIB) at 2.1–2.2 Gy per fraction to deliver a conformal dose to lymph nodes that would not receive a full dose from a brachytherapy implant. This ensures the completion of radiotherapy in a shorter time frame than a sequential boost, though doses to adjacent normal tissues need to be carefully considered.

HDR brachytherapy (hypofractionated)

Timing	Start brachytherapy after 10–20 Gy EBRT or as soon as there is tumor response to be amenable for implantation. Alternatively, brachytherapy may begin following the completion of EBRT. Intracavitary brachytherapy is typically performed once weekly during EBRT and twice a week when EBRT is completed. Alternatively, multiple fractions may be delivered with a single implant during a hospitalization In patients with absolute neutrophil counts less than 500 mm^3, brachytherapy should be held until count recovery [8]
Analgesia	Analgesia options for cervical cancer brachytherapy include general, spinal, intravenous sedation and/or oral pain medication. Our practice is to use titrated doses of fentanyl, starting with 50 μg IV, and lorazepam with 1 mg IV, 20–30 min prior to the start of the procedure
Position	Dorsal lithotomy position
Pelvic exam	Examination under anesthesia—a bimanual examination to document any residual nodularity, the cervix size, and the size of the vaginal fornices (i.e., disease extension/response to treatment). The uterus is sounded to aid in the selection of the appropriate tandem applicator. Insertion of radiopaque markers in the cervix aids localization of the cervix on imaging.

Preparation and procedure	• A Foley catheter is inserted into the bladder, and the balloon is inflated with dilute contrast • The ABS/GEC-ESTRO recommendations can be used for guidance in choosing the appropriate applicator according to the patient's anatomy and target geometry, but familiarity and experience with the applicator are essential for providing appropriate treatment [7, 9]. Applicator options include tandem and ovoids, tandem and ring, tandem and cylinder, and tandem and ovoid or ring with guides for interstitial needles. Interstitial catheters can be used to allow full coverage in cases such as poorly fitting intracavitary applicators, bulky residual tumor, parametrial involvement, and lower vaginal involvement • After the selection of appropriate applicators (including the angle of the intrauterine tandem and the size of the ring or ovoids), the applicators are placed. A tenaculum may be placed on the upper lip of the cervix to provide countertraction for the placement of the intrauterine tandem. Supplemental interstitial catheters may be placed to improve dosimetry by increasing the dose to the high-risk clinical target volume (HR-CTV) and reducing the dose to adjacent organs at risk • Radio-opaque vaginal packing or vaginal packing balloons are used to displace the bladder base anteriorly and the anterior rectal wall posteriorly away from the intracavitary applicator. Packing also serves to prevent the displacement of the tandem from the uterus and to secure the positioning of the entire applicator • A Smit sleeve can be useful for anatomically difficult implants • Imaging (CT, MRI) is done for each implant immediately following the placement of the applicator and is essential for treatment planning of each procedure. 3D imaging allows for accurate contouring of the tumor, cervix, uterus, and OAR. While the OARs can be readily visualized on CT, MRI is superior for delineating the tumor for image-guided brachytherapy, particularly in the setting of parametrial involvement [8]
Treatment planning	**Image-guided brachytherapy:** • Typically starts with standard applicator loading, and then source dwell times can be optimized based on 3D images (CT or MRI) of the implant and anatomy • We recommend using the GEC-ESTRO guidelines for target delineation/definition (Fig. 32.1) [8, 9] with prescription to the high-risk CTV (HR-CTV) • OARs that should be contoured include the bladder, rectum, and sigmoid, with consideration of vaginal points and ureters **2D (X-ray) planning:** • Prescribe to point A: 2 cm superior to external cervical os and 2 cm lateral to central canal/tandem • Point B: 5 cm lateral from a point 2 cm superior to the cervical os along the patient's midline (represents the location of parametrial/obturator nodes) • Bladder point: the posterior surface of Foley balloon on lateral X-ray and center of the balloon on AP film • Rectal point: 5 mm posterior to the posterior vaginal wall between ovoids • Vaginal point: the mid-ovoid on lateral X-ray film and the lateral edge of ovoid on AP film

Documentation	Documentation of brachytherapy is essential and should include the type of isotope and source; description of the target (including size and shape), target dose, dose per fraction, and the fractionation plan; the applicator type and size features and the treatment plan documentation (dose distributions to the target and OAR). Even if 3D planning is used, the dose for point A (2 cm superior to the cervical os and 2 cm lateral to the intrauterine tandem) should be recorded per ICRU system [8]

32.5.2 *Modified ABS Checklist for Brachytherapy [7, 8]*

Procedure checklist for brachytherapy
☐ Consents present in the chart
☐ IV access obtained
☐ "Timeout" to identify the patient's treatment prescription and session number
☐ Anesthesia administered
☐ Examination under anesthesia
☐ Document disease extension in drawing
☐ Dilation of cervical os; use ultrasound if insertion is difficult
☐ Smit sleeve placement if preferred
☐ Applicator placement
☐ Caution that the applicator does not slip
☐ Packing
☐ Imaging (CT, MRI, plain radiographs)
☐ Prescription
☐ Treatment planning
☐ Documentation of OAR (sigmoid, rectum, bladder) doses in the chart
☐ QA checks
☐ Timeout to confirm treatment prescription and session number prior to treatment delivery
☐ Treatment delivery
☐ Dictation of treatment administered
☐ Applicator removed
☐ Post-treatment care
☐ Follow-up scheduled

32.6 Commonly Used Dose/Fractionation Schemes

32.6.1 *Definitive Treatment*

- **EBRT + intracavitary brachytherapy:** EBRT to pelvis (using either a four-field technique or IMRT). Daily dose of 1.8–2 Gy × 25–28 fractions to a total of 45–50.4 Gy. A split-pelvis field with a midline block can be considered (with higher dose delivered by brachytherapy). If there is common iliac or para-aortic lymph node involvement, an extended treatment field is utilized with IMRT. Pelvic sidewall boost to a total dose of 50–54 Gy can be considered for Stage IIB and higher. Gross nodal disease can be boosted to a total dose of 60–70 Gy [6, 7].

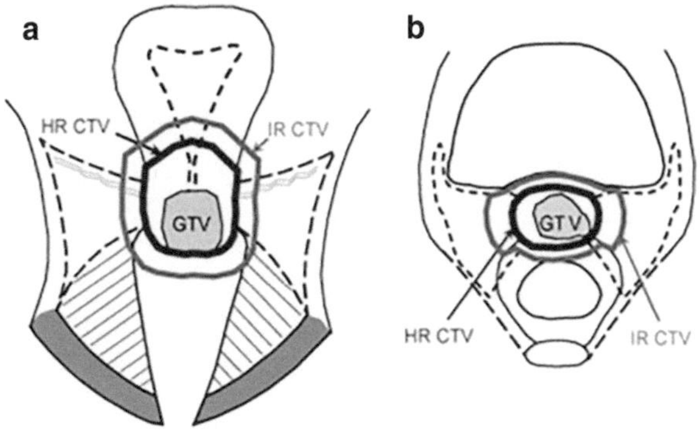

Fig. 32.1 GEC-ESTRO guidelines for 3D-target delineation for cervix cancer. Coronal view (**a**) and transverse view (**b**) of limited disease with partial remission after EBRT. A low-risk clinical target volume (LR-CTV) corresponds to EBRT targets, comprising all potentially involved tissues (not shown in this figure). A high-risk CTV (HR-CTV) includes the whole cervix and presumed residual disease at the time of brachytherapy (determined by visualization, palpation, and MRI). An intermediate-risk CTV (IR-CTV) encompassing the HR-CTV with directional margins (usually 5–15 mm), and at least the initial volume at diagnosis [10, 11]

Nodal boost may be sequential (occurring after completion of pelvic EBRT), or a simultaneous integrated boost (SIB). An SIB allows a shorter time to completion of EBRT by delivering a higher (2.1–2.2 Gy/day), moderately hypofractionated dose to involved nodes during each day of pelvic EBRT. IMRT allows this conformal dose to be delivered safely to adjacent organs at risk.

- Concurrent chemotherapy with weekly cisplatin is recommended for Stages IB2–IVA in patients with adequate renal function. The ABS recommends that chemotherapy be administered the day that EBRT is delivered, and not on a day of a brachytherapy treatment [6, 7].
  - Dose reporting for cervical brachytherapy is typically converted to a biologically equivalent dose in 2-Gy fractions (EQD2). This aids in the conversion between different fractionation regimens and in summing EBRT and brachytherapy doses.
  - Classic tandem and ovoid geometry is based on the dose to point A, and this should be recorded even when 3D planning is used.
  - The DVH parameter typically used to describe target coverage is the dose received by at least 90% of the target volume (HR-CTV D90 using GEC-ESTRO definition).
  - In cases of complete response or a partial response (<4 cm residual disease) to EBRT, the target D90 should be greater than 80 Gy (EQD2).
  - In cases of residual tumors >4 cm at the time of brachytherapy, target D90 of at least 85–90 Gy EQD2 is recommended. Interstitial needle application may be needed to provide optimal coverage.

Common intracavitary brachytherapy-HDR doses (combined with EBRT, 1.8 Gy × 25 fx) [7, 8]

Fractionation to point A	Total EQD2(Gy) to the tumor inclusive of EBRT (point A with $\alpha/\beta = 10$ Gy)	Comments
5.5 Gy × 5	79.8	Complete response or <4 cm of residual disease after chemoradiation
5 Gy × 6	81.8	
7 Gy × 4	83.9	
6 Gy × 5	84.3	Patients with tumors >4 cm after EBRT

32.6.2 Postoperative Treatment

- Postoperative pelvic radiation with EBRT to a total dose of 45–50.4 Gy should be considered in high-risk cases [12]. Vaginal brachytherapy (as a vaginal cuff boost) is not routinely given but should be considered in patients with a less than radical hysterectomy, close or positive margins, large or deeply invasive tumors, parametrial or vaginal involvement, or extensive LVI. Vaginal brachytherapy dosing ranges from 5 Gy × 5 fractions to 7 Gy × 3 fractions (total dose to vaginal mucosa 45–80 Gy when combined with EBRT) [10].

32.6.3 Palliative Treatment

- In the setting of metastatic disease, a single fraction (8–10 Gy) of external beam radiotherapy can be delivered to the pelvis using AP-PA fields or a four-field arrangement for palliation of pelvic pain or bleeding [11–13].

32.7 Normal Tissue Tolerance

OAR	Radiographic (ICRU point)	3D imaging (D2 cc)	Comments
Bladder	5× < 3.7 Gy	<90 Gy[a]	
Rectum	5× < 3.7 Gy	<70–75 Gy[a]	Dose–volume effect relationship for late rectal morbidity was published by the EMBRACE collaborative group [14, 15] Rectal D2cc > 75 Gy was associated with grade 2–4 rectal toxicity (fistula) in 3 years A D2cc ≤ 65 Gy was associated with less frequent and severe rectal morbidity [14, 15]
Sigmoid		<70–75 Gy[a]	

OAR	Radiographic (ICRU point)	3D imaging (D2 cc)	Comments
Ureters		<70 Gy	
Uterus		<100 Gy	
Ovaries			Sterilization after 2–3 Gy; ovarian failure with 5–10 Gy. Patients who are over 35 years or receive chemotherapy are at greater risk for ovarian failure
Vagina		<50–60 Gy	Doses above 50–60 Gy can cause fibrosis and stenosis High doses (>100 Gy) may cause fistulization with adjacent organs. High doses to the vaginal mucosa are often inevitable; the dose to the vagina should be limited according to the extent of the disease. Upper vaginal mucosa limit usually <120 Gy, midvaginal mucosa <80–90 Gy, and lower vaginal mucosa <60–70 Gy [10] The EMBRACE study reported that a higher recto-vaginal reference point dose, EBRT dose of more than 45 Gy in 25 fx, and tumor extension in the vagina were risk factors for vaginal stenosis [14, 15]. Based on the model curve, the risk for vaginal stenosis was 20% at 65 Gy, 27% at 75 Gy, and 34% at 85 Gy (recto-vaginal reference point dose). Therefore, the authors recommended keeping the EBRT dose <45 Gy in 25 fx and planning aim of <65 Gy EQD2 (EBRT + brachytherapy dose) to the recto-vaginal reference point [15, 16]

The cumulative dose delivered by EBRT and brachytherapy needs to be integrated during treatment planning to avoid significant overexposure to midline structures, particularly the bladder and rectum

[a] Max point dose defined as <0.035 cc

32.8 Patient Management Considerations

32.8.1 Acute Toxicity

- Acute urinary symptoms such as urgency and frequency occur in more than 40% of the patients and are usually minor [8]. Urinary tract infection should be excluded and if present treated according to culture sensitivity.
- Mild or occasional diarrhea can be managed with loperamide. For persistent and/or severe diarrhea, evaluate patients for *Clostridium difficile* infection prior to initiation of loperamide. Patients should undergo dietary consultation. Loperamide dosing: initial 4 mg orally once followed by 2 mg orally after each loose stool, not exceeding 16 mg per 24 h. Loperamide maintenance: daily dosage between 4 and 8 mg.

- At the time of intracavitary applicator placement, uterine perforation can occur. It typically occurs in the posterior cervix but it may also occur at the fundus. If a uterine perforation is suspected, the applicator should be removed immediately without initiating treatment, and the applicator should be reinserted to obtain proper positioning. The patient should be started on broad-spectrum antibiotics [6]. An unrecognized uterine perforation with subsequent radiation treatment delivery with the tandem outside the uterus and close to or in the bowel or bladder may result in significant toxicity [6].
- In patients with absolute neutrophil counts less than 500 mm^3, brachytherapy should be held until count recovery [8].

32.8.2 Late Toxicity

- Common late effects include vaginal stenosis (minimized by vaginal dilator use and resumption of sexual activity) and vaginal dryness (treat with topical estrogen).
  - A rate of 3.6% grade $\geq$ 3 late vaginal morbidity (at 2 years) in patients who were treated by IGRT plus brachytherapy was reported by the EMBRACE study. The majority of the patients experienced mild and moderate vaginal symptoms (grade $\geq$ 1, 89%; grade $\geq$ 2, 29%), of which the majority developed within 6 months. The most frequent vaginal toxicity observed was vaginal stenosis, followed by vaginal dryness [15].
- Rare complications: urethral stricture (<3%), vesico-vaginal or recto-vaginal fistula (<2.5%), and femoral head fracture (risk after EBRT to pelvis).
- The risk of developing major urinary toxicity is greatest in the first 3 years following radiation (0.7% per year) [8, 17].

32.9 Follow-Up

- H&P includes bimanual, pelvic, and rectal examination every 3 months for the first 2 years, every 6 months for years 3–5, and then annually.
- At the authors' institution, we recommend performing cervical and/or vaginal cytology annually for detection of genital tract malignancies. However, the value may be limited due to post-radiation changes. Abnormal high-grade cytology should be followed by colposcopy and biopsy for histologic confirmation.
- Post-treatment imaging with PET-CT is routinely performed at 3 months following completion of definitive chemoradiotherapy. If there is a metabolic complete response, further imaging is typically performed only with abnormal pelvic examinations or symptoms.
- Laboratory assessment: CBC, BUN, and creatinine as indicated based on baseline function, symptom, or examination findings suspicious for recurrence.

32.10 Relevant Literature

- A Cochrane collaboration review of HDR versus LDR for locally advanced uterine cervix cancer did not find significant differences between HDR and LDR intracavitary brachytherapy when considering overall survival, disease-free survival, recurrence-free survival and local control rate, recurrence, metastasis, and treatment-related complications [18]. The authors recommend the use of HDR intracavitary brachytherapy for all clinical stages of cervix cancer due to the potential advantages of HDR intracavitary brachytherapy: outpatient treatment, patient convenience, accuracy of source and applicator positioning, and individualized treatment planning.
- Brachytherapy is an integral component of therapy and should be a component of all definitive treatments. Cervical SBRT (or other EBRT techniques) boost in lieu of brachytherapy is not standard of care due to suboptimal dosimetry and worse overall survival in comparison with brachytherapy. Most earlier randomized trials for advanced cervical cancer (i.e., RTOG 9001 [19] and GOG 120 [20]) utilized LDR brachytherapy, which is beyond the scope of this chapter.

Select retrospective and prospective studies of hypofractionation for gynecological malignancies

Study	Patients	Treatments	Median follow-up	Outcome
HDR brachytherapy plus EBRT as definitive treatment				
Potter 2021 [21]	1416	EBRT 45–50 Gy plus MRI-guided brachytherapy HR-CTV D90 85–94 Gy total (combined with EBRT) 42% pulsed dose rate brachytherapy 57% HDR brachytherapy	51 months	• 5-year LC 92% • 5-year pelvic control 87% • 5-year DFS 68% • 5-year OS 74% • 5-year G3–5 toxicity GU 6.8% GI 8.5% Vaginal 5.7% Fistula 3.2%
*SBRT plus EBRT as definitive treatment (*Note: the authors do not recommend SBRT in lieu of brachytherapy)*				
Albuquerque 2019 [22] Phase 2	15	EBRT 45 Gy (10 Gy simultaneous integrated boost to involved LN), plus SBRT boost 7 Gy × 4 fx	19 months	• 2-year LC 70.1% • 2-year PFS 46.7% • 2-year OS 53.3% • grade >3 toxicity, 26.7%

Study	Patients	Treatments	Median follow-up	Outcome
Hsieh 2013 [23] Retrospective	9	EBRT 50.4 Gy, plus SBRT boost 15–27 Gy in 5–9 fx	36 months	• LC 78% • Grade 3 (18%): diarrhea and thrombocytopenia
Jorcano 2010 [24] Retrospective	9 cervix 17 uterine	EBRT 45–50.4 Gy, plus SBRT boost 7 Gy × 2 fx	47 months	• 3-year OS 96% • 3-year LC 96% • grade > 2 toxicity GU 4% GI 12% Sexual function disturbances 29.4%
SBRT for recurrence				
Kunos 2012 [25] Phase 2	Total 50 • 9 cervix • 18 uterine • 25 ovary • 2 vulva	SBRT sites: PALN (38%), pelvis (28%) 8 Gy × 3 fx	15 months	• LC 100% • grade 3–4 toxicity (6%): diarrhea, fistula
Dewas 2011 [26] Retrospective	Total 16 • 4 cervix • 1 uterine • 11 non-gyn cancers	SBRT sites: Pelvic side wall 6 Gy × 6 fx	10.6 months	• 1-year LC 51% • median PFS 8.3 months • No grade 3 toxicity
Choi 2009 [27] Retrospective	Total 28 • 26 cervix • 2 uterine	SBRT sites: PALN 11–15 Gy × 3 fx (24 pts) EBRT + SBRT boost (4 pts) Chemotherapy sequencing varied	Not reported	• 4-year OS 50% • 4-year LC 68% • 4-year PFS 45% • grade 3–4 toxicity 21%
Mesko 2017 [28] Retrospective	Total 28 (47 targets) • 2 cervix • 8 uterine • 15 ovary • 2 vagina • 1 uterine carcinosarcoma	SBRT sites: 17% liver, 21% lung, 17% PALN, 26% other LNs, 19% pelvic soft tissue Median 8 Gy (range, 5–18) × 5 fx (range, 1–10)	12.8 months	• OS 86% • median PFS 10.8 months • No failures occurred in lung or nodal targets • grade 3 toxicity 3% (GU toxicity in a previously irradiated site)

Study	Patients	Treatments	Median follow-up	Outcome
SBRT for oligometastatic cancer				
Hasan 2016 [29] Retrospective	Total 30 • 11 cervix • 12 endometrial • 3 ovarian • 2 uterine-serous • 2 carcinosarcoma	Median 27.5 Gy (range, 15–40) in 5 fx (range, 3–5) SBRT sites: pelvic and PALN	60 months	• 5-year OS 42% • 5-year LC 67% • 3-year DFS 52% • median DFS 47 months • median OS 43.3 months • No grade 3–4 toxicity
Smile 2021 [30] Retrospective	Total 34 • 7 cervix • 12 ovarian • 11 uterine • 2 fallopian tube • 3 primary peritoneal	Median 24 Gy (range 18–54 Gy) in 3 fx (range 3–6) SBRT sites: pelvic and PALN	12 months	• 1-year LC 92.5% • 2-year LC 92.5% • 1-year systemic control 60.2% • 1-year OS 85.0% • 2-year OS 70.2% • No grade 3–4 toxicity
HDR for central pelvic re-irradiation				
Badakh 2009 [31] Retrospective	22	HDR interstitial 4–6 Gy × 6–10 fx, BID	9.2 months	• median OS 9.2 months • grade 4 toxicity 18%: fistulas, soft tissue
Zolciak-Siwinska 2014 [32] Retrospective	20	HDR interstitial, cylinder, or IORT With/without EBRT and/or Hyperthermia	31 months	• 3-year OS 68% • 3-year LC 45% • 3-year DFS 42% • Acute toxicity: no grade > 3 toxicity • Late toxicity: grade 3 toxicity GU (10%), GI (5%); grade 4 obliteration of the vagina (40%)
Mabuchi 2014 [33] Retrospective	52	HDR interstitial 6 Gy × 7 fx; BID	55.6 months	• 5-year OS 52.6% • Late grade 3–4 toxicity 25%: fistulas, bowel obstruction, and ulceration
Palliation				
Kim 2013 [34] Retrospective	17	EBRT 5 Gy × 4–5 fx daily	12.2 months	• median OS 7.8 months • Vaginal bleeding control 93.8% • Pelvic pain control 66.7% • Acute toxicity: grade 3 diarrhea (5.9%)

Study	Patients	Treatments	Median follow-up	Outcome
Grigsby 2002 [35] Retrospective	15	Cervical ring HDR 5 Gy × 2 fx prescribed to surface Administered one week apart for emergent bleed prior to definitive EBRT and intracavitary brachytherapy	32 months	• Vaginal bleeding control 93% • Mean rectal dose 1.75 Gy, mean bladder dose 1.65 Gy, mean point A dose 0.85 • No acute toxicity • All patients went on to complete definitive therapy (chemotherapy with EBRT and brachytherapy)
Halle 1986 [11] Retrospective	42	EBRT 10 Gy × 1–2 fx Administered monthly	12.8 months	• Vaginal bleeding control 90% • Pelvic pain control 44% • Five late toxicities: fistulas, ulceration, tissue necrosis

Abbreviations: *HDR* high dose rate, *EBRT* external beam radiotherapy, *HR-CTV* high-risk clinical target volume, *LC* local control, *DFS* disease-free survival, *OS* overall survival, *GU* genitourinary, *GI* gastrointestinal, *LN* lymph node, *SBRT* stereotactic body radiotherapy, *PFS* progression-free survival, *PALN* para-aortic lymph node, *BID* twice daily, *IORT* intraoperative radiotherapy

References

1. American Cancer Society. American Cancer Society: cancer facts & figures 2021. Atlanta; 2021.
2. Han K, Milosevic M, Fyles A, Pintilie M, Viswanathan AN. Trends in the utilization of brachytherapy in cervical cancer in the United States. Int J Radiat Oncol Biol Phys. 2013;87(1):111–9.
3. Tanderup K, Fokdal LU, Sturdza A, et al. Effect of tumor dose, volume and overall treatment time on local control after radiochemotherapy including MRI guided brachytherapy of locally advanced cervical cancer. Radiother Oncol. 2016;120(3):441–6.
4. Fyles A, Keane TJ, Barton M, Simm J. The effect of treatment duration in the local control of cervix cancer. Radiother Oncol. 1992;25(4):273–9.
5. Bhatla N, Berek JS, Cuello Fredes M, et al. Revised FIGO staging for carcinoma of the cervix uteri. Int J Gynaecol Obstet. 2019;145(1):129–35.
6. Viswanathan AN, Thomadsen B, American Brachytherapy Society Cervical Cancer Recommendations Committee; American Brachytherapy Society. American Brachytherapy Society consensus guidelines for locally advanced carcinoma of the cervix. Part I: general principles. Brachytherapy. 2012;11(1):33–46.
7. Viswanathan AN, Beriwal S, De Los Santos JF, et al. American Brachytherapy Society consensus guidelines for locally advanced carcinoma of the cervix. Part II: high-dose-rate brachytherapy. Brachytherapy. 2012;11(1):47–52.
8. Potter R, Haie-Meder C, Van Limbergen E, et al. Recommendations from gynaecological (GYN) GEC ESTRO working group (II): concepts and terms in 3D image-based treatment

planning in cervix cancer brachytherapy-3D dose volume parameters and aspects of 3D image-based anatomy, radiation physics, radiobiology. Radiother Oncol. 2006;78(1):67–77.
9. Haie-Meder C, Potter R, Van Limbergen E, et al. Recommendations from Gynaecological (GYN) GEC-ESTRO Working Group (I): concepts and terms in 3D image based 3D treatment planning in cervix cancer brachytherapy with emphasis on MRI assessment of GTV and CTV. Radiother Oncol. 2005;74(3):235–45.
10. Small W Jr, Beriwal S, Demanes DJ, et al. American Brachytherapy Society consensus guidelines for adjuvant vaginal cuff brachytherapy after hysterectomy. Brachytherapy. 2012;11(1):58–67.
11. Halle JS, Rosenman JG, Varia MA, Fowler WC, Walton LA, Currie JL. 1000 cGy single dose palliation for advanced carcinoma of the cervix or endometrium. Int J Radiat Oncol Biol Phys. 1986;12(11):1947–50.
12. Boulware RJ, Caderao JB, Delclos L, Wharton JT, Peters LJ. Whole pelvis megavoltage irradiation with single doses of 1000 rad to palliate advanced gynecologic cancers. Int J Radiat Oncol Biol Phys. 1979;5(3):333–8.
13. Chafe W, Fowler WC, Currie JL, Davis ML, Walton LA, Montana G. Single-fraction palliative pelvic radiation therapy in gynecologic oncology: 1,000 rads. Am J Obstet Gynecol. 1984;148(5):701–5.
14. Mazeron R, Fokdal LU, Kirchheiner K, et al. Dose-volume effect relationships for late rectal morbidity in patients treated with chemoradiation and MRI-guided adaptive brachytherapy for locally advanced cervical cancer: results from the prospective multicenter EMBRACE study. Radiother Oncol. 2016;120(3):412–9.
15. Kirchheiner K, Nout RA, Lindegaard JC, et al. Dose-effect relationship and risk factors for vaginal stenosis after definitive radio(chemo)therapy with image-guided brachytherapy for locally advanced cervical cancer in the EMBRACE study. Radiother Oncol. 2016;118(1):160–6.
16. Adams LB, Richmond J, Corbie-Smith G, Powell W. Medical mistrust and colorectal cancer screening among African Americans. J Community Health. 2017;42:1044.
17. Liberman D, Mehus B, Elliott SP. Urinary adverse effects of pelvic radiotherapy. Transl Androl Urol. 2014;3(2):186–95.
18. Liu R, Wang X, Tian JH, et al. High dose rate versus low dose rate intracavity brachytherapy for locally advanced uterine cervix cancer. Cochrane Database Syst Rev. 2014;2014(10):CD007563.
19. Eifel PJ, Winter K, Morris M, et al. Pelvic irradiation with concurrent chemotherapy versus pelvic and para-aortic irradiation for high-risk cervical cancer: an update of radiation therapy oncology group trial (RTOG) 90-01. J Clin Oncol. 2004;22(5):872–80.
20. Rose PG, Bundy BN, Watkins EB, et al. Concurrent cisplatin-based radiotherapy and chemotherapy for locally advanced cervical cancer. N Engl J Med. 1999;340(15):1144–53.
21. Potter R, Tanderup K, Schmid MP, et al. MRI-guided adaptive brachytherapy in locally advanced cervical cancer (EMBRACE-I): a multicentre prospective cohort study. Lancet Oncol. 2021;22(4):538–47.
22. Albuquerque K, Hrycushko BA, Harkenrider MM, et al. Compendium of fractionation choices for gynecologic HDR brachytherapy-an American Brachytherapy Society Task Group report. Brachytherapy. 2019;18(4):429–36.
23. Hsieh CH, Tien HJ, Hsiao SM, et al. Stereotactic body radiation therapy via helical tomotherapy to replace brachytherapy for brachytherapy-unsuitable cervical cancer patients—a preliminary result. Onco Targets Ther. 2013;6:59–66.
24. Jorcano S, Molla M, Escude L, et al. Hypofractionated extracranial stereotactic radiotherapy boost for gynecologic tumors: a promising alternative to high-dose rate brachytherapy. Technol Cancer Res Treat. 2010;9(5):509–14.
25. Kunos CA, Brindle J, Waggoner S, et al. Phase II clinical trial of robotic stereotactic body radiosurgery for metastatic gynecologic malignancies. Front Oncol. 2012;2:181.
26. Dewas S, Bibault J, Mirabel X, et al. Robotic image-guided reirradiation of lateral pelvic recurrences: preliminary results. Radiat Oncol. 2011;6(1):77.

27. Choi CW, Cho CK, Yoo SY, et al. Image-guided stereotactic body radiation therapy in patients with isolated para-aortic lymph node metastases from uterine cervical and corpus cancer. Int J Radiat Oncol Biol Phys. 2009;74(1):147–53.
28. Mesko S, Sandler K, Cohen J, Konecny G, Steinberg M, Kamrava M. Clinical outcomes for stereotactic ablative radiotherapy in oligometastatic and oligoprogressive gynecological malignancies. Int J Gynecol Cancer. 2017;27(2):403–8.
29. Hasan S, Ricco A, Jenkins K, et al. Survival and control prognosticators of recurrent gynecological malignancies of the pelvis and para-aortic region treated with stereotactic body radiation therapy. Front Oncol. 2016;6:249.
30. Smile TD, Reddy CA, Qiao-Guan G, et al. Stereotactic body radiotherapy for the treatment of oligometastatic gynecological malignancy in the abdomen and pelvis: a single-institution experience. J Radiosurg SBRT. 2021;7(3):189–97.
31. Badakh DK, Grover AH. Reirradiation with high-dose-rate remote afterloading brachytherapy implant in patients with locally recurrent or residual cervical carcinoma. J Cancer Res Ther. 2009;5(1):24–30.
32. Zolciak-Siwinska A, Bijok M, Jonska-Gmyrek J, et al. HDR brachytherapy for the reirradiation of cervical and vaginal cancer: analysis of efficacy and dosage delivered to organs at risk. Gynecol Oncol. 2014;132(1):93–7.
33. Mabuchi S, Takahashi R, Isohashi F, et al. Reirradiation using high-dose-rate interstitial brachytherapy for locally recurrent cervical cancer: a single institutional experience. Int J Gynecol Cancer. 2014;24(1):141–8.
34. Kim DH, Lee JH, Ki YK, et al. Short-course palliative radiotherapy for uterine cervical cancer. Radiat Oncol J. 2013;31(4):216–21.
35. Grigsby PW, Portelance L, Williamson JF. High dose ratio (HDR) cervical ring applicator to control bleeding from cervical carcinoma. Int J Gynecol Cancer. 2002;12(1):18–21.

Chapter 33
Endometrial Cancer

Brittaney-Belle E. Gordon, Mahesh Varia, and Ashley A. Weiner

33.1 Introduction

Hypofractionation in the radiotherapeutic management of endometrial cancer has an important but selective role in post-operative vaginal cuff HDR brachytherapy. SBRT is used for oligometastatic disease, rarely as a boost technique with EBRT, and for palliation. These data have mostly been reported from retrospective cohorts that include other gynecological malignancies as discussed in the cervical cancer chapter. Surgery [total hysterectomy with bilateral salpingo-oophorectomy (BSO)] with or without nodal assessment (sentinel lymph node biopsy or nodal dissection) is the primary treatment of endometrial cancer. Recommendations for adjuvant radiotherapy are based on surgical pathology. Factors considered include depth of invasion, grade, lymphovascular space invasion, and nodal involvement. The use of postoperative vaginal cuff brachytherapy for high-intermediate risk early-stage endometrial cancer is increasing in recent years after reports indicating its efficacy in local control and favorable toxicity profile in comparison with pelvic EBRT. There is ongoing research assessing the efficacy and toxicity of hypofractionated pelvic EBRT; however, these fractionation strategies are not standardly used in clinical practice.

B.-B. E. Gordon
University of Pittsburgh Medical Center, Pittsburgh, PA, USA

Hillman Comprehensive Cancer Center, Pittsburgh, PA, USA

M. Varia · A. A. Weiner (✉)
University of North Carolina, School of Medicine, Chapel Hill, NC, USA

Department of Radiation Oncology, University of North Carolina, School of Medicine, Chapel Hill, NC, USA
e-mail: ashley_weiner@med.unc.edu

O. Kaidar-Person, R. Chen (eds.), *Hypofractionated and Stereotactic Radiation Therapy*, https://doi.org/10.1007/978-3-031-47701-0_33

33.2 Pearls

- Uterine cancer is the most common gynecologic malignancy in the United States and the sixth most common cancer diagnosis in women worldwide.
- Mostly diagnosed in post-menopausal women (median age 60 years); 4% of the women are younger than 40 years. The incidence is most common among American Indian, Alaskan Native, and African-American women followed by Caucasian, Hispanic, and Asian women, respectively. Notably, African-American women experience poorer prognoses, regardless of stage, pathology, socioeconomic status, and treatment [1].
- Risk factors include excess (unopposed) estrogen exposure: early age at menarche, nulliparity, late age at menopause, obesity, estrogen-secreting tumors, tamoxifen therapy, and estrogen-progestin postmenopausal hormone therapy. Diabetes mellitus and high-fat diet are also considered risk factors.
- Genetic predisposition: Lynch syndrome, BRCA1 mutation.
- The most common presenting symptom is postmenopausal uterine bleeding (75–90%).
- Most diagnoses occur at an early stage: disease confined to the uterus (67–80%), spread to regional lymph nodes and organs (21%), and distant metastases (12%).
- Histology: Adenocarcinoma (i.e., endometrioid cancer) is the most common subtype (90–95%). Type 1 endometrioid cancers (75–80%) are estrogen-dependent, low-grade, and uterus-confined cancers that typically occur in post-menopausal women and have a favorable prognosis. Type 2 endometrioid cancers (10–20%) are estrogen-independent, non-endometrioid (serous, clear cell, mixed histology, undifferentiated, carcinosarcoma) cancers with poorer prognosis. Uterine sarcoma ~5% [2].
- **Local Anatomy and patterns of spread:**
  - The uterus is located posterior to the urinary bladder, anterior to the rectum, and superior to the uterine cervix and vagina.
  - Local spread is through invasion of the myometrium or the cervix and less commonly to uterine serosa, parametria, or vagina.
  - Extrauterine spread of endometrioid cancer primarily occurs through lymphatic drainage to locoregional lymph nodes (pelvic, iliac, obturator, presacral, and paraaortic) and the adnexa.
  - Surgical series have described several pathologic risk factors for lymphatic spread including depth of invasion, tumor grade [3], tumor size [4], and LVSI [5].
  - Hematogenous dissemination to the lungs and liver is less common. Uterine sarcoma can spread to the lungs.
- **Medical workup:**
  - Physical exam including a pelvic exam with speculum and bimanual examination.

- For women with post-menopausal vaginal bleeding, the American College of Obstetricians and Gynecologists recommends initial evaluation with either endometrial biopsy or transvaginal ultrasonography. Endometrial thickness of greater than 4 mm on ultrasound requires a biopsy. Non-diagnostic endometrial biopsy should be followed by dilation and curettage.
- Laboratory tests: CBC, serum chemistries, LFTs, and renal function tests. CA-125 is optional for high-grade endometrioid histology, serous or clear cell histology, and advanced stage.
- Though the majority of women diagnosed are postmenopausal, fertility consultation should be considered for patients of childbearing age.

- **Imaging studies:**
  - For patients who will have surgical staging and primary treatment, preoperative imaging is reserved for those with high-grade or non-endometrioid cell type or suspected advanced stage on clinical evaluation. Chest X-ray can be considered.
  - Suspected/gross cervical involvement: contrast abdomen and pelvis MRI is recommended to evaluate the extent of the disease.
  - Suspected extrauterine disease: MRI/CT/PET as clinically indicated.
- Operable patients undergo initial hysterectomy (open, laparoscopic, or robotic) with BSO ± adjuvant treatment based on age, stage, and pathologic risk factors.
- The highest risk site of disease recurrence after surgery is at the vaginal cuff.
- Regardless of tumor type, the estimated 5-year OS is 85–90% for Stage I, 75–85% for Stage II, 50–65% for Stage III, and 20–25% for Stage IV (FIGO 26th report).
- Evaluation of the genetic foundation of endometrial cancer has yielded specific molecular subgroups that are associated with tumor mutagenicity and aggressiveness beyond the typical stage and grade (Fig. 33.1). DNA polymerase-epsilon (POLE) mutation is associated with a favorable prognosis, while mismatch repair (MLH1, PMS2, MSH2, and MSH6) deficiency (MMRd) is associated with an intermediate prognosis. No specific molecular profile (NSMP) group can be separated into two groups: NSMP with beta (β) catenin (CTNNB1) mutation and NSMP without CTNNB1 mutation. CTNNb1 is associated with distant recurrence such that NSMP without CTNNB1 mutation is associated with a favorable prognosis and NSMP with CTNNB1 mutation has an intermediate prognosis. TP53 when mutated allows unrestricted cancer growth and confers a poor prognosis. L1 cell adhesion molecule (L1CAM) overexpression is a significant risk factor for both pelvic and distant recurrences and confers a poor prognosis [6–9].

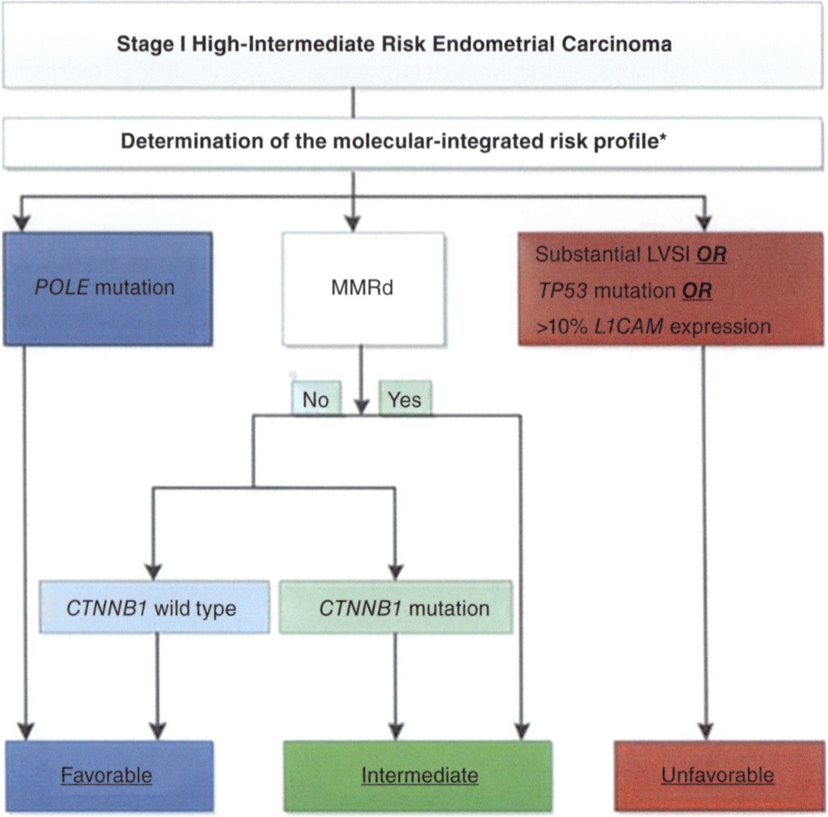

*Patients with multiple characteristics (double classifiers) were designated intermediate risk. MMRd= Mismatch repair-deficiency.

Fig. 33.1 Molecular-integrated risk profile (Reprinted with permission of the publisher, Elsevier [6])

33.3 Patient Selection

33.3.1 Adjuvant Setting (After Hysterectomy/BSO)

FIGO Stage I–II

- Surgical pathology must be fully assessed to determine recommendations for adjuvant radiotherapy.
- For patients with FIGO Stage I endometroid cancer, three risk factors are typically considered: high grade (grade 2–3), deep myometrial invasion, and LVSI. Adjuvant treatment is recommended for patients with age <50 years with all three risk factors; 50–69 years with two risk factors; and 70 years and older with any one risk factor. These risk factors for recurrence were initially described in GOG 99 [10].

- Low-risk patients who do not meet the above criteria are recommended for close surveillance only.
- Patients meeting the above high-intermediate risk criteria are recommended to receive adjuvant EBRT or VBT.
- Many of these patients are candidates for VBT alone; however, some patients have a substantial risk of occult nodal involvement (i.e., grade 3 disease with deep myometrial invasion, or extensive LVSI) warranting EBRT to target the at-risk nodal basins in addition to the vaginal cuff.
- Occasionally, a patient may have risk factors that warrant EBRT and have additional risk factors for recurrence at the vaginal cuff (high-grade histology, positive surgical margins, or FIGO stage II—cervical stromal invasion) and a VBT boost is administered.
- Initiate brachytherapy after the vaginal cuff is healed, usually at least 4–6 weeks post-surgery (within 12 weeks postoperatively).

FIGO Stage IIIC

- Patients with lymph node involvement will typically receive 6 cycles of chemotherapy ± pelvic EBRT. EBRT typically is administered at the time of completion of chemotherapy, if recommended. VBT boost may be warranted if there are additional risk factors for vaginal cuff recurrence (e.g., high-grade histology, positive surgical margins, or cervical stromal invasion).

33.3.2 Definitive Setting

- Medically inoperable patients with early stage disease without risk factors per MRI (positive LN, deep myometrium involvement) can be treated by intracavitary brachytherapy alone, while patients with risk factors can be treated with EBRT + brachytherapy [11, 12]. Hormone therapy (either systemic or via a hormonal intrauterine device) alone can be considered for unfit patients.
- Patients with unresectable disease (e.g., invasion of the vagina, bladder, and rectum) or with extrauterine pelvic disease are candidates for EBRT + brachytherapy ± chemotherapy, or neoadjuvant chemotherapy or chemoradiotherapy followed by surgical resection, or chemotherapy alone [11–13].

33.3.3 Recurrent Disease

- Patients with recurrent disease should only be considered for surgery if gross tumor resection can be achieved. RT with curative intent is indicated in patients with isolated pelvic relapse after surgery alone to the initial disease [13].

- Brachytherapy technique for vaginal cuff recurrence (intracavitary vs. interstitial) is based on the depth of vaginal wall invasion and the distribution of the disease. In cases of superficial (<5–7 mm) recurrences, VBT may be selected. For lesions invading >5–7 mm, VBT provides an inadequate dose at depth compared with interstitial techniques [11, 14, 15]. For recurrences in the pelvic lymph nodes or pelvic sidewall not amenable for brachytherapy, pelvic EBRT is given with a boost to the region of gross involvement.

33.4 Treatment Planning

33.4.1 Vaginal Brachytherapy

Timing	Brachytherapy should be started within 12 weeks after surgery. We recommend once weekly intracavitary brachytherapy if administered during EBRT. VBT can be administered twice weekly as a monotherapy or after EBRT completion
Analgesia	Consider premedication with anxiolytics, pain medication, or mild sedation [11]. These are often not necessary with VBT
Position	Dorsal lithotomy position
Pelvic exam	Perform a visual inspection and manual examination with care to ensure that the vaginal cuff is well healed and that there is no recurrence at the vaginal apex or vaginal cuff dehiscence. In a subset of patients for whom the placement of a vaginal applicator may be difficult (postoperative changes, pain, etc.), prior discussion with the patient, relaxation techniques, and/or lubrication of the applicator can aid in the insertion
Preparation and procedure	• Placement of a radio-opaque marker at the vaginal cuff can assist in verifying that the applicator is in contact with the vaginal mucosa • The choice of applicator depends on patient's anatomy and physician's experience. In many patients, the postoperative vagina is cylindrical and it can be treated adequately with a properly sized vaginal cylinder. In some situations, ovoids may provide better dosimetry due to the remnants of the vaginal fornices • The applicator should be lubricated prior to placement. After placement of the applicator, a visual check is done to verify that the applicator is midline, and not tilted laterally, anteriorly, or posteriorly • The treatment target is the submucosal lymphatics of the vagina, and in most situations only the upper 1/3—1/2 (about 3–5 cm) vagina must be targeted [11, 16–19]. Increased treatment length can result in increased toxicity • To allow an optimal dose distribution, the vaginal mucosa needs to be in contact with the applicator surface (no air gaps). The ABS recommends the use of the largest diameter cylinder that can comfortably fit into the apex of the vagina to reduce mucosal dose [11]
Treatment planning:	Treatment planning can be 2D (X-ray) and/or 3D (CT, MRI) based. For treatment planning optimization, points should be placed around both the apex and the lateral aspects of the applicator [19]
Documentation	Documentation of brachytherapy is essential and should include the type of isotope and source, description of the target (including size and shape), prescription depth, target dose, dose per fraction, fractionation plan, applicator type and size features, and the treatment plan documentation (dose distribution to the target and OAR)

33.4.2 Intact Uterus

Timing	Brachytherapy should be started as soon as possible. We recommend once weekly intracavitary brachytherapy if administered during EBRT. Brachytherapy can be administered twice weekly as a monotherapy or after EBRT completion
Analgesia	Analgesia options include general, spinal, intravenous sedation, and/or oral pain medication. Our practice is to use titrated doses of fentanyl, starting with 50 μg IV, and lorazepam with 1 mg IV, 20–30 min prior to the start of the procedure
Position	Dorsal lithotomy position
Pelvic exam	Examination under anesthesia—a bimanual examination to document uterine size, the cervix size, and the size of the vaginal fornices (i.e., disease extension/response to treatment). The uterus is sounded to aid in the selection of the appropriate tandem applicator. Insertion of radiopaque markers in the cervix can aid localization of the cervix on imaging
Procedure	• A Foley catheter is inserted into the bladder, and the balloon is inflated with dilute contrast • Tandem and ovoids are commonly used for brachytherapy in this setting. Other applicators include tandem and ring applicators or a Rotte Y applicator. Simon-Heyman capsules or multiple intrauterine tandems can be used to further distribute the dose to the uterus • After the selection of appropriate applicators (including the angle of the intrauterine tandem and the size of the ring or ovoids), cervical os is dilated to enable accommodation of Simon-Heyman capsules (if used). Ultrasound guidance can be used during applicator insertion to help guide the dilation of the endocervical canal and evaluate the placement of the uterine applicators. A tenaculum may be placed on the upper lip of the cervix to provide countertraction for the placement of the intrauterine tandem. A ring or ovoids can be used if lateral cervical dosing is needed • It is important that the tandem extends to the uterine fundus to ensure that the entire endometrial lining is treated • Radio-opaque vaginal packing is used to displace the bladder base anteriorly and the anterior rectal wall posteriorly away from the intracavitary applicator. Packing also serves to prevent the displacement of the tandem from the uterus and to secure the positioning of the entire applicator • A Smit sleeve can be useful for anatomically difficult implants • Imaging (CT, MRI) is done for each implant immediately following the placement of the applicator and is essential for treatment planning of each procedure • 3D imaging allows for accurate contouring of the tumor, cervix, uterus, and OAR
Treatment planning	Using 3D treatment planning, brachytherapy is prescribed to the uterine serosa
Documentation	Documentation of brachytherapy is essential and should include the type of isotope and source, description of the target (including size and shape), prescription depth, target dose, dose per fraction, fractionation plan, applicator type and size features, and the treatment plan documentation (dose distribution to the target and OAR)

33.5 Common Dose/Fractionation Schemes

33.5.1 Vaginal Brachytherapy

- At the authors' institution, VBT is typically prescribed to a dose of 7 Gy at 0.5 cm depth × 3 fractions for VBT alone after hysterectomy. The goal is to achieve an LDR equivalent of 30 Gy at 0.5 cm depth and 65 Gy at the surface. VBT alone is typically completed for patients with early-stage high-intermediate-risk endometrial cancer.

Common vaginal brachytherapy doses [11, 20, 21]

Dose/fx	Prescription depth
7 Gy × 3	0.5 cm depth
4 Gy × 6	Vaginal surface
6 Gy × 5	Vaginal surface
5.5 Gy × 4	0.5 cm depth

33.5.2 EBRT Followed by Vaginal Brachytherapy

- EBRT is typically 45–50.4 Gy. Midline block (at ~40 Gy) can be used if brachytherapy is planned [11].
- Involved unresected lymph nodes can be boosted during EBRT with 1.8 Gy daily [11] fractions for a total of 59.4 Gy (sequential boost). Alternatively, a simultaneous integrated boost (SIB) can be utilized to deliver 2.1–2.2 Gy per fraction to the involved lymph nodes during the initial 25–28 EBRT fractions.
- At the authors' institution, VBT is typically prescribed to a dose of 5 Gy to the vaginal surface × 3 fractions when administered in conjunction with EBRT.

Common vaginal brachytherapy doses (combined with EBRT, 1.8 Gy × 25–33 fractions) [11, 22]

Dose/fx	Prescription depth
5 Gy × 3	Vaginal surface or 0.5 cm depth
6 Gy × 2	Vaginal surface or 0.5 cm depth
6 Gy × 3	Vaginal surface

33.5.3 RT for Medically Inoperable Patients

- Patients with Stage I grade 1–2 disease with minimal myometrial invasion can be treated with brachytherapy alone. All other patients should receive EBRT in conjunction with brachytherapy. The CTV encompasses the whole uterus extending to the serosal surface and should receive an EQD2 of at least 48 Gy for brachytherapy alone and at least 65 Gy for the combination of EBRT plus VBT. A GTV may also be defined using T2-weighted MRI and may be prescribed a dose of >80 Gy [12].

Common brachytherapy doses (without EBRT) for inoperable endometrial cancer [12]

Dose/fx Prescribed to uterine serosa	EQD2(Gy) to the tumor (point A with $\alpha/\beta = 10$ Gy)	Comments
6 Gy × 6 6.4 Gy × 6 7.3 Gy × 5 8.5 Gy × 4	48 52.5 52.6 52.4	Consider heavier loading in the tandem compared to cervical tandem and ovoids and/or utilization of Simen-Heyman capsules. Prescription depth in myometrium is modified according to the imaging findings of uterine size and proximity of small bowel and sigmoid colon

Common brachytherapy doses (combined with EBRT, 1.8 Gy × 25 fractions) for inoperable endometrial cancer [12]

Dose/fx Prescribed to uterine serosa	EQD2(Gy) to the tumor (point A with $\alpha/\beta = 10$ Gy)	Comments
6.5 Gy × 3 5.2 Gy × 4 5 Gy × 5	71.1 70.6 75	Consider heavier loading in the tandem compared to cervical tandem and ovoids and/or utilization of Simen-Heyman capsules. Prescription depth in myometrium is modified according to the imaging findings of uterine size and proximity of small bowel and sigmoid colon

33.5.4 Hypofractionated Pelvic Radiation

- Traditionally, radiation oncologists have been apprehensive about the use of hypofractionated radiotherapy to treat primary gynecological cancers due to the perceived increased toxicities associated with higher doses per fraction. However, with recent literature demonstrating the safety and efficacy of hypofractionated radiotherapy in other cancers, such as breast and lung cancer, there has been renewed interest in investigating the safety and efficacy of hypofractionated radiotherapy in gynecological malignancies. Accordingly, several prospective clinical trials examining the safety, tolerability, and efficacy of hypofractionated radiotherapy in endometrial cancer have been initiated with results expected in the next 3–5 years [23–26].
- The Stereotactic Pelvic Adjuvant Radiation Therapy in Cancers of the Uterus (SPARTACUS) was a prospective phase I/II clinical trial that examined the safety profile of SBRT in endometrial cancer. Forty-one patients with Stage 1–3 endometrial cancers were treated with adjuvant radiation 30 Gy in 5 fractions, every other day or once weekly. Patients primarily experienced grade 1 and 2 (gastro-

intestinal or genitourinary) toxicities, 63% and 24% respectively, with no documented grade ≥ 3 toxicities. There was no identified locoregional recurrence over a median of 9 months of follow-up. The study concluded that hypofractionated RT is feasible and tolerable [27].

- Ultimately, randomized controlled trials investigating the safety, tolerability, and efficacy of hypofractionated radiotherapy vs. conventional radiotherapy regimens will determine the best treatment options for patients with gynecologic malignancies.

33.5.5 Stereotactic Body Radiotherapy (SBRT) for Oligometastatic Disease

- SBRT is increasingly used for the treatment of oligometastatic gynecologic malignancies. SBRT is associated with good locoregional control of oligometastatic disease, thereby improving progression-free and potentially overall survival in patients with good response to systemic therapies. SBRT dosages are dependent on the extent and location of the disease but typically range 18–48 Gy total in 3–6 fractions [28, 29].

33.6 Normal Tissue Tolerance

- EBRT+ VBT total EQD2 dose:
  - Upper vagina mucosa 150 Gy, mid-vagina mucosa 80–90 Gy, lower vagina mucosa 60–70 Gy. (NOTE: the proximal vagina is a target in VBT)
  - Small bowel <45–50.5 Gy
  - Rectal point dose <70 Gy
  - Bladder <75 Gy

Dose constraints to OARs for brachytherapy

OAR	Radiographic (ICRU point)	3D imaging (D2cc)
Bladder	5× < 3.7 Gy	<90 Gy[a]
Rectum	5× < 3.7 Gy	<70–75 Gy[a]
Sigmoid	–	<70–75 Gy[a]
Ureters	–	<70 Gy

[a] Max point dose defined as <0.035 cc

33.7 Patient Management Considerations

- After the completion of treatment, patients should be given a vaginal dilator to prevent scar tissue and adhesions within the vagina. Patients are instructed to place the dilator within the vagina for 10–15 min several times per week.

33.7.1 Acute Toxicity

- Due to the conformal dosimetry of vaginal cuff brachytherapy, toxicity rates to bowel, bladder, and rectum are low. There is generally minimal acute toxicity during treatment with vaginal cuff brachytherapy alone.

33.7.2 Late Toxicity

- Late toxicity is also rare with vaginal cuff brachytherapy alone. The most common side effect is stenosis and atrophy of the vagina, which can result in vaginal shortening or narrowing. Rare incidences of severe bowel, rectum, and bladder toxicity (e.g., rectovaginal fistula, radiation colitis or cystitis, vaginal or bladder necrosis) could occur when VBT is administered with EBRT.

33.8 Follow-Up

- H&P including pelvic exam should be completed every 3–6 months for the first 2–3 years, then every 6 months for 5 years, and then annually.
- CA-125 is useful if the pre-operative level was elevated.
- Imaging only if clinically indicated and/or if extra-uterine spread was present at initial surgery.

33.9 Relevant Literature

For patients with FIGO stage I endometroid cancer, three pathologic risk factors are considered: high-grade, deep myometrial invasion, and LVSI. Adjuvant treatment with radiotherapy is recommended for patients with age <50 years with all three risk factors; 50–69 years with two risk factors; and 70 years and older with any one risk factor. These risk factors for recurrence were initially described in GOG 99 [10]. Adjuvant radiotherapy has been shown in multiple trials [10, 30] to provide a benefit in terms of locoregional recurrence without an overall survival benefit. Most locoregional recurrences occur at the vaginal cuff. In select patients with a low risk of nodal recurrence, VBT can be used instead of pelvic EBRT with a similar reduction in vaginal cuff recurrences and improved toxicity profile.

Prospective randomized phase 3 trials of EBRT and VBT

VBT alone vs. VBT + EBRT

Study	rm 1: VBT-alone	rm 2: VBT + EBRT	edian follow-up	utcomes
Onsrud (2013) [31] Stage 1	($N = 280$) 60 Gy LDR	($n = 288$) 60 Gy LDR + 40 Gy EBRT	20.5 years	Median OS 20.48 years VBT vs. 20.5 years EBRT + VBT (NS)
Aalders (1980) [32] Stage I	($n = 277$) 60 Gy LDR	($n = 263$) 60 Gy LDR + 40 Gy EBRT	3–10 years	5-year OS VBT 91% vs. EBRT + VBT 89% (NS) Vaginal/pelvic recurrence VBT 6.9% vs. EBRT + VBT 1.9% ($p < 0.01$) grade 3+ toxicity VBT 0.7% vs. EBRT + VBT 1.1%
Sorbe (2012) [33] Stage I	($n = 263$) HDR 3 Gy × 6 or 5.9 Gy × 3 or LDR 20 Gy × 1	($n = 285$) VBT + 46 Gy EBRT	62 months	5-year OS VBT 90% vs. EBRT + VBT 89% (NS) Pelvic recurrence VBT 5.3% vs. EBRT + VBT 0.4% ($p < 0.0006$) Vaginal recurrence VBT 2.7% vs. EBRT + VBT 1.9% (NS) grade 3 toxicity VBT 0.8% vs. EBRT + VBT 1.9%

VBT vs. EBRT

Study	Arm 1: VBT	Arm 2: EBRT	Median follow-up	Outcomes
Nout (2010) [34] PORTEC-2 Stage I–II	($n = 213$) HDR 7 Gy × 3 at 0.5 cm or LDR 30 Gy at 0.5 cm	($n = 214$) 46 Gy EBRT	45 months	5-year OS VBT 84.8% vs. EBRT 79.6% (NS) Pelvic recurrence VBT 3.8% vs. EBRT 0.5% ($p = 0.02$) Vaginal recurrence VBT 1.8% vs. EBRT 1.6% (NS) grade 3 toxicity VBT <1% vs. EBRT 3% grade 1–2 GI toxicity VBT 12.6% vs. EBRT 53.8% ($p < 0.05$)

Abbreviations: *VBT* vaginal brachytherapy, *EBRT* external beam radiation therapy, *Gy* gray, *LDR* low dose rate, *OS* overall survival, *HDR* high dose rate

Selected studies of postoperative HDR-VBT alone

Study	*N*	Treatments	Median follow-up	Outcomes
Prospective				
Sorbe (1990) [35] Stage I	404	5.0 Gy × 6 4.5 Gy × 6 6.0 Gy × 5 9.0 Gy × 4	NA	5-year OS 92% Pelvic/vaginal recurrence 1.7% Vaginal recurrence 0.7% Acute toxicity 30.9%, late toxicity 15.8% The high-dose group 9 Gy × 4 had a higher rate and grade of late complications
Retrospective				
Weiss (1998) [36] Stage IA–II	122	7.0 Gy × 3	25.6 months	Pelvic recurrence 4.1% Vaginal recurrence 1.6% Recurrence occurred in 3.8% of patients with moderate risk and in 20.5% of patients with high risk No grade 3–4 toxicity
Petereit (1999) [37] Stage IB	191	16.2 Gy × 2 prescribed to surface	38 months	4-year OS 95% Pelvic recurrence 0.5% Vaginal recurrence 0% 0.5% grade 5 (colo-vaginal fistula) 4% asymptomatic vaginal cuff necrosis
Horowitz (2002) [38] Stage IB–II	164	7 Gy × 3 at 0.5 cm	65 months	5-year OS 87% Pelvic recurrence 0.6% Vaginal recurrence 1.2% No grade 3–4 toxicity
Alektiar (2005) [18] Stage IB–IIB	382	6.0–7.0 Gy × 3	48 months	5-year OS 93% Pelvic recurrence[a] 3% Vaginal recurrence 0.8% No grade 3–4 toxicity
Diavolitsis (2012) [39] Stage IA	169	7.0 Gy × 3 5.5 Gy × 4 at 0.5 cm	103 months	5-year OS 95.5% 5-year RFS 94.4% Pelvic recurrence 0.5% Vaginal recurrence 0.5% No grade 3–4 toxicity

Abbreviations: *Gy* gray, *OS* overall survival, *RFS* relapse-free survival
[a] Pelvic recurrences included patients with distant recurrence and paraaortic lymph nodes
Selected studies of postoperative pelvic EBRT and VBT

Study	*N*	Treatmentsa	Median follow-up	Outcomes
Retrospective				
Lybeert (1989) [40] Stage I–IV	291	40 Gy EBRT + 5 Gy × 4 at 0.5 cm HDR	NA	5-year RFS Stage I: 88% Stage II: 68% Stage III/IV: 50% Pelvic recurrence 2.7% Vaginal recurrence 2.7% No grade 3–4 toxicity
Nori (1994) [41] Stage I	300	40 Gy EBRT + 7 Gy × 3 at 0.5 cm HDR	12 years	PFS 96.6% Pelvic recurrence 0.3% Vaginal recurrence 2% No grade 3–4 toxicity
Algan (1996) [42] Stage I/II	81	45 Gy EBRT + 4 Gy × 3 at 0.5 cm HDR or 30 Gy LDR to surface	NA	5-year OS 83% Pelvic recurrence 3% Vaginal recurrence 4% grade 3 toxicity 3%
Cannon (2009) [43] Stage II	50	45–51 Gy EBRT + more than four different fractionations for HDR. 60% were 5 Gy × 5 or 7.8 Gy × 2	5.2 years	5-year OS 82% 5-year DFS 82% Pelvic recurrence 4% Vaginal recurrence 0% Toxicity grade 3 (2%), grade 4 (2%)

Abbreviations: *Gy* gray, *fx* fraction(s), *EBRT* external beam radiation therapy, *HDR* high dose rate, *RFS* relapse-free survival, *PFS* progression-free survival, *LDR* low dose rate, *OS* overall survival, *DFS* disease-free survival

[a] Median doses of radiation are reported in the table

Selected studies evaluating SBRT in oligometastatic gynecologic cancers

Study	Patients	Treatments	Median follow-up	Outcomes
Retrospective				
Hasan (2016) [28]	(*n* = 30) Endometroid, cervical, ovarian Uterine-serous, carcinosarcoma	Median 27.5 Gy (range 15–40 Gy) in 5 fx (range: 3–5)	5 years	OS: 1 year (85%), 5 years (42%), median 43.3 months LC: 3 years (73%), 5 years (67%) DFS: median 47 months No grade 3–4 toxicity
Smile (2021) [29]	(*N* = 34) Endometrial, cervical, ovarian	Median 24 Gy (range 18–54 Gy) in 3 fx (range 3–6)	12 months	OS: 1 year (85%), 2 years (70.2%) LC: 1 year (92.5%), 2 years (92.5%) No grade 3–4 toxicity

Abbreviations: *Gy* gray, *LC* local control, *OS* overall survival, *DFS* disease-free survival, *fx* fraction(s)

References

1. Siegel RL, Miller KD, Fuchs HE, Jemal A. Cancer statistics, 2022. CA Cancer J Clin. 2022;72(1):7–33. https://doi.org/10.3322/caac.21708.
2. Morice P, Leary A, Creutzberg C, Abu-Rustum N, Darai E. Endometrial cancer. Lancet. 2016;387(10023):1094–108. https://doi.org/10.1016/S0140-6736(15)00130-0.
3. Creasman WT, Morrow CP, Bundy BN, Homesley HD, Graham JE, Heller PB. Surgical pathologic spread patterns of endometrial cancer. A Gynecologic Oncology Group Study. Cancer. 1987;60(8 Suppl):2035–41.
4. Schink JC, Rademaker AW, Miller DS, Lurain JR. Tumor size in endometrial cancer. Cancer. 1991;67(11):2791–4. https://doi.org/10.1002/1097-0142(19910601)67:11<2791::aid-cncr2820671113>3.0.co;2-s.
5. Cohn DE, Horowitz NS, Mutch DG, Kim SM, Manolitsas T, Fowler JM. Should the presence of lymphvascular space involvement be used to assign patients to adjuvant therapy following hysterectomy for unstaged endometrial cancer? Gynecol Oncol. 2002;87(3):243–6. https://doi.org/10.1006/gyno.2002.6825.
6. Wortman BG, Bosse T, Nout RA, et al. Molecular-integrated risk profile to determine adjuvant radiotherapy in endometrial cancer: evaluation of the pilot phase of the PORTEC-4a trial. Gynecol Oncol. 2018;151(1):69–75. https://doi.org/10.1016/j.ygyno.2018.07.020.
7. Leon-Castillo A, de Boer SM, Powell ME, et al. Molecular classification of the PORTEC-3 trial for high-risk endometrial cancer: impact on prognosis and benefit from adjuvant therapy. J Clin Oncol. 2020;38(29):3388–97. https://doi.org/10.1200/JCO.20.00549.
8. O'Hara AJ, Bell DW. The genomics and genetics of endometrial cancer. Adv Genomics Genet. 2012;2012(2):33–47. https://doi.org/10.2147/AGG.S28953.
9. van den Heerik A, Horeweg N, Nout RA, et al. PORTEC-4a: international randomized trial of molecular profile-based adjuvant treatment for women with high-intermediate risk endometrial cancer. Int J Gynecol Cancer. 2020;30(12):2002–7. https://doi.org/10.1136/ijgc-2020-001929.
10. Keys HM, Roberts JA, Brunetto VL, et al. A phase III trial of surgery with or without adjunctive external pelvic radiation therapy in intermediate risk endometrial adenocarcinoma: a Gynecologic Oncology Group study. Gynecol Oncol. 2004;92(3):744–51. https://doi.org/10.1016/j.ygyno.2003.11.048.
11. Small W Jr, Beriwal S, Demanes DJ, et al. American Brachytherapy Society consensus guidelines for adjuvant vaginal cuff brachytherapy after hysterectomy. Brachytherapy. 2012;11(1):58–67. https://doi.org/10.1016/j.brachy.2011.08.005.
12. Schwarz JK, Beriwal S, Esthappan J, et al. Consensus statement for brachytherapy for the treatment of medically inoperable endometrial cancer. Brachytherapy. 2015;14(5):587–99. https://doi.org/10.1016/j.brachy.2015.06.002.
13. Colombo N, Creutzberg C, Amant F, et al. ESMO-ESGO-ESTRO consensus conference on endometrial cancer: diagnosis, treatment and follow-up. Int J Gynecol Cancer. 2016;26(1):2–30. https://doi.org/10.1097/IGC.0000000000000609.
14. Jhingran A, Burke TW, Eifel PJ. Definitive radiotherapy for patients with isolated vaginal recurrence of endometrial carcinoma after hysterectomy. Int J Radiat Oncol Biol Phys. 2003;56(5):1366–72. https://doi.org/10.1016/s0360-3016(03)00414-0.
15. Lin LL, Grigsby PW, Powell MA, Mutch DG. Definitive radiotherapy in the management of isolated vaginal recurrences of endometrial cancer. Int J Radiat Oncol Biol Phys. 2005;63(2):500–4. https://doi.org/10.1016/j.ijrobp.2005.02.004.
16. Wahl AO, Gaffney DK, Jhingran A, et al. ACR Appropriateness Criteria(R) adjuvant management of early-stage endometrial cancer. Oncology (Williston Park). 2016;30(9):816–22.
17. Harkenrider MM, Grover S, Erickson BA, et al. Vaginal brachytherapy for postoperative endometrial cancer: 2014 Survey of the American Brachytherapy Society. Brachytherapy. 2016;15(1):23–9. https://doi.org/10.1016/j.brachy.2015.09.012.

18. Alektiar KM, Venkatraman E, Chi DS, Barakat RR. Intravaginal brachytherapy alone for intermediate-risk endometrial cancer. Int J Radiat Oncol Biol Phys. 2005;62(1):111–7. https://doi.org/10.1016/j.ijrobp.2004.09.054.
19. Harkenrider MM, Block AM, Alektiar KM, et al. American Brachytherapy Task Group report: adjuvant vaginal brachytherapy for early-stage endometrial cancer: a comprehensive review. Brachytherapy. 2017;16(1):95–108. https://doi.org/10.1016/j.brachy.2016.04.005.
20. Albuquerque K, Hrycushko BA, Harkenrider MM, et al. Compendium of fractionation choices for gynecologic HDR brachytherapy—an American Brachytherapy Society Task Group report. Brachytherapy. 2019;18(4):429–36. https://doi.org/10.1016/j.brachy.2019.02.008.
21. Alban GM, Buscariollo DL, Cheng T, et al. Low-dose adjuvant cylinder brachytherapy for endometrioid endometrial cancer. Pract Radiat Oncol. 2020;10(2):95–103. https://doi.org/10.1016/j.prro.2019.11.004.
22. Viswanathan AN, Moughan J, Miller BE, et al. NRG oncology/RTOG 0921: a phase 2 study of postoperative intensity-modulated radiotherapy with concurrent cisplatin and bevacizumab followed by carboplatin and paclitaxel for patients with endometrial cancer. Cancer. 2015;121(13):2156–63. https://doi.org/10.1002/cncr.29337.
23. University of Chicago. Study of pelvic hypofractionated radiotherapy in endometrial cancer. 2021. https://ClinicalTrials.gov/show/NCT04683653.
24. University of Utah, NC Institute. Hypofractionated radiotherapy for the treatment of cervical or endometrial cancer. 2021. https://ClinicalTrials.gov/show/NCT05139368.
25. Meier T, University of Cincinnati. Adjuvant hypofractionated whole pelvis radiation therapy in endometrial cancer. 2021. https://ClinicalTrials.gov/show/NCT04458402.
26. Centre SHS, Princess Margaret Hospital C, Royal Victoria Hospital C, Hospital CV, London Regional Cancer Program C. Stereotactic pelvic adjuvant radiation therapy in cancers of the uterus II. 2021. https://ClinicalTrials.gov/show/NCT04890912.
27. Leung EW, Gladwish AP, Davidson MTM, et al. Stereotactic pelvic adjuvant radiation therapy in cancers of the uterus (SPARTACUS): a multicenter prospective trial evaluating acute toxicities and patient reported outcomes. Int J Radiat Oncol Biol Phys. 2021;111(3):S18–9. https://doi.org/10.1016/j.ijrobp.2021.07.072.
28. Hasan S, Ricco A, Jenkins K, et al. Survival and control prognosticators of recurrent gynecological malignancies of the pelvis and para-aortic region treated with stereotactic body radiation therapy. Front Oncol. 2016;6:249. https://doi.org/10.3389/fonc.2016.00249.
29. Smile TD, Reddy CA, Qiao-Guan G, et al. Stereotactic body radiotherapy for the treatment of oligometastatic gynecological malignancy in the abdomen and pelvis: a single-institution experience. J Radiosurg SBRT. 2021;7(3):189–97.
30. Creutzberg CL, Nout RA, Lybeert ML, et al. Fifteen-year radiotherapy outcomes of the randomized PORTEC-1 trial for endometrial carcinoma. Int J Radiat Oncol Biol Phys. 2011;81(4):e631–8. https://doi.org/10.1016/j.ijrobp.2011.04.013.
31. Onsrud M, Cvancarova M, Hellebust TP, Trope CG, Kristensen GB, Lindemann K. Long-term outcomes after pelvic radiation for early-stage endometrial cancer. J Clin Oncol. 2013;31(31):3951–6. https://doi.org/10.1200/JCO.2013.48.8023.
32. Aalders J, Abeler V, Kolstad P, Onsrud M. Postoperative external irradiation and prognostic parameters in stage I endometrial carcinoma: clinical and histopathologic study of 540 patients. Obstet Gynecol. 1980;56(4):419–27.
33. Sorbe BG, Horvath G, Andersson H, Boman K, Lundgren C, Pettersson B. External pelvic and vaginal irradiation versus vaginal irradiation alone as postoperative therapy in medium-risk endometrial carcinoma: a prospective, randomized study—quality-of-life analysis. Int J Gynecol Cancer. 2012;22(7):1281–8. https://doi.org/10.1097/IGC.0b013e3182643ba0.
34. Nout RA, Smit VT, Putter H, et al. Vaginal brachytherapy versus pelvic external beam radiotherapy for patients with endometrial cancer of high-intermediate risk (PORTEC-2): an open-label, non-inferiority, randomised trial. Lancet. 2010;375(9717):816–23. https://doi.org/10.1016/S0140-6736(09)62163-2.

35. Sorbe BG, Smeds AC. Postoperative vaginal irradiation with high dose rate afterloading technique in endometrial carcinoma stage I. Int J Radiat Oncol Biol Phys. 1990;18(2):305–14. https://doi.org/10.1016/0360-3016(90)90094-z.
36. Weiss E, Hirnle P, Arnold-Bofinger H, Hess CF, Bamberg M. Adjuvant vaginal high-dose-rate afterloading alone in endometrial carcinoma: patterns of relapse and side effects following low-dose therapy. Gynecol Oncol. 1998;71(1):72–6. https://doi.org/10.1006/gyno.1998.5155.
37. Petereit DG, Tannehill SP, Grosen EA, Hartenbach EM, Schink JC. Outpatient vaginal cuff brachytherapy for endometrial cancer. Int J Gynecol Cancer. 1999;9(6):456–62. https://doi.org/10.1046/j.1525-1438.1999.99061.x.
38. Horowitz NS, Peters WA 3rd, Smith MR, Drescher CW, Atwood M, Mate TP. Adjuvant high dose rate vaginal brachytherapy as treatment of stage I and II endometrial carcinoma. Obstet Gynecol. 2002;99(2):235–40. https://doi.org/10.1016/s0029-7844(01)01672-6.
39. Diavolitsis V, Rademaker A, Lurain J, Hoekstra A, Strauss J, Small W Jr. Clinical outcomes in international federation of gynecology and obstetrics stage IA endometrial cancer with myometrial invasion treated with or without postoperative vaginal brachytherapy. Int J Radiat Oncol Biol Phys. 2012;84(2):415–9. https://doi.org/10.1016/j.ijrobp.2011.12.010.
40. Lybeert ML, van Putten WL, Ribot JG, Crommelin MA. Endometrial carcinoma: high dose-rate brachytherapy in combination with external irradiation; a multivariate analysis of relapses. Radiother Oncol. 1989;16(4):245–52. https://doi.org/10.1016/0167-8140(89)90036-4.
41. Nori D, Merimsky O, Batata M, Caputo T. Postoperative high dose-rate intravaginal brachytherapy combined with external irradiation for early stage endometrial cancer: a long-term follow-up. Int J Radiat Oncol Biol Phys. 1994;30(4):831–7. https://doi.org/10.1016/0360-3016(94)90357-3.
42. Algan O, Tabesh T, Hanlon A, Hogan WM, Boente M, Lanciano RM. Improved outcome in patients treated with postoperative radiation therapy for pathologic stage I/II endometrial cancer. Int J Radiat Oncol Biol Phys. 1996;35(5):925–33. https://doi.org/10.1016/0360-3016(96)00188-5.
43. Cannon GM, Geye H, Terakedis BE, et al. Outcomes following surgery and adjuvant radiation in stage II endometrial adenocarcinoma. Gynecol Oncol. 2009;113(2):176–80. https://doi.org/10.1016/j.ygyno.2008.12.029.

Part XI
Celiac SBRT

Chapter 34
Celiac Plexus SBRT

Yaccov R. Lawrence and Maoz Ben Ayun

34.1 Introduction

Severe upper abdominal/lower back pain is a defining characteristic of pancreatic cancer. Celiac plexus radiosurgery is an experimental palliative treatment developed at the Sheba Medical Center, Israel, and is part of an ongoing prospective trial. High-dose radiation is targeted to the retroperitoneal celiac plexus, from the levels of the 12th thoracic to the level of the second lumbar vertebrae, inclusive. The preliminary positive results of an international phase II trial have been reported in abstract form.

34.2 Pearls

- Severe upper abdominal/lower back pain is a defining characteristic of pancreatic cancer: The majority of patients suffer pain and one-third grade their pain as moderate to severe [1]. This pain syndrome is associated with decreased mood, decreased functional status, and poor prognosis [2].
- Perineural invasion, whereby a cancer cell invades the perineural spaces surrounding nerves, is thought to be responsible for both pancreatic cancer's aggressive behavior and also pancreatic cancer-induced pain [3].
- Similar pain syndromes are seen in other cancers invading the celiac axis region.

Y. R. Lawrence (✉) · M. B. Ayun
Department of Radiation Oncology, Sheba Medical Center, Ramat Gan, Israel
e-mail: yaacov.lawrence@sheba.health.gov.il

O. Kaidar-Person, R. Chen (eds.), *Hypofractionated and Stereotactic Radiation Therapy*, https://doi.org/10.1007/978-3-031-47701-0_34

- Afferent nerve endings are located within the pancreas. The nerves pass through the celiac ganglion, the splanchnic nerves, the sympathetic trunk, and finally into the dorsal horn of the spinal cord. Nociceptive signals are subsequently relayed upward to the spinothalamic tract, the thalamus, and higher cortical centers [4].
- Opioid medications are the first-line treatment for pancreatic pain, but many patients require high doses associated with unacceptable systemic side effects.
- There are a wide range of techniques used to target the celiac plexus nerve pathway including celiac plexus block, celiac plexus neurolysis, EUS-guided radiofrequency ablation, high-intensity focused ultrasound, and splanchnicectomy. The relative effectiveness of these different techniques is unclear [5–8]. One recent randomized trial found *celiac plexus neurolysis combined with opioids* to be no more effective than opioids alone [9].
- Contemporary surveys of pancreatic cancer patients have repeatedly shown that their pain is frequently poorly controlled [1, 10].
- Radiosurgery targeted to the trigeminal cranial nerve is used in the treatment of trigeminal neuralgia. Typically, a dose of 70–90 Gy is prescribed [11].

34.3 Treatment Planning Considerations

Simulation instructions	• Supine, hands above the head or placed on the chest • Administer intravenous and oral contrast if tolerated • Motion management should be used
Contouring	• Contour adjacent critical structures (lower esophagus, stomach, bowel, liver, kidneys, and spinal cord) • Particular care needs to be taken not to miss the third part of the duodenum which may be very thin on axial slices and difficult to locate • Likewise in the post-Whipple scenario, care must be taken to contour the small bowel used to reconstruct the extrahepatic bowel ducts • The celiac plexus itself is not visible on CT or MRI scans. Hence, contour the anterior and lateral walls of the abdominal aorta, from the level of the 12th thoracic to the second lumbar vertebrae inclusive, as a surrogate structure using a 0.5-cm diameter brush • Adjacent primary tumor may or may not be treated based upon physician and patient preferences (Figs. 34.1 and 34.2)

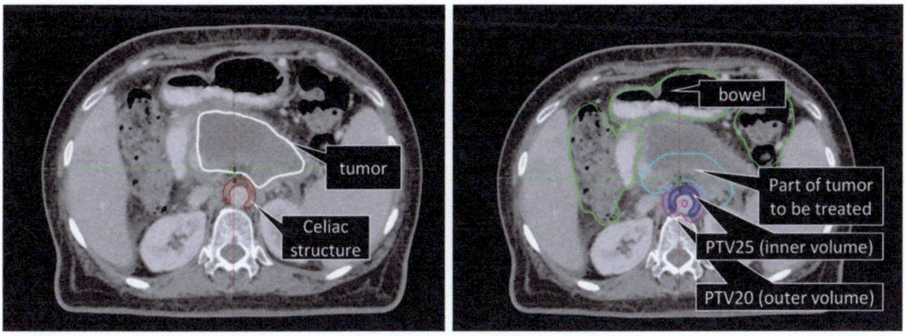

Fig. 34.1 An axial view of the CT simulation demonstrating the celiac plexus structure. *Left*: The celiac plexus structure is contoured using the lateral and anterior abdominal aorta walls as a surrogate structure; the adjacent pancreatic tumor is also contoured. *Right*: The PTV25Gy (the celiac contour) and PTV20Gy (a 0.5 cm expansion of the celiac contour) are demonstrated. In this case, the physician decided to treat part of the abutting primary tumor to a dose of 15 Gy

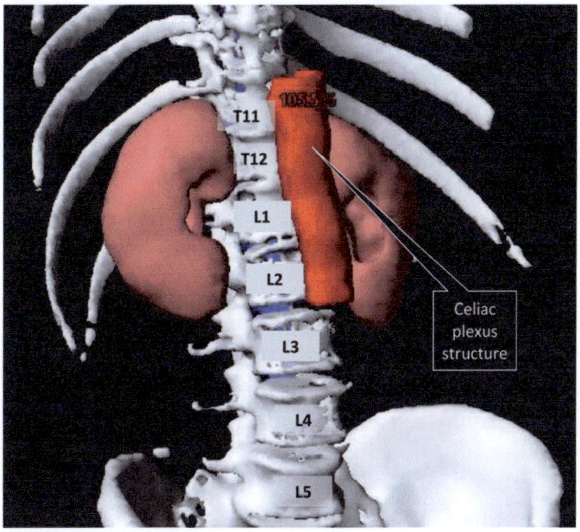

Fig. 34.2 Three-dimensional representation of the celiac plexus structure. Generally, the structure commences at the level of the superior border of the 12th thoracic vertebra and finishes at the level of the caudal border of the second lumbar vertebra. In this case, the celiac axis had an unusually high anatomical location, necessitating the celiac plexus contour to start at the level of the 11th thoracic vertebra

34.4 Prescription Dose

Prescription dose	• The treatment is delivered as a single fraction (Figs. 34.3 and 34.4) • Prescription dose (in the context of IRB-approved clinical protocol): – Celiac plexus 25 Gy – 0.5 cm uniform expansion around celiac plexus 20 Gy – Adjacent primary tumor (if treated) 12–15 Gy – For patients with a poor performance status, a lower dose of 12 Gy may be considered

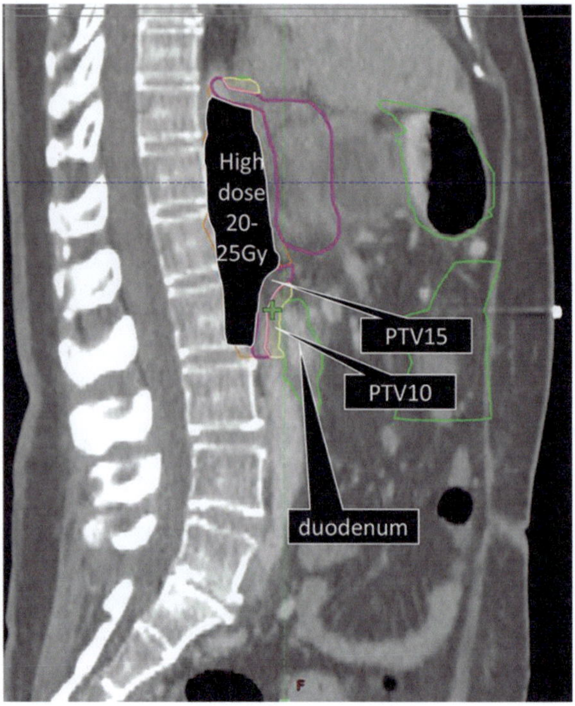

Fig. 34.3 A sagittal view of the CT simulation demonstrating the celiac plexus structure. The third part of the duodenum is seen lying immediately anterior to the abdominal aorta. This necessitates a dose-painting approach in order to respect the duodenum's constraint

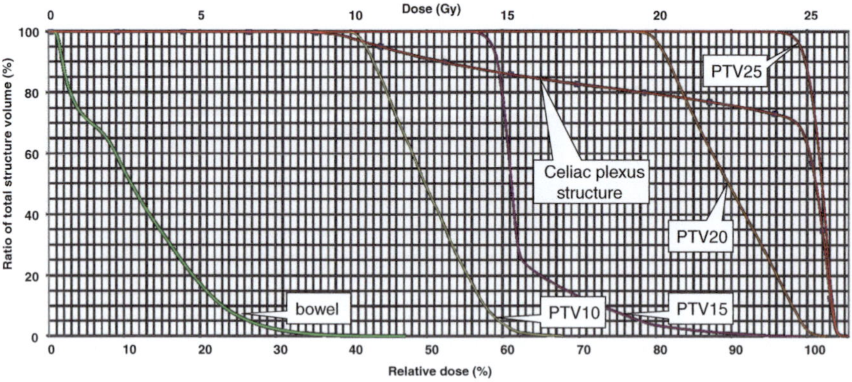

Fig. 34.4 A typical dose-volume histogram (DVH) of celiac plexus radiosurgery. The physician has defined four discreet PTV structures: PTV25Gy, PTV20Gy, PTV15GY, and PTV10Gy with the latter representing the part of the celiac plexus abutting the bowel. The dose-painting strategy results in the "celiac plexus structure" being partly under-dosed

34.5 Dose Constraints

Kidney	Kidney: Dmean ≤5.5 Gy • If there is only one functional kidney or renal function is impaired, Dmean ≤5 Gy • Acceptable deviation—one individual kidney has a mean dose of <7.5 Gy, but both kidneys together have a mean dose of ≤5.5 Gy (this is conditional upon both kidneys being functional) – Acceptable deviation—one individual kidney has a mean dose of <7.5 Gy, but both kidneys together have a mean dose of ≤5.5 Gy (this is conditional upon both kidneys being functional)
Bowel	For the purposes of dose constraints, esophagus, stomach, and small and large bowel are all considered bowel Less than 1 cc receives 11 Gy Acceptable deviation—no more than 5 cc receives over 12 Gy. Max 15 Gy
Liver	700 cc of healthy liver receives less than 10 Gy
Spinal cord	Max dose 10 Gy Acceptable deviation—<1 cc receive 11 cc

- Treatment planning
  - The isocenter is typically placed anterior to the T12 vertebra, near the aorta.
  - Priority is given to normal tissue constraints over target coverage.
  - To aid with treatment planning, typically, a dose-painting approach is used. PTV25Gy, PTV20Gy, PTV15Gy, and PTV10Gy are defined based on relative distance to celiac plexus vs. bowel.
  - At the Sheba Medical Center, treatment is planned using three VMAT arcs with varied collimator rotational angles, calculated using AAA version 15.6. The treatment is delivered on a Varian TrueBeamSTx LINAC equipped with a high-definition multileaf collimator (HD-MLC) and a couch with six degrees of freedom. A dose rate of 1400 monitor unit (MU)/min is chosen, delivered in 6 MV flattening filter-free (FFF) photon mode. The total MU is typically 10,000.
- Treatment delivery.
  - Prior to treatment, the patient receives anti-emetic medication: 8 mg dexamethasone PO combined with a tablet of Netupitant/palonosetron, (brand name *Akynzeo)*. Serotonin 5-HT3 receptor antagonists (e.g., ondansetron) combined with dexamethasone are an alternative. Proton pump inhibitors should be administered daily from the day of treatment for 4 weeks.
  - The patient is given oral contrast 20–30 min prior to treatment to aid with visualization of the duodenum.
  - A cone-beam CT is performed to visualize the soft tissue structures. It is important to ensure that the small bowel is outside of the high-dose regions.
  - Treatment typically takes 15–20 min, with beam-on-time of approximately 7 min.
  - Patients should be advised that pain relief may take 2–3 weeks to take effect and that sometimes there is a mild worsening of pain initially.

34.5.1 Preliminary Results of a Pilot Clinical Trial [12]

- Pain was assessed on the 11-point pain Numerical Rating Scale (NRS).
- Pain interference with activities of daily living was assessed with the Brief Pain Inventory (Short Form).
- The primary endpoint was NRS pain 3 weeks post-treatment.
- Seventeen patients were evaluable, with a median age of 68 years.
- Toxicity was limited to CTCAE v4.0 grade 1–2: nausea, fatigue, and occasional transient worsening of pain being the main side effects.
- Median baseline pain was 6/10 (IQR 5–7), was reduced to 2.3/10 (IQR 0.9–3.6) ($p < 0.0005$) at 3 weeks, and to 2.5/10 (IQR 0–3.1) at 6 weeks post-treatment, for both $p < 0.001$.
- Median opioid consumption numerically decreased: baseline 52.9 morphine milligram equivalents, 3 weeks 43.9 morphine milligram equivalents, and 6 weeks 37.5 morphine milligram equivalents (NS).
- BPI pain interference improved significantly: median baseline score of 7.1 dropped to 1.1 at 3 weeks and 0 at 6 weeks ($p < 0.01$ for both time points).

34.5.2 International Study Results [13, 14]

- A phase II trial tested the technique in Israel, USA, Canada, Poland, and Portugal. The trial closed in early 2022.
- A total of 125 patients were treated during the trial. Secondary endpoints include a range of pain and quality of life indices.
- ClinicalTrials.gov Identifier: NCT03323489.
- Results, as reported in abstract form:
- Average pain decreased by a mean of 2.5 points at 3 weeks (86 reported) and 3.2 points at 6 weeks (67 reported), both $p < 0.001$.
- Opioid usage decreased by 0.6 mg/day at 3 weeks (NS) and 16.9 mg/day at 6 weeks ($p = 0.005$).
- Pain interference scores improved significantly across all domains at both 3 and 6 weeks, aside from walking at 3 weeks.
- Treatment was well tolerated; among 125 treated patients there were 6 SAEs considered "possibly related" to treatment, all of which are commonly associated with advanced cancer.
- The FACT-Hep total health-related quality of life (HRQOL) score increased by 7.8 points at 3 weeks (54/90 reported, NS diff. from 8) and 16.6 points at 6 weeks (45/90 reported, sig. >8, $p = 0.01$), showing an improvement in patients' HRQOL. Changes in FACT-Hep were especially noted in the Physical Well-Being subscale.

References

1. Damm M, Weniger M, Kölsch AK, Lampert C, Ceyhan GO, Beer S, et al. The quality of pain management in pancreatic cancer: a prospective multi-center study. Pancreatology. 2020;20(7):1511–8.
2. Dobosz Ł, Kaczor M, Stefaniak TJ. Pain in pancreatic cancer: review of medical and surgical remedies. ANZ J Surg. 2016;86(10):756–61.
3. Liang D, Shi S, Xu J, Zhang B, Qin Y, Ji S, et al. New insights into perineural invasion of pancreatic cancer: more than pain. Biochim Biophys Acta. 2016;1865(2):111–22.
4. Kang CM, Lee HY, Yang HJ, Jang HJ, Gil YC, Kim KS, et al. Bilateral thoracoscopic splanchnicectomy with sympathectomy for managing abdominal pain in cancer patients. Am J Surg. 2007;194(1):23–9.
5. Bang JY, Sutton B, Hawes RH, Varadarajulu S. EUS-guided celiac ganglion radiofrequency ablation versus celiac plexus neurolysis for palliation of pain in pancreatic cancer: a randomized controlled trial (with videos). Gastrointest Endosc. 2019;89(1):58–66.e3.
6. Marinova M, Rauch M, Mücke M, Rolke R, Gonzalez-Carmona MA, Henseler J, et al. High-intensity focused ultrasound (HIFU) for pancreatic carcinoma: evaluation of feasibility, reduction of tumour volume and pain intensity. Eur Radiol. 2016;26(11):4047–56.
7. Masuda T, Kuramoto M, Shimada S, Ikeshima S, Yamamoto K, Nakamura K, et al. Splanchnicectomy for pancreatic cancer pain. Biomed Res Int. 2014;2014:941726.
8. O'Reilly D, Fou L, Hasler E, Hawkins J, O'Connell S, Pelone F, et al. Diagnosis and management of pancreatic cancer in adults: a summary of guidelines from the UK National Institute for Health and Care Excellence. Pancreatology. 2018;18(8):962–70.
9. Kanno Y, Koshita S, Masu K, Ogawa T, Kusunose H, Murabayashi T, et al. Efficacy of EUS-guided celiac plexus neurolysis compared with medication alone for unresectable pancreatic cancer in the oxycodone/fentanyl era: a prospective randomized control study. Gastrointest Endosc. 2020;92(1):120–30.
10. Beesley VL, Wockner LF, O'Rourke P, Janda M, Goldstein D, Gooden H, et al. Risk factors for current and future unmet supportive care needs of people with pancreatic cancer. A longitudinal study. Support Care Cancer. 2016;24(8):3589–99.
11. Wilson TA, Karlsson B, Huang L, Ramanathan D, Oyoyo U, Boling W. Optimizing radiosurgery for trigeminal neuralgia: impact of radiation dose and anatomic target on patient outcomes. World Neurosurg. 2020;143:e482–91.
12. Hammer L, Hausner D, Ben-Ayun M, Shacham-Shmueli E, Morag O, Margalit O, Boursi B, Yarom N, Jacobson G, Katzman T, Abrams R, Dicker A, Golan T, Symon Z, Lawrence YR. Single-fraction celiac plexus radiosurgery: a preliminary proof-of-concept phase 2 clinical trial. Int J Radiat Oncol Biol Phys. 2022;113(3):588–93. https://doi.org/10.1016/j.ijrobp.2022.02.038. Epub 2022 Mar 4. PMID: 35257800.
13. Lawrence Y, Miszczyk M, Dawson LA, Barry AS, Pardo DD, Aguiar A, Limon D, Pfeffer RM, Buckstein M, Gnessin H, Fluss R. Celiac plexus radio-surgery for pain management in advanced cancer: an international phase II trial. Int J Radiat Oncol Biol Phys. 2022;114(5):1060–1.
14. Lawrence YR, Miszczyk M, Barry AS, Diaz Pardo DA, Aguiar A, Limon D, Pfeffer RM, Buckstein M, Margalit O, Fluss R, Meron T. Celiac plexus radiosurgery for pain management in advanced cancer: an international phase II trial, health-related quality of life (HRQOL) outcomes. J Clin Oncol. 2023;41(4_suppl):662.

Appendix. Timmerman Tables

Reprint with permission, Robert Timmerman MD, International Journal of Radiation Oncology, Biology, Physics, 2022, Volume 112, Issue 1, Pages 4–21, Copyright © 2021 Elsevier Inc (Tables A.1, A.2, A.3, A.4, A.5, A.6, A.7, A.8, and A.9).

O. Kaidar-Person, R. Chen (eds.), *Hypofractionated and Stereotactic Radiation Therapy*, https://doi.org/10.1007/978-3-031-47701-0

Table A.1 Timmerman tables, one fraction

Serial tissue	**Volume (cm³)**	**Volume max (Gy)**	**Max point dose (Gy)[a]**	**Toxicity endpoint (grade ≥3)**
Optic pathway	<0.2	8	10	Neuritis
Cochlea			9	Hearing loss
Brain stem (not medulla)	<0.5	10	15	Cranial neuropathy
Spinal Cord	<0.35	10	14	Myelitis
Cauda equina	<5	14	16	Neuritis
Sacral plexus	<5	14.4	16	Neuropathy
Esophagus[b]	<5	20	24	Esophagitis
Brachial plexus	<3	13.6	16.4	Neuropathy
Peripheral (named) nerve	<2 cm length	16	20	Neuropathy
Heart/pericardium	<15	16	22	Pericarditis
Great vessels	<10	31	37	Aneurysm
Trachea and large bronchus[b]	<4	27.5	30	Impairment of pulmonary toilet
Bronchus, smaller airways	<0.5	17.4	20.2	Stenosis with atelectasis
Rib	<5	28	33	Pain or fracture
Skin	<10	25.5	27.5	Ulceration
Stomach	<5	17.4	22	Ulceration/fistula
Bile duct			30	Stenosis
Duodenum[b]	<5	17.4	22	Ulceration
Jejunum/ileum[b]	<30	17.6	20	Enteritis/obstruction
Colon[b]	<20	20.5	31	Colitis/fistula
Rectum[b]	<3.5	30	33.7	Proctitis/fistula
	<20	23		
Ureter			35	Stenosis
Bladder wall	<15	12	25	Cystitis/fistula
Penile bulb	<3	16		Erectile dysfunction
Femoral heads	<10	15		Necrosis
Renal hilum/ vascular trunk	15	14		Malignant hypertension
Parallel tissue	**Critical volume (cm³)**	**Critical volume dose max (Gy)**	**Max point dose (Gy)[a]**	**Toxicity endpoint (grade ≥3)**
Lung (right and left)	1500 for males and 950 for females[c]	7.2		Basic lung function
Lung (right and left)			V-8 Gy <37%	Radiation pneumonitis
Liver	700[c]	11.6		Basic liver function
Renal cortex (right and left)	200[c]	9.5		Basic renal function

[a] "Point" defined as ≤0.035 cm³

[b] Avoid circumferential irradiation

[c] One-third of the "native" total organ volume (before any resection or volume reducing disease), whichever is greater

Table A.2 Timmerman tables, 2 fx

Serial tissue	Volume (cm^3)	Volume max (Gy)	Max point dose (Gy)[a]	Toxicity endpoint (grade ≥3)
Optic pathway	<0.2	11.7	13.7	Neuritis
Cochlea			11.7	Hearing loss
Brain stem (not medulla)	<0.5	13	19.1	Cranial neuropathy
Spinal Cord	<0.35	13	18.3	Myelitis
Cauda equina	<5	18	20.8	Neuritis
Sacral plexus	<5	18.5	20.8	Neuropathy
Esophagus[b]	<5	24.3	28.3	Esophagitis
Brachial plexus	<3	17.8	21.2	Neuropathy
Peripheral (named) nerve	<2 cm length	21	25.5	Neuropathy
Heart/pericardium	<15	20	26	Pericarditis
Great vessels	<10	35	41	Aneurysm
Trachea and large bronchus[b]	<4	34.5	38	Impairment of pulmonary toilet
Bronchus, smaller airways	<0.5	21.6	25.1	Stenosis with atelectasis
Rib	<5	34	41.5	Pain or fracture
Skin	<10	28.3	30.3	Ulceration
Stomach	<5	20	26	Ulceration/fistula
Bile duct			33	Stenosis
Duodenum[b]	<5	20	26	Ulceration
Jejunum/ileum[b]	<30	19.2	24	Enteritis/obstruction
Colon[b]	<20	25.8	39	Colitis/fistula
Rectum[b]	<3.5	38	41.3	Proctitis/fistula
	<20	26.7		
Ureter			37.5	Stenosis
Bladder wall	<15	14.5	29	Cystitis/fistula
Penile bulb	<3	20.5		Erectile dysfunction
Femoral heads	<10	19.5		Necrosis
Renal hilum/ vascular trunk	15	16.8		Malignant hypertension
Parallel tissue	**Critical volume (cm^3)**	**Critical volume dose max (Gy)**	**Max point dose (Gy)[a]**	**Toxicity endpoint (grade ≥3)**
Lung (right and left)	1500 for males and 950 for females[c]	9.4		Basic lung function
Lung (right and left)			V-10 Gy <37%	Radiation pneumonitis
Liver	700[c]	15.1		Basic liver function
Renal cortex (right and left)	200[c]	12.5		Basic renal function

[a] "Point" defined as ≤0.035 cm^3

[b] Avoid circumferential irradiation

[c] One-third of the "native" total organ volume (before any resection or volume reducing disease), whichever is greater

Table A.3 Timmerman tables, 3 fx

Serial tissue	Volume (cm^3)	Volume max (Gy)	Max point dose (Gy)[a]	Toxicity endpoint (grade ≥3)
Optic pathway	<0.2	15.3	17.4	Neuritis
Cochlea			14.4	Hearing loss
Brain stem (not medulla)	<0.5	15.9	23.1	Cranial neuropathy
Spinal Cord	<0.35	15.9	22.5	Myelitis
Cauda equina	<5	21.9	25.5	Neuritis
Sacral plexus	<5	22.5	25.5	Neuropathy
Esophagus[b]	<5	27.9	32.4	Esophagitis
Brachial plexus	<3	22	26	Neuropathy
Peripheral (named) nerve	<2 cm length	25.5	30.6	Neuropathy
Heart/pericardium	<15	24	30	Pericarditis
Great vessels	<10	39	45	Aneurysm
Trachea and large bronchus[h]	<5	39	43	Impairment of pulmonary toilet
Bronchus, smaller airways	<0.5	25.8	30	Stenosis with atelectasis
Rib	<5	40	50	Pain or fracture
Skin	<10	31	33	Ulceration
Stomach	<5	22.5	30	Ulceration/fistula
Bile duct			36	Stenosis
Duodenum[b]	<5	22.5	30	Ulceration
Jejunum/ileum[b]	<30	20.7	28.5	Enteritis/obstruction
Colon[b]	<20	28.8	45	Colitis/fistula
Rectum[b]	<3.5	43	47	Proctitis/fistula
	<20	30.3		
Ureter			40	Stenosis
Bladder wall	<15	17	33	Cystitis/fistula
Penile bulb	<3	25		Erectile dysfunction
Femoral heads	<10	24		Necrosis
Renal hilum/vascular trunk	15	19.5		Malignant hypertension
Parallel tissue	**Critical volume (cm^3)**	**Critical volume dose max (Gy)**	**Max point dose (Gy)[a]**	**Endpoint (grade ≥3)**
Lung (right and left)	1500 for males and 950 for females[c]	10.8		Basic lung function
Lung (right and left)			V-11.4 Gy <37%	Radiation pneumonitis
Liver	700[c]	17.7		Basic liver function
Renal cortex (right and left)	200[c]	14.7		Basic renal function

[a] "Point" defined as ≤0.035 cm^3

[b] Avoid circumferential irradiation

[c] One-third of the "native" total organ volume (before any resection or volume reducing disease), whichever is greater

Table A.4 Timmerman tables, 4 fx

Serial tissue	**Volume (cm^3)**	**Volume max (Gy)**	**Max point dose (Gy)[a]**	**Toxicity endpoint (grade ≥3)**
Optic pathway	<0.2	19.2	21.2	Neuritis
Cochlea			18	Hearing loss
Brain stem (not medulla)	<0.5	20.8	27.2	Cranial neuropathy
Spinal Cord	<0.35	18	25.6	Myelitis
Cauda equina	<5	26	28.8	Neuritis
Sacral plexus	<5	26	28.8	Neuropathy
Esophagus[b]	<5	30.4	35.6	Esophagitis
Brachial plexus	<3	24.8	29.6	Neuropathy
Peripheral (named) nerve	<2 cm length	28.8	34.8	Neuropathy
Heart/pericardium	<15	28	34	Pericarditis
Great vessels	<10	43	49	Aneurysm
Trachea and large bronchus[b]	<5	42.4	47	Impairment of pulmonary toilet
Bronchus, smaller airways	<0.5	28.8	34.8	Stenosis with atelectasis
Rib	<5	43	54	Pain or fracture
Skin	<10	33.6	36	Ulceration
Stomach	<5	25	33.2	Ulceration/fistula
Bile duct			38.4	Stenosis
Duodenum[b]	<5	25	33.2	Ulceration
Jejunum/ileum[b]	<30	22.4	31.6	Enteritis/obstruction
Colon[b]	<20	30.8	48.5	Colitis/fistula
Rectum[b]	<3.5	47.2	51.6	Proctitis/fistula
	<20	34		
Ureter			43	Stenosis
Bladder wall	<15	18.5	35.6	Cystitis/fistula
Penile bulb	<3	27		Erectile dysfunction
Femoral heads	<10	27		Necrosis
Renal hilum/ vascular trunk	15	21.5		Malignant hypertension
Parallel tissue	**Critical volume (cm^3)**	**Critical volume dose max (Gy)**	**Max point dose (Gy)[a]**	**Toxicity endpoint (grade ≥3)**
Lung (right and left)	1500 for males and 950 for females[c]	12		Basic lung function
Lung (right and left)			V-12.8 Gy <37%	Radiation pneumonitis
Liver	700[c]	19.6		Basic liver function
Renal cortex (right and left)	200[c]	16		Basic renal function

[a] "Point" defined as ≤0.035 cm^3

[b] Avoid circumferential irradiation

[c] One-third of the "native" total organ volume (before any resection or volume reducing disease), whichever is greater

Table A.5 Timmerman tables, 5 fx

Serial tissue	Volume (cm³)	Volume max (Gy)	Max point dose (Gy)[a]	Toxicity endpoint (grade ≥3)
Optic pathway	<0.2	23	25	Neuritis
Cochlea			22	Hearing loss
Brain stem (not medulla)	<0.5	23	31	Cranial neuropathy
Spinal Cord	<0.35	22	28	Myelitis
Cauda equina	<5	30	31.5	Neuritis
Sacral plexus	<5	30	32	Neuropathy
Esophagus[b]	<5	32.5	38	Esophagitis
Brachial plexus	<3	27	32.5	Neuropathy
Peripheral (named) nerve	<2 cm length	31.5	38	Neuropathy
Heart/pericardium	<15	32	38	Pericarditis
Great vessels	<10	47	53	Aneurysm
Trachea and large bronchus[b]	<5	45	50	Impairment of pulmonary toilet
Bronchus, smaller airways	<0.5	32	40	Stenosis with atelectasis
Rib	<5	45	57	Pain or fracture
Skin	<10	36.5	38.5	Ulceration
Stomach	<5	26.5	35	Ulceration/fistula
Bile duct			41	Stenosis
Duodenum[b]	<5	26.5	35	Ulceration
Jejunum/ileum[b]	<30	24	34.5	Enteritis/obstruction
Colon[b]	<20	32.5	52.5	Colitis/fistula
Rectum[b]	<3.5	50	55	Proctitis/fistula
	<20	37.5		
Ureter			45	Stenosis
Bladder wall	<15	20	38	Cystitis/fistula
Penile bulb	<3	30		Erectile dysfunction
Femoral heads	<10	30		Necrosis
Renal hilum/ vascular trunk	15	23		Malignant hypertension
Parallel tissue	**Critical volume (cm³)**	**Critical volume dose max (Gy)**	**Max point dose (Gy)[a]**	**Toxicity endpoint (grade ≥3)**
Lung (right and left)	1500 for males and 950 for females[c]	12.5		Basic lung function
Lung (right and left)			V-13.5 Gy <37%	Radiation pneumonitis
Liver	700[c]	21.5		Basic liver function
Renal cortex (right and left)	200[c]	17.5		Basic renal function

[a] "Point" defined as ≤0.035 cm³

[b] Avoid circumferential irradiation

[c] One-third of the "native" total organ volume (before any resection or volume reducing disease), whichever is greater

Table A.6 Timmerman tables, 8 fx

Serial tissue	Volume (cm^3)	Volume max (Gy)	Max point dose (Gy)[a]	Toxicity endpoint (grade ≥3)
Optic pathway	<0.2	27.2	29.6	Neuritis
Cochlea			26.4	Hearing loss
Brain stem (not medulla)	<0.5	27.2	37.6	Cranial neuropathy
Spinal Cord	<0.35	26.4	33.6	Myelitis
Cauda equina	<5	34	38.4	Neuritis
Sacral plexus	<5	34	38.4	Neuropathy
Esophagus[b]	<5	36.8	43.2	Esophagitis
Brachial plexus	<3	32.8	39.2	Neuropathy
Peripheral (named) nerve	<2 cm length	37	43	Neuropathy
Heart/pericardium	<15	34.4	40	Pericarditis
Great vessels	<10	55.2	62	Aneurysm
Trachea and large bronchus[b]	<5	50	56	Impairment of pulmonary toilet
Bronchus, smaller airways	<0.5	38.4	48.8	Stenosis with atelectasis
Rib	<5	50	63	Pain or fracture
Skin	<10	43.2	45.6	Ulceration
Stomach	<5	31.2	42	Ulceration/fistula
Bile duct			48	Stenosis
Duodenum[b]	<5	31.2	42	Ulceration
Jejunum/ileum[b]	<30	28.8	40	Enteritis/obstruction
Colon[b]	<20	35.2	57.5	Colitis/fistula
Rectum[b]	<3.5	56	61.5	Proctitis/fistula
	<20	45		
Ureter			53	Stenosis
Bladder wall	<15	22.4	44.8	Cystitis/fistula
Penile bulb	<3	35		Erectile dysfunction
Femoral heads	<10	35		Necrosis
Renal hilum/vascular trunk	15	28		Malignant hypertension
Parallel tissue	**Critical volume (cm^3)**	**Critical volume dose max (Gy)**	**Max point dose (Gy)[a]**	**Toxicity endpoint (grade ≥3)**
Lung (right and left)	1500 for males and 950 for females[c]	14.4		Basic lung function
Lung (right and left)			V-15.2 Gy <37%	Radiation pneumonitis
Liver	700[c]	24.8		Basic liver function
Renal cortex (right and left)	200[c]	20		Basic renal function

[a] "Point" defined as ≤0.035 cm^3
[b] Avoid circumferential irradiation
[c] One-third of the "native" total organ volume (before any resection or volume reducing disease), whichever is greater

Table A.7 Timmerman tables, 10 fx

Serial tissue	Contouring instructions	Volume (cm³)	Volume max (Gy)	Max point dose (Gy)	Toxicity endpoint (grade ≥3)
Optic pathway	One structure both sides from posterior globe, including chiasm, to proximal optic radiations	<0.5	30.6	33.1	Neuritis
Eye (retina)	Each side separately, entire globe	Mean dose	<26	30	Retinitis
Lens	Each side separately			7	Cataract
Eyelid, meibomian glands (one side)	Each side separately, upper and lower lid as one structure			21.3	Dry eye syndrome
Lacrimal gland (one side)	Each side separately	<1	14.1	23.6	Lack of tears
Cochlea	Each side separately, include at least three CT slices	<0.5	25	27	Hearing loss
Brain stem (not medulla)	Superiorly from incisura, midbrain and pons only, one structure	<5	32	38	Cranial neuropathy
Spinal cord	Entire bony canal including at least 10 cm superior and inferior to PTV	<5	31	36	Myelitis
Salivary gland (one side)	Each parotid gland separately	<7 Mean dose	14.1 <17.7	21.3	Xerostomia
Larynx	Starting 1 cm above first appearance of true vocal cord, include entire cord, arytenoid muscles, corniculate and arytenoid cartilages, and portions of thyroid cartilage abutting these structures ending at the first appearance of the cricothyroid ligament	<3	30	45	Necrosis/ edema
TM joint	Each side separately starting at the superior articular surface near the zygoma bone and ending at the notch at the superior part of the ramus of the mandible	<1	37.7	41.4	Inflammation
Cauda equina	Based on the bony limits of the spinal canal starting superiorly at the bottom of the spinal cord (typically around L2) and ending at the inferior extent of the thecal sac (typically S3)	<5	35	41	Neuritis

Table A.7 (continued)

Sacral plexus	Outlining the space defined medially by the sacral foramina from S1 to S3, including contouring within the sacral foramina, posteriorly along the limits of the true pelvis, laterally to 2–3 cm lateral to the sacral foramina, and anteriorly about 3–5 mm from the posterior limits of the contour	<5	35	41	Neuropathy
Esophagus	Include the mucosal, submucosa, and all muscular layers out to the fatty adventitia at least 10 cm superior and inferior to PTV	<5	40	48	Esophagitis
Brachial plexus	Each side separately from the spinal nerves exiting the neuro-foramina from around C5 to T2 to include only the major trunks of the brachial plexus using the subclavian and axillary vessels as a surrogate for identifying its location, extending proximally at the bifurcation of the brachiocephalic trunk into the jugular/subclavian veins (or carotid/subclavian arteries) and following along the route of the subclavian vein to the axillary vein ending after the neurovascular structures cross the second rib	<3	37	43	Neuropathy
Heart/ pericardium	Contoured along with the pericardial sac; the superior aspect (or base) for purposes of contouring will begin at the level of the inferior aspect of the aortic arch (aorto-pulmonary window) and extend inferiorly to the apex of the heart	<15	36.6	42.5	Pericarditis
Great vessels	The wall and lumen of the named vessel at least 10 cm superior and inferior to PTV	<10	55.7	62.9	Aneurysm
Trachea and large bronchus	Contour the trachea and cartilage rings starting 10 cm superior to the PTV and extending inferiorly to the bronchi, ending at the first bifurcation of the named lobar bronchus	<5	52	59	Impairment of pulmonary toilet

(continued)

Table A.7 (continued)

Skin	The outer 0.5 cm of the body surface anywhere within the whole-body contour	<10	46.3	48.9	Ulceration
Stomach	The entire stomach wall and the gastric contents included from the GE junction to the proximal duodenum at the pylorus	<50	33.9	45	Ulceration/ fistula
Duodenum	The entire duodenal wall and lumen from the pylorus to the duodenojejunal flexure	<5	33.9	45	Ulceration
Jejunum/ ileum	Any and all loops of small bowel as one structure within 10 cm of the PTV in any direction	<120	33.9	41	Enteritis/ obstruction
Renal hilum/ vascular trunk	Each side separately, including major calyces, renal pelvis, and proximal renal artery medial to the aorta	15	30.7		Malignant hypertension
Colon	One structure, including wall and contents of lumen starting 10 cm superior to PTV and ending 10 cm below PTV	<20	47	60	Colitis/fistula
Rectum (including stool)	One structure, including wall of rectum and all contents in lumen; start contouring 10 cm superior to PTV and then inferior to anal sphincter	<10	52	65	Proctitis/ fistula
		<20	49		
		<30	46		
		<40	43		
Bladder (with urine)	Contour the bladder wall and all urine ending inferiorly at the base of the prostate	<90	48	53	Cystitis/ fistula
		<125	45		
Bladder (suprapubic wall)	Contour the anterior inferior wall resting above and around the superior aspect of the pubic bone starting at the prostate inferiorly and extending 2–3 cm superiorly from there	<5	23	42	Dysuria
Penile bulb	Contour starting superiorly at the inferior aspect of the pelvic diaphragm (urethral sphincter) and extending inferiorly and anteriorly up to 3 cm	<3	38	44	Erectile dysfunction
Femoral heads	Contour both right and left separately	<10	38	43.5	Necrosis

Table A.7 (continued)

Parallel tissue	Contouring instructions	Critical volume (cm³)	Critical volume dose max (Gy)	Other constraints	Toxicity endpoint (grade ≥3)
Lung (right and left) minus GTV	Contour right and left lung as one structure, including all parenchymal lung tissue but excluding the GTV and major airways (trachea and main/lobar bronchi)	1500 for males and 950 for females[a]	15		Basic lung function
Lung (right and left) minus GTV	Contour right and left lung as one structure, including all parenchymal lung tissue but excluding the GTV and major airways (trachea and main/lobar bronchi)			V-16 Gy <37%	Radiation pneumonitis
Liver minus GTV	Contour right and left lobes as one structure, including all parenchymal liver tissue but excluding the GTV and major draining ducts, extrahepatic portal vein, and gall bladder	700[a]	27		Basic liver function
Renal cortex (right and left)	Contour right and left kidney as one structure, including all parenchymal capsular tissue but excluding the renal hilum/vascular trunk (see above)	200[a]	21		Basic renal function

Abbreviations: *CT* computed tomography, *GE* gastroesophageal, *GTV* gross target volume, *PTV* planning target volume, *TM* temporomandibular

[a] One-third of the "native" total organ volume (before any resection or volume reducing disease), whichever is greater

Table A.8 Timmerman tables, 15 fx

Serial tissue	Contouring instructions	Volume (cm^3)	Volume Max (Gy)	Max point dose (Gy)	Toxicity endpoint (grade ≥3)
Optic pathway	One structure both sides from posterior globe, including chiasm, to proximal optic radiations	<0.5	39	42	Neuritis
Eye (retina)	Each side separately, entire globe	Mean dose	<33	37.5	Retinitis
Lens	Each side separately			9	Cataract
Eyelid, meibomian glands (one side)	Each side separately, upper and lower lid as one structure			27	Dry eye syndrome
Lacrimal gland (one side)	Each side separately	<1	18	30	Lack of tears
Cochlea	Each side separately, include at least three CT slices	<0.5	30	33	Hearing loss
Brain stem (not medulla)	Superiorly from incisura, midbrain and pons only, one structure	<5	40	44	Cranial neuropathy
Spinal cord	Entire bony canal including at least 10 cm superior and inferior to PTV	<5	39	42	Myelitis
Salivary gland (one side)	Each parotid gland separately	<7	18	27	Xerostomia
		Mean dose	<22.5		
Larynx	Starting 1 cm above first appearance of true vocal cord, include entire cord, arytenoid muscles, corniculate and arytenoid cartilages, and portions of thyroid cartilage abutting these structures ending at the first appearance of the cricothyroid ligament	<3	34.5	52.5	Necrosis/ edema
TM joint	Each side separately starting at the superior articular surface near the zygoma bone and ending at the notch at the superior part of the ramus of the mandible	<1	48	52.5	Inflammation
Cauda equina	Based on the bony limits of the spinal canal starting superiorly at the bottom of the spinal cord (typically around L2) and ending at the inferior extent of the thecal sac (typically S3)	<5	40.5	48	Neuritis

Table A.8 (continued)

Sacral plexus	Outlining the space defined medially by the sacral foramina from S1 to S3, including contouring within the sacral foramina, posteriorly along the limits of the true pelvis, laterally to 2–3 cm lateral to the sacral foramina, and anteriorly about 3–5 mm from the posterior limits of the contour	<5	40.5	48	Neuropathy
Esophagus	Include the mucosal, submucosa, and all muscular layers out to the fatty adventitia at least 10 cm superior and inferior to PTV	<5	45	54	Esophagitis
Brachial plexus	Each side separately from the spinal nerves exiting the neuroforamina from around C5 to T2 to include only the major trunks of the brachial plexus using the subclavian and axillary vessels as a surrogate for identifying its location, extending proximally at the bifurcation of the brachiocephalic trunk into the jugular/subclavian veins (or carotid/subclavian arteries) and following along the route of the subclavian vein to the axillary vein ending after the neurovascular structures cross the second rib	<3	48	52.5	Neuropathy
Heart/pericardium	Contoured along with the pericardial sac; the superior aspect (or base) for purposes of contouring will begin at the level of the inferior aspect of the aortic arch (aorto-pulmonary window) and extend inferiorly to the apex of the heart	<15	42	48.9	Pericarditis
Great vessels	The wall and lumen of the named vessel at least 10 cm superior and inferior to PTV	<10	57	65	Aneurysm
Trachea and large bronchus	Contour the trachea and cartilage rings starting 10 cm superior to the PTV and extending inferiorly to the bronchi, ending at the first bifurcation of the named lobar bronchus	<5	55.5	63	Impairment of pulmonary toilet

(continued)

Table A.8 (continued)

Skin	The outer 0.5 cm of the body surface anywhere within the whole-body contour	<10	54	57	Ulceration
Stomach	The entire stomach wall and the gastric contents included from the GE junction to the proximal duodenum at the pylorus	<50	39	51	Ulceration/ fistula
Duodenum	The entire duodenal wall and lumen from the pylorus to the duodenojejunal flexure	<5	39	51	Ulceration
Jejunum/ ileum	Any and all loops of small bowel as one structure within 10 cm of the PTV in any direction	<120	39	46.5	Enteritis/ obstruction
Renal hilum/ vascular trunk	Each side separately, including major calyces, renal pelvis, and proximal renal artery medial to the aorta	15	37.5		Malignant hypertension
Colon	One structure, including wall and contents of lumen starting 10 cm superior to PTV and ending 10 cm below PTV	<20	47	64.5	Colitis/fistula
Rectum (including stool)	One structure, including wall of rectum and all contents in lumen; start contouring 10 cm superior to PTV and then inferior to anal sphincter	<10	60	70.5	Proctitis/ fistula
		<20	57		
		<30	52.5		
		<40	49.5		
Bladder (with urine)	Contour the bladder wall and all urine ending inferiorly at the base of the prostate	<90	55.5	61.5	Cystitis/ fistula
		<125	52.5		
Bladder (suprapubic wall)	Contour the anterior inferior wall resting above and around the superior aspect of the pubic bone starting at the prostate inferiorly and extending 2–3 cm superiorly from there	<5	26	48	Dysuria
Penile bulb	Contour starting superiorly at the inferior aspect of the pelvic diaphragm (urethral sphincter) and extending inferiorly and anteriorly up to 3 cm	<3	42	48	Erectile dysfunction
Femoral heads	Contour both right and left separately	<10	40	46.5	Necrosis

Table A.8 (continued)

Parallel tissue	Contouring instructions	Critical volume (cm^3)	Critical volume dose max (Gy)	Other constraints	Toxicity endpoint (grade ≥3)
Lung (right and left) minus GTV	Contour right and left lung as one structure, including all parenchymal lung tissue but excluding the GTV and major airways (trachea and main/lobar bronchi)	1500 for males and 950 for females[a]	16.5		Basic lung function
Lung (right and left) minus GTV	Contour right and left lung as one structure, including all parenchymal lung tissue but excluding the GTV and major airways (trachea and main/lobar bronchi)			V-18 Gy <37%	Radiation pneumonitis
Liver minus GTV	Contour right and left lobes as one structure, including all parenchymal liver tissue but excluding the GTV and major draining ducts, extrahepatic portal vein, and gall bladder	700[a]	30		Basic liver function
Renal cortex (right and left)	Contour right and left kidney as one structure, including all parenchymal capsular tissue but excluding the renal hilum/vascular trunk (see above)	200[a]	24		Basic renal function

Abbreviations: *CT* computed tomography, *GE* gastroesophageal, *GTV* gross target volume, *PTV* planning target volume, *TM* temporomandibular

[a] One-third of the "native" total organ volume (before any resection or volume reducing disease), whichever is greater

Table A.9 Timmerman tables, 20 fx

Serial tissue	Contouring instructions	Volume (cm³)	Volume max (Gy)	Max point dose (Gy)	Toxicity endpoint (grade ≥3)
Optic pathway	One structure both sides from posterior globe, including chiasm, to proximal optic radiations	<0.5	42	48	Neuritis
Eye (retina)	Each side separately, entire globe	Mean dose	<36	42	Retinitis
Lens	Each side separately			10	Cataract
Eyelid, meibomian glands (one side)	Each side separately, upper and lower lid as one structure			30	Dry eye syndrome
Lacrimal gland (one side)	Each side separately	<1	18	32	Lack of tears
Cochlea	Each side separately, include at least three CT slices	<0.5	32	36	Hearing loss
Brain stem (not medulla)	Superiorly from incisura, midbrain and pons only, one structure	<5	44	50	Cranial neuropathy
Spinal Cord	For medulla: starting at inferior pons to foramen magnum; for cord: entire bony canal including at least 10 cm superior and inferior to PTV	<5	42	46	Myelitis
Salivary gland (one side)	Each parotid gland separately	<7	18	30	Xerostomia
		Mean dose	<24		
Larynx	Starting 1 cm above first appearance of true vocal cord, include entire cord, arytenoid muscles, corniculate and arytenoid cartilages, and portions of thyroid cartilage abutting these structures, ending at the first appearance of the cricothyroid ligament	<3	36	58	Necrosis/ edema
TM joint	Each side separately starting at the superior articular surface near the zygoma bone and ending at the notch at the superior part of the ramus of the mandible	<1	52	58	Inflammation
Cauda equina	Based on the bony limits of the spinal canal starting superiorly at the bottom of the spinal cord (typically around L2) and ending at the inferior extent of the thecal sac (typically S3)	<5	44	52	Neuritis

Table A.9 (continued)

Sacral plexus	Outlining the space defined medially by the sacral foramina from S1 to S3, including contouring within the sacral foramina, posteriorly along the limits of the true pelvis, laterally to 2–3 cm lateral to the sacral foramina, and anteriorly about 3–5 mm from the posterior limits of the contour	<5	44	52	Neuropathy
Esophagus	Include the mucosal, submucosa, and all muscular layers out to the fatty adventitia at least 10 cm superior and inferior to PTV	<5	48	58	Esophagitis
Brachial plexus	Each side separately from the spinal nerves exiting the neuroforamina from around C5 to T2 to include only the major trunks of the brachial plexus using the subclavian and axillary vessels as a surrogate for identifying its location, extending proximally at the bifurcation of the brachiocephalic trunk into the jugular/subclavian veins (or carotid/subclavian arteries) and following along the route of the subclavian vein to the axillary vein ending after the neurovascular structures cross the second rib	<3	54	58	Neuropathy
Heart/ pericardium	Contoured along with the pericardial sac; the superior aspect (or base) for purposes of contouring will begin at the level of the inferior aspect of the aortic arch (aorto-pulmonary window) and extend inferiorly to the apex of the heart	<15	46	52	Pericarditis
Great vessels	The wall and lumen of the named vessel at least 10 cm superior and inferior to PTV	<10	60	70	Aneurysm
Trachea and large bronchus	Contour the trachea and cartilage rings starting 10 cm superior to the PTV and extending inferiorly to the bronchi, ending at the first bifurcation of the named lobar bronchus	<5	58	66	Impairment of pulmonary toilet

(continued)

Table A.9 (continued)

Skin	The outer 0.5 cm of the body surface anywhere within the whole-body contour	<10	60	64	Ulceration
Stomach	The entire stomach wall and the gastric contents included from the GE junction to the proximal duodenum at the pylorus	<50	42	54	Ulceration/ fistula
Duodenum	The entire duodenal wall and lumen from the pylorus to the duodenojejunal flexure	<5	42	54	Ulceration
Jejunum/ Ileum	Any and all loops of small bowel as one structure within 10 cm of the PTV in any direction	<120	42	50	Enteritis/ Obstruction
Renal hilum/ vascular trunk	Each side separately, including major calyces, renal pelvis, and proximal renal artery medial to the aorta	15	40		Malignant hypertension
Colon	One structure, including wall and contents of lumen starting 10 cm superior to PTV and ending 10 cm below PTV	<20	50	66	Colitis/fistula
Rectum (including stool)	One structure, including wall of rectum and all contents in lumen; start contouring 10 cm superior to PTV and then inferior to anal sphincter	<10	66	74	Proctitis/ fistula
		<20	62		
		<30	58		
		<40	54		
Bladder (with urine)	Contour the bladder wall and all urine ending inferiorly at the base of the prostate	<90	60	66	Cystitis/ fistula
		<125	56		
Bladder (suprapubic wall)	Contour the anterior inferior wall resting above and around the superior aspect of the pubic bone starting at the prostate inferiorly and extending 2–3 cm superiorly from there	<5	28	52	Dysuria
Penile bulb	Contour starting superiorly at the inferior aspect of the pelvic diaphragm (urethral sphincter) and extending inferiorly and anteriorly up to 3 cm	<3	44	52	Erectile dysfunction
Femoral heads	Contour both right and left separately	<10	44	50	Necrosis

Table A.9 (continued)

Parallel tissue	Contouring instructions	Critical volume (cm^3)	Critical volume dose max (Gy)	Other constraints	Toxicity endpoint (grade ≥3)
Lung (right and left) minus GTV	Contour right and left lung as one structure, including all parenchymal lung tissue but excluding the GTV and major airways (trachea and main/lobar bronchi)	1500 for males and 950 for females[a]	18		Basic lung function
Lung (right and left) minus GTV	Contour right and left lung as one structure, including all parenchymal lung tissue but excluding the GTV and major airways (trachea and main/lobar bronchi)			V-19 Gy <37%	Radiation pneumonitis
Liver minus GTV	Contour right and left lobes as one structure, including all parenchymal liver tissue but excluding the GTV and major draining ducts, extrahepatic portal vein, and gall bladder	700[a]	32		Basic liver function
Renal cortex (right and left)	Contour right and left kidney as one structure, including all parenchymal capsular tissue but excluding the renal hilum/vascular trunk (see above)	200[a]	26		Basic renal function

Abbreviations: *CT* computed tomography, *GE* gastroesophageal, *GTV* gross target volume, *PTV* planning target volume, *TM* temporomandibular

[a] One-third of the "native" total organ volume (before any resection or volume reducing disease), whichever is greater

Index

O. Kaidar-Person, R. Chen (eds.), *Hypofractionated and Stereotactic Radiation Therapy*, https://doi.org/10.1007/978-3-031-47701-0

MIX
Papier aus verantwortungsvollen Quellen
Paper from responsible sources
FSC® C105338

If you have any concerns about our products,
you can contact us on
ProductSafety@springernature.com

In case Publisher is established outside the EU,
the EU authorized representative is:
Springer Nature Customer Service Center GmbH
Europaplatz 3, 69115 Heidelberg, Germany

Printed by Libri Plureos GmbH
in Hamburg, Germany